Sustainable Health and Long-Term Care Solutions for an Aging Population

Ben Fong
The Hong Kong Polytechnic University, Hong Kong

Artie Ng
The Hong Kong Polytechnic University, Hong Kong

Peter Yuen
The Hong Kong Polytechnic University, Hong Kong

A volume in the Advances in Medical Diagnosis, Treatment, and Care (AMDTC) Book Series

IGI Global
DISSEMINATOR OF KNOWLEDGE

Published in the United States of America by
IGI Global
Medical Information Science Reference (an imprint of IGI Global)
701 E. Chocolate Avenue
Hershey PA, USA 17033
Tel: 717-533-8845
Fax: 717-533-8661
E-mail: cust@igi-global.com
Web site: http://www.igi-global.com

Library of Congress Cataloging-in-Publication Data

Names: Fong, Ben, 1954- editor. | Ng, Artie, 1966- editor. | Yuen, Peter, 1953- editor.
Title: Sustainable health and long-term care solutions for an aging population / Ben Fong, Artie Ng, and Peter Yuen, editors.
Description: Hershey PA : Medical Information Science Reference, [2018]
Identifiers: LCCN 2017007446| ISBN 9781522526339 (hardcover) | ISBN 9781522526346 (ebook)
Subjects: | MESH: Health Services for the Aged--economics | Long-Term Care--economics | Health Services for the Aged--organization & administration | Health Policy--trends | Far East
Classification: LCC RA564.8 | NLM WT 31 | DDC 362.1084/6--dc23 LC record available at https://lccn.loc.gov/2017007446

This book is published in the IGI Global book series Advances in Medical Diagnosis, Treatment, and Care (AMDTC) (ISSN: 2475-6628; eISSN: 2475-6636)

British Cataloguing in Publication Data
A Cataloguing in Publication record for this book is available from the British Library.

Advances in Medical Diagnosis, Treatment, and Care (AMDTC) Book Series

ISSN:2475-6628
EISSN:2475-6636

Mission

Advancements in medicine have prolonged the life expectancy of individuals all over the world. Once life-threatening conditions have become significantly easier to treat and even cure in many cases. Continued research in the medical field will further improve the quality of life, longevity, and wellbeing of individuals.

The **Advances in Medical Diagnosis, Treatment, and Care (AMDTC)** book series seeks to highlight publications on innovative treatment methodologies, diagnosis tools and techniques, and best practices for patient care. Comprised of comprehensive resources aimed to assist professionals in the medical field apply the latest innovations in the identification and management of medical conditions as well as patient care and interaction, the books within the AMDTC series are relevant to the research and practical needs of medical practitioners, researchers, students, and hospital administrators.

Coverage

- Medical Procedures
- Disease Management
- Critical Care
- Patient Interaction
- Internal Medicine
- Alternative Medicine
- Disease Prevention
- Experimental Medicine
- Cancer Treatment
- Diagnostic Medicine

IGI Global is currently accepting manuscripts for publication within this series. To submit a proposal for a volume in this series, please contact our Acquisition Editors at Acquisitions@igi-global.com or visit: http://www.igi-global.com/publish/.

The Advances in Medical Diagnosis, Treatment, and Care (AMDTC) Book Series (ISSN 2475-6628) is published by IGI Global, 701 E. Chocolate Avenue, Hershey, PA 17033-1240, USA, www.igi-global.com. This series is composed of titles available for purchase individually; each title is edited to be contextually exclusive from any other title within the series. For pricing and ordering information please visit http://www.igi-global.com/book-series/advances-medical-diagnosis-treatment-care/129618. Postmaster: Send all address changes to above address.

Titles in this Series

For a list of additional titles in this series, please visit: www.igi-global.com/book-series

Emerging Applications, Perspectives, and Discoveries in Cardiovascular Research
Ashim Malhotra (Pacific University, USA) and Shivani Soni (California State University, Fullerton, USA & Chapman University, USA & Alabama State University, USA)
Medical Information Science Reference • copyright 2017 • 439pp • H/C (ISBN: 9781522520924) • US $225.00 (our price)

Healthcare Community Synergism between Patients, Practitioners, and Researchers
Valerie C. Bryan (Florida Atlantic University, USA) and Jennifer Lynne Bird (Florida Atlantic University, USA)
Medical Information Science Reference • copyright 2017 • 348pp • H/C (ISBN: 9781522506409) • US $210.00 (our price)

Transformative Healthcare Practice through Patient Engagement
Guendalina Graffigna (Catholic University of the Sacred Heart, Italy)
Medical Information Science Reference • copyright 2017 • 382pp • H/C (ISBN: 9781522506638) • US $215.00 (our price)

Promoting Patient Engagement and Participation for Effective Healthcare Reform
Guendalina Graffigna (Catholic University of the Sacred Heart of Milan, Italy)
Medical Information Science Reference • copyright 2016 • 357pp • H/C (ISBN: 9781466699922) • US $220.00 (our price)

Effective Methods for Modern Healthcare Service Quality and Evaluation
Panagiotis Manolitzas (Technical University of Crete, Greece) Evangelos Grigoroudis (Technical University of Crete, Greece) Nikolaos Matsatsinis (Technical University of Crete, Greece) and Denis Yannacopoulos (Piraeus University of Applied Sciences, Greece)
Medical Information Science Reference • copyright 2016 • 315pp • H/C (ISBN: 9781466699618) • US $190.00 (our price)

Handbook of Research on Trends in the Diagnosis and Treatment of Chronic Conditions
Dimitrios I. Fotiadis (University of Ioannina, Greece)
Medical Information Science Reference • copyright 2016 • 659pp • H/C (ISBN: 9781466688285) • US $385.00 (our price)

IGI Global
DISSEMINATOR OF KNOWLEDGE

701 East Chocolate Avenue, Hershey, PA 17033, USA
Tel: 717-533-8845 x100 • Fax: 717-533-8661
E-Mail: cust@igi-global.com • www.igi-global.com

Editorial Advisory Board

List of Reviewers

Table of Contents

Detailed Table of Contents

The U.S. population is living longer, placing a demand on long-term care services. In the U.S., Medicaid is the primary player in funding costly long-term care for the aged poor. As a major health reform law, the 2010 Patient Protection and Affordable Care Act, Public Law 111-148, gives financial incentive for states to expand Medicaid, transitioning long-term care services from facilities toward community care. Facing other funding obligations and recent recessions, not all states expanded their Medicaid long-term care program using the financial incentives. Some states continue to spend more dollars on traditional nursing facility care despite legislation. This chapter explores why some states spend more revenue on nursing facility long-term care despite enhanced federal funding to reform, while others are spending more on home and community-based services. Regression analysis and 50 state-level data is used.

This chapter examines the continuum of care in use at the Yee Hong Centre for Geriatric Care in Toronto, Ontario, Canada. The service continuum is a response to the needs of a diverse Chinese Canadian population, where services in the appropriate language and culture are limited. Within the funding context, service coordination for seniors within Ontario can be characterized as fragmented, with over-use of acute care hospitalization and long-term care institutionalization. Community agencies must find a way to adapt to changing systems as the Ontario government moves away from institutionalization and toward community care. This chapter explores challenges that are faced by a socially-minded organization within a medically-minded funding system. It also addresses ways to cope with the constraints.

People are living longer but not, unfortunately, living longer healthy lives as there is an increasing number of years spent in ill-health from the age of 65 years onwards. Rates of chronic non-communicable diseases are increasing. This purpose of this chapter is to describe how modern healthcare aims to involve patients more in their care (so called self-management) to reduce the incidence of complications linked to chronic disease while attempting to promote healthy ageing. Support for patients' self-management is multifaceted but patients require support from healthcare professionals and this will be discussed as well as the educational requirements of the healthcare professionals who support those patients. How well nurses are prepared for giving patients health promotion advice will be described using an example of research from the United Kingdom. The chapter will conclude with an outline of how healthcare professionals are considered as role models for healthy living.

An exponential growth in elderly population reflects a proportional increase in recourses that are unaffordable and unsustainable to the economy. This rapid demand for health services and long-term care not only leads to non-financial implication like shortage of manpower and long waiting time, but this also creates a large burden on health and related services in the public sector. Involving the private sector to provide better and more efficient facilities and services and to encourage innovation will enhance productivity, speed up project and service delivery, and increase opportunities for investment in health. This chapter examines existing problems within health care systems in aging populations such as Hong Kong, explores the advantages and challenges of Public Private Partnership (PPP), identifies successful factors in establishing PPPs models, reviews the PPP projects in Hong Kong and elsewhere and recommends methods in promoting PPP in health and long-term care as sustainable solutions.

The purpose of this book chapter is to explore the similarities and differences in the development of performance measures and accreditation systems for the quality assurance of elderly care service providers of Asian and Western origins, focusing on Hong Kong, Macau, Australia and Canada. Building on a proposed theoretical framework, this study utilizes a multiple-case study method to examine the influencing factors for the accreditation approach adopted by a jurisdiction. The findings suggest that the quality assurance of the elderly care service operators of the Asian origins as selected appears to lag behind those of the Western countries and undergo their own peculiar paths of development. Thus, Hong Kong and Macau could learn from the practical experience of Australia and Canada in terms of their concerted approaches for funding, accreditation and assessments under an increasingly market-driven service sector in which the well-being of the end-users needs to be adequately protected.

A rapidly aging population is an international challenge. Although much has been done, senior citizens today are not experiencing better health than our ancestors. This chapter reviews evidence on the current international good practices, the positive clinical and economic impact of integrated care, and how

Operations Research/Management Science (OR/MS) methodologies add value to the implementation of integrated care. In the second half of the chapter, three enablers of implementing integrated care are reviewed: 1) a common technological platform, 2) service-restructuring with the introduction of new job roles and recruitment, and 3) creation of a financial model that incentivizes integrated care. In conclusion, while research has shown that integrated care is effective in fostering aging in place, challenges remain as to how it could be implemented given that population aging has increased the demands on healthcare resources. This chapter reviews how OR/MS methodologies can facilitate the implementation of integrated care.

The objective of this chapter is to propose a framework examining the impacts of technological, organizational and environmental factors on the innovation adoption of knowledge management (KM) in long-term care context. This chapter begins with the definition, rationale and importance of KM. Secondly, KM stories, KM in long-term care, prior frameworks in long-term care and knowledge barriers in health care settings will be reviewed. Furthermore, the KM for long-term care in Technology-Organization-Environment (TOE) framework is discussed and proposed. The technology dimension includes security, complexity and costs. Besides, organizational dimension is composed of top management support, firm size, nursing leadership and the readiness. For environmental dimensions, this chapter will focus on competitive pressure and vendor support. As KM is proven to understand performance in long-term care organizations, the proposed framework provides insight to health care organization leaders on how to enhance the effectiveness of KM system.

Statistics have shown that not only the proportion of elderly as part of the world's population is growing, but there also is a growing deficit of the working population compared to the retired population. Therefore, the provision for age-related medical conditions will put a heavy pressure on the healthcare system. This chapter discusses how pervasive computing can be used to help to achieve sustainability in healthcare for the elderly. Mobile devices can facilitate old adults to actively seek for health and nutrition information, beware of their vital signs, and follow an active life style in a safe manner. Light-weight wearable electronic devices can provide acute care and rehabilitation services to the elderly without causing a big impact to their quality of life. A model is suggested to integrate the use of pervasive computing in health education, health management, doctor support, and monitored rehabilitation at home.

This chapter attempts to construct a framework for Long-Term Care (LTC) service providers to utilize Corporate Social Responsibility (CSR) concepts as the guiding principles for improving management and operations in a socially responsible manner. The framework adopts selected dimensions of the ISO 26000:2010 standard and the Triple Bottom Line framework in the economic, social, and ethical perspectives. LTC service providers need to understand CSR and can benefit from adopting best practices of CSR. Application of the proposed framework for LTC service providers are discussed. This chapter concludes by proposing future research directions on the relation between LTC and CSR.

With the efforts of Social Welfare Department, voluntary works in Hong Kong become systemic and popular. Volunteers have been involved in developing local elderly services in many organisations in recent years. Contributions of volunteers related to elderly services in some organisations have been reviewed in this chapter, introducing the scope of services among the volunteers. Training and rewarding systems are also highlighted in order to examine the engagement of volunteers. The case of a local welfare organisation is used to discuss the operational issues encountered in Hong Kong. With a view to relieve the shortage of manpower and demand of the healthcare system, suggestions of further enhancing the ability of volunteers and extending their scope of services in the home of elderly people are proposed. Pertinent issues in sustaining trained volunteers in the voluntary long-term care work are also presented.

This chapter introduces the SSLD (Strategies and Skills Learning and Development) System as a comprehensive model for practice in psychosocial service for seniors. The challenges and issues associated with aging are complex, and involve physical, biological, psychological, social, existential and spiritual dimensions. In order to address them in a comprehensive and balanced manner, we need to draw on an extensive set of knowledge, experience and skills taken from various healthcare and human service professions. The SSLD system is built on a meta-theoretical structure that interfaces well with both analytic and holistic conceptualizations of the human person within his or her life-world, or being-in-the-world. Principles and methods of SSLD practice are described through phases of intervention: engagement and problem translation, N3C assessment, 6D (domains of being-in-the-world) formulation, implementation, review and evaluation. These are illustrated with practice examples. Issues related to practice research and knowledge production are also explored.

Aging is a function of time and is a natural and integral part of the life cycle. Aging process differs among individuals and brings all kinds of changes, affecting not just the physical body and its functions, but also to the social, psychological and financial situations to individuals. Aging in place (AIP) is a common preference among older people for remaining in their local community and maintaining their social networks throughout the aging process. Issues about appropriateness of aging in place, long-term care, and residential homes are discussed. Some models and recommendations are discussed, completed with thoughts on future studies.

The research on patients' preferred place of care and death has received increasing attention in recent decades. In palliative care, one of the main goals is to facilitate patients to stay in their preferred place of care, and to die in the place of their choice. Although 'home' is often quoted as the most preferred place of care and death among the terminally-ill in other places, local studies suggested otherwise. In Hong Kong, death is highly institutionalized with the vast majority of deaths occurring in public hospitals. Local culture, health care system and its provision and accessibility, presence of public health care policy on palliative care and care for the terminally-ill are among the factors affecting patients' preferred and actual place of care and death. This chapter is going to provide an overview of the recent studies and to discuss the topic from the Asian perspectives, and to highlight on the debates on the related policies.

Community care is one of the worldwide strategies for governments to manage contemporary healthcare challenges and long-term care. In response to an ageing population, the Hong Kong government has been promoting the concepts of community care and made initiatives, inter alia, in community-based rehabilitation (CBR). Despite these new drives, there is insufficient supply of CBR services. Provisions of CBR are currently fragmented, project-based, or on a self-financed basis. The authors argue that there is a lack of longer-term plan on CBR and that the government still relies on the heavily subsidized public hospital system. In this chapter, the authors share their views on the opportunities and challenges of CBR in Hong Kong.

Foreword

In Hong Kong, we are proud of health indices such as longevity, low infant and maternal mortality. Now our life expectancy has taken over Japan ranking almost top globally. While it has been our dream that our seniors would enjoy longer living to share the success of society, ageing population has also become a pressing public issue and also be labeled as burden to society. I am finding very hard to live with this paradoxical view. We need a sustainable health and long-term care solutions for an aging population. We can then take pride of our achievements in health and enjoy our social life with our seniors and this would include me as it is not too far ahead. This book comes very timely not only providing solutions for elderly care but also the way forward of our health care delivery system

Currently we do not have good understanding of the economics in financing long term care nor understanding the importance of universal health coverage. Chapters by Yuen and Luk have enlightened our understanding of these two aspects respectively. We lack evidence on impact of home and community based on elderly to convince our policy makers the financial incentives of de-institutionalization of elderly services. Chapter by Schmeida and McNeal have made use of regression analysis and 50 state-level data to unfold the mystery. Moreover, an effective model of public-private partnership can no longer be delayed. It should be encouraged to develop further as discussed in chapter by Ho and Fong. The chapters of the section on policies and systems would put us on the right track as solid policies and robust systems would assure sustainable development.

We need to move away from fragmented services by putting community based rehabilitation as main stream services rather than ad hoc basis. Chapter by Tong and Fong share their views on the current opportunities and limitations. We also need to investigate models to facilitate continuum of long-term care with better co-ordination and integration not only prolongation of living but quality of living as active citizens. Chapter by Liu, Wong, Chu and Leung makes use of the model in Canada to explore the challenges faced by a socially-minded organization within a medically-minded funding system, and addresses ways to cope with the constraints. Chapter by Leung, Chau, Lee, Chen and Lee provides a review of evidence on the positive clinical and health economic impact of integrated care.

Good management is essential to ensure maintenance of policy and system to be sustained. Excellent management and solutions should be reflected by performance measures which are needed for accreditation of quality elderly care centers as discussed in chapter by Ng, Leung and Ho. Lo and Ng propose a framework examining the impacts of technological, organizational and environmental factors on the innovation adoption of knowledge management (KM) in long-term care context which would help to understand performance in long-term care organizations. Technology such as the use of pervasive computing in health education, health management, doctor support, and monitored rehabilitation at home for the elderly would be an option to relieve the pressure on health care systems as discussed in the chapter by Wong and Lo. Different types of management and practices would be considered as solutions.

Apart from policy, legislative and management measures, one would turn to frameworks for corporate social responsibility as described by Law and Ng, "Strategies and Skills Learning and Development System" as a comprehensive model for practice in psychosocial service for seniors described by Tsang and Ip, and proposal by Lau and Chan in enhancing the ability of volunteers and extending their scope of services in the home of elderly people. We cannot forget the role of Chinese Herbal Medicine in managing health conditions of the elderly in health care systems. Chapter by Chan, Seto, Au Yeung and Chan reviews existing therapeutics for the treatment of cardiovascular disease, Most of all, one cannot also avoid discussing how the elder people spend the last journey and chapter by Woo, Kwok and Tse provides an overview of the recent studies and discusses the topic from the Asian perspectives, and highlighting on the debates on the related policies.

Professional and Higher education needs to have a new perspective on sustainable long-term care for aging population as raised by Cheung and Dwakes in their chapters. They propose the educational requirements of the healthcare professionals in supporting the elderly in self-management. Higher education institution should be the hub for knowledge transfer and putting evidence into practice and policy. It is also important to discuss good practices and explore how the good practices can be translated into good evidence. This book is '*Anatomy*' and '*Physiology*' textbook of aging and health as it dissects the issues comprehensively in a holistic way, and also describes how the systems should function effectively.

Albert Lee
The Chinese University of Hong Kong, Hong Kong & National Academy of Medicine, USA

Preface

The initiative to develop this book was inspired by the conclusions of the Health Conference organized by College of Professional and Continuing Education of The Hong Kong Polytechnic University in 2016. The theme of the conference was “Aging, Health and Long-term Care: Integrity, Innovation and Sustainability”. The Keynote Speech, “The Future Cost of Health and Care”, was delivered by Sir James Mirrlees, Nobel Laureate in Economic Sciences (1996) and Master of Morningside College of the Chinese University of Hong Kong. While Sir James pointed out that “It is likely that future costs of care and medical treatment of the elderly need not rise much, if at all, as a proportion of GDP”, there were considerable opposing views about economic sustainability under an aging population associated with concerns over limitations of public expenditures, the acute-centric health care system, the misalignment of public policies, the continued improvement in life expectancy and the need for quality.

Sustainable development of an aging society is gaining the attention of policy makers throughout the world and is becoming an imperative goal of public policy. But how can the world be better prepared for its aging societies? How could institutions and other stakeholders’ concerns be addressed in a practical and feasible way? Status quo is unlikely to be adequate in tackling this structural change in demographics.

Against such a background, this book aims to addresses the issues of health and long term care for the aging population of the world. It explores potential mitigating measures at the policy level as well as interdisciplinary and managerial solutions on care and services that are relevant to policy makers, managers and health care professionals for the planning, development and delivery of quality health and long-term care around the world.

OBJECTIVE OF THE BOOK

The pursuit of quality health and long-term care is likely to result in a significant financial and social burden for both the emerging and advanced economies. The objectives of this book are to explore issues pertinent to health and long term care costs and to find alternative ways of financing care, as well as the development of innovative service models to meet the increased demands in a quality, cost-effective and more humanistic manner. The book covers topics such as the redesigning of service provision patterns, the collection and utilization of data for performance and quality improvement, the use of technology in the planning and provision of care, and the setting new framework for training and research in health and long-term care. Our objective is to share the latest practices, knowledge, research findings and philosophy of the subject from different countries with various stakeholders in the health and long term care sector. While the majority of the authors, and consequently cases and examples used, are from Hong Kong, there are also contributors and studies from the Canada, Chinese Mainland, U.K., U.S.A., and other countries, providing a global perspective to the problem.

STRUCTURE OF THIS BOOK

The book is structured into three main sections: (1) Policies and Systems, (2) Management and Solutions, and (3) Innovation in Practices. Section 1 provides a context to the issues examined in the rest of the book with respect to public policy and governance system in dealing with aging societies. Section 2 then looks into a variety of management issues in relation to delivering solutions to the challenges. Section 3 explores emerging innovations in practice by different types of professionals in the provision of health and long-term care services.

Section 1: Policies and Systems

Section 1 of this book comprises six chapters that set the context for the materials in the remainder of the book through the lenses of economics, policy and systems. It is a collection of articles that look into challenges in financing and delivering health and long-term care faced by various economic jurisdictions around the world, including Canada, China, Hong Kong, U.K., and U.S.A.

In Chapter 1, Peter Yuen articulates key concepts of economics relevant to the financing and delivery of long term care services. It examines the magnitude of population aging in developed economies, and the associated implications for long term care. Key economic concepts relating to the demand, supply and financing of long term care services are then discussed. Policies, practices and major models of financing of long term care are explored and a conceptual framework for reform is presented.

Chapter 2 by Ching Yuen Luk examines the complex interplay of forces that shape the health insurance reform in China and identifies problems that impede the government from achieving true universal health coverage (UHC). It shows that China's multi-layered social health insurance system has so far failed to provide insured people with access to a range of essential services. To achieve true UHC, the government has to overcome significant hurdles in the design of its existing social health insurance system.

In Chapter 3, Mary Schmeida and Ramona Sue McNeal examine the challenges of long-term care financing in the U.S. It looks into the U.S Medicaid system as the primary player in funding costly long-term care for the aged poor. The authors attempt to explain why some states spent more on nursing homes, while others spent more on home and community-based services.

The case of Yee Hong Centre for Geriatric Care of Canada is explained by Kwong Yuen Liu, Bonnie H. Y. Wong, Maria Chu, and William Y. W. Leung in Chapter 4. It presents the continuum of care concept practiced at the Yee Hong Centre for Geriatric Care in Toronto, Ontario, Canada. The service continuum is a response to the needs of a diverse Chinese Canadian population, where services in the appropriate language and culture are limited. This chapter explores the challenges faced by a socially-minded organization within a medically-minded funding system.

In Chapter 5, Susan Dawkes and Simon Cheung review the U.K. Health Promotion Initiatives for Healthy Aging. This chapter explores how best to involve patients in their care to reduce incidence of complications linked to chronic disease in an attempt to promote healthy ageing. The authors opine that patients' self-management requires support from healthcare professionals who in turn need to be trained to become role models of healthy living. How nurses are prepared for giving patients health promotion advice is described using a study from the U.K.

The experience of Public Private Partnership in Health and Long-Term Care in Hong Kong is shared by Wing Tung Ho and Ben Fong in Chapter 6. This chapter examines the advantages and challenges of the Public Private Partnership (PPP) scheme, identifies successful factors in establishing PPPs models, and recommends methods in promoting PPP in health and long-term care as sustainable solutions.

Section 2: Management and Solutions

Section 2 of this book comprises six chapters that focus on managerial issues and possible solutions in addressing increasing demand for quality health and long-term care services. These proposed solutions include the adoption of an accreditation system for quality assurance, the use of integrated care, the application of information technology and knowledge management, the deployment of volunteers, as well as the enhancement of accountability among operators through embedding social responsibility in their corporate management.

Chapter 7 by Artie Ng, Tiffany Leung and Jack Ho explores the similarities and differences in the development of performance measures and accreditation systems for the quality assurance of elderly care service providers in Hong Kong, Macau, Australia and Canada. The study utilizes a multiple-case study method to examine the influencing factors for the accreditation approach adopted by a jurisdiction. It suggests that the quality assurance of the elderly care service operators in Hong Kong and Macau appear to lag behind those of the Western countries.

Eman Leung and his co-authors explore how operations research and management science methodologies could add value to the implementation of integrated care in Chapter 8. The authors also discuss three enablers for implementing integrated care: 1) a common technological platform, 2) service-restructuring, and 3) a financial model for integrated care.

Chapter 9 by Man Fung Lo and Peggy Ng proposes a framework for the adoption of knowledge management (KM) in the long-term care context. Prior frameworks in long-term care and knowledge barriers are presented. KM for long-term care in a Technology-Organization-Environment (TOE) framework is constructed and proposed.

In Chapter 10, Adam Wong and Man Fung Lo examine how pervasive computing can be used to help to achieve sustainability in health care provision for the elderly. It explores how mobile devices can facilitate old adults to follow an active life style in a safe manner, and how light-weight wearable electronic devices can enhance care and rehabilitation to the elderly. A model is presented integrating the use of pervasive computing in health education, health management, doctor support, and rehabilitation at home.

In Chapter 11, Vincent Law and Candace Ng present a framework for Long Term Care (LTC) service providers to utilize Corporate Social Responsibility (CSR) concepts as the guiding principles for improving management and operations in a socially responsible manner. The framework integrates selected dimensions of the ISO 26000:2010 standard with the economic, social and ethical perspectives embedded in the Triple Bottom Line concept. Potential applications of the proposed framework for LTC service providers are explored.

In Chapter 12, Ting-leung Lau and Kin-yee Chan document how volunteers have been involved in developing local elderly services. Contributions of volunteers and the associated training and reward systems are discussed. The case of a local welfare organisation is used to highlight the operational issues encountered. Suggestions for further enhancing the ability of volunteers and extending their scope of services in the home of elderly people are proposed.

Section 3: Innovation in Practices

Section 3 of this book comprises six chapters introducing various innovative practices for the delivery of health and long-term care. In these chapters, the authors share their insights from their different professional perspectives, embracing psychological, medical, nutritional, cultural and social-community approaches.

In Chapter 13, Ka Tat Tsang and Linus Chui introduce the SSLD (Strategies and Skills Learning and Development) System as a comprehensive model for practice in psychosocial service for seniors. Principles and methods of SSLD practice are described through the different phases of intervention.

In Chapter 14, Ben Fong and Vincent Law discuss aging as a natural and integral part of life cycle. Issues relating to the appropriateness of aging in place, long-term care, and residential homes are discussed. Some innovative models and recommendations for future studies are presented.

In Chapter 15, Raymond Woo and his co-authors look into the case of Hong Kong where death is highly institutionalized with the vast majority of deaths occurring in public hospitals. The chapter examines the factors affecting patients' preferred and actual place of care and death.

Kar-wai Tong and Kenneth Fong in Chapter 16 share their views on the opportunities and challenges of community-based rehabilitation (CBR) in Hong Kong. The author argues that despite the various drives for CBR in Hong Kong, there is still insufficient supply of CBR services, and the provisions of CBR are currently fragmented, project-based, and operating on a self-financing basis.

Enoch Chan and his co-authors in Chapter 17 review existing therapeutics for the treatment of cardiovascular disease, and discuss the use of Traditional Chinese Medicine (TCM) in the treatment of the disease, and the potentials and challenges of incorporating TCM into the mainstream healthcare system.

In the last chapter, Simon Cheung and Susan Dawkes investigate the determinants of fruits and vegetables consumption behavior among university students in Hong Kong and their relevance to healthy aging. They point out that those who consume fruits and vegetables regularly have a reduced risk of many chronic diseases.

TARGET AUDIENCE

The editors hope that this text will stimulate ideas for the pursuit of integrity, innovation and sustainability for the financing and delivery of health and long term care in this rapidly aging context, and that policy makers, academicians, researchers, students, long-term care service providers, health care professionals, health service managers, and government officials will find the materials interesting and useful.

Acknowledgment

The book is made possible through the efforts of the contributing authors, editorial advisors, reviewers, and colleagues of the publisher, IGI Global, in particular Courtney Tychinski, Kayla Wolfe, Jan Travers, and Katie Shearer. The Editors are grateful to them all. The Editors also wish to thank colleagues, who are not named in this book, but have given valuable advice to the publication. It is a great honor to have Professor Albert Lee, Professor (Clinical) at the Jockey Club School of Public Health and Primary Care of The Chinese University of Hong Kong to write the Foreword for the book. The Editors wish to thank him for his support.

Ben Fong
The Hong Kong Polytechnic University, Hong Kong

Artie Ng
The Hong Kong Polytechnic University, Hong Kong

Peter Yuen
The Hong Kong Polytechnic University, Hong Kong

Section 1

Policies and Systems

Chapter 1
The Economics of Long-Term Care:
Key Concepts and Major Financing and Delivery Models

Peter P. Yuen
The Hong Kong Polytechnic University, Hong Kong

ABSTRACT

This chapter presents key concepts of economics relevant to the financing and delivery of long term care services. It first examines the magnitude of population aging in developed economies, and the associated implications for long term care. Key economic concepts relating to the demand, supply and financing of long term care services are then discussed. Policies, practices and major models of financing of long term care are further explored followed by a presentation of the conceptual framework for reform. It concludes that in view of the magnitude of the problem, incremental changes in the existing systems are unlikely to be adequate. A clear understanding of the economic concepts to underpin major transformation of existing systems and policies that do not align with populations trends is urgently needed.

INTRODUCTION

Economics is "the study of how men and society end up choosing…to employ scarce productive resources that could have alternative uses to produce various commodities and distribute them for consumption…. It analyses the costs and benefits of improving patterns of resource allocation" (Samuelson 1976).

The economics of long term care, therefore, refers to the use of economic concepts, theories and tools to analyze how resources are allocated in the financing and delivery of different types of long term care services, as well as how they should be reallocated to achieve more desirable outcomes.

Long term care (often also referred to as social care or aged care) consists of a mix of services to assist an impaired person to function in activities of daily living (ADL), include bathing, transferring, toileting, and dressing, as well as incidental activities to daily living (IADLs), which include cooking, housekeeping, moving around, and managing personal finances (Spector & Fleishman 2001). It does

DOI: 10.4018/978-1-5225-2633-9.ch001

not include the medical care that the impaired person requires. Long term care covers both community services and residential services. Community services include services delivered to the home of the individual (such as home-helpers' services, visiting nursing services), and services provided at day care centres. Residential services include a range of residential facilities depending on the severity of disability (such as self-care homes, care and attention homes, nursing homes and infirmaries) (Yuen 2014). The care is generally provided over a long period of time, and often until death. While the unit cost of care is relatively low compare to acute care, the total cost of care can be very high in view of the high number of persons requiring care and the fact that it is necessary to provide care over a long period of time.

This chapter first examines the magnitude of population aging in developed economies, and the associated implications for long term care. Concepts and issues relating to the demand, supply and financing of long term care services are then discussed. Policies, practices and major models of financing as well as a conceptual framework for reform are presented towards the end.

BACKGROUND

As a result of longer life-expectancies, the elderly population is rising at a speed, which is unprecedented in the history of mankind. It is a global phenomenon affecting every country and region, with industrialized economies experiencing the highest ageing growth rate at the present time. The share of the population aged 80 years and over is expected to more than double in coming decades across the OECD, growing from 4% in 2010 to close to 10% by 2050 (Colombo & Mercier, 2011).

This ageing process is widespread and enduring, because of the ubiquitous and sustaining nature of the trend of longer life expectancies and lower fertility rate of developed economies. The world is not likely to return to the kind of age structure that the previous generations experienced (United Nations Population Division, 2001).

Associated with ageing is the increasing need for long term care for a significant percentage of the elderly population. Long term care expenditure has been on the increase for most countries, and is expected to increase at a much greater rate in the coming decades. In the USA, it was estimated that 25% of its population age 65 and above requires some form of long term care (Feldstein). In the United Kingdom it was found that while, on average, people could expect to live to age 77, 15 of these years would be spent with some form of disability (WHO, 2015). In Australia, it was found that three quarters of the elderly persons who died used some form of long term care during the twelve months before death, and around half of them used long term care services more than four years before death (Australian Institute of Health and Welfare 2015). In Hong Kong, it has been projected long term care spending will increase from 1.4 percent of GDP (in 2011) to 3 percent of GDP by 2036, with an average growth rate of 3.1% (Chung et al, 2009).

A very significant form of disability relating to aging is dementia. In 2015, dementia affected more than 47 million people worldwide. By 2030, it is estimated that more than 75 million people will be living with dementia, and the number is expected to triple by 2050. In one Australian study, it was estimated that around 10% of the expected increase in health-care costs during the next 20 years would come from demand for care for this condition alone (Vos, Goss, Begg & Mann, 2007; WHO, 2015)

While the notion that longer life expectancy inevitably translates into higher health care expenditure is challenged by some – some studies indicate that expenditures for the 65-74 age group for hospital care as well as for outpatient visits actually fell (Oliver, Foot & Humphries 2014, Kingsley 2015, Rolden, van Bodegom & Westendorp 2014) -- few would dispute that long term care expenditures will increase as the population ages. A clear understanding of the economics of long term care is therefore essential in formulating appropriate strategies to tackle this serious problem.

KEY CONCEPTS RELATING TO THE ECONOMICS OF LONG TERM CARE

The following sections examine a number of commonly used economic concepts and apply them to the long term care sector. Concepts relating to demand and supply are first examined. Financing and payment systems are then explored, follow by analyses of major financing models and the conceptual model for financing reform.

Demand for Long Term Care

The term "demand" is often used liberally in everyday life which may or may not mean the same as the economic term. Three related concepts --"Needs", "Wants", and "Demand" -- for services are elaborated below within the context of both institutional and community-based long term care.

Needs

"Needs" are professionally defined, generally refer to the quantity of a particular service which health care professionals believe ought to be consumed. For long term care, there are generally accepted measurements to determine the degree of impairment a person suffers in carrying out ADL and IADL in determining the need for a particular type of service.

There are assessment tools to measure the patient's functional performance, sensory performance, mental health, continence, communication, behavioural symptoms, mood symptoms, pain symptoms, pressure ulcers etc. (Lou et al, 2011). Commonly used measurements include:

- **Barthel Index (BI):** Measures the level of independence in daily activities, including personal hygiene, bathing, feeding, toileting, mobility, bowel control, and bladder control (Mahoney & Barthel, 1965; Collin et al, 1988);
- **Instrumental Activities of Daily Living Index (IADL):** Assesses the level of dependency of an elderly person on more complex daily living activities, including the ability to prepare meals, take medication, communicate with others, do laundry, perform housekeeping tasks, do grocery shopping, handle finances etc (Lawton & Brody, 1969; Tong & Man, 2002);
- **Time Up-and-Go Test (TUG) and Elderly Mobility Scale (EMS):** Measures basic mobility, which is a commonly used predictor of functional dependence (Cheung, Au, Lam and Jones, 2008, Yu; Chan & Tsim, 2007);
- **Norton Scale:** Assesses risk for pressure sore development (Norton et al, 1979);
- **Berg Balance Scale (BBS) and Morse Fall Scale (MFS):** Measures balance impairment and can be used to predict the risk of fall (Berg et al 1992, Morse et al 1986);
- **Mini-Mental State Examination (MMSE):** Assesses cognitive impairment, covering time/place orientation, attention, short-term memory, language etc and is often used to assess dementia (Folstein et al, 1975);

- **Geriatric Depression Scale (GDS):** Screens elderly persons for depressive symptoms (Yesavage et al, 1983).

These types of assessment are often carried out to determine the type of services needed and/or the eligibility to receive benefits either in kind or in cash. It is important that public financial support should be targeted where the need is the highest. The basket of subsidized services should strategically address users' needs and cost-effectiveness considerations. Benefits should be tied to the need-level. Patients with cognitive impairment, for example, should be given high priority because of the intensity of care required.

Want

"Want" refers to the quantity of service which the patient and/or his family would like to consume at zero price. "Wants" tend to vary from one population to another because of cultural or other reasons. What may be deemed to be "needed" by professionals may or may not be wanted by consumers. On the other hand, what may be deemed as unnecessary by professionals could be "wanted" by the consumer. For example, based on an objective assessment of the patient's condition, health care professionals may decide that the patient should be best cared for at home or on at a day care centre, but family members might still "want" the patient to continue to stay in a hospital. This is quite common, as hospital care is often heavily subsidised by government or paid for by insurance, whereas caring for the patient at home or at a day care centre is not, or the government subsidy is not as generous (Chee & Phua, 2016). Apart from the payment issue, some family members do not "want" to assume the responsibility to care for the patient at home, even though the patient's disability could be mild and "need" not go to a residential facility.

"Need" is often assessed by asking consumers whether or not they want the service (often without indicating to them the price or the full cost of the service) through questionnaire survey. Politicians sometimes survey residents in their constituency and asked them if they would like government to open a particular type of care facility in their neighbourhood. Signature campaigns for a particular type of service by pressure groups are also manifestations of "want".

Demand

"Demand" is an economic term – the quantity that consumers are willing to consume at a given price. It is related to but not synonymous with "need' or "want". It is dependent on price (own price and price of substitutes), as well as the income and taste of the consumer.

Price

The impact of price on demand is affected to a large extent by its elasticity. A service that is highly price elastic implies that a small change in either its own price or the price of its substitute will result in a big change in the quantity demanded. On the contrary, a service that is price inelastic means that changes in its own price or the price of its substitute will have little impact on the demand. Less skilled long term care services (for example, bathing, toileting etc) for the less dependent elderly are generally more price elastic than more skilled care required for the more dependent elderly. Coverage by long term care insurance will reduce the price at the point of consumption for users and hence will impact significantly on demand.

The price of substitutes also affects demand. Different co-payment rates for different types of long term care service can drive demand from one type of care to another. For example, day care and home care are substitutes for residential care for many elderlies. In an attempt to encourage greater use of day care and home care services, many countries are now requiring higher copayment for residential care and at the same time providing free non-residential care services. In Hong Kong, because a high percentage of residential care are heavily subsidized by government and community based services are not, the percentage of elder persons in residential facilities is much higher than those receiving community based care as well as those in neighouring countries like Japan and Singapore (Chiu et.al 2009).

The demand for voluntary long term care insurance also tends to be highly price elastic. Take-up rate is generally much higher if there are government subsidies or tax incentives to defray part of the premium expenses.

Income

Given a same price level, demand can also vary as a result of the income of the user. Similar to the case of price, the impact of income on the demand for a particular type of long term care service is dependent on the elasticity of the demand. Long term care services are generally income elastic. High income families are generally more likely to purchase services that enhance comfort for the patient and convenience for family members, whereas lower income families often will have to forgo them, and rely more on free care provided by family members.

Taste

Factors other than price and income that affect demand are collectively known as "taste". This generally refers to cultural norms and lifestyle preferences. In some cultures, for example, sending your frail elderly parents to a residential old age home is a norm, while in some cultures it would be considered unfilial to do so. The propensity of a population to purchase insurance is another example that will affect the demand for long term care insurance. Risk-avoidance culture tend to have a higher percentage of population buying voluntary insurance than population in a risk-taking culture (Yuen 1992)

SUPPLY OF LONG TERM CARE

Long term care services can be roughly divided into non-residential services and residential services. Non-residential services include services delivered to the patient's home (home-based care), care provided at day care centers (day care), and integrated programmes (Lou, Kwan & Chan, 2011). As for residential services, there are different types of facilities depending on the severity of the disability, and can be grouped under the following major categories (in order of the impairment levels of the resident): hostels and homes for the elderly; care and attention homes; nursing homes; infirmaries; and hospices (Chung et al, 2009). Non-residential services generally cost less than residential services, and are generally considered better for the patient. For non-residential services to be more effective, some countries have formal programmes to integrate them with primary health care services, targeting people at low risk of death, enabling patients to stay at home and yet receive all the necessary care and treatment in the community (Atun, 2004; Chappell et.al, 2004; Stuck et.al, 2002; WHO, 2015; Lou, Kwan & Chan, 2011; Chin & Phua, 2016).

Delivery entities for long term care services include government units, quasi-nongovernment organizations (QUANGOs), not-for-profit non-governmental organizations (NGOs), private for-profit organizations and informal carers. Direct provision by government units are less common these days, and provision by NGOs seems to be the general trend. Provision by private for-profit operators is common is some countries – in Japan, over 40 percent of home care is provided by private for-profit providers (Chin & Phua, 2016). Informal carers, mostly family members, with or without the assistance of domestic helpers, are always very important providers of care in most countries.

Similar to demand, supply is affected by price and price elasticity. Inelastic supply means that a big increase rise in price results only in a small increase in the quantity supplied. An inelastic supply is therefore highly undesirable. An understanding of factors affecting supply elasticity is important. Major factors affecting supply elasticity for long term care services include: manpower, land, capital, and local legal requirements.

Manpower

The workforce for long term care comprises of a wide spectrum of individuals, ranging from unpaid, untrained informal carers (often family members) to the highly trained, highly paid formal professional carers. Manpower shortage is a common problem hindering the supply of adequate places in long term care facilities.

Formal Carers

For formal carers, the existing service care model for most countries tends to be highly "acute care-centric", in terms of the training as well as job opportunities of the formal care providers (Woo, 2007). Training programmes for doctors, nurses and allied health professions all tend to put emphasis on acute inpatient care, resulting in silos of highly specialized professions all wanting to work in the acute care sector.

The compartmentalized arrangement for health care vs long term care in many countries often lead to inability of long term care agencies to recruit adequate number of nursing and allied health staff to their facilities, as well as to frequent loss of qualified staff to acute care facilities because of the lack of promotion prospect in these agencies for these professional staff. The lack of medical staff in long term care facilities have also resulted in frequent visits to high cost hospitals' accident and emergency departments and hospital admissions of residents from long term care institutions. The strict division of labour among the different types of health care professionals and their inpatient focused training further aggravate the elderly care manpower problem (Yuen, 2014).

There is an urgent need to move away from the current "acute care-centric" and "institutionalization focused" system (Woo, 2007) to a patient oriented, community based, holistic and multitasking approach (Atun, 2004; Chu & Chi, 2006; Coulson et al., 2000) in basic training as well as in-service development of knowledge and skills for service providers. A training project for home care staff in London has found that a bottom-up approach, focusing not purely on clinical knowledge, but more on interactions between staff, patients and families, quality of life and emotion of the clients and their families issues is more appropriate (Cooper et al, 2009; King, 2012).

Informal Carers

While everyone agrees that enabling elderly to "age in place" in their homes with support of their family members is most desirable, the fact is that in most developed countries, because of low fertility rates and other social factors, the number of younger family members able and willing to care for their elderly parents continue to shrink. Informer carers often faces a great deal of stress and do not receive much support from their government (Kua, 1997; Metha, 2005). Many countries have resorted to the employment of foreign domestic helpers to provide care for the elderly in their homes (Yeo & Huang, 2009).

Land

In urban areas, high land price is often a major barrier for the supply of long term care facilities, especially for commercial operators. Some governments grant land at reduced or nil premium to nonprofit NGOs delivering long term care services.

Apart from hindering the supply of places, high cost of space can also affect quality of care, particularly residential care. High land price also results in many families having to live in very crammed space, which also renders caring for their elderly members at home difficult.

Capital

The lack of startup capital is a common problem for NGOs. In Japan, for example, shortly after the implementation of long term care insurance, there were not enough long term care facilities even though funding was available for families to purchase the care (Ichien, 2000). To mitigate this problem, the Singaporean government has schemes (Community Silver Trust and Eldercare Fund) which provides grants to NGOs wanting to provide long term care services in the community (Ministry of Health, 2000, 2012).

In many other countries, it is not uncommon to find that there are more than one government bodies to oversee both health care and long-term care. In Hong Kong, for example, the funding of health care services comes from the Food and Health Bureau and the funding for long-term care services comes from the Labour and Welfare Bureau. It is difficult to divert resources from the relatively well funded acute health care sector to the less well funded long-term care sector to tackle some obvious problems such as the early discharge of elderly patients, who stay at acute hospitals inappropriately (Yuen, 2014).

Local Legal Requirements

Laws and regulations governing long term care facilities and manpower can affect the supply elasticity for long term care. Stringent requirements on the operators and facilities can deter or hinder the supply of services. Stringent requirements on training programmes for health care professions can also have an adverse effect.

LONG TERM CARE FINANCING

A country/region's long term care financing can be broadly described by the following equation:

T + CI + VI + OPP + FF = P*Q

where

T stands for taxes. It includes general taxation, special taxes and levies.
CI stands for compulsory long term care insurance.
VI stands for voluntary long term care insurance.
OPP stands for out of pocket payment by users, mainly from personal savings. It includes current and fixed assets of the patient.
FF stands future fund of the government. It included all kinds of investment tools set up by government to secure stable returns for the future to mitigate the impact of population ageing.
P stands for price of service.
Q stands for quantity of service.

Components on the left hand side of the equation are sources of fund to finance long term care. Components on the left hand side of the equation represent how the funds are being used. Long term care financing reform involves changing the weighting of different components in the equation. Elaborations on each of the components are provided below.

Tax

This includes all forms of government general revenue, such as income tax, sales tax, special taxes, and different types of levies. Tax is generally a very important source of financing for long term care services, even for countries with mandatory long term care insurance. In some countries, tax revenues are used to build facilities and to subvent services from NGOs. In countries with compulsory long term care insurance, tax revenues are often used to subsidise the insurance so as to keep the premium low, as well as to pay for the premium of the unemployed and those in low income. The reliance on taxation to pay for long term care services is highly problematic for most countries with an ageing population, as revenue from direct taxation normally declines with a shrinking working population. Some form of tax broadening might be necessary by levying special taxes on either individuals or businesses to help pay for the ever increasing long term care expenses.

Compulsory Long Term Care Insurance

This is either a part of the mandatory social insurance, or a standalone government programme, requiring all working adults or only those reaching a certain age (such as 40 years old in Japan) to participate. A certain percentage of a person's income is deducted to go into a central insurance fund. In the event of disability, long term care expenses will be covered in part or in full by the insurance after assessment. Similar to tax, revenue from premium diminishes with an aging population, requiring a constant increase in premium rate for the working population, creating problems of intergeneration equity.

A variant of compulsory long term care insurance is savings-insurance arrangement, in which working adults are required to contribute a percentage of income to a long term care savings account. Upon reaching a certain age, 65 for example, the balance, in part or in full, will be used as a lump payment for long term care insurance for the individual (The Harvard Team, 1999). This arrangement migrates the problem of intergeneration equity, as each elderly person carries with him/her accumulated savings as contribution to the insurance premium.

Voluntary Long a Term Care Insurance

Voluntary private long term care insurance is generally available in most countries. In the event of disability, benefits will be paid out in the form of either a lump sum or reimbursement for services up to a certain amount after assessment. Premium can also be paid annually or in form of a lump sum, depending on the plan. However, for various reasons, the market for voluntary private long term care insurance is small in most countries. In OECD countries, long term care expenditure paid by private insurance is less than two percent of total long term care expenditure (OECD, 2011a), and in the USA, where private insurance is so common, it is still less than four percent (Brown & Finkelstein, 2007).

Out of Pocket Payment/Co-Payment

This refers to users fees, charged to patients either on a partial or full cost recovery basis. Patients'/families' income and savings, included current and fixed assets, are the sources for such payment.

Most systems require some cost-sharing on long term care benefits. Almost no long term care system is entirely free. In USA, out-of-pocket payment accounts for one-third of total long term care expenditure, which is very significant (Brown & Finkelstein, 2007).

The rate of copayment can be linked to income as well as to needs. In France, for example, a long term care cash benefit pays up to €1,235 per month for a high-need/low-income user, but only €27 per month for the highest- income users, while in Sweden there is a cap for cost-sharing on home-help services of €180 per month. Paying higher benefits to low-income dependents as in France and other countries ensures access to care for those who need it without excessive public expenditures (Colombo and J Mercier 2011).

Paying for long term care using fixed asset of the patient is becoming more common. There are a number of possible mechanisms to help users with low and moderate incomes but have accumulated assets to turn some of these assets (for example, a house) into cash to pay for such expenses. An example from Ireland is the Irish Nursing Home Loans under which a resident can defer to the time of his or her death their nursing home contribution set on the basis of the value of their non-financial assets, such as their home (Colombo & Mercier, 2011).

Futures Fund

This is a form of pre-funding or a collective savings account (Savings Working Group Final Report to the Minister of Finance, 2011) whereby government set aside some funds to pay for future obligations. Some futures funds are general in nature, and are intended to increase government's future revenue in general to offset government's unfunded superannuation liability in the future. Some are even used to fund infrastructural projects, in hopes that these projects will contribute to more government revenue in the future, enabling government to spend more on social welfare services then (Tsang, 2014). They can also be earmarked for specific purposes, for example for health and long term care. These earmarked funds can provide more reliable funding to the intended services, as these services do not need to compete with other forms of public service. The competition from all forms of public service is expected to be acute as the population ages.

Prices and Quantity

Price times quantity of long term care services represent the total expenditure on long term care. Given the total amount is determined by the factors in the left hand side of the equation, high price charged by providers would limit the quantity of services to be available, resulting in long waiting list for the needed services. The price charged is determined largely by the wage level of different types of care workers, and the cost for the use of the space for the facilities. Skilled health care professionals, such as doctors, nurses, physiotherapists, occupational therapists, are generally well paid and will be reflected in the price charged for the care. A well planned mix of health care professionals leading teams of less-trained carers can reduce costs. In expensive cities, if private facilities are required to pay market price for the use of space, and the charges for their service would bound to be prohibitively high. NGOs for long term care are often provided space at nil or greatly reduced rental by government in order to keep their price level low.

PAYING SYSTEMS FOR LONG TERM CARE

Paying systems for long term care providers vary. It includes block grants, per diem rates, fee-for-service, case mix payments, and pay for outcome (Jacobs & Rapoport, 2014). Liang (1991) advocates a system that gives financial power to the elderly to safeguard their independence and a system that could promote supply-side innovations and diversity of services.

Block Grants

This is the most traditional payment system, whereby government or some funding body provides a block grant to a government unit or to an NGO in the form of subvention for the delivery of long term care services. This is common for tax-based systems. Some form of contractual agreement is made between the funder and the provider. This type of funding does not encourage the provider to be consumer oriented, as money does not follow patients under this system. There is a need to monitor quality closely. There is also little financial incentives for the provider under this type of funding to be efficient.

Fee-for-Service

This is less common for long term care providers, but can be found for certain selected services provided by some commercial providers as well as by NGOs providing services on a self-financing basis. Supply side moral hazards exist under this mode of payment – there is a tendency for providers to provide more than what is necessary. Providers paid by such system are generally more eager to please consumers than those funded by the block grant system.

Per Diem Payment

Providers are paid based on the average daily or sessional cost for providing care. It can be based on a flat per diem rate or facility specific per diem rates (e.g. one rate for skilled nursing care and a different rate for intermediate care). This is common for insurance based systems. The advantage of this payment is that institutions have incentives to minimize costs, while the disadvantages include providers cherry picking healthier patients and the tendency for them to compromise on quality.

Case Mix Payment

Under this payment systems, patients are charged based on groups associated with the patients' ADL scores and the associated services required such as the degree of cognition impairment, rehabilitation requirements etc. (Schlenker, 1986). If condition of the patient changes, the payment rate will change accordingly. A commonly used case mix payment system is the Resource Utilisation Groups (RUG) (Fries & Conney, 1985), which has subsequently been updated as RUG II (Micheletti & Shlala, 1986) and RUG III (Fries et al, 1994).

The advantage of this type of payment system is that the payment to providers reflects closely accurate cost for the services without the incentives to deliver unnecessary services. The disadvantage is that the system provides no incentives to help improve the condition of the patient, as payment will decrease when the patient dependency is reduced.

Pay for Outcome

This payment system attempts to address the perverse incentives described above. Institution will receive a higher payment if the outcome is achieved – i.e. when the patient's dependency improves. As the implementation is more complicated and requires close monitoring of the patient's condition and the quality of care provided, adoption of such payment system is still uncommon.

MAJOR FINANCING MODELS

The section examines existing models of long term care financing of various countries and the associated advantages and disadvantages of each model. There are different ways to categories major models of long term care financing systems. OECD has grouped different countries' long term care systems into three main clusters: (1) universal coverage within a single programme; (2) means-tested safety-net schemes; and (3) mixed systems (OECD, 2011b). This chapter categories long term care systems according to their main source of financing. Accordingly, long term care financing systems are classified as either: (a) mainly tax-based; (b) mainly insurance based; or (3) a combination of both.

Tax-Based Systems

For tax-based systems (e.g. UK, Nordic countries, Australia, New Zealand, Hong Kong), LTC services are heavily subsidized by different levels of government from general taxation without the creation of a separate long term care fund. Copayment for services is common. Services can be provided directly by government units or through NGOs. Long waiting time for services is quite common. Some countries also provide cash payment or vouchers for selected services in lieu of direct service provision. Universal coverage is common, although some countries limit the benefits to the elderly age group and/or persons below certain income (means-tested). For example, Nordic countries -- Denmark, Finland, Norway and Sweden -- generally provide universal coverage, while the UK requires mean-testing for personal care, but not for services for the severely disabled. Hong Kong's publicly funded LTC services are nonmeans-tested, but waiting time to access them could be long, and many families have no choice but to purchase services in the self-financing sector. The advantage of such non-earmarked approach to funding is the simplicity and the relatively low administration costs required. The major disadvantage of such system is the lack of reliable funding, as there will always be fierce competition for funding from general taxation, especially for countries with a rapidly ageing population, in which tax revenue is likely to shrink because of the shrinking working population. Underfunding is quite common under such mode of financing (OECD 2011b, Chu & Chi 2006, Social Welfare Department 2013, South China Morning Post 2014, Yuen 2014).

Insurance-Based Systems

Long term care services under such systems could be funded by a standalone compulsory, universal coverage for the elderly, long term care insurance scheme (e.g. Germany), or a compulsory scheme with universal access as part of the social insurance or mandatory health insurance scheme (e.g. Belgium, Netherlands), or a mean-tested scheme as part of the health insurance scheme (Medicaid in USA) (OECD 2011b). There are also voluntary private long term care insurance plans, but no countries adopt them as the dominant funding source for long term care services. They tend to be supplementary plans. Even for the USA, where private health insurance is the dominant form of financing for health care, only 4 percent of total long termcare costs are paid for by private insurance (Brown and Finkelstein 2008).

The comprehensiveness of coverage (i.e. the basket of services covered) and the level of copayment vary quite significantly among different types of schemes as well as within the same type.

Standalone programmes tend to be more comprehensive in terms of coverage and lower in terms of copayment, as they create a sense of entitlement for the enrollees. The disadvantage of the separation of health care and long term care funding is the possible creation of barriers to continuity of care as well as tendencies to shift costs from one sector to another.

Mixed Systems

While most countries tend to have a mix of funding sources for the financing of LTC services, countries with "mixed systems" refer to those with tax and LTC Insurance both playing a very significant role in terms of the share of financing. For example, in Japan, tax and mandatory long term care insurance each constitute around 45 percent of the total long term care payments. In Korea, the share is 37 percent from tax and 52 Percent from mandatory long term care insurance (OECD, 2011; Ichien, 2000; Kwon, 2009). In Singapore, all citizens over the age of 40, are automatically enrolled, with opt-out option, on Eldershield, a long term care insurance scheme. The Singaporean Government also uses tax revenue to subsidized middle to low income households (covering two-thirds of all households) to offset part of the copayment expenses for long term care services (Chee & Phua, 2016). In addition, Eldercare Fund and Community Silver Trust Fund are funds set up by the Singaporean Government using tax money to provide grants to NGOs.

In short, mixed systems permit long term care insurance premium level to remain low, as tax revenues are used to subsidize the long term care insurance schemes. Tax revenue can also be used to provide direct subsidies to patients for systems with high copayment. Finally, tax revenue is also used to provide capital grants to NGOs to facilitate supply.

CONCEPTUAL FRAMEWORK IN REFORMING LONG TERM CARE SYSTEMS

The above sections indicate that arrangements for the financing and delivery of long term care services vary greatly from country to country. Economists are interested in finding a resource allocation pattern which is optimum. Who should provide the service? Who should pay for the service? What pattern of financing and care is cheaper to operate? What pattern produces better quality? What pattern is more equitable? What pattern promotes greater efficiency?

The above questions suggest that there are two dimensions involved: financing and provision.

Each of the dimension of a long term care service can be described by a public/private mix continuum as shown in Box 1.

The entire long term care system is combination of the different types of services – (1) residential care, (2) day care and (3) home care -- each with its own pattern of public/private financing and delivery. The position on the continuum could be different for three different of types of long term care services. For example, for the financing dimension, residential care are heavily subsidized publicly in some countries, while most community based services have to be paid for privately. In other countries, government subsidizes community based services in an attempt to incentives community based care, and require higher co-payment on the part of the patient for residential services. As for the provision dimension, variations also exit as to whether the service is provided by government, NGOs, or private for profit organizations.

While the continuum is a theoretical one, the type of system that exists in most countries tend to lie somewhere in between the two extremes.

Incorporating the financing and delivery dimensions, long term care systems can best be described by the following Figure for a given type of service.

Square 1 represents a system that is predominantly private in both financing and delivery: e.g. a patient paying for a services out of pocket or through private insurance in a private nursing home;

Square 2 represents a system that is paid for publicly but delivered by private providers: e.g. a public voucher system in which a patient can choose a private provider and pay for the service using a government voucher;

Square 3 represents a system that is predominantly public in both financing and delivery: e.g. a patient paying very little for services in a publicly owned and financed institution;

Box 1.

100% Private	100% Public

Figure 1.

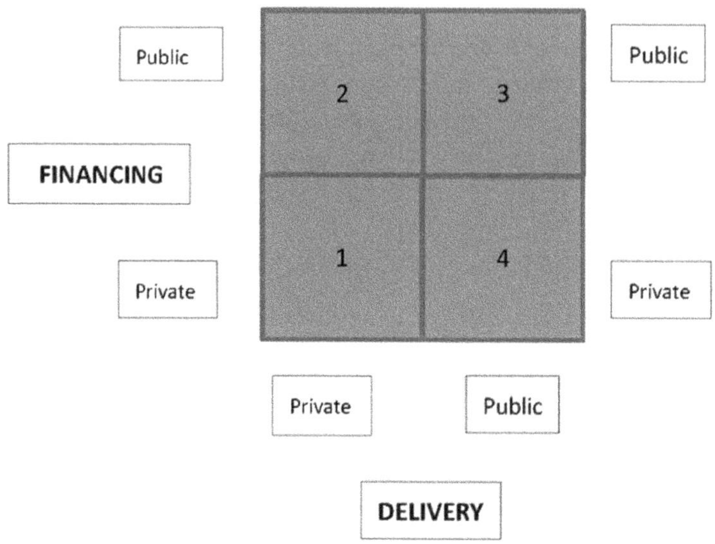

Square 4 represents a user pay system in which government provides most of the care, but the patient is required to pay for the full cost or a significant percentage of the actual cost.

Reforming the long term care system would involve examining the impact and desirability of moving from one position to another in the graph – e.g. should government provide more or less subsidies to a particular type of long term care; should more or less private organizations be involved in the provision. In general, greater public financing promotes greater equity, while more private financing and delivery can lead to a faster supply of services. Directions of reform should be based on the characteristics of the system as well as the values of its residents.

CONCLUSION

Building an equitable long term care system that delivers high quality care and is sustainable is the goal of most government. However, in view of the speed of population aging and the magnitude of the problem, status quo or even incremental changes to the existing systems are not likely to be adequate to achieve that goal. A more revolutionary response to population ageing is needed to transform systems and policies that are fundamentally misaligned with population trends. Achieving such alignment will require a clear understanding of the above-mentioned economics associated with older age and a focused conceptualization of what needs to be done to cope with this serious situation which is best suited to the historical and cultural context of the country/region.

Presently, the workforce in most countries is too acute-centric, resources are directed disproportionately to inpatient care, high out-of-pocket expenditure for the consumer is common (the majority of whom do not have regular income), the financing system seldom empowers the elderly to purchase the kind of service that he/she desires, and most of these systems do not appear to be sustainable in light of the rapidly shrinking working population.

The transformation of the financing and delivery systems of such magnitude is not likely to be able to evolve naturally on their own. Government stewardship is crucial and necessary. More evidence based inquiries into the forces of supply and demand, and into the incentive systems associated with financing and payment are required to underpin policy reform initiatives that are urgently needed.

REFERENCES

Atun, R. (2004). *What are the advantages and disadvantages of restructuring a health care system to be more focused on primary care services?* Copenhagen: WHO Regional Office for Europe. Retrieved from http://www.euro.who.int/document/e82997.pdf

Australian Institute of Health and Welfare. (2015). *Use of aged care services before death. Data linkage series no. 19. Cat. no. CSI 21*. Canberra: AIHW.

Berg, K., Wood-Dauphinee, S., Williams, J. I., & Makki, B. E. (1992). Measuring balance in the elderly: Validation of an instrument. *Canadian Journal of Public Health*, *83*, S7–S11. PMID:1468055

Brown, J., & Finkelstein, A. (2007). Why is the market for long-term care insurance so small? *Journal of Public Economics*, *91*(10), 1967–1991. doi:10.1016/j.jpubeco.2007.02.010

Brown, J., & Finkelstein, A. (2008). The interaction of public and private insurance: Medicaid and long-term care insurance market. *The American Economic Review*, *98*(3), 1083–1102. doi:10.1257/aer.98.3.1083

Chappell, N. L., Dlitt, B. H., Hollander, M. J., Miller, J. A., & McWilliam, C. (2004). Comparative Costs of Home Care and Residential Care. *The Gerontologist*, *44*(3), 389–400. doi:10.1093/geront/44.3.389 PMID:15197293

Cheung, K. K. W., Au, K., Lam, W. W. S., & Jones, A. Y. M. (2008). Effects of a structured exercise programme on functional balance in visually impaired elderly living in a residential setting. *Hong Kong Physiotherapy Journal*, *26*(1), 45–28. doi:10.1016/S1013-7025(09)70007-7

Chin, C. W. W., & Phua, K. (2016). Long Term Care Policy: Singapores Experience. *Journal of Aging & Social Policy*, *28*(2), 113–129. doi:10.1080/08959420.2016.1145534 PMID:26808468

Chin, C. W. W., & Phua, K. H. (2016). Long-term care policy: Sinagapores Experience. *Journal of Aging & Social Policy*, *28*(2), 113–129. doi:10.1080/08959420.2016.1145534 PMID:26808468

Chu, L. W., & Chi, I. (2006). Long-Term Care and Hospital Care for the Elderly. In G. M. Leung & J. Bacon-shone (Eds.), *Hong Kong's Health System* (pp. 223–252). Hong Kong: Hong Kong University Press.

Chui, W. E., Chan, K., Chong, M. A., Ko, S. L., ... Ng, Y. S. (2009). Elderly Commission's Study on Residential Care Services for the Elderly: Final Report. The University of Hong Kong.

Chung, R. Y., Tin, K. Y. K., Cowling, B. J., Chan, K. P., Chan, W. M., Lo, S. V., & Leung, G. M. (2009). Long-term care cost drivers and expenditure projection to 2036 in Hong Kong. *BMC Health Services Research*, *9*(1), 172. doi:10.1186/1472-6963-9-172 PMID:19775476

Collin, C., Wade, D. T., Davies, S., & Horne, V. (1988). The Barthel ADL Index: A Reliability Study. *International Disability Studies*, *10*(2), 61–63. doi:10.3109/09638288809164103 PMID:3403500

Colombo F. and J Mercier (2011). Balancing fair protection and financial sustainability in long-term care. *Eurohealth, 17*(2–3), 3-6.

Coulson, I., Minichiello, V., Kao, R. S., Lin, F., & Wan, C. C. (2000). Developing collaborative gerontology programs offshore: A case study. *Educational Gerontology*, *26*, 387–400. doi:10.1080/036012700407866

Feldstein, P. J. (1993). *Health Care Economics*. Albany, NY: Delmar Publishers.

Folstein, M. F., Fostein, S. E., & McHugh, P. R. (1975). Mini-mental state: A practical method for grading the cognitive state of patients for the clinician. *Journal of Psychiatric Research*, *12*(3), 189–198. doi:10.1016/0022-3956(75)90026-6 PMID:1202204

Fries, B. E., & Cooney, L. M. (1985). Validation and use of resource utilization groups as a case-mix measure for long-term care. *Medical Care*, *23*(2), 123–132. doi:10.1097/00005650-198502000-00003 PMID:3919223

Fries, B. E., Schneider, D. P., Foley, W. J., Gavazzi, M., Burke, R., & Cornelius, E. (1994). Redefining a case mix measure for nursing homes: Resouce utilization groups (RUG-III). *Medical Care*, *32*(7), 668–685. doi:10.1097/00005650-199407000-00002 PMID:8028403

Harvard Team. (1999). *Improving Hong Kong Health Care System: Why and for Whom?* Hong Kong: HKSAR Government Printer.

Ichien, M. (2000). Introduction of Long-term Care Insurance in Japan. *International Review of Public Administration*, *5*(2), 23–36. doi:10.1080/12294659.2000.10804953

Kingsley, D. E. (2015). Aging and health care costs: Narrative versus reality. *Poverty & Public Policy*, *7*(1), 3–21. doi:10.1002/pop4.89

Kua, E. H., & Tan, S. L. (1997). Stress of caregivers of dementia patients in the Sinagore Chinese family. *International Journal of Geriatric Psychiatry*, *12*(4), 466–469. doi:10.1002/(SICI)1099-1166(199704)12:4<466::AID-GPS517>3.0.CO;2-U PMID:9178051

Kwon, S. (2009). *Introduction of Long-Term Care Insurance in Korea*. Paper presented at the Asian Social Protection in Comparative Perspective Conference, Singapore.

Lawton, M., & Brody, E. (1969). Assessment of older people: Self-maintaining and instrumental activities of daily living. *The Gerontologist*, *9*(3 Part 1), 179–186. doi:10.1093/geront/9.3_Part_1.179 PMID:5349366

Liang, W. (1991). *Empowering The Elderly: Direct Consumer Funding of Care Services. Choice in Welfare Series No. 6*. London: IEA Health & Welfare Unit.

Lou, Kwan, & Chan. (2011). *A Study on the Effectiveness of Community Care Services in Hong Kong*. The University of Hong Kong.

Mahoney, F. I., & Barthel, D. W. (1965). Functional evaluation: The barthel index. *Maryland State Medical Journal*, *14*, 61–65. PMID:14258950

Metha, K. K. (2005). A critical review of Singapore's policies aimed at supporting families caring for older members. *Journal of Aging & Social Policy, 18*, 43–57. PMID:17135094

Micheletti, J., & Shlala, T. J. (1986). RUGsII: Implications for management and quality in long-term care. *Quality Review Bulletin, 12*(7), 236–242. doi:10.1016/S0097-5990(16)30049-5 PMID:3092161

Ministry of Health. (2000). Eldercare Fund. *Ministry of Health.* Retrieved from: https://www.moh.gov.sg/content/moh_web/home/pressRoom/pressRoomItemRelease/2000/establishment_of_eldercare_fund.html

Ministry of Health. (2012). Community Silver Trust. *Ministry of Health.* Retrieved from: https://www.moh.gov.sg/content/moh_web/home/pressRoom/Parliamentary_QA/2012/community_silvertrust.html

Morse, J. M., Morse, B. M., & Tylko, S. (1986). Development of a scale to identify the fall-prone patient. *Canadian Journal on Aging, 8*, 66–77.

Norton, D., McLaren, R., & Exton-smith, A. N. (1979). *An investigation of Geriatric problems in hospital* (3rd ed.). London: Churchill Livingstone.

OECD. (2001a). *Private long term care insurance: A niche or a "Big Tent"?* OECD.

OECD. (2011b). *Public Long-term Care Financing Arrangements in OECD Countries in Help Wanted. Providing and Paying for Long Term Care.* OECD.

Oliver, D., Foot, C., & Humphries, R. (2014). *Making our health and care systems fit for an ageing population.* London: The King's Fund.

Rolden, H. J. A., van Bodegom, D., & Westendorp, R. G. J. (2014). RGJ. Variation in the costs of dying and the role of different health services, socio-demographic characteristics, and preceding health care expenses. *Social Science & Medicine, 120*, 110–117. doi:10.1016/j.socscimed.2014.09.020 PMID:25238558

Samuelson, P. A. (1976). *Economics.* Tokyo: McGraw Hill.

Savings Working Group Final Report to the Minister of Finance. (2011). *Saving New Zealand: Reducing Vulnerabilities and Barriers to Growth and Prosperity.* Retrieved from http://purl.oclc.org/nzt/r-1348

Schlenker, R. E. (1986). Case mix reimbursement for nursing homes. *Journal of Health Politics, Policy and Law, 11*(3), 445–461. doi:10.1215/03616878-11-3-445 PMID:3098827

Social Welfare Department. (2013). *Legislative Council Paper CB(2)673/12-13(01) Long-term Care Policy for the Elderly and Persons with Disabilities.* Paper presented to the Joint Subcommittee on Long Term Care Policy.

South China Morning Post. (2014). *Hong Kong faces challenge ensuring the elderly feel right at home.* Retrieved from http://www.scmp.com/news/hong-kong/article/1433787/hong-kong-faces-challenge-ensuring-elderly-feel-right-home

Spector, W. D., & Fleishman, J. A. (2001). *The Characteristics of Long-Term Care Users.* U.S. Department of Health and Human Services, Agency for Healthcare Research and Quality Research Report.

Stuck, A.E., Egger, M., Hammer, A., Minder, C.E., & Beck, J.C. (2002). Home visits to prevent nursing home admission and functional decline in elderly people: systematic review and meta-regression analysis. *JAMA, 287*(8), 1022–8.

Tong, A. Y., & Man, D. W. (2002). The validation of the Hong Kong Chinese version of Lawton instrumental activities of daily living scale for institutionalized elderly persons. *The Occupational Therapy Journal of Research*, *22*, 132–142.

Tsang, J. C. (2014). The 2014-15 Budget. Speech by the Financial Secretary, the Hon John C Tsang moving the Second Reading of the Appropriation Bill 2014, 26 February 2014, Hong Kong.

United Nations Population Division. (2001). New York: World Population Ageing.

Vos, T., Goss, J., Begg, S., & Mann, N. (2007). *Projection of health care expenditure by disease: a case study from Australia*. New York: United Nations.

WHO. (2015). *World Report on Aging and Health*. Retrieved from: http://www.who.int/ageing/events/world-report-2015-launch/en/

Woo, J. (2007). Development of elderly care services in Hong Kong: Challenges and creative solutions. *Clinical Medicine*, *6*(6), 548–550. doi:10.7861/clinmedicine.7-6-548 PMID:18193700

Yeo, B., & Huang, S. (2009). Foreign domestic workers and home-based care for elders in Singapore. *Journal of Aging & Social Policy*, *22*(1), 69–88. doi:10.1080/08959420903385635 PMID:20390713

Yesavage, J. A., Brink, T. L., Rose, T. L., Lum, O., Huang, V., Adey, M., & Leirer, V. O. (1983). Development and validation of a geriatric depression screening scale: A preliminary report. *Journal of Psychiatric Research*, *17*(1), 37–49. doi:10.1016/0022-3956(82)90033-4 PMID:7183759

Yuen, P. P. (1992). The Privatization of Hospital Services: An Empirical Study of the Determinants of the Public/Private Mix. Hong Kong Public Administration, 1(1), 24-64.

Yuen, P. P. (2014). Financing Health Care and Long-term Care in a Rapidly Ageing Context: Assessing Hong Kong's Readiness. *Public Policy and Administration*, *17*(1), 56–64.

Chapter 2
Moving Towards Universal Health Coverage:
Challenges for the Present and Future in China

Ching Yuen Luk
Nanyang Technological University, Singapore

ABSTRACT

This study uses a refined version of historical institutionalism to critically examine the complex interplay of forces that shape the health insurance reform trajectory in China since the mid-1980s and identifies problems that impede the government from achieving universal health coverage (UHC). It shows that China's multi-layered social health insurance system has covered more than 95 percent of its population, but failed to provide insured people with access to a range of essential services and make health care affordable. To achieve UHC, the government has to overcome significant hurdles, which include the inherently discriminatory design of the social health insurance system, disorder in the drug distribution system, deficits in the funding of health insurance, and insufficient medical protection for the old people.

INTRODUCTION

Since the mid-1980s, the problem of rising medical costs and the combing forces of population ageing and the burden of non-communicable diseases (NCDs) have driven the Chinese government to establish a multi-layered social health insurance system with an aim of providing affordable and sustainable health care for its population. At present, the social health insurance system has covered more than 95 percent of population (Asia Insurance Review, 2015). However, many insured people still have difficulties in accessing a range of essential services and face high out-of-pocket medical expenses. Meanwhile, the uninsured people lack access to basic and affordable health care. The government still has a long way to go to achieve universal health coverage (UHC), which refers to all people having access to needed health services without suffering financial hardship (World Health Organization, 2013, p. xi).

DOI: 10.4018/978-1-5225-2633-9.ch002

Health insurance reform in China has been explored and examined in many Western and Chinese studies. But the processes of health insurance reform and forces that shape the reform trajectory have not been completely understood. The relationship between UHC and health insurance reform has not been explored clearly. In order to fill the existing research gaps, this study uses a refined version of historical institutionalism to examine the forces that have shaped the trajectory of health insurance reforms in China since the mid-1980s, the problems that have impeded the government from achieving UHC and solutions adopted by the government to solve such problems.

BACKGROUND

Rapidly ageing population (Hsu et al., 2015), rising medical costs (Augustovski et al., 2011) and the burden of NCDs (Bristol, 2014, p.1) have driven governments worldwide to find ways to achieve UHC. According to the World Health Organization (WHO), there are three dimensions of UHC: (i) the breadth of coverage; (ii) the depth of coverage; and (iii) the height of coverage (World Health Organization, 2008, pp. 25-6). The breadth of coverage refers to 'the proportion of the population that enjoys social health protection' (World Health Organization, 2008, p. 25). The depth of coverage refers to the provision of the range of essential services that can effectively address people's health needs (World Health Organization, 2008, p. 26) while the height of coverage refers to the portion of healthcare costs covered by pooled funding and pre-payment mechanisms (World Health Organization, 2008, p. 26). In recent years, UHC has become a key global health objective advocated by WHO and the World Bank (Cheng, 2015, p.1) and has been adopted by many countries as a national aspiration (Reich et al., 2016, p. 811). It is believed that UHC can improve the health and well-being of people (World Health Organization, 2013, p. xi), and "is necessary for economic growth and development" (Cheng, 2015, p. 2).

However, there is neither a single model nor a single correct path to achieve UHC. Due to resource constraints and differences in political, economic, social and historical contexts, the timetable, the pace, the process and the approach to achieve UHC vary among developed and developing countries. International evidence shows that UHC is achieved gradually and over many decades (Carrin et al., 2008; Savedoff & Smith, 2011). The study of Savedoff and Smith (2011, p. 45) found that Chile and Malaysia achieved UHC at least 20 years later than Sweden and Japan, but they reached comparable levels of population health by spending smaller shares of their income on health services. The study of Reich et al. (2016) categorized 11 countries into four groups based on their pace of attaining UHC. Bangladesh and Ethiopia belonged to Group 1 countries because they were still in the agenda-setting stage of attaining UHC (Reich et al., 2016, p. 812). Indonesia, Vietnam, Ghana and Peru belonged to Group 2 countries, which had initial programmes in place but "coverage gaps remained in access to services and financial protection" (Reich et al., 2016, p. 812). Thailand, Brazil and Turkey belonged to Group 3 countries, which had achieved many UHC policy goals but faced the challenges in sustaining coverage (Reich et al., 2016, pp. 811-2). Japan and France belonged to Group 4 countries, which had achieved UHC but continuously adjusted their national policies to meet changing circumstances and solve the problem of rising costs (Reich et al., 2016, pp. 811-2). The above studies show that achieving UHC is a long term process and an ongoing task with different development stages.

Like its country counterparts, China puts UHC high on its reform agenda. Its effort to reform the health care financing system began in the mid-1980s when the central government encouraged local government to explore different payment methods to reduce skyrocketing medical costs. In 1994, the pilot medical insurance model implemented in the cities of Zhenjiang in Jiangsu province and Jiujiang in Jiangxi province paved the way for the establishment of the multi-layered basic medical insurance system. The multi-layered basic medical insurance system consists of four schemes: (i) a mandatory Urban Employee Basic Medical Insurance (UEBMI) Scheme; (ii) a voluntary New Rural Cooperative Medical System (NRCMS); (iii) a voluntary Urban Resident Basic Medical Insurance (URBMI) Scheme; and (iv) the Critical Illness Insurance Scheme (CIIS). By the end of 2014, China's coverage rate of basic medical insurance exceeded 95 percent (Asia Insurance Review, 2015). However, China still lags behind in terms of the depth and the height of coverage.

MAIN FOCUS OF THE CHAPTER

Issues, Controversies, Problems

In China, rising medical costs, a rapidly ageing population and the burden of NCDs are the three main reasons for the government to implement health care financing reform. Since the 1980s, the implementation of pro-market economic reforms drastically raised medical costs. Fiscal decentralization emphasized self-sufficiency, "with very few resources transferred from higher levels of government to facilities at the lower levels to support recurrent costs" (Shen et al., 2014, p. 142). Government subsidies to hospitals were reduced to "basic salaries and minimal administrative costs" (Pang, 2003, p. 67), which "accounted for only about 10 percent of average public hospital revenues" (The World Bank, 2010, p. ix). Hospitals became profit-driven and cost recovery institutions (Feng, 2016, p.102). They recovered their operation costs through sales of services and drugs (Langenbrunner & Somanathan, 2011, p. 214). The bonus system for hospital doctors was also introduced, which linked the performance of doctors to "the revenue generated by doctors through provision of services and drugs over a revenue target" (Liu & Mills, 2005, p.11). This provided a strong incentive for hospital doctors to "induce patient demand for both services and drugs" (Liu & Mills, 2005, p. 11). Overprescribing and overcharging became a widespread practice in hospitals (Langenbrunner & Somanathan, 2011, p. 214). It drove up medical costs. Meanwhile, the free health care enjoyed by urban population through Labor Insurance Scheme (LIS) and Government Funded Health Care Scheme (GHS) encouraged waste and abuse in the health care system (Huang, 2013, p. 63). From 1986 to 1992, the spending of LIS and GHS "together grew at an annual average of 25 percent" (Duckett, 2001, p. 293). The combined medical care expenditure from LIS and GHS drastically increased from Reminbi (RMB) 3.16 billion in 1978 to RMB 56 billion in 1994 (Huang, 2013, p. 63). Rising medical costs drove the government to reform the urban health care financing system. In rural areas, the Cooperative Medical System (CMS), which provided peasants with basic medical care through their contribution to a commune-based medical fund, collapsed in the 1990s because the transition from agricultural collectives to the household responsibility system under the economic reforms weakened the financial base of the CMS (Liu, 2004, p. 159). The collapse of the CMS led to almost 80 percent of the rural population having no medical coverage (Li et al., 2015, p. 1079). "Since then, medical expenses [in rural areas] sky-rocketed along with high-rate economic growth, which outstripped the growth of personal income" (Li et al., 2015, p. 1079). Health care in rural areas became unaffordable and peasants suffered from medical impoverishment (Li et al., 2015, p. 1079).

In China, population ageing "has emerged too early and too rapidly, under circumstances of relative socio-economic under-development" (Permanent Mission of the People's Republic of China to the United Nations, 2008). In 1985, China had the largest number of elderly in their population. They accounted for 20 percent of the world elderly population (Wu, 1991, p. 18). In 1999, China officially became an 'ageing society' when its population aged 60 and over reached 10 percent of its total population (Zhu, 2011, p. 431). In 2015, the number of elderly population aged 60 and over passed 220 million, which accounted for 16 per cent of the total population in China (finance.china.com.cn, 2016 March 8). Population aging in China did not go hand-in-hand with economic growth. Per capita Gross Domestic Product (GDP) of China was only US$806 in 1999 (Zhang, 2013, p. 344). It was very much lower than per capita GDP of developed countries. Developed countries had already attained high socio-economic development when becoming an 'ageing society', with per capita GDP ranging between US$5000 and US$10,000 (Kaufman et al., 2013, p. 45). In this sense, China has the characteristics of 'getting old before getting rich', which refers to the situation of achieving a high aging degree on a lower income level (Cai, 2015, p. 128) while developed countries get rich first before getting old (Haber, 2013, p. 376). Consequently, China's phenomenon of 'getting old before getting rich' brings pressures and burden to economy and society because the country lacks money and resources to provide medical services for the elderly. According to Ministry of Health (MOH), chronic disease incidence and physical disability rate of old people aged over 60 years was respectively 3.2 times and 3.6 times that of the total population in the nation (Li 2006 September 29). MOH reported that health resource depletion by old people aged over 60 years was 1.9 times the national average (Li, 2006 September 29). Per capita health care expenditure for the elderly in China was three to five times higher than that of young adults and average annual per capita health care expenditure for the elderly was 2.56 times the national average (Qiu, 2015, p. 96). Under this circumstance, the health care system will be increasingly under pressure to cope with the increasing demand by ageing population.

The burden of NCDs is another reason why the government wants to implement health insurance reform and achieve UHC. When the People's Republic of China (PRC) was founded in October 1949, China carried a heavy burden for communicable diseases, such as tuberculosis, dysentery and smallpox (The China Health Care Study Group, 1974), due to decades of war, polluted water supplies and poor sanitary conditions (Banister, 1987, p. 50). By the mid-1970s, many communicable diseases had been eliminated or greatly decreased in incidence through vaccination, environmental sanitation and hygiene, patriotic public health campaigns, health education, disease screening and the provision of community-level health care (Hipgrave, 2011, pp. 225-9). Since the late 1970s, China has experienced rapid economic growth due to modernization and its transformation to a market economy. Its population enjoyed better living standards and had higher disposable income. They shifted away from the traditional consumption of grain products toward high-fat, low-carbohydrate and low-fiber diets (Zhang et al., 2015, p. 4661). Their physical activity levels decreased due to improvement in public transport system, workers' transitions from heavy industry to service industry jobs (Zang & Ng, 2016), "higher community urbanicity, vehicle ownership, [television] TV and computer ownership" (Zang & Ng, 2016, p. 40). Physical inactivity and unhealthy diet led to more Chinese people suffering from and dying of chronic NCDs. Data from Global Burden of Disease showed that 65 percent of the worldwide mortality in 2010 was caused by NCDs (Min et al., 2015, p. 840); whereas in China, 85 percent of the mortality in 2010 was caused by NCDs, with cardiovascular diseases (38 percent of deaths), malignant neoplasms (26 percent of deaths), and cerebrovascular disease (21 percent of deaths) being the leading causes of death (Min et al., 2015, p. 840). Consequently, NCDs lead to serious financial loss of the Chinese economy (Sun et al., 2009). In 2003, the estimated economic burden of chronic diseases in China accounted for 7.3 percent of Gross Domestic Product (GDP) and 71.5 percent of the total economic burden of all diseases (Sun et al., 2009, p. 42). NCDs also lead to "indirect economic loss due to lost employment, disability, or premature deaths" (Tang et al., 2013, p. 7). Besides, NCDs "impose a substantial financial burden on many households" (Kankeu et al., 2013, p. 31). For example, about 11.6 percent of households in Central and Western China were pushed under the US$ 1.08 poverty line due to outpatient expenses incurred by chronic diseases (Kankeu et al., 2013, p. 31). In sum, the problems of ageing population, rising medical costs and the burden of NCDs have driven the Chinese government to attain UHC.

The Chinese government strives to provide equitable and affordable health care services for its people through a multi-layered basic medical insurance system. A review of literature shows that many studies examined the effects of individual medical insurance scheme in China. Most of these studies analyzed the UEBMI, the URBMI and the NRCMS in specific places in China. For the UEBMI, there were studies examining the impact of the pilot experiment of urban health insurance scheme on equity in health care access (Liu et al., 2002), the impact of the UEBMI on equity in health care financing (Yi et al., 2005), hospital expenditure containment (Meng et al., 2004), cost containment and access to care (Dong, 2008). Studies on the URBMI are relatively scant, which included those examining the impact of the URBMI on health care utilization and expenditure (Liu & Zhao, 2014), health services access (Chen et al., 2014), health status, relieving financial burden and satisfaction rate of participants (Lin et al., 2009). For the NRCMS, there were studies examining the impact of the NRCMS on primary health care (Babiarz et al., 2010), health service utilization and out-of-pocket spending (Wagstaff et al., 2009), accessibility and affordability of health care services (Wang et al., 2014) and satisfaction of participants (Chen et al., 2015). There were also studies examining inpatient reimbursement from the NRCMS (Wang et al., 2012) and the achievement of policy goals of the NRCMS (Li et al., 2015). Meanwhile, some studies used a comparative perspective to examine the impact of UEBMI and URBMI on the hospitalization services utilization (Feng et al., 2013), inpatient and outpatient health service utilization (Zhou et al., 2014), or the impact of the UEBMI, the URBMI, the NRCMS on health outcomes among the elderly in 20 provinces (Liu et al., 2016). Literature review shows that most of these studies are quantitative studies that use multi-year data and economic models to examine health insurance schemes in China. The strengths of these studies lie in providing numeric estimates and deriving important trends from research data. However, the weakness of these studies is that most of the correlations produced by such studies only examine the closeness of the variables, but ignore underlying causes. Moving towards UHC is a long process, fraught with challenges and requiring patience. A review of literature review shows that previous studies examined specific health insurance scheme(s) in a specific place and in a specific period. Besides, they used different methodologies to collect data and different perspectives to analyze health insurance scheme. As a result, they fail to provide a clear picture about the way China moves towards UHC and forces that shape the developmental trajectory towards UHC. In order to fill the existing research gaps, this study uses a refined version of historical institutionalism as a unifying logic to analyze the process of health insurance reforms in China since the mid-1980s and critically examines forces that shape the reform trajectory over time. It examines the problems that impede the government from achieving UHC and the government's solutions to solve such problems.

THEORETICAL FRAMEWORK: THE REFINED VERSION OF HISTORICAL INSTITUTIONALISM

The traditional version of historical institutionalism is characterized by its emphasis on the roles of institutions and path dependency in shaping the goals, preferences, strategies and behavior of political actors and generating distinctive policy trajectory of a nation (Hall & Taylor, 1996; Lecours, 2000; Pierson & Skocpol, 2002). Institutions are defined by historical institutionalists as "the formal and informal procedures, routines, norms and conventions embedded in the organizational structure of the polity" (Hall & Taylor, 1996, p. 938). Emphasis is put on asymmetric power relations (Hall & Taylor, 1996, p. 940; Saurugger, 2014, p. 91) that some groups win while others lose (Hall & Taylor, 1996, p. 941). Path dependence refers to the dynamics of self-reinforcing processes in a political system (Pierson, 2000a, p. 74) that "[d]ecisions made and structures introduced in the past generate irreversibilities" (Kirchner, 2013, p. 45). "[A]ctors have strong incentives to focus on a single alternative and to continue down a specific path once initial steps are taken in that direction" (Pierson, 2000b, p. 254).

Understandably, historical institutionalism is a useful approach to explain policy continuity (James, 2015, p. 218). Nevertheless, it is "less equipped to explain policy changes" (Weir, 2006, p. 172) or path-breaking reforms (James, 2015, p. 218). In many historical institutionalist accounts, the concept of critical junctures is used to explain rapid policy changes (Moore, 1966; Collier & Collier, 1991; Thelen, 1999; Mahoney, 2001). Critical junctures refer to change points where big, exogenous shocks (such as cleavages or crises) disrupt the existing institutional equilibrium and consequently set institutions onto a new path or new equilibrium state that will be reproduced through increasing return processes. Junctures are 'critical' because "once an option is selected, it becomes progressively more difficult to return to the initial point when multiple alternatives were still available" (Mahoney, 2001, p. 7). Nevertheless, using the concept of critical junctures to explain policy change contains three conceptual shortcomings. Firstly, it ignores the possibility that change can be endogenously generated (Streeck & Thelen, 2005, p. 19). Secondly, transformative policy change often results from "an accumulation of gradual and incremental change" (Streeck & Thelen, 2005, p. 19). Thirdly, institutional or policy change becomes purely a product of fate (Steinmo, 2008, p. 129) because critical junctures are often unpredictable and unforeseeable based on prior events (Flynn, 2015, p. 10).

Recognizing the fact that the traditional version of historical institutionalism has limitation to explain policy or institutional change, this study adopts the refined version of historical institutionalism, which was developed by the author in her book entitled *Health Insurance Reforms in Asia* (2014), to examine China's transformation to a multi-layered health insurance system. The refined version of historical institutionalism identifies three sources of change -- environmental triggers, institutional entrepreneurs and ideas – and examines how these three sources of change interact with institutions and path dependency over time to produce a particular policy trajectory and lead to policy change. As an open system, institutions interact with their external environments in a back-and-forth manner (Burke, 2011, p. 71). They must respond to or adapt to changes in external environments for the purposes of survival and prosperity, "which can result in changing the mission and shifting priorities and goals" (Lussier, 2009, p. 53). Political, economic, social and technological are four macro forces that frequently affect institutions and the changes that institutions pursue (Auster et al., 2005, p. 21). In order to examine the interaction between institutions and the shifting contextual conditions, the refined version of historical institutionalism brings in the concept of environmental triggers, which was developed by Cortell and Peterson (1999).

Environmental triggers refer to unexpected international or domestic events, crises or gradual pressures, alone or in combination, that produce pressure for institutional or policy changes (Cortell & Peterson, 1999, pp. 183-4). International triggers include geopolitical conflict, war, changing balance of power, macroeconomic change, technological change, shocks, and international treaties (Cortell & Peterson, 1999, p. 185). Domestic triggers include election, change of government, coup d'état, revolution, civil war, social movement, social conflict, economic change and demographic change (Cortell & Peterson, 1999, p. 185). External environments only "act as stimulant or trigger for [institutional] change" (Bratton, 2015, p. 504). It still requires institutional entrepreneurs to exploit windows of opportunities opened by external environment in order to enact change (Luk, 2014, p. 13). Institutional entrepreneurs are the agents of change (DiMaggio, 1988). They are agents of legitimacy who "support the creation of new institutions and reform existing institutions in ways that they deem to be appropriate and aligned with their interests" (Haunschild & Chandler, 2008, p. 633). To bring about institutional change depends on institutional entrepreneurs' willingness and ability to act (Battilana & Leca, 2009, p. 263). While willingness to act is dependent on the interests of institutional entrepreneurs, ability to act is mostly determined by tangible resources (e.g. employees, material and financial assets) and intangible resources (e.g. reputation, knowledge, social capital) institutional entrepreneurs possess or to which they have access (Battilana & Leca, 2009, p. 263). Institutional entrepreneurs must alter "deeply embedded norms, values and practices" (Hardy & Maguire, 2008, p. 209) and then legitimate and establish the new rules or practices as the expected, important and valued ones for the institutional field (Hinings et al., 2004, p. 309). To do so, they need to use new ideas as catalyst for change. Ideas are causal beliefs that "posit connections between things and between people in the world" (Béland & Cox, 2011, p. 3). They are important because "they are simultaneously the media through which agents understand the world and the material that constitutes it" (Blyth, 2011, p. 84). They "shape the content of policy proposals and the perception of interests at the heart of political struggles" (Béland, 2007, p. 23). They provide interpretive frameworks (Béland & Cox, 2011, p. 3) for policy actors to prioritize certain concerns of policy over others and strategically craft frames to make policies politically feasible and acceptable (Luk, 2014, p. 14). New ideas can take hold when old ideas are discredited and push aide. It happens when old ideas become unfit for the changing environment or less responsive to policy problems, and "are perceived to fail for some reasons" (Campbell, 2002, p. 33). This opens a window of opportunity for institutional entrepreneurs to introduce new ideas. Institutional entrepreneurs who are in a strong position to campaign for new ideas can generate support for such ideas and new practice.

To sum up, the refined version of historical institutionalism brings in environmental triggers, institutional entrepreneurs and ideas to explain how their interaction with institutions and path dependency can lead to institutional change. Meanwhile, the refined version of historical institutionalism has a core assumption that institutions remain key influences on policy outcomes because political institutions can either reinforce or upset the effects of environmental pressures, enable or constrain the behavior of institutional entrepreneurs, and filter ideas (Luk, 2014, pp. 16-7).

HEALTH CARE FINANCING SYSTEM IN THE PRE-REFORM ERA

On 1 October 1949, the PRC was founded by the Chinese Communist Party (CCP) under the leadership of Mao Zedong. In the context of the Cold War, the world was divided into two hostile camps: the capitalist camp led by the United States and the socialist camp led by the Soviet Union (Chen, 2001, p. 50). Mao chose to lean to the side of the Soviet Union. Against this background, China adopted the Soviet-style political system that emphasized "absolute single-party rule by a disciplined and hierarchical party organization" (Walder, 2015, p. 83) and "an economic model that mandated complete state ownership and control over the economy" (Walder, 2015, p. 83). A healthy workforce was crucial to developing the economy and society. But the lack of health resources and the Soviet model of economic development that strongly emphasized heavy industry led to an urban bias in health care financing system in China. Two types of free health care programs were implemented in urban areas: the LIS in 1951 and the GHS in 1952. The LIS was part of the wider labor insurance system that was modeled after the Soviet Union. Following the Soviet model, the LIS did not require employees' contributions; it put the trade unions in charge of its administration; and it copied many details concerning eligibility and benefits (Hu, 2016, pp. 96-7). Although the term 'insurance' was used to describe the scheme, the LIS did not contain any insurance elements (Luk, 2014). It had no premium contribution. Instead, it required state and collective enterprises to initially contribute 3 percent, and then 4.5 to 5.5 percent in 1957 of the payroll to the labor insurance fund (Li, 2009, pp. 34-5). The LIS provided medical coverage for employees and their direct dependents. For eligible employees, the LIS covered all their charges for diagnosis, treatment, generic drugs and hospitalization (Li, 2009, p. 35). As to their direct dependent, they could consult doctors free of charge at designated hospitals, with the LIS covering one-half of their fees for generic drugs and surgery (Li, 2009, p. 35). In the midst of the Cultural Revolution (1966-1976), the LIS was no longer administered by the trade unions but was handed over to enterprises (Duckett, 2001, p. 292). The LIS was then funded by the enterprises' employee welfare funds (Duckett, 2001; Li, 2009). As regards the GHS, it was funded by the state budget to provide medical coverage for government employees and retirees, personnel employed by institutions engaged in cultural, educational, health, and economic-construction activities, cadres, disabled military personnel, university and college students (Li, 2009; Wong et al., 2006). It covered both outpatient and inpatient expenses of eligible persons (Li, 2009, p. 36). For urban population who were not covered by the LIS or GHS, they had to pay on their own when seeking medical care. Nevertheless, hospitals were nationalized and prices for medical services and drugs were set below actual costs in order to "allow the average uninsured or poor Chinese to access basic health services" (Yip & Eggleston, 2004, p. 269). "The revenue shortfall was subsidized by government budgets, which made up more than 60 percent of total hospital operating revenue" (Yip & Eggleston, 2004, p. 269). Health care during Mao's era aimed to achieve Mao's objective of providing accessible and affordable health care services.

Due to urban bias in health care financing, most of the rural population had to pay on their own when seeking medical care before 1955 (Liu & Cao, 1992, p. 503). In the mid-1950s, the development of collective economy in rural areas provided the basis for the development of CMS. The CMS was a pre-payment health plan which collected funding from three sources: individual contribution, collective welfare fund and government subsidy (Liu et al., 1995, p. 1086). CMS participants enjoyed free visits and certain drugs free of charge at the village clinic, enjoyed 70 to 90 percent discount rate for buying certain drugs, copayment for referred hospital visits at township or higher-level and copayment for referred hospitalization (Liu & Cao, 1992, pp. 502-3). The CMS was promoted after the Sino-Soviet Split in 1960 and developed rapidly during the Cultural Revolution. The participation rate drastically increased to 80 percent in the late 1960s and reached the peak of 90 percent in 1979 (Liu & Cao, 1992, p. 504).

HEALTH CARE FINANCING REFORM SINCE THE MID-1980S

Due to rapid increase in health care costs, local governments in the mid-1980s were encouraged to carry out experiments on demand-side and supply-side cost containment. According to the study of Zheng (2009), there were three types of demand-side cost containment measures: copayment policy, financial contracting with the GHS participants, and the social pooling of the LIS. Under the copayment policy, the LIS participants were required by their working units to bear 15 percent of their medical expenses (Zheng, 2009, p. 263). As to the GHS participants, they were required to bear 5 to 20 percent of their outpatient and inpatient medical expenses (Zheng, 2009, p. 262). The copayment policy was intended to make the LIS and GHS participants more cost conscious. As regards financial contracting with the GHS participants, certain amount of health care funds was appropriated by local governments to cover participants' outpatient medical expenses only or all of their medical expenses (Zheng, 2009, p. 262). The implementation of the social pooling account of the LIS required employers' and employees' financial contribution to pay for medical expenses of certain types of critical illnesses (Zheng, 2009, p. 263). As to the pre-payment scheme in hospitals, a lump sum was given by work units to hospitals to pay for the medical expenses of their employees (Dong, 2001; Gu, 2001). Hospitals were "allowed to retain their residual revenues when the costs of health care were less than the specified amount" (Dong, 2001, p. 7). But they had to bear the financial burden if there was cost overrun. Health care financing reform at this stage remained limited by its narrow scope (Dong, 2001; Gu, 2001) and failed to tackle the fundamental weaknesses that were rooted in financing, payment and management of the LIS and GHS (Dong, 2001, p. 8).

In November 1994, the government selected Zhenjiang in Jiangsu Province and Jiujiang in Jiangxi Province as pilot reform cites to implement a health insurance model that was later known as the two-*jiang* model. The two-*jiang* model was characterized by combining an individual Medical Savings Account (MSA) and a social pooling fund (SPF). It required both the employers and employees to have mandatory contribution, with the former contributing 10 percent of their total annual payroll and the latter contributing 1 percent of their annual salary to the health insurance fund (Zheng, 2009, p. 266). Premium contributions were then split into the MSA and the SPF to pay for medical expenses of insured employees. Medical expenses were funded through three tiers (Cheung, 2001, p. 69; Liu et al., 2004, p. 48; Zheng, 2009, p. 266). The first tier was the MSA. The second tier was out-of-pocket payment for medical expenses that exceeded the amount in the MSA. The third tier was the SPF with copayment schedules (Liu et al., 2004, p. 48) when the out-of-pocket payment exceeded 5 percent of an employee's annual salary (Zheng, 2009, p. 266). The merits of the two-*jiang* model were that it was able to increase individual cost consciousness by introducing cost-sharing components and strengthen risk pooling. In 1996, the pilot reform on the basis of the two-*jiang* model was extended to 57 cities in the nation.

On the basis of experience from the pilot reform, the government in December 1998 introduced a nationwide health care financing reform through the implementation of the UEBMI Scheme. The UEBMI Scheme, which was designed on the basis of the two-*jiang* model, consisted of an individual MSA and a SPF. It required the mandatory contribution from employers and employees in both the public and private sectors. But retired employees could participate in the UEBMI Scheme without any premium contribution. Employers were required to contribute 6 percent of their total wage bills while employees were required to contribute 2 percent of their total wage bills to the Basic Medical Insurance (BMI) Fund

(The State Council, 1998). Premium contributions were then split into the MSA and the SPF. The MSA covered the general outpatient medical expenses and drug fees at designated medical institutions (Li, 2009, p. 46). The SPF covered inpatient medical expenses that were above the threshold or below the ceiling, with the rest being paid out-of-pocket by the insured employees (Li, 2009, p. 46). The threshold was about 10 percent of the average local wages while the ceiling was about four times the average annual local wages (The State Council, 1998). Health insurance cards were issued to the UEBMI participants to seek medical care at designated medical institutions. *The Drug Formulary for National Basic Medical Insurance* was also issued by the government to specify essential medicines that could be reimbursed by the UEBMI Scheme (Luk, 2014, p. 49). Local governments could adjust premium contribute rate, threshold and ceiling of the SPF according to the economic condition and the principle of balancing revenue and expenditure (The State Council, 1998). On the other hand, retired cadres, old Red Army and disabled military personnel could still enjoy free health care (The State Council, 1998), with their medical expenses paid by the SPF of the UEBMI Scheme (Luk, 2014).

In 2003, the government implemented the NRCMS to reduce rural population's financial burden caused by illnesses and improve their health (General Office of the State Council, 2003). Based on the spirit of mutual aid, the NRCMS was a voluntary scheme that provided rural households with medical protection against catastrophic illnesses. It was financed through three sources: individual contribution, local government subsidies, and central government subsidies (General Office of the State Council, 2003). An individual annually contributed RMB 10, with local and central government each providing subsidies of RMB 10 per enrolled individual (General Office of the State Council, 2003). The NRCMS was administered in county level that "county administrators [were] encouraged to define benefits packages on the basis of local needs and resources" (Babiarz et al., 2010, p. c5617). In July 2003, the NRCMS was implemented in 310 of China's more than 2,800 rural counties (Bai & Wu, 2014, p. 452). The coverage was further extended to 1,451 counties in 2006 and 2,729 counties in 2008 (Li, 2009, p. 65). The participation rate reached 91.5 percent in 2008 and 98.7 percent in 2013 (National Bureau of Statistics of China, 2014).

In July 2007, the government implemented the URBMI Scheme to provide non-working urban residents with medical protection against catastrophic illnesses treated at outpatient and inpatient settings (The State Council, 2007). Non-working urban residents referred to young children, primary and secondary school students, unemployed urban residents, the severely disabled and the elderly from low-income families (The State Council, 2007). The URBMI Scheme "adopts voluntary enrolment, a decision that was made after weighing the high administrative costs and the risk of adverse selection" (Chen et al., 2014, p. 278). It was funded by individual contributions and government subsidies. According to the State Council (2007), the government would provide subsidies of not less than RMB 40 per enrolled individual.

In August 2012, the government implemented the CIIS, which provided the NRCMS and URBMI participants with an extra layer of medical protection against catastrophic illnesses (National Development and Reform Commission et al., 2012). The CIIS was bought from a qualified commercial insurer by using the surplus of the NRCMS and the URBMI or increasing the funds collected from the NRCMS and the URBMI (National Development and Reform Commission et al., 2012). Those insured by the CIIS would be compensated for at least half of their out-of-pocket medical expenses that exceeded the average annual per capita disposable income, on top of their basic medical insurance reimbursement (National Development and Reform Commission et al., 2012).

FORCES THAT SHAPED THE HEALTH CARE FINANCING REFORM TRAJECTORY

The establishment of the multi-layered health insurance system demonstrates the government's ongoing effort to provide affordable and accessible health care for its population. This study reveals that there is a complex interplay of forces shaping the health care financing reform trajectory in China, which included (i) a highly centralized political institution, (ii) domestic environmental triggers, (iii) the introduction of new ideas by institutional entrepreneurs, and (iv) the lock-in effects of health insurance model.

China is run by a party-state system. The CCP, which has been the ruling party in China, is a highly centralized political institution that emphasizes "concentration of power in the hands of its top leaders" (Larus, 2012, p. 108). It "enforced strict discipline and had tentacles that reached into the state governing apparatus and the military" (Larus, 2012, p. 107). It "entrusts implementation of its policies and day-to-day administration of the country to the institution of the State, headed by the State Council" (Lawrence & Martin, 2013, p. 4). "The top State officials at every level of administration usually concurrently hold senior Party posts, to ensure Party control" (Lawrence & Martin, 2013, p. 4). The highly centralized political structure enables the top leaders to enjoy the monopoly on implementing health care financing reforms without having any political opposition.

Windows of opportunity for implementing health care financing reforms are mainly created by domestic environmental triggers. When Deng Xiaoping succeeded Mao to become the new political leader in 1978, he transformed China from a centrally planned economy to a market-oriented one. The market-oriented economy reduced the government's role in hospital financing while giving hospitals greater financial autonomy to charge medical fees. Hospitals became profit-driven. They regarded patients as consumers and medicine as a commodity (Pang, 2003, p. 42). Their profit-seeking behavior led to the collapse of the LIS and GHS systems because the government and the employers were unable to pay the drastically increased medical expenses of their employees. The changing economic context caused by change in political leadership triggered the experimental reform in containing medical costs in demand-side and supply-side in the mid-1980s. Economic reforms were continuously pursued by Jiang Zemin, who was the successor to Deng. This further drove up medical costs and compelled the government to introduce a two-*jiang* model in the pilot health insurance reform in 1994 and eventually implement a nationwide health insurance reform that led to the UEBMI Scheme replacing the old LIS and GHS schemes. Meanwhile, the changing social context due to the combining forces of rapidly aging population and the burden of NCD also created windows of opportunity for institutional entrepreneurs to implement health care financing reforms.

The opening of policy windows provides the opportunities for institutional entrepreneurs to introduce new ideas into the policy environment and transform such ideas into the two-*jiang* model. New ideas became politically prominent because the old ideas were seen as failing and new ideas were more responsive to the problem of rising medical costs. The old ideas of free health care and egalitarianism endorsed by Mao were discredited during Deng's era because they failed to fit into the market-oriented economic environment. In particular, the idea of free health care encouraged overuse of medical services and both demand-side and supply-side moral hazard, which led to drastic increase in medical costs and the collapse of the LIS and GHS systems. This provided an opportune time for political leaders to advocate a replacement set of ideas: individual responsibility, social solidarity, cost sharing and risk pooling. These new ideas were then transformed into the two-*jiang* model. The successful experience of the two-*jiang* model in reducing medical costs created a lock-in effect, which led to the path of subsequent health insurance reforms following the same direction of promoting the ideas of individual responsibility, social solidarity, cost sharing and risk pooling, and introducing health insurance schemes for different segments of population. The lock-in effect created a transformative effect on the health care financing system that a multi-layered health insurance system was established to replace the LIS-GHS system.

The use of refined version of historical institutionalism shows that health insurance reform in China is shaped by a complex interplay of forces. Among these forces, window of opportunity alone is not enough to bring changes if institutional entrepreneurs who are the agents of change do not exploit windows of opportunities. Meanwhile, institutional entrepreneurs who have political will to implement health insurance reform also need to have a highly centralized political system that put them in an advantageous position to promote new ideas and reforms. Political institutions remain the most dominant force in shaping health insurance reforms because political institutions can reinforce or upset the effects of environmental triggers, filter ideas, enable or constrain the behaviour of institutional entrepreneurs.

PROBLEMS IN THE CURRENT HEALTH INSURANCE SYSTEM

Based on the principle of 'basic medical protection, wide population coverage' (*bao ji ben, guang fu gai*), the government since 1998 has gradually established a multi-layered medical insurance system to provide medical coverage for different segments of population. However, the medical insurance system contains several problems: (i) the inherently discriminatory design of the social health insurance system; (ii) disorder in the drug distribution system; (iii) deficits in the medical insurance fund and (iv) the fragmented design of the social health insurance system.

Firstly, the inherently discriminatory design of the multi-layered medical insurance system creates deep structural inequality between different population groups. It is similar to a feudal hierarchy in ancient China (Luk, 2014, p. 74), which divides people into different classes, with different rights. The retired cadres, old Red Army and disabled military personnel are the privileged few enjoying free health care, with their medical expenses paid by the SPF of the UEBMI. Free health care is a way for the Chinese government to repay for the continuing loyalty of these special groups of people who served the country and fought for the country (Luk, 2014, p. 74). The UEBMI Scheme is the most comprehensive scheme in the multi-layered medical insurance system because it covers both outpatient and inpatient medical expenses while the NRCMS and the URBMI Scheme only cover medical expenses for catastrophic illnesses. The NRCMS and the URBMI Scheme are unable to alleviate participants' financial burden of health care expenditure that many participants have to pay medical expenses on their own. According to Mr. Hong Huang, Vice-President of China Insurance Regulatory Commission, insured peasants still had to bear rather high out-of-pocket medical expenses because the NCRMS only reimbursed half of their medical expenses (Lu, 2015 February 10). In 2012, there were more than 1 million URBMI patients whose inpatient fees exceeded catastrophic household expenditure for health care (China Social Insurance Net, 2015). Catastrophic household expenditure for health care was defined as out-of-pocket payments for health care that exceeded 40 percent of annual household non-food expenditure (Su et al., 2006; Gotsadze et al., 2009). The average catastrophic household expenditure for health care in China was RMB 9,826 in 2012 (China Social Insurance Net, 2015). On the other hand, inequality between the retired and incumbent employees is found within the UEBMI system. It is because retired employees do not have to pay any insurance premium, with their medical expenses paid by the SPF of the UEBMI Scheme. Besides, they enjoy higher reimbursement rate but lower self-payment rate than incumbent employees. At present, migrant workers are still excluded from joining the basic medical insurance system because their rural *hukou* do not grant them any rights or access to participate in the UEBMI. Since they are engaged in low-wage, low-skill jobs, most of them can only afford to go to 'black clinics' that are unlicensed clinics with poor hygiene to seek medical care (Xinhua Net, 2013 March 28).

Secondly, money in the individual MSA and the SPF was inappropriately depleted due to high drug prices and physician-induced demand. In China, "on average 40-50 per cent of hospital revenues come from drug prescriptions" (Brombal, 2014, p. 107) while "medicines account for less than 15 percent of total healthcare expenditure across Europe" (European Federation of Pharmaceutical Industries and Association, 2014, p. 20). It shows that drug prices are unreasonably high in China and impose heavy financial burden on insured and uninsured people. Drug prices have risen quickly since the mid-1980s when the government let market forces determine drug prices. Drug prices have been marked up for many times after going through the complex pharmaceutical distribution system that contains six to nine manufacturer-wholesaler-retailer layers (Li, 2013, p. 19). For example, the retailing price of a cancer drug was seven times higher than the wholesaling price and 14 times higher than the manufacturing price, generating a profit of 1,300 percent (Kong et al., 2011, p. 1069). High drug prices were also caused by the practice of drug manufacturers and wholesalers offering kickbacks to hospitals and doctors to ensure the sale of certain types of expensive drugs (Li, 2013, p. 18). Since 1998, the government has imposed price caps on drugs for more than 30 times (Beijing Business Today, 2014a December 9). But the result was that price-cut drugs quickly disappeared from the market because their profit margin was too small in the eyes of drug manufacturers and health care providers (Henan Business Daily, 2013 December 31). In 2010, a survey found that 342 of more than 500 types of essential medicines were in severe shortage in 40 major hospitals in China (Wang & Chen, 2015 October 12). Doctors ended up prescribing the more expensive drugs that accelerated the depletion of medical insurance fund. Besides, the practice of physician-induced demand through doctor ordering unnecessary tests, performing unnecessary surgeries, asking patient to have inpatient treatment, and prescribing unnecessary drugs (e.g. antibiotics and imported drugs) also led to the inappropriate depletion of basic medical insurance funds and unnecessary waste of medical resources (Lei & Wu, 2014, p. 10).

Thirdly, medical insurance fund deficit has been reported in many places that people may face the risk of being 'underinsured' or 'uninsured'. According to Mr. Wei-gang Jin, Head of the Social Security Institute, the Ministry of Human Resources and Social Security, some regions had already experienced a deficit in the medical insurance fund due to the growth rate in expenditure exceeding the growth rate in revenue of different medical insurance funds (Beijing Business Today, 2014b December 9). According to Mr. Jin, a total of 225 districts in China in 2013 experienced a deficit in the UEBMI funds and a total of 108 districts experienced a deficit in the URBMI funds (Beijing Business Today, 2014b December 9). Meanwhile, places such as Beijing experienced a deficit in the NRCMS fund in 2012 (Li, 2015 February 13). *Green Book of Health Reform and Development 2014* estimated that there would be deficit in all the NRCMS funds in 2017 (Nanfang Metropolis Daily, 2015 February 10). Paying the rising medical expenses of retired employees, over-prescription and paying expensive examination fees of hospitals and health insurance fraud were regarded as three main reasons for putting increasing pressure on the country's health insurance fund (China Business News, 2015 November 30).

Fourthly, the fragmented design of the social health insurance system fails to provide sufficient medical protection for the old people. At present, China does not have a health insurance scheme tailored for the elderly. According to *the 2013 Analysis Report of National Health Services Survey in China*, 45.1 percent of 61,057 old people surveyed participated in NRCMS, 32.4 percent participated in the

UEBMI Scheme, and 10.8 per cent participated in the URBMI Scheme in 2013 (Center for Health Statistics and Information, 2015, p. 95). But the medical services and drugs covered by these health insurance schemes are not specific for treating common diseases in old age. Unlike young people, old people usually have greater medical need and suffer from NCDs that have higher prevalence rate, a longer period in treatment and higher medical expenses. The two-week prevalence, "an index of health service need and one of the morbidity indicators used to investigate inequalities in health status" (Zhu et al., 2015, e008441) drastically increased from 25 percent in 1993 to 56.9 percent in 2013 (Center for Health Statistics and Information, 2015, p. 98). In 2013, high blood pressure and diabetes were top two diseases for the two-week prevalence (Center for Health Statistics and Information, 2015, p. 100). In the same year, NCDs, including cerebrovascular disease, high blood pressure, ischemic heart disease, chronic obstructive pulmonary disease (COPD) and diabetes, were top five diseases that required urban and rural old people aged 60 or above to receive inpatient treatment (Center for Health Statistics and Information, 2015, p. 111). In 2013, the average number of inpatient days for the old people was 12.8 days (Center for Health Statistics and Information, 2015, p. 111) and the average inpatient cost for old people was RMB 9,506 (Center for Health Statistics and Information, 2015, p. 113). Since the current fragmented health insurance system only provides basic medical coverage for the participants, many old people have to pay their medical expenses on their own. Out-of-pocket medical expenditures impose a heavy financial burden on old people (Ma & Sun, 2014, p.29). Due to the problem of 'getting old before getting rich', many old people do not have enough money to pay for their medical expenses. The lack of financial means becomes a barrier for old people to seek medical treatment. For example, having financial difficulty was the main reason for old people who needed inpatient treatment ended up not receiving any inpatient treatment in 2013 (Center for Health Statistics and Information, 2015, p. 113). But for old people who really seek medical treatment, they may possibly fall into poverty or fall back into poverty due to illnesses (Wu & Li, 2006, p.121).

SOLUTIONS AND RECOMMENDATIONS

At present, many insured participants, in particular the URBMI and NRCMS ones, still find it difficult and expensive to seek medical care due to having partial medical coverage, bearing high out-of-pocket expenses and facing a continuous increase in medical costs. To alleviate the financial burden of these groups of people and reduce health inequality, the State Council in January 2016 issued *Opinions on Integrating the Basic Medical Insurance Systems for Urban and Rural Residents* (hereafter the 2016 Opinions), which aimed at gradually establishing a unified basic medical insurance system through the integration of the URBMI Scheme and the NRCMS (The State Council, 2016). According to *the 2016 Opinions*, the URBMI and NRCMS participants will have the same payment standards and enjoy the same medical insurance coverage. The new system will be mainly financed by individual contribution and government subsidies and cover medical expenses of outpatient and inpatient services, with a reimbursement rate of up to 75 percent for inpatient stay (The State Council, 2016). A unified drug formulary and medical service item catalogue will be issued for insurance reimbursement (The State Council, 2016). It is expected that the unified medical insurance system can break the urban-rural dichotomy, strengthen the efficiency of risk pooling, provide better financial protection and achieve equal medical treatments.

Migrant workers finding it difficult and expensive to seek medical treatment is still a pressing issue at this stage. In February 2016, Premier Li Keqiang said that 100 million migrant workers would be granted urban residence permits in an orderly way by 2020 (Xinhua Net, 2016 February 1) and might have full right and access to urban social services in future. Over the past few years, some local governments have carried out different measures to reduce the medical inequality of migrant workers. For example, county government in Sichuan starting in 2015 provided free medical checkup for migrant workers (Xinhua Net, 2016 January 15). Starting in 2012, the Zhengzhou government established Migrant Worker Basic Medical Insurance System, which provided inpatient medical coverage for about 100,000 migrant workers (Xinhua Net, 2016 January 15). Starting on January 1 2014, the Shenzhen government expanded Local Supplementary Medical Insurance Scheme to cover migrant workers' treatment costs for catastrophic illnesses at outpatient clinics (Shenzhen News, 2013 October 18). However, there is yet to establish a unified medical protection system for migrant workers.

The medical expenses of retired employees would deplete medical insurance fund quickly and affect the financial sustainability of medical insurance fund in the long run. In face of a rapidly ageing population, the government were examining the feasibility of retired employees paying premium contribution for health care (Guo, 2016 January 4). At present, it is too early to tell whether the base premium should be determined by the pension fund received by retired employees per month or the average monthly salary before retirement; and how insurance premium should be paid or what the level of medical coverage should be (Guangzhou Daily, 2016 January 5). But one thing is for sure, retiree contribution for health care requires amending *The Social Insurance Law of the People's Republic of China*, which states that retired employees do not need to pay any premium contribution for health care (Guo, 2016 January 4; Guangzhou Daily, 2016 January 5).

The ineffective mechanism to reduce health providers' moral hazard is one of the reasons for a considerable unnecessary drain on medical insurance fund and the inefficient and unnecessary use of medical resources. Restraining health providers' moral hazard does not mean that health care providers should be prohibited from earning profits. After all, health care providers receive inadequate subsidies from the government and need to generate enough revenues to keep up their operations. Nevertheless, a line should be drawn between earning profits and protecting the interests of patients. To ensure that money accumulated in the individual MSA and the SPF are appropriately used, the government has carried out several measures to reduce hospitals' reliance on drug sales as the main source of revenue and the practice of physician-induced demand. Since 2012, the government has introduced a pilot program of the zero-markup policy for essential drugs in primary health care institutions, county hospitals and urban public hospitals, "with the aim of delinking the financial relationship between medical services and medicine delivery" (Mao & Chen, 2015, p. 10). Under the zero-markup policy, public hospitals abolish the 15 percent mark-up they charge on drug sales but are compensated by receiving government subsidies and increasing charges for consultation, hospital beds, surgery and medical tests. The zero-markup policy for drugs has brought mixed results for patients and hospitals. The policy helps patients greatly reduce their financial burden if their medical treatment simply relies on taking medicines (Zhou, 2016 February 1). For patients who require surgical treatment and hospitalization, however, they may face higher medical expenses. On the other hand, some hospitals in Zhejiang had deficit due to the financial incapability of local government to compensate the hospitals with enough subsidies (Time-weekly, 2014 April 10). Some hospitals in Guangzhou had deficit of over RMB 6 to 7 million because government subsidies were not enough to compensate their loss of drug revenues (Zhou, 2016 February 1).

In order to restrain the profit-seeking behavior of health care provider, the Ministry of Human Resources and Social Security in August 2014 imposed penalties on health care providers that breached the terms of agreement or committed fraudulent activities. They included the government refusing to pay the bills for services provided in medical institutions, temporarily suspending settlement of health insurance claims and ordering rectification within a prescribed time period or terminating service agreement (Ministry of Human Resources and Social Security, 2014). Another measure is that, starting from June 1, 2015, the government lifted price controls for most of the drugs and let the market determine drug retail price (National Development and Reform Commission et al., 2015). Maximum ex-works prices and maximum retail prices of narcotics drugs and Class I psychotropic drugs would still be subject to the government's price control while ex-work price or retail price of other drugs would be determined by the market (National Development and Reform Commission et al., 2015). The government would strengthen its role in monitoring drug prices and conduct investigations when necessary if there are frequent or significant drug price fluctuations (National Development and Reform Commission et al., 2015).

The problem of ageing population has become more serious. In response to this problem, the government can consider establishing a health insurance scheme tailored for the old people, especially for the needy and disabled ones. In Singapore, the government introduces two health care financing schemes for the old people. One of the schemes is called Medifund Silver, which provides financial assistance for needy elderly patients aged 65 or above that have problems paying their medical bills (Ministry of Health, 2008). Another scheme is called ElderShield, which is a voluntary and affordable severe disability insurance scheme that provides basic financial protection to those who need long-term care, especially during old age (Ministry of Health, 2016). "All Singapore Citizens and Permanent Residents with Medisave accounts are automatically enrolled in ElderShield at the age of 40" (Ministry of Health, 2016) and can receive a monthly cash payout in the event of a severe disability (Ministry of Health, 2016). The Chinese government can learn from the Singaporean government in order to reduce the financial burden of old people. Meanwhile, the Chinese government has proposed the idea of integrating medical and nursing care for the elderly, which aims to achieve the important goal of 'healthy aging' through the provision of all-round care for the elderly (The National Committee of the Chinese People's Political Consultative Conference, 2014). By integrating medical and nursing care for the elderly, the government wants to allow senior care facilities to provide medical service legally and emphasizes prevention of diseases, maintaining good physical and mental health, rehabilitation services and sense of security. Emphasis on the prevention of disease can reduce the old people's financial burden caused by medical treatment. This can also reduce their demand for medical services in public hospitals.

FUTURE RESEARCH DIRECTIONS

It is undeniable that the Chinese government has made great efforts to reduce rising medical costs and finance health care through a multi-layered health insurance system. But the government's effort to achieve UHC still has a long way to go. To achieve the real sense of UHC, the ongoing health insurance reform should be accompanied by reforms on drug prices and hospital management. Besides, these reforms need regular review and assessment in order to see if they can meet the original policy goals. At the time of this study, the data for assessing the CIIS is still unavailable and specific plans for integrating the URBMI Scheme and the NRCMS have not been formulated. Future studies can examine the impact of the CIIS or the unified health insurance system on reducing medical expenses. Future studies can also examine the financial sustainability of social insurance system in China or compare the financial sustainability of China's social insurance system with that of social insurance system in other Asian or Western countries.

CONCLUSION

To conclude, China's health insurance reform is an ongoing process responding to changing political and socio-economic circumstances. Three decades of health insurance reforms show that China's transformation to a multi-layered social health insurance system was due to the complex interaction between political institutions and three sources of institutional change: environmental triggers, institutional entrepreneurs and ideas. China is moving towards UHC and is moving towards the right direction. Nevertheless, the government has to overcome significant hurdles, in particular the inherently discriminatory design of the social health insurance system, disorder in the drug distribution system,deficit in the funding of health insurance, and insufficient medical protection for the old people in order to achieve a real sense of UHC.

REFERENCES

Asia Insurance Review. (2015). *China: 1 bln+ people to have state-run critical illness cover.* Retrieved June 12, 2016, from http://www.asiainsurancereview.com/News/View-NewsLetter-Article?id=33334&Type=edaily

Augustovski, F., Martí, S. G., Riviere, A. P., & Rubinstein, A. (2011). Universal coverage with rising healthcare costs; health outcomes research value in decision making in Latin America. *Expert Review of Pharmacoeconomics & Outcomes Research, 11*(6), 657–659. doi:10.1586/erp.11.83 PMID:22098279

Auster, E. R., Wylie, K. K., & Valente, M. S. (2005). *Strategic organizational change: building change capabilities in your organization*. Basingstoke, UK: Palgrave Macmillan. doi:10.1057/9780230508064

Babiarz, K. S., Miller, G., Yi, H., Zhang, L., & Rozelle, S. (2010). New evidence on the impact of Chinas New Rural Cooperative Medical Scheme and its implications for rural primary healthcare: Multivariate difference-in-difference analysis. *BMJ (Clinical Research Ed.), 341*(2), c5617. doi:10.1136/bmj.c5617 PMID:20966008

Bai, C., & Wu, B. (2014). Health insurance and consumption: Evidence from Chinas New Cooperative Medical Scheme. *Journal of Comparative Economics, 42*(2), 450–469. doi:10.1016/j.jce.2013.07.005

Banister, J. (1987). *China's changing population.* Stanford, CA: Stanford University Press.

Battilana, J., & Leca, B. (2009). The role of resources in institutional entrepreneurship: insights for an approach to strategic management that combines agency and institutions. In L. A. Costanzo & R. B. MacKay (Eds.), *Handbook of research on strategy and foresight* (pp. 260–274). Cheltenham, UK: Edward Elgar. doi:10.4337/9781848447271.00022

Beijing Business Today. (2014a, December 9). *Price caps on drugs has little effectiveness,* Chinese version. Retrieved July 15, 2016, from http://finance.sina.com.cn/chanjing/cyxw/20141209/012021026167.shtml

Beijing Business Today. (2014b, December 9). *Some regions experience a deficit in the medical insurance fund,* Chinese version. Retrieved July 15, 2016, from http://www.cn-healthcare.com/article/20141209/content-465355.html

Béland, D. (2007). Ideas and institutional change in social security: Conversion, layering, and policy drift. *Social Science Quarterly*, *88*(1), 20–38. doi:10.1111/j.1540-6237.2007.00444.x

Béland, D., & Cox, R. H. (2011). Introduction: ideas and politics. In D. Béland & R. H. Cox (Eds.), *Ideas and Politics in Social Science Research* (pp. 3–20). New York: Oxford University Press.

Blyth, M. (2011). Ideas, uncertainty, and evolution. In D. Béland & R. H. Cox (Eds.), *Ideas and Politics in Social Science Research* (pp. 83–104). New York: Oxford University Press.

Bratton, J. (2015). *Introduction to work and organizational behaviour* (3rd ed.). New York: Palgrave Macmillan. doi:10.1007/978-1-137-43206-3

Bristol, N. (2014). *Global action toward universal health coverage*. Retrieved June 1, 2016, from https://www.ciaonet.org/attachments/24280/uploads

Brombal, D. (2014). Health sector reforms in contemporary China: a political perspective. In K. E. Brodsgaard (Ed.), *Globalization and Public Sector Reform in China* (pp. 100–124). Abingdon, UK: Routledge.

Burke, D. D. (2011). *Organization change: theory and practice* (3rd ed.). Thousand Oaks, CA: SAGE Publications.

Cai, F. (2015). Demystifying China's Economy Development. Berlin: Springer Berlin Heidelberg. doi:10.1007/978-3-662-46103-7

Campbell, J. L. (2002). Ideas, politics, and public policy. *Annual Review of Sociology*, *28*(1), 21–38. doi:10.1146/annurev.soc.28.110601.141111

Carrin, G., Mathauer, I., Xua, K., & Evans, D. B. (2008). Universal coverage of health services: Tailoring its implementation. *Bulletin of the World Health Organization*, *86*(11), 857–863. doi:10.2471/BLT.07.049387 PMID:19030691

Center for Health Statistics and Information. (2015). *The 2013 Analysis Report of National Health Services Survey in China, Chinese version*. Retrieved February 26, 2017, from http://www.nhfpc.gov.cn/mohwsbwstjxxzx/s8211/201610/9f109ff40e9346fca76dd82cecf419ce.shtml

Chen, D., Tang, K. K., Zhao, L., & Zhang, Y. (2015). Will China's Cooperative Medical System fail again? Insight from farmer satisfaction survey. *Health Promotion International*, *30*(2), 251–261. doi:10.1093/heapro/dat032 PMID:23669160

Chen, G., Liu, G. G., & Xu, F. (2014). The Impact of the urban resident basic medical insurance on health services utilisation in China. *PharmacoEconomics*, *32*(3), 277–292. doi:10.1007/s40273-013-0097-7 PMID:24178373

Chen, J. (2001). *Mao's China and the Cold War*. Chapel Hill, NC: University of North Carolina Press.

Cheng, T. (2015). Universal health coverage: An overview and lessons from Asia. *Harvard Public Health Review*, *4*, 1–12.

Cheung, A. B. L. (2001). Health policy reform. In L. Wong & N. Flynn (Eds.), *The market in Chinese social policy* (pp. 63–87). Houndmills, UK: Palgrave. doi:10.1057/9781403919939_4

China Business News. (2015 November 30). *Expenditures of medical insurance funds exceeded revenues of medical insurance funds in many regions in China,* Chinese version. Retrieved July 14, 2016, from http://finance.sina.com.cn/china/20151130/005723882229.shtml

China Social Insurance Net. (2015). *Analysis on personal financial burden among inpatients who were covered by the Urban Resident Basic Medical Insurance Scheme*, Chinese version. Retrieved July 14, 2016, from http://www.spicezee.com/zhishi/yiliao/108433.html

Collier, R. B., & Collier, D. (1991). *Shaping the political arena: critical junctures, the labor movement, and regime dynamics in Latin America*. Princeton, NJ: Princeton University Press.

Cortell, A. P., & Peterson, S. (1999). Altered states: Explaining domestic institutional change. *British Journal of Political Science*, *29*(1), 177–203. doi:10.1017/S0007123499000083

DiMaggio, P. (1988). Interest and agency in institutional theory. In L. G. Zucker (Ed.), *Institutional patterns and organizations: culture and environment* (pp. 3–21). Cambridge, MA: Ballinger Pub. Co.

Dong, W. (2001). *Health care reform in urban China*. Retrieved July 7, 2016, from http://munkschool.utoronto.ca/cphs/wp-content/uploads/2012/03/Weizhen_Dong-2001-02.pdf

Dong, W. (2008). Cost containment and access to care: The Shanghai health care financing model. *The Singapore Economic Review*, *53*(1), 27–41. doi:10.1142/S0217590808002823

Duckett, J. (2001). Political interests and the implementation of China's urban health insurance reform. *Social Policy and Administration*, *35*(3), 290–306. doi:10.1111/1467-9515.00234

European Federation of Pharmaceutical Industries and Association. (2014). *Health & Growth: Working Together for a Healthy Europe*. Retrieved July 17, 2016, from www.efpai.eu

Feng, Y., Xiong, X., Xue, Q., Yao, L., Luo, F., & Xiang, L. (2013). The impact of medical insurance policies on the hospitalization services utilization of people with schizophrenia: A case study in Changsha, China. *Pakistan Journal of Medical Sciences*, *29*(3), 793–798. doi:10.12669/pjms.293.3273 PMID:24353630

Feng, Z. (2016). Marginalisation and health provision in transitional China. In H. X. Zhang, B. Wu, & R. Sanders (Eds.), *Marginalisation in China: perspectives on transition and globalization* (pp. 97–116). Aldershot, UK: Ashgate.

finance.china.com.cn. (2016 March 8). *Li Bin: China's elderly population aged 60 and over passed 220 million in 2015*, Chinese version. Retrieved June 18, 2016, from http://finance.huanqiu.com/roll/2016-03/8672801.html

Flynn, M. B. (2015). *Pharmaceutical autonomy and public health in Latin America: state, society, and industry in Brazil's AIDS program*. New York, NY: Routledge.

General Office of the State Council. (2003). *Opinions on Establishing the New Rural Cooperative Medical System,* Chinese version. Retrieved July 12, 2016, from http://www.law-lib.com/law/law_view.asp?id=43058

Gotsadze, G., Zoidze, A., & Rukhadze, N. (2009). Household catastrophic health expenditure: Evidence from Georgia and its policy implications. *BMC Health Services Research, 9*(1), 69. doi:10.1186/1472-6963-9-69 PMID:19400939

Gu, E. (2001). Market transition and the transformation of the health care system in urban China. *Policy Studies, 22*(3/4), 197–215. doi:10.1080/01442870120112692

Guangzhou Daily. (2016 January 5). *Do retired employees need to pay premium contribution for health care?* Chinese version. Retrieved July 16, 2016, from http://jiankang.163.com/16/0105/08/BCI6N50N0038002S.html

Guo, J. (2016 January 4). *How long does it last for 720 million retired employees not paying premium contribution for medical care?* Chinese version. Retrieved July 16, 2016, from http://www.yicai.com/news/4733894.html

Haber, D. (2013). *Health promotion and aging: practical applications for health professionals* (6th ed.). New York, NY: Springer Publishing Company, LLC.

Hall, P. A., & Taylor, R. C. R. (1996). Political science and the three new institutionalisms. *Political Studies, 44*(5), 936–957. doi:10.1111/j.1467-9248.1996.tb00343.x

Hardy, C., & Maguire, S. (2008). Institutional entrepreneurship. In R. Greenwood, C. Oliver, K. Sahlin, & R. Suddaby (Eds.), *The SAGE handbook of organizational institutionalism* (pp. 198–217). Los Angeles, CA: SAGE. doi:10.4135/9781849200387.n8

Haunschild, P., & Chandler, D. (2008). Institutional-level learning: learning as a source of institutional change. In R. Greenwood, C. Oliver, K. Sahlin, & R. Suddaby (Eds.), *The SAGE handbook of organizational institutionalism* (pp. 624–649). Los Angeles, CA: SAGE. doi:10.4135/9781849200387.n27

Henan Business Daily. (2013, December 31). *The reasons for cheap essential drugs disappearing from the market in China,* Chinese version. Retrieved July 15, 2016, from http://www.cb.com.cn/investigation/2013_1231/1031072.html

Hinings, C. R., Greenwood, R., Reay, T., & Suddaby, R. (2004). Dynamics of change in organizational fields. In M. S. Poole & A. H. Van de Ven (Eds.), *Handbook of organizational change and innovation* (pp. 304–323). New York: Oxford University Press.

Hipgrave, D. (2011). Communicable disease control in China: From Mao to now. *Journal of Global Health, 1*(2), 224–238. PMID:23198121

Hsu, M., Huang, X., & Yupho, S. (2015). The development of universal health insurance coverage in Thailand: Challenges of population aging and informal economy. *Social Science & Medicine, 145*, 227–236. doi:10.1016/j.socscimed.2015.09.036 PMID:26452699

Hu, A. (2016). *China's social insurance in the twentieth century: a global historical perspective*. Leiden, Germany: Brill.

Huang, Y. (2013). *Governing Health in Contemporary China. Milton Park.* Abingdon, UK: Routledge.

James, K. (2015). *The rise of the value-added tax*. New York, NY: Cambridge University Press. doi:10.1017/CBO9781107358522

Kankeu, H. T., Saksena, P., Xu, K., & Evans, D. B. (2013). The financial burden from non-communicable diseases in low- and middle-income countries: A literature review. *Health Research Policy and Systems*, *11*(1), 31. doi:10.1186/1478-4505-11-31 PMID:23947294

Kaufman, S. R., Livingston, J., Zhang, H., & Lock, M. (2013). Transforming concepts of ageing: three case studies from anthropology. In T. Dening & A. Thomas (Eds.), *Oxford Textbook of Old Age Psychiatry* (2nd ed.; pp. 39–56). Oxford University Press. doi:10.1093/med/9780199644957.003.0004

Kirchner, S. (2013). How organizations become enduring: disentangling the organizational identity paradox. In J. Sydow & G. Schreoygg (Eds.), *Self-reinforcing processes in and among organizations* (pp. 33–54). Houndmills, UK: Palgrave Macmillan. doi:10.1057/9780230392830_3

Kong, X., Li, Z., & Kong, Y. (2011). The formation basis of high drug prices, Chinese version. *China Pharmacy*, *22*(12), 1069–1071.

Langenbrunner, J. C., & Somanathan, A. (2011). *Financing health care in East Asia and the Pacific: best practices and remaining challenges*. Washington, DC: World Bank.

Larus, E. F. (2012). *Politics and society in contemporary China*. Boulder, CO: Lynne Rienner Publishers.

Lawrence, S. V., & Martin, M. F. (2013). *Understanding China's Political System*. Retrieved July 18, 2016, from https://www.fas.org/sgp/crs/row/R41007.pdf

Lecours, A. (2000). Theorizing cultural identities: Historical institutionalism as a challenge to the culturalists. *Canadian Journal of Political Science*, *33*(3), 499–522. doi:10.1017/S0008423900000172

Lei, P., & Wu, Z. (2014). Analysis on over-medication in hospitals in China, Chinese version. *Chinese Health Economics*, *33*(5), 9–11.

Li, C., Hou, Y., Sun, M., Lu, J., Wang, Y., Li, X., & Hao, M. et al. (2015). An evaluation of China's new rural cooperative medical system: Achievements and inadequacies from policy goals. *BMC Public Health*, *15*(1), 1079. doi:10.1186/s12889-015-2410-1 PMID:26494015

Li, Q. (2009). The study on realizing the path to universal health insurance in China, Chinese version. Beijing: People's Publishing House.

Li, S. (2006, September 29). *Population aging brings three types of pressure to China*, Chinese version. Retrieved June 24, 2016, from http://www.huaxia.com/xw/zh/2006/00516600.html

Li, T. (2015, February 13). *Individual premium contribution of the New Rural Cooperative Medical System (NRCMS) will increase to Renminbi 120, but some regions still have the problem of expenditure exceeding revenue of the NRCMS fund*, Chinese version. Retrieved July 14, 2016, from http://news.xinhuanet.com/politics/2015-02/13/c_127491063.htm

Li, Y. (2013). Analysis on high drug prices, the practice of drug kickbacks, and the centralized bidding and procurement for drugs, Chinese version. *Contemporary Economics*, *23*, 17–19.

Lin, W., Liu, G. G., & Chen, G. (2009). The urban resident basic medical insurance: A landmark reform towards universal coverage in China. *Health Economics, 18*(S2), S83–S96. doi:10.1002/hec.1500 PMID:19551750

Liu, G. G., Yuen, P., Hu, T., Li, L., & Liu, X. (2004). Urban health insurance reform: what can we learn from the pilot experiment? In A. Chen, G.G. Liu, & K.H. Zhang (Eds.), Urbanization and social welfare in China (pp. 38-62). Aldershot, UK: Ashgate.

Liu, G. G., Zhao, Z., Cai, R., Yamada, T., & Yamada, T. (2002). Equity in health care access to: Assessing the urban health insurance reform in China. *Social Science & Medicine, 55*(10), 1779–1794. doi:10.1016/S0277-9536(01)00306-9 PMID:12383462

Liu, H., & Zhao, Z. (2014). Does health insurance matter? Evidence from China's urban resident basic medical insurance. *Journal of Comparative Economics, 42*(4), 1007–1020. doi:10.1016/j.jce.2014.02.003

Liu, X., & Cao, H. (1992). China's cooperative medical systems: Its historical transformation and the trend of development. *Journal of Public Health Policy, 13*(4), 501–511. doi:10.2307/3342538 PMID:1287043

Liu, X., & Mills, A. (2005). The effect of performance-related pay of hospital doctors on hospital behaviour: A case study from Shandong, China. *Human Resources for Health, 3*(1), 11. doi:10.1186/1478-4491-3-11 PMID:16253137

Liu, X., Wong, H., & Liu, K. (2016). Outcome-based health equity across different social health insurance schemes for the elderly in China. *BMC Health Services Research, 16*(1), 9. doi:10.1186/s12913-016-1261-5 PMID:26762146

Liu, Y. (2004). Development of the rural health insurance system in China. *Health Policy and Planning, 19*(3), 159–165. doi:10.1093/heapol/czh019 PMID:15070864

Liu, Y., Hsiao, W. C. L., Li, Q., Liu, X., & Ren, M. (1995). Transformation of China's rural health care financing. *Social Science & Medicine, 41*(8), 1085–1093. doi:10.1016/0277-9536(95)00428-A PMID:8578331

Lu, X. P. (2015, February 10). *Government official from China Insurance Regulatory Commission: Individuals currently still have to bear a relatively high medical expenses*, Chinese version. Retrieved July 14, 2016, from http://finance.sina.com.cn/stock/t/20150210/111321518553.shtml

Luk, S. (2014). *Health Insurance Reforms in Asia.* London: Routledge.

Lussier, R. N. (2009). *Management fundamentals: concepts, applications, skill development* (4th ed.). South Western College.

Ma, Y., & Sun, S. (2014). Analysis on the medical insurance system for the elderly, Chinese version. *China Social Security, 9*, 28–29.

Mahoney, J. (2001). *The legacies of liberalism: path dependence and political regimes in Central America.* Baltimore, MD: Johns Hopkins University Press.

Mao, W., & Chen, W. (2015). *China: The zero mark-up policy for essential medicines at primary level facilities*. Retrieved July 17, 2016, from http://www.who.int/health_financing/documents/Efficiency_health_systems_China/en/

Meng, Q., Rehnberg, C., Zhuang, N., Bian, Y., Tomson, G., & Tang, S. (2004). The impact of urban health insurance reform on hospital charges: A case study from two cities in China. *Health Policy (Amsterdam), 68*(2), 197–209. doi:10.1016/j.healthpol.2003.09.010 PMID:15063019

Min, Y., Jiang, L., Yan, L. L., Wang, L., Basu, S., Wu, Y., & Stafford, R. S. (2015). Tackling China's noncommunicable diseases: Shared origins, costly consequences and the need for action. *Chinese Medical Journal, 128*(6), 839–843. doi:10.4103/0366-6999.152690 PMID:25758283

Ministry of Health. (2008). *Medifund Silver*. Retrieved February 26, 2017, from https://www.moh.gov.sg/content/moh_web/home/pressRoom/pressRoomItemRelease/2008/medifund_silver.html

Ministry of Health. (2016). *ElderShield Fast Facts*. Retrieved February 26, 2017, from https://www.moh.gov.sg/content/dam/moh_web/Publications/Educational%20Resources/2016/ElderShield%20Fast%20Facts%20Brochure.pdf

Ministry of Human Resources and Social Security. (2014). *Opinions on Further Strengthening the Supervision and Management of Medical Services for the Basic Medical Insurance*, Chinese version. Retrieved July 17, 2016, from http://www.law-lib.com/law/law_view.asp?id=460883

Moore, B. (1966). *Social origins of dictatorship and democracy: lord and peasant in the making of the modern world*. Boston: Beacon Press.

Nanfang Metropolis Daily. (2015 February 10). *Green Book of Health Reform and Development 2014 said that medical insurance funds are faced with risks and will have a deficit in 2017*, Chinese version. Retrieved July 12, 2016, from http://www.nandu.com/html/201502/10/1050767.html

National Bureau of Statistics of China. (2014). *China Statistical Yearbook 2014*. Retrieved July 12, 2016, from http://www.stats.gov.cn/tjsj/ndsj/2014/indexch.htm

National Development and Reform Commission, Ministry of Health, Ministry of Finance, Ministry of Human Resources and Social Security, Ministry of Civil Affairs, and China Insurance Regulatory Commission. (2012). *The Guiding Opinions on the Launch of the Work on Critical Illness Insurance for Urban and Rural Residents,* Chinese version. Retrieved July 12, 2016, from http://www.gov.cn/gzdt/2012-08/31/content_2214223.htm

National Development and Reform Commission, National Health and Family Planning Commission, Ministry of Human Resources and Social Security, Ministry of Industry and Information Technology, Ministry of Finance, Ministry of Commerce, and China Food and Drug Administration. (2015). *Opinions on Proceeding with the Reform on Drug Pricing,* Chinese version. Retrieved July 17, 2016, from http://www.sdpc.gov.cn/zcfb/zcfbtz/201505/W020150505398057890638.pdf

Pang, S. M. (2003). *Nursing ethics in modern China: conflicting values and competing role requirements*. Amsterdam: Rodopi.

Permanent Mission of the People's Republic of China to the United Nations. (2008). *Preventing neglect and abuse in a rapidly ageing society*. Retrieved June 18, 2016, from http://www.china-un.org/eng/chinaandun/socialhr/aging_disabilities/t531015.htm

Pierson, P. (2000a). Not just what, but when: Timing and sequence in political processes. *Studies in American Political Development, 14*(1), 72–92. doi:10.1017/S0898588X00003011

Pierson, P. (2000b). Increasing returns, path dependence, and the study of politics. *The American Political Science Review, 94*(2), 251–267. doi:10.2307/2586011

Pierson, P., & Skocpol, T. (2002). Historical institutionalism in contemporary political science. In I. Katznelson, & H. V. Milner (Eds.), Political science: The state of the discipline (pp.693-721). New York: American Political Science Association.

Qiu, Y. (2015). The impact of aging population on health care expenditures in China, Chinese version. *Journal of Nanjing College for Population Programme Management, 31*(2), 95–102.

Reich, M. R., Harris, J., Ikegami, N., Maeda, A., Cashin, C., Araujo, E. C., & Evans, T. G. et al. (2016). Moving towards universal health coverage: Lessons from 11 country studies. *Lancet, 387*(10020), 811–816. doi:10.1016/S0140-6736(15)60002-2 PMID:26299185

Saurugger, S. (2014). *Theoretical approaches to European integration*. Basingstoke, UK: Palgrave Macmillan.

Savedoff, W. D., & Smith, A. L. (2011). *Achieving universal health coverage: learning from Chile, Japan, Malaysia and Sweden*. Retrieved June 5, 2016, from http://www.resultsfordevelopment.org/knowledge-center/achieving-universal-health-coverage-learning-chile-japan-malaysia-and-sweden

Shen, C., Zhao, X., & Zou, H. (2014). Fiscal decentralization and public services provision in China. *Annals of Economics and Finance, 15*(1), 135–160.

Shenzhen News. (2013, October 18). *Shenzhen will implement new medical insurance measure starting on January 1 next year; Local Supplementary Medical Insurance Scheme will cover migrant workers*, Chinese version. Retrieved July 16, 2016, from http://www.sznews.com/news/content/2013-10/18/content_8641375.htm

Steinmo, S. (2008). Historical institutionalism. In D. D. Porta & M. Keating (Eds.), *Approaches and methodologies in the social sciences: a pluralist perspective* (pp. 118–138). Cambridge, UK: Cambridge University Press. doi:10.1017/CBO9780511801938.008

Streeck, W., & Thelen, K. (2005). Introduction: institutional change in advanced political economies. In W. Streeck & K. Thelen (Eds.), *Beyond continuity: institutional change in advanced political economies* (pp. 3–39). Oxford, UK: Oxford University Press.

Su, T. T., Kouyaté, B., & Flessa, S. (2006). Catastrophic household expenditure for health care in low–income society: A study from Nouna District, Burkina Faso. *Bulletin of the World Health Organization, 84*(1), 21–27. doi:10.2471/BLT.05.023739 PMID:16501711

Sun, Q., Liu, X., Meng, Q., Tang, S., Yu, B., & Tolhurst, R. (2009). Evaluating the financial protection of patients with chronic disease by health insurance in rural China. *International Journal for Equity in Health*, *8*(1), 42. doi:10.1186/1475-9276-8-42 PMID:20003188

Tang, S., Ehiri, J., & Long, Q. (2013). Chinas biggest, most neglected health challenge: Non-communicable diseases. *Infectious Diseases of Poverty*, *2*(1), 7. doi:10.1186/2049-9957-2-7 PMID:23849054

The China Health Care Study Group. (1974). *Health Care in China, an introduction: The report of a study group in Hong Kong*. Geneva: Christian Medical Commission.

The National Committee of the Chinese People's Political Consultative Conference. (2014). *Integrating medical and nursing care for the elderly,* Chinese version. Retrieved February 26, 2017 from http://www.cppcc.gov.cn/zxww/2014/12/30/ARTI1419900481141424.shtml

The State Council. (1998). *The Decision of the State Council Concerning the Establishment of the Urban Employee Basic Medical Insurance,* Chinese version. Retrieved July 8, 2016, from http://www.gov.cn/banshi/2005-08/04/content_20256.htm

The State Council. (2007). *The Guiding Opinions on Piloting Urban Resident Basic Medical Insurance,* Chinese version. Retrieved July 13, 2016, from http://www.gov.cn/zwgk/2007-07/24/content_695118.htm

The State Council. (2016). *Opinions on Integrating the Basic Medical Insurance Systems for Urban and Rural Residents,* Chinese version. Retrieved July 16, 2016, from http://www.gov.cn/zhengce/content/2016-01/12/content_10582.htm

The World Bank. (2010). *Fixing the public hospital system in China.* Retrieved June 26, 2016, from http://siteresources.worldbank.org/HEALTHNUTRITIONANDPOPULATION/Resources/281627-1285186535266/FixingthePublicHospitalSystem.pdf

Thelen, K. (1999). Historical institutionalism in comparative politics. *Annual Review of Political Science*, *2*(1), 369–404. doi:10.1146/annurev.polisci.2.1.369

Time-weekly. (2014). *The Zero-mark-up Policy for Drugs in Public Hospitals in Zhejiang,* Chinese version. Retrieved July 17, 2016, from http://money.163.com/14/0410/07/9PF0NPUI00252G50.html

Wagstaff, A., Lindelow, M., Gao, J., Xu, L., & Qian, J. (2009). Extending health insurance to the rural population: An impact evaluation of Chinas new cooperative medical scheme. *Journal of Health Economics*, *1*(1), 1–19. doi:10.1016/j.jhealeco.2008.10.007 PMID:19058865

Walder, A. G. (2015). *China under Mao: a revolution derailed.* Cambridge, MA: Harvard University Press. doi:10.4159/9780674286689

Wang, J., & Chen, G. (2015 October 12). *Cheap essential drugs disappear from the market: 342 of more than 500 drugs are in severe shortage,* Chinese version. Retrieved July 15, 2016, from http://news.sciencenet.cn/htmlnews/2015/10/328428.shtm

Wang, J., Zhou, H., Lei, Y., & Wang, X. (2012). Financial protection under the New Rural Cooperative Medical Schemes in China. *Medical Care*, *50*(8), 700–704. doi:10.1097/MLR.0b013e318249d8bf PMID:22354207

Wang, X., He, X., Zheng, A., & Ji, X. (2014). The effects of Chinas New Cooperative Medical Scheme on accessibility and affordability of healthcare services: An empirical research in Liaoning Province. *BMC Health Services Research, 14*(1), 388. doi:10.1186/1472-6963-14-388 PMID:25217224

Weir, M. (2006). When does politics create policy? The organizational politics of change. In I. Shapiro, S. Skowronek, & D. Galvin (Eds.), *Rethinking political institutions: the art of the state* (pp. 171–186). New York: New York University Press.

Wong, C., Lo, V. I., & Tang, K. (2006). *China's urban health care reform: from state protection to individual responsibility*. Lanham, MD: Lexington Books.

World Health Organization. (2008). *Primary health care: now more than ever*. Retrieved February 19, 2016, from http://www.who.int/whr/2008/whr08_en.pdf

World Health Organization. (2013). *The world health report 2013: research for universal health coverage*. Retrieved June 1, 2016, from http://apps.who.int/iris/bitstream/10665/85761/2/9789240690837_eng.pdf?ua=1

Wu, C. (1991). *The aging of population in China*. Retrieved June 21, 2016, from http://www.cicred.org/Eng/Publications/pdf/c-d16.pdf

Wu, G., & Li, W. (2006). New Health Revolution, Chinese version. Beijing: Tsinghua University Press.

Xinhua Net. (2013, March 28). *Mass media in the West said that the presence of structural defects in China's health insurance system had pushed migrant workers to visit black clinics,* Chinese version. Retrieved July 14, 2016, from http://news.qq.com/a/20130328/000824.htm

Xinhua Net. (2016, January 15). *The Chinese Communist Party's newspaper reported that migrant workers find it difficult to see a doctor,* Chinese version. Retrieved July 16, 2016, from http://finance.sina.com.cn/china/2016-01-15/doc-ifxnrahr8315304.shtml

Xinhua Net. (2016, February 1). *China to orderly urbanize migrant workers: Premier Li*. Retrieved July 16, 2016, from http://news.xinhuanet.com/english/2016-02/01/c_135065434.htm

Yi, Y., Maynard, A., Liu, G., Xiong, X., & Lin, F. (2005). Equity in health care financing: Evaluation of the current urban employee health insurance reform in China. *Journal of the Asia Pacific Economy, 10*(4), 506–527. doi:10.1080/13547860500291745

Yip, W., & Eggleston, K. (2004). Addressing government and market failures with payment incentives: Hospital reimbursement reform in Hainan, China. *Social Science & Medicine, 58*(2), 267–277. doi:10.1016/S0277-9536(03)00010-8 PMID:14604613

Zang, J., & Ng, S. W. (2016). Age, period and cohort effects on adult physical activity levels from 1991 to 2011 in China. *The International Journal of Behavioral Nutrition and Physical Activity, 13*(1), 40. doi:10.1186/s12966-016-0364-z PMID:27094983

Zhang, R., Wang, Z., Fei, Y., Zhou, B., Zheng, S., Wang, L., & Yu, Y. et al. (2015). The difference in nutrient intakes between Chinese and Mediterranean, Japanese and American diets. *Nutrients, 7*(6), 4661–4688. doi:10.3390/nu7064661 PMID:26066014

Zhang, Y. (2013). Meeting the ageing challenge: China's social care policy for the elderly. In G. Wang, & Y. Zheng (Eds.), China: Development and governance (pp. 343-350). Singapore: World Scientific Pub. Co.

Zheng, G. C. (2009). *The development of social security system with Chinese characteristics*. Beijing: China Labour & Social Security Publishing House.

Zhou, Q. (2016, February 1). *The zero mark-up policy leads to hospitals having difficulty in earning revenues,* Chinese version. Retrieved July 17, 2016 from http://news.youth.cn/sh/201602/t20160201_7591716.htm

Zhou, Z., Zhu, L., Zhou, Z., Li, Z., Gao, J., & Chen, G. (2014). The effects of Chinas urban basic medical insurance schemes on the equity of health service utilization: Evidence from Shaanxi Province. *International Journal for Equity in Health, 13*(1), 23. doi:10.1186/1475-9276-13-23 PMID:24606592

Zhu, C., Sun, X., Geng, Q. F. R., Yang, H., & Jiang, W. (2015). Self-rated chronic conditions and 2-week prevalence in adults in Zhongshan, China: An epidemiological survey. *BMJ Open*, *5*(11), e008441. doi:10.1136/bmjopen-2015-008441 PMID:26560055

Zhu, Z. (2011). Whither China in the 21st century? In Z. Zhu (Ed.), *The People's Republic of China Today: Internal and External Exchanges* (pp. 429–440). Hackensack, NJ: World Scientific.

KEY TERMS AND DEFINITIONS

Ageing Population: A population with an increasing proportion of people over 65 years old.

Basic Medical Insurance: A form of public insurance that covers medical costs of the Chinese population. But its reimbursement for medical care is quite limited that participants still have to pay high out-of-pocket medical expenses.

Drug Formulary: A list of approved prescription drugs that are selected for coverage by a medical insurance plan based on their reported medical efficacy, safety and cost effectiveness.

Historical Institutionalism: An approach that centers on political institutions and past events to explain political or policy outcomes.

Non-Communicable Disease: A disease that is not contagious among people.

Physician-Induced Demand: A phenomenon whereby a doctor provides excess medical treatment for a patient in order to earn more revenues.

Universal Health Coverage: A form of medical insurance that is provided to all citizens of a country.

Chapter 3
Long-Term Care Spending Relevant to U.S. Medicaid Expansion:
Medicaid Long-Term Care Spending

Mary Schmeida
Kent State University, USA

Ramona Sue McNeal
University of Northern Iowa, USA

ABSTRACT

The U.S. population is living longer, placing a demand on long-term care services. In the U.S., Medicaid is the primary player in funding costly long-term care for the aged poor. As a major health reform law, the 2010 Patient Protection and Affordable Care Act, Public Law 111-148, gives financial incentive for states to expand Medicaid, transitioning long-term care services from facilities toward community care. Facing other funding obligations and recent recessions, not all states expanded their Medicaid long-term care program using the financial incentives. Some states continue to spend more dollars on traditional nursing facility care despite legislation. This chapter explores why some states spend more revenue on nursing facility long-term care despite enhanced federal funding to reform, while others are spending more on home and community-based services. Regression analysis and 50 state-level data is used.

INTRODUCTION

Longevity has increased in high-income countries (World Health Organization, 2014). In the U.S., those 65 years and older are living longer, placing a demand on long-term care services. Nearly 82.3 million seniors are expected in the U.S. by 2040, over twice that in 2000 (U.S. Dept. of Health and Human Services, 2014, p. 3). "With the percentage of our population who are elderly or disabled increasing faster than that of the younger groups, the need for long-term care is expected to increase" (Centers for Medicare

DOI: 10.4018/978-1-5225-2633-9.ch003

and Medicaid Services [CMS], November 16, 2015, p. 31). Medicaid long-term care service(s) are an option for those American seniors facing poverty, yet, need substantive care (Schmeida & McNeal, 2015).

The history of Medicaid funding for community-based long-term healthcare is over 30 years. In 2010, U.S. legislation in support of Medicaid expanded to fit the needs of many poor population groups, including the fast growing aged poor with long-term care needs. Reforming healthcare, the 2010 Patient Protection and Affordable Care Act (ACA) offers financial incentive for states to increase their Medicaid enrollment including long-term care (Public Law 111–148, 2010). It builds upon the Deficit Reduction Act of 2005 (Public Law 109-171, 2005) to "rebalance state Medicaid long-term care spending" from nursing facility care to home and community-based services, allowing the recipient to remain in a beneficial community setting, less costly to government (Mathematica, 2014, p. 2; Public Law 111-148, 2005; Schmeida & McNeal, 2015). The idea of home and community-based long-term care is growing, made "doable" as financial support improves, political ideological values promote, and caregivers make it a realization (Schmeida & McNeal, 2015). In Fiscal Year 2015, Medicaid enrollment increased by 13.8% (on average) across the 50 states, and total Medicaid spending increased 13.9% on average (Kaiser Family Foundation [KFF], October 2015, p. 1).

How states in the U.S. attempt to meet their many financial obligations while addressing a demand for long-term care is becoming a delicate balancing act. There are many issues state leaders consider when providing long-term care including how to best maximize Medicaid dollars. This chapter explores why some states continue to spend more revenue on traditional nursing facility care despite federal incentives to reform, while other states are spending more on home and community-based services. Specifically, what factors (state economic [supply and demand], political, and need/ demand) explain the differences in Medicaid long-term care spending across the 50 states? This chapter answers this question using multivariate regression analysis and 50 state-level data.

POLICY BACKGROUND

A timeline of the 1935 Social Security Act (SSA) and its amendments reveals how U.S. social policies have evolved into the modern day reform effort. Federal benefits for the aged did not become law until the Roosevelt Administration signing of the 1935 Social Security Act (Public Law 74-271, 1935). This Act (SSA) offered federal old age grants, helping states with provisions for "aged persons, blind persons, dependent and crippled children, maternal and child welfare, public health, and the administration of their unemployment compensation laws" and other purposes. It created the "Old-Age Reserve" account, now known as Social Security under its Title II. This was a venue for today's private nursing home industry by prohibiting social security payout to recipients residing in substandard public poor homes (P.L. 74-271, p. 620-622; KFF, August 2015, p. 1). Since inception, the SSA of 1935 has grown in scope. Once a worker's "retirement program" is now a family security program (CQ, 2015); nursing homes now receive the medical payments for care not beneficiaries; and Medicare and Medicaid programs were added in 1965 (Public Law 89-97). Unlike Medicare that covers medical care for the aged, Medicaid is the U.S. social insurance program for the poor. As a redistributive program, it manipulates the allocation of property rights, wealth, and other value among social classes (Ripley & Franklin, 1980). Medicaid is a federal-state means tested insurance program (CMS, 2014), with the federal government giving states financial assistance (cost sharing) as an incentive to subsidize care and service its residents (Public Law 111-148, 2005). As an open-ended matching program, states must provide services for mandatory "categorically needy" populations, such as the aged, blind, and disabled to receive any federal matching funds (CMS, November 16, 2015, p. 24).

The Social Security Amendments of 1965 biased Medicaid toward institutional nursing home care (Public Law 89-97, 1965; KFF, December 2015), but this has changed. In 1981, a SSA amendment (Section 1915c) allows states to offer home and community-based services (HCBS) as an alternative to traditional nursing home care (KFF, August 2015), with the state of Oregon first to use HCBS waivers (Kane, 2012). In 1999, the Supreme Court in *Olmstead v. L.C.* ruled it a violation of the Americans with Disability Act of 1990 (requiring the disabled be provided with appropriate accommodations in housing, employment and public service) not to open up HCBS to the disabled (Public Law 101-336; Kane, 2012). With time more changes are made to policies for the aged. Under the George W. Bush Administration, the Deficit Reduction Act of 2005 gave states federal monies to further expand HCBS (Public Law 109-171, 2005). To date, states have the option to offer HCBS to residents, while the traditional nursing home from the original 1965 Act remains as a mandatory back-up. In 2010, the Patient Protection and Affordable Care Act (ACA), considered key reform, gave states even more Medicaid long-term care options (Public Law 111–148, 2010; KFF, August 2015). Provisions include expanding eligibility; improving nursing home transparency; more expansion of HCBS long-term care; de-institutionalizing the disabled; and funding aging and disability centers (Public Law 111–148, 2010; National Conference of State Legislatures, 2011; KFF, December 2015, p. 6). Most of ACA's long-term care provisions have money inducement. In ACA's Balancing Incentive Payments Program, for example, "states may receive additional Medicaid matching funds when they meet certain requirements for expanding the percentage of long-term care spending for home- and community-based services" (National Conference of State Legislatures, November, 2011, p. 1). Politically, response to ACA's Medicaid expansion has varied across federal and state leadership. In January 2016, the U.S. Congress passed legislation to phase it out, but was vetoed by former President Barack Obama. Change may yet occur since recent U.S. elections have brought in a new presidential administration (Donald Trump) differing in party and ideology. Although Medicaid is redistributive, change may occur since the characteristics of ACA are regulatory. Regulatory policy brings conflict within the policy community, and usually transferred to a higher level (Ripley and Franklin, 1980) for resolution.

Medicaid long-term care stakeholders include recipients, industry, and government. The U.S. Department of Health and Human Services and its Centers for Medicare and Medicaid Services are major players in program implementation (CMS, 2015). Interest groups, e.g. the Americans with disabilities have played a role in moving long-term care dollars from traditional nursing homes to home and community-based settings, expanding HCBS waivers for the aged (Kane, 2012).

MEDICAID LONG-TERM CARE FINANCING

As a federal-state matching program with shared responsibility, the federal government guarantees one dollar for every state dollar spent on Medicaid, with enhanced matching rates for particular services (KFF, May, 2015). The state's share of Medicaid spending largely depends on tax revenue. Personal income, corporate income, and largely property taxes are big sources, with local sales tax the second largest in the "total" local tax revenue (Rockefeller Institute of Government, March, 2016). However, not all states are alike. Alaska e.g. differs in having neither personal income tax nor sales tax, mostly funding its state budget from oil taxes and royalties (KFF, October 15, 2015a).

State Fiscal Stress

The state share of the federal-state matching formula has been challenged by recession budget deficits (2001 and 2007) and other state obligations external to Medicaid (Pew, December 10, 2015; United States Government Accountability Office [GAO], 2011). With greater enrollment and lesser state funds, funding was a stretch for most, and state policy action was taken to stimulate state revenue. California e.g. implemented "a number" of policies to decrease spending and increase revenue when budget shortfall was multi-billion (KFF, October 15, 2015b). Also, the U.S. Congress enacted the American Recovery and Reinvestment Act of 2009 giving states "general fiscal relief," temporarily increasing the federal share of the matching rate or Federal Medical Assistance Percentage (Public Law 111-5, 2009; GAO, 2011, p. 1). To prevent deficit cut-backs on government programs, the GAO (a Congressional arm) recommended a prototype formula for temporary increases in the FMAP providing an automatic, timely, and targeted state assistance, using the U.S. labor market as trigger for the increases (GAO, July, 2015).

State recession recovery has not been uniform. The 2015 total end-of-year budget balance (in dollars and a share of expenditures) "was lower than at the pre-recession peak" across states (Pew, January 5, 2016, p. 1), with a few still facing a budget deficit. Alaska for example, has faced a deficit since 2013 (KFF, October 15, 2015a), while others---Arizona, California, Minnesota, and Virginia have a budget surplus (Pew, January 27, 2016). Many states are cautious to commit spending their recession recovery on pricey projects, such as Medicaid, as "recent volatility and losses in the stock market foreshadow less income tax revenue. And the trend in sales tax receipts is weakening, as consumers turn to untaxed Internet sales and cautious buying habits" (Pew, January 27, 2016, p. 2). States have forecasted a slow tax revenue growth for 2016 and 2017 (Rockefeller Institute of Government, March 2016, p.18). The GAO projects Medicaid spending to increase about 60% by fiscal year 2023 (GAO, July, 2015).

Long-Term Care Expenditure

Government healthcare spending is largely driven by ACA's expansion of Medicaid (CMS, November 16, 2015, p. 6). In fiscal year 2015, 29 states expanded and "spending growth in expansion states far exceeded growth in non-expansion states" (p. 1). Hikes in provider costs, health services including drug costs explained the total spending increases, on average 13.9% (KFF, October, 2015, p. 1). Fully funded by the federal government, ACA temporarily raised physician reimbursement for particular Medicaid fees and primary care services, included are internists and family physicians (Urban Institute, 2014, p. 1). This was done as an inducement to physicians to cover projected Medicaid enrollee increases. Some provider rate increases (Alaska), however, were done prior to ACA (Kaiser Family Foundation, October 15, 2015a).

Long-term care expenditures are led by nursing home facilities or "institutions." The CMS (2014) reports, 2013 long-term care expenditures led all Medicaid costs with nursing facility expenditures at $38.3 billion, managed care at $10.7 billion, home and community-based waivers at $5 billion, and inpatient hospital at $3.4 billion (pp. 45-46). As a percent of total Medicaid long-term care spending, between 2002 (32%) and 2013 (46%) there was a 14% increase, largely from community-based services such as home health, and states waiving the Title XIX federal nursing home requirement so as to use community-based services (KFF, December, 2015, p. 5, 8). Noted, home and-community-based-service recipients spend less on long-term care than those institutionalized (MACPAC, June, 2014).

While politicians often emphasize the financial savings on moving away from the traditional nursing facility toward home and community-based services, other actors frame the debate differently. Citizens of the 1970s demanded an alternative to nursing facilities that were poor in quality, while the disabled in the 1990s argued discrimination and segregation for limiting them to a facility setting. Today, states have choices in how they distribute Medicaid spending on long-term care (Public Law 111–148, 2010). While many states are following the federal lead allocating more money on home and community-based services, other states continue to spend monies primarily on nursing facilities.

State Revenue Opportunity

Expanding Medicaid long-term care services can be a money opportunity for states, not necessarily a cost burden. Under ACA (Public Law 111–148), Medicaid expansion can generate state revenue. States are responding to Medicaid's matching cost obligation with alternative sources of financing. According to the GAO, there has been an increase in state use of healthcare provider tax (such as nursing homes) and local governments to supplement state general funds in covering costs. In state fiscal year 2012, 26% or over $46 billion of "total nonfederal share of Medicaid payments" was generated from health provider taxes ($18.8 billion) and local government funds ($18.1 billion); and can result in an increase of federal matching funds (December, 2015, p. 8, 10). State Medicaid spending can have a "multiplier effect" on state economy, bringing payment to health providers and indirectly effecting businesses and industries (KFF, May, 2015, p. 9), such as the medical goods industry. In effect, Medicaid can be a source of federal revenue to states (KFF, May, 2015) adopting expansion, but also a growing expenditure as the guaranteed 100% federal matching for adopting states levels off at 90% by 2020, leaving adopters responsible for the 10%. As an inducement to expand long-term care, ACA gives several enhanced funding options for long-term care home and community-based services. States can choose among the options to increase their funding (KFF, December, 2015, p. 6).

POLICY IMPLEMENTATION: THE COMMUNICATIONS MODEL

In exploring variation to state compliance with the Obama Administration's health reform policy (ACA), this study turns to the Goggin, Bowman, Lester, and O'Toole (1990) Communications Model designed to frame intergovernmental policy, such as the U.S. Medicaid program. The goal of this model is to depict implementation over time and determine why there is variation in how states implement federal laws. Goggin et al. (1990) argue that communication is center in policy implementation. Policy content and message, in addition to the level of communication federal agencies have with state and local agencies, is likely to affect the success or failure of implementation. If state and local policy implementers regard the message and content as credible, implementation of the law is more likely to mirror its original intent.

The dependent variable under this framework is the extent to which the state has carried out federal policy. Depending on the state, implementation may be categorized as delay, defiance, compliance, or strategic delay (1990). The main independent variables under the Communication Model are federal-level and state-level inducements and constraints. The federal government can compel the states to act through *inducements* such as offering states financial incentive to expand Medicaid enrollment and long-term care services, *constraints* such as mandating nursing facility care upon all states, *sanctions* or a combination of both. In the case of long-term care, the federal government is compelling states to "rebalance state Medicaid long-term care spending" from nursing home institutional care to home and community-based services (Mathematica, 2014). The Obama Administration relied on inducements to promote state compliance to expand Medicaid in the form of an enhanced federal funding matching rate for new enrollees of select populations. Specifically, a 100% guaranteed federal match rate inducement for states adopting expansion from 2014-2016, leveling off at 90% by 2020 (leaving adopting states responsible for 10%), but no enhanced funding for non-expansion states (KFF, May, 2015). State-level inducements and constraints often take the form of pressure from state and local groups. Depending on how the policy impacts stakeholders at the state and local level, they may either help or hinder its implementation. The intervening variables are state organizational and ecological capacities, or resources which allow state officials to ignore messages from other political actors. State organizational capacity refers to items such as a state's administrative personnel and financial commitment to a program. State ecological capacity refers to factors such as public opinion and the economic well-being of the state (Goggin et al, 1990).

Other have applied the Communication Model but across different policy domains, such as environmental, telecommunication, and education policy areas. Using Goggin et al (1990), Cline (2003) analyzed the State Environmental Protection Agency Superfund program for environmental cleanup from 1987 to 1994 at the state-level using a pooled cross-sectional time-series analysis with an event-count model. This study found organizational capacity, and state-local level inducements and constraints can influence EPA Superfund program implementation. Using the Communication Model, McNeal (2012) explored state response to federal funding initiatives for improving high-speed broadband infrastructure and local government ownership of broadband facilities. Using multivariate regression analysis and 50 state data, McNeal found state-local inducements and constraints (good government interest group strength) and ecological capacity (Republican Party control of state government) mattered in implementation. Dotterweich-Bryan and McNeal (2004) studied state response to the No Child Left Behind Act of 2002. Using the Communication Model, 50 state data, and multivariate methods they found the greatest impact was state political ecological capacity (including state minority diversity, legislative professionalism and professional networks). Contrary to other studies, state-local inducements and constraints (education interest groups) did not have a significant impact on implementing the Act.

Applying the Communication Model, we explore why some states continue to spend more revenue on traditional nursing facility care despite federal financial incentives to reform, whereas other states are expanding their home and community-based services. We explore this question using empirical analysis.

EMPIRICAL MODEL: DATA AND MEASUREMENT

Data

This chapter uses secondary data analysis to explore why some states spend more revenue on nursing facility long-term care despite enhanced federal funding to reform, while others are spending more on home and community-based services. The dataset for this study was compiled using a number of sources including state and government websites as well as nonprofit organizations, among other groups. Among these sources are the U.S. Census Bureau, the U.S. Bureau of Commerce, the Kaiser Family Foundation and the Pew Charitable Trust. Most of the study variables are common to implementation research, while a few are unique to this policy area.

Determinants of Spending on Long-Term Healthcare

The exploration of why certain states favor nursing facilities over home and community-based services begins with an examination of state factors that influence the amount of money each state dedicates to each alternative healthcare delivery strategy. The literature on policy adoption suggests there are factors that explain the differences in state spending. Early research found socio-economic factors including state wealth are important to policy adoption (Gray, 1973; Hwang & Gray, 1991), while other studies point to politics (Mooney & Lee, 1995). In addition, the literature shows that greater demand or need for a policy increases the chance for adoption (Meier, 1994; Mooney & Lee; 1995). Although each of these factors matter in policy adoption, their relative importance depends on the policy area being examined. Medicaid, like other forms of public assistance, is a redistributive policy. Since these policies provide benefits to one group at the expense of another, they are known for policy conflict. It is expected that political factors will play a central role in state funding of long-term healthcare options (Lowi, 1964).

Dependent variables were created for monies allocated to Medicaid dollars distributed to nursing facilities and home healthcare. Each dependent variable was calculated by dividing the FY 2014 spending for each category (Kaiser Family Foundation, 2015a) by the 2014 gross state product (U.S. Department of Commerce, 2015) to get the percentage of the state's gross state product spent on each program. The selection of independent or control variables was based on policy adoption literature. This framework argues that policy adoption is contingent on politics, state resources, and demand or need within the state. When exploring the impact of politics on policy adoption, there are number of political actors to consider including local officials and agencies. Each of these actors may either work to encourage or discourage the adoption of a particular legislation depending on how they perceive the impact.

A number of factors can influence policymaker action(s) including both institutional ideology (elected official ideology) and citizen ideology. Support for increased public assistance funding is more associated with a liberal ideology. It is expected that states where state legislatures and citizens are more liberal, more funding would be allocated to Medicaid programs in the state. In order to control for citizen ideology and institutional ideology two indices were added each ranging from 0 to 100 with higher scores indicating greater liberalism (Fording, 2012). These indices are updated versions of those first proposed by Berry et al (1998). The measure for institutional ideology is constructed using a weighted average of ideological scores for the governor, and the 2 major parties in both houses of the state legislature. Citizen ideology is constructed by averaging ideological scores for incumbents and challengers (or hypothetical challenger) for each state congressional district (Berry et al, 1998, pp. 331-332). Governors can have a significant impact on funding for state programs through institutional powers including their control over the state budget, veto powers and appointment powers. The strength of these institutional powers is measured on a five-point scale where 1 indicates weak and 5 indicates strong (Donovan, Mooney & Smith, 2013). State agencies represent a final set of political actors who have influence over whether a policy is adopted (Goggin et al, 1990). It may be easier to adopt policy if a state has greater control over the resources of the implementing agency. As an indicator of control over state agencies, an index measuring state legislative oversight of the bureaucracy was included. It was constructed using a four-point scale where 1 indicates that the state legislature has no oversight power of the bureaucracy and 4 indicates that the legislature can impose costs and / or suspend rules (Gerber, Maestas & Dometruis, 2005).

Several measures of state resources were added including urbanization, recession recovery and Medicaid expansion. Urbanization is measured by the percent of the population living in urban areas (United States Census Bureau, 2012a). Recession recovery is an indicator of the extent to which a state has "bounced back" from the Great Recession and is operationally defined as the percent difference in state tax revenues between the 3rd quarter of 2009 and the fourth quarter of 2014 (Pew Charitable Trusts, December 10, 2015). Markell (1993) expands the definition of resources to include a strong record of policy implementation of an issue area. As an indicator of whether a state has a record of implementation, a dummy variable was added for whether or not the state adopted to expand Medicaid, coded 1 for yes and 0 for no (Pew Charitable Trusts, July 1, 2014). Finally, Mooney & Lee (1995) argue that public demand or the need for a policy/ program is an important factor in predicting policy adoption. The first measure of need is the change in Medicaid fees, measured as cumulative percent change in Medicaid primary care physician fees 2008-2012 (Kaiser Family Foundation, 2013). It is expected that in states where these fees have risen, the percentage of the gross state product (GSP) earmarked for healthcare programs will be higher. State obligations to non-healthcare policies represent a competing demand for healthcare dollars. It is expected that states with higher obligations, measured (in dollars) as the combined level of unfunded retirement costs and unfunded retiree healthcare costs (Pew Charitable Trusts, May 17, 2016) will have fewer resources to allocate to the Medicaid program. Medicaid enrollment rate for the aged / disabled (Pew Charitable Trusts, July 1, 2014) and the percent increase in citizens age 65+ from 2003 to 2013 (United States Census Bureau, 2014) are demand indicators of the numbers or citizens who need long-term care services as well as a future demand.

Impact of Medicaid Expansion on Home Health Services

In Table 2, the Communication Model will act as a blueprint for examining if Medicaid expansion under the Americans with Disability Act of 1990 (ADA) has been instrumental in reallocating more of the Medicaid dollars from nursing facilities to home and community-based services. The dependent variable is the percentage of Medicaid spending on long-term care distributed to home health and personal care for the year 2014 (Kaiser Family Foundation, 2015a). The main independent variables under the Communication Model are federal-level and state-level inducements and constraints. The federal government can compel the states to act through inducements, constraints or a combination of both. Most recently, provisions under the 2010 Patient Protection and Affordable Care Act (ACA) encourage more long-term spending to be allocated toward home and community-based services, emphasized by inducements. In addition to the federal government's impact on Medicaid long-term care, other stakeholders ranging from the nursing home industry to Americans living with disabilities have played a significant role in shaping state long-term care policy. To control for the possible influence of state-level interests groups, a measure for the overall impact of interest group on the state political system was included. This four-point scale indicates the overall impact that interest groups have in a state political system as related to other groups. A score of 5 indicates that interest groups are dominating in the political system as compared to other groups, and a score of 1 indicates that they are complementary / subordinate (Nownes, Thomas & Hrebenar, 2008).

State government officials may choose to ignore "messages" from stakeholders both in and outside of government, based on resources. The ability to ignore these messages is referred to as state capacity (Goggin et al, 1990). There are two forms of state resources: ecological capacity and organizational capacity. Ecological capacity concerns the "contextual environment in which state government operates" (Goggin et al, 1990, p. 911). Similarly, organizational capacity refers to the resources available to the state agency that oversees the policy implementation (Goggin et al, 1990, p. 911). There are three categories of ecological capacity: economical, political, and situational. Economical capacity concerns the availability of monetary resources. Several measures of state resources were added including recession recovery and education attainment. Educational attainment is measured as the percent of the state population over the age of 25 with a bachelor's degree or higher (U.S. Census Bureau, 2012b). Measures for governor's institutional power, citizen ideology and ideology of elected officials (institutional ideology) were added to control for the political capacity. In addition, a measure of female legislators was added since they are more interested in certain policy areas including education, health and welfare as compared to their male counterparts (Bratton & Haynie, 1999). The presence of women legislators is measured using the percent women in a state legislature for each year (Center for American Women and Politics, 2014). The final area of ecological capacity is state situational capacity which refers to citizen demand or need. The percent increase in citizens age 65+ from 2003 to 2013 was used as an indicator of need. Two measures were included for organizational capacity (agency resource); legislative control over the resources of the implementing agency, and state-funded Medicaid expenditures as a percent of state's own source revenue for the year 2012 (Pew Charitable Trusts, July 1, 2014).

FINDINGS AND DISCUSSION

Determinants of Spending on Long-Term Healthcare

In Table 1, the dependent variables are coded so that higher scores are associated with greater allocation of Medicaid funds to long-term healthcare. Since the dependent variables are continuous, multivariate regression analysis is used. The findings in Table 1 suggest that circumstances that lead to Medicaid funds being used for nursing facilities (nursing homes) are quite different from that of home and community-based services (home health and personal care). Specifically, the findings suggest that spending decisions on community-based care is similar to most redistributive type policies in that political factors play the biggest role. On the other hand, political factors do not play a role in state spending decisions for nursing facilities, instead a limited number of state resources and indicators of public need help to predict funding for nursing facilities.

The only variables found to be statistically significant in the model for nursing facility funding (Table 1) were state urbanization, state recession recovery, state Medicaid enrollment rate for the aged / disabled, and the percent increase in residents age 65+ from 2003 to 2013. The finding that no political factors were significant for the regression model on nursing facility Medicaid funding is not the only result that was unexpected. While the policy adoption literature argues that greater state wealth is associated with policy action, the findings suggest that poorer states were more likely to provide greater Medicaid funding to their nursing facilities. Urbanism is an indicator of state wealth (Walker, 1969), but the model indicated that rural states were more likely to provide greater funding for costly nursing facilities. One explanation is that rural states have both fewer care providers and established community care industries to provide home health services, due to geography issues (Schmeida, 2005). Although recession recovery was added as an indicator of state wealth, the finding that it is negatively associated with nursing facility spending suggests it is acting as a measure of need. States who have "bounced back" from the Great Recession are allocating fewer Medicaid dollars to nursing facilities. It is likely that recovered economy states have fewer people in need of public assistance, including Medicaid. As predicted, as more seniors / disabled citizens are Medicaid enrolled, greater spending is made by the state to nursing facilities. However, it is counterintuitive that as the percent of people age 65+ increases that less Medicaid money is allocated.

Table 1. State Medicaid spending on long-term care (2014)

Variables	Nursing Facilities		Home Health and Personal Care	
	β (se)	p>|t|	β (se)	p>|t|
State Political Constraints				
Governor's institutional power	-.33(.24)	.185	**.50(.26)**	**.065**
Institutional ideology (liberal)	-.01(.01)	.568	**.02(.01)**	**.035**
Ideology of citizens (liberal)	-.00(.02)	.956	**-.04(.02)**	**.041**
Legislative oversight of bureaucracy	.20(.17)	.238	.17(.18)	.360
State Resources				
Recession recovery	**-.02(.01)**	**.083**	-.02(.01)	.170
Medicaid expansion	.81(.58)	.170	.53(.62)	.399
Urban population (%)	**-.04(.02)**	**.081**	-.02(.02)	.375
State Needs/Demands				
Change in Medicaid physician fees	1.78(1.84)	.340	**4.43(1.99)**	**.031**
State obligations	1.72E-08(1.42E-08)	.235	1.77E-08(1.53E-08)	.254
Medicaid enrollment rate	**.11(.05)**	**.041**	**.10(.05)**	**.083**
Percent increase population 65+	**-.06(.02)**	**.013**	.03(.02)	.181
Constant	5.06(2.64)	.063	-.23(2.85)	.935
Adjusted R2	.4546	**.0002**	.3729	
F(11, 38)	4.65		3.65	**.0014**
N	50		50	

Note: Multivariate regression estimates with standard errors in parentheses. Reported probabilities are based on two-tailed tests. Statistically significant coefficients at .10 or less in bold.

One possible explanation is that there is a "tipping point" where once public spending to costly nursing facilities reaches a certain percentage of the state budget, public officials look into less costly policy alternatives, such as home and community based long-term care services.

Unlike funding to nursing facilities, state political factors were found to play an important role in Medicaid funding of community home health and personal care services, see Table 1. The political factors relevant to funding include governor's institutional power, citizen ideology and institutional ideology. At first glance, it seems puzzling that states with conservative citizens and liberal legislators would allocate more long-term Medicaid dollars to community-based care. A possible explanation is framing. Groups who want a particular policy to be adopted or rejected may try to influence how it is depicted or framed in order to get a preferred outcome. There are a number of groups involved in the battle over how to best address the growing demand for long-term care, ranging from the nursing home industry to persons with disabilities. Their strong arguments (cost containment and civil right to choose the care setting) are encouraging the transition into community-based care. These arguments appeal to individuals on both the left and right. The finding that states with more powerful governors are associated with more spending toward community-based care emphasizes their role in the budget making process. Unlike spending on nursing home facilities, state resources were not found to play a role in community-based care spending. In addition, only two need / demand factors were found to be statistically significant.

As found with the public spending on nursing facilities regression model, as more seniors / disabled citizens are Medicaid enrolled there is greater state spending on community home health and personal care. Finally, the fee change for primary physicians was found to be positively associated with greater spending on community-based care. This suggests that costly physician service plays an important part in long-term care spending decisions made by states. As physician costs increases, states are shifting public funding to less expensive long-term care alternatives.

Impact of the Medicaid Expansion on Home Health and Personal Care Services

In Table 2, the dependent variable is coded so that higher scores are associated with a greater percent of Medicaid long-term care funding being allocated to community home health and personal care services. Since the dependent variables are continuous, multivariate regression analysis is used. The findings suggest that for this policy area, the state-level interest groups and ecological capacity are dominating "communication" with regard to long-term care policy discussion.

Table 2. Percent of Medicaid long-term care spending distributed to home health and personal care (2014)

Variables	Percent of Spending on Home Health and Personal Care	
	β (se)	p>|t|
Federal-Level Inducements and Constraints		
Medicaid expansion	-1.97(6.11)	.749
State-Level Inducements and Constraints		
Overall interest group impact	**5.48(2.95)**	**.071**
Ecological Capacity		
Political		
Institutional ideology (liberal)	**.31(.09)**	**.002**
Ideology of citizens (liberal)	-.07(.23)	.754
Percent women in the state legislature	**-1.19(.56)**	**.042**
Governor's institutional power	**6.47(2.26)**	**.007**
Economical		
Percent with a high school degree	**1.68(.88)**	**.063**
Recession recovery	.17(.11)	.119
Situational		
Percent increase population 65+	**.98(.23)**	**.000**
Organizational Capacity		
State legislative oversight of bureaucracy	-2.86(1.71)	.102
State funded Medicaid expenditures	1.13(1.12)	.320
Constant	**-139.40(71.71)**	**.059**
Adjusted R^2	.4087	
F(11, 38)	4.08	**.0006**
N	50	

Note: Multivariate regression estimates with standard errors in parentheses. Reported probabilities are based on two-tailed tests. Statistically significant coefficients at .10 or less in bold.

Expanding Medicaid long-term care services was not found to be a statistically significant predictor of whether states spend more of their overall long-term care Medicaid dollars on community-based care or traditional nursing facilities. This occurs despite several enhanced funding options provided by ACA for home and community-based services (HCBS). There are several possible explanations for this finding. First, as Goggin et al. (1990) argue, states may elect to ignore the messages from other political actors and choose to enact their own policy preferences. In the long-term care issue area, the states may be listening to other powerful actors, such as the nursing home industry. At the state-level, the nursing home industry has become an increasingly powerful lobbying force. In 1985, hospitals / nursing homes were ranked 17th among the 20 most influential interests at the state-level; by 2007 this industry rose to 5th in the rankings (Nownes, Thomas & Hrebenar, 2008, p. 117). As a second explanation, this study used a fairly rudimentary measure for the Goggin et al. (1990) concept of state-level inducements and constraints. A dummy variable was used to indicate whether the state had expanded Medicaid. Whereas, a measure of the amount of enhanced funding received under the Americans with Disability Act of 1990 for long-term care HCBS may have shown a relationship between Medicaid expansion and spending on community-based care. Although the federal government was found not related to how Medicaid spending was allocated, state-level actors were related. In states where interests groups are more powerful, states spent a greater percent of their long-term care Medicaid dollars on community-based care. This is not surprising, given the history of interest group advocacy related to this policy.

Although states may decide to ignore messages from other political actors, their ability to do so is based on state resources (state capacity). Four measures were included to control for the state political environment. Consistent with findings in Table 1, liberal state legislatures and powerful governors were found to be associated with a greater percent of long-term funding being allocated to community home health and personal care. Unexpected was the finding that citizen ideology was not related to spending allocations, and the percent of women in the state legislature was negatively related. Possibly, states with more women in their state legislature tend to be ones where the legislature is less powerful (Squire, 1992). In these states, the executive branch will have greater control over policy. Two measures were included for state wealth with mixed results. States with higher education attainment among their citizens were found more likely to allocate more monies to community home health and personal services, whereas there was no relationship between spending and recession recovery. These findings are consistent with Table 1 that shows funding decisions on community care is characteristic of redistributive policy where political factors take a lead over other factors. The percent increase in citizens age 65+ from 2003 to 2013 was included as an indicator of need (situational capacity) and found to be positively associated with the percent of Medicaid dollars allocated to long-term care home health and personal services. This is supported by findings in Table 1 suggesting there is a "tipping point" where once public spending to nursing homes becomes untenable, state public officials explore alternative less costly policy solutions. Finally, unlike ecological capacity, none of the measures of organizational resources were found related to long-term care spending decisions.

Our findings are similar to other intergovernmental social policy research. Goggin (1999) studied the State Children's Health Insurance Program (Public Law 105-33, 1997) for poor children and pregnant women. Much like ACA Medicaid expansion, it also has federal financial incentives for states to expand coverage (P.L. 105-33; NSCL, 2017). He found the state political environment to play the biggest role in whether states chose to implement the program, which is consistent with our study on state expansion of Medicaid coverage for long-term healthcare. One possible explanation for the similarity is the political realities of the U.S. Even though government health insurance exists, healthcare insurance has been mostly treated as a private good in the U.S. with employer-based insurance being the dominant. Today, there is a significant division between the Democratic and Republican Parties on the proper role of the government in ensuring access to healthcare.

Monte Carlo Simulations

To further explore the impact of factors suggested by the Communication Model on how states are distributing Medicaid spending on long-term care, the predicted percentage (probability estimates) of Medicaid long-term care spending allocated to home health and personal care from Table 2 are presented in Tables 3 and 4. While the findings in Table 2 show a number of state-level variables played a significant role in how states distributed their long-term care spending, we chose interest group strength, institutional ideology and the increase in population 65+ years for further study. Variables selected were limited to those found as statistically significant. Non-selected were those under the categories of federal-level inducements and constraints or organizational capacity since they were not significant. Interest group strength was included because it was the only variable in the model for state-level inducement and constraints, in addition to being statistically significant. Whereas, there were a number of variables under the category of ecological capacity found to be significant with state spending on community home health and personal care. We selected institutional ideology and increase in population 65+ years for further analysis because they had the lowest p-value.

To illustrate the impact of these variables, the coefficients reported in Table 2 were converted to predicted percentage (probability estimates) of state Medicaid long-term care spending allocated to home health and personal care using the Clarify; one of many examples of Monte Carlo simulation approaches (King, Tomz, & Wittenberg, 2000). Monte Carlo simulation describes computer algorithms that draw a large numbers of random samples from probability distributes and uses these samples to help generate estimates (King, Tomz, & Wittenberg, 2000, p. 349). Table 3 explores the impact of interest group strength and the institutional ideology on predicted percentage of Medicaid long-term care spending (on community home health and personal care). Table 4 considers the impact of interest group strength and increase in population 65+ years on the predicted percentage of the Medicaid long-term care community spending.

IMPACT OF INTEREST GROUP STRENGTH AND THE INSTITUTIONAL IDEOLOGY

Table 3 presents the predicted percentages (probability estimates) of Medicaid long-term care spending allocated to community home health and personal care with varying levels of state-level interest group strength and institutional ideology. Institutional ideology was set at one standard deviation above the mean, the mean, and one standard deviation below the mean while interest group strength was set at its four categories ranging from complementary/subordinate to dominant. The remaining control variables were set at their mean if they are continuous variables and categorical variables were set at their median. The probability estimates show in states where the legislature is more liberal and interest groups strength relative to other actors (including political parties) is stronger, state allocation of Medicaid long-term care spending to community home health and personal care is more likely to be higher. The percentage of funds allocated to home health and personal care increases by roughly 17% when comparing states

Table 3. The impact of interest group strength and institutional ideology on the predicted percentage of Medicaid long-term care spending on community home health and personal care (2014)

Interest Group Strength/ Institutional Ideology	Complementary/ Subordinate	Complementary	Dominant/ Complementary	Dominant
High (liberal)	40.4% (7.06)	46.0% (5.58)	51.6% (5.43)	57.2% (6.71)
Mean	30.9% (6.59)	36.5% (4.82)	42.1% (4.49)	47.7% (5.85)
Low(conservative)	29.8% (6.61)	35.4% (24.84)	41.0% (4.49)	46.6% (5.83)
Difference (high-low)	10.6%	10.6%	10.6%	10.6%

where interest groups are dominant to those where interest groups are complementary/ subordinate. Similarly, in states where the legislature is more liberal (set at one standard deviation above the mean on the ideological scale), the percent of funds dedicated to home health and personal care increases by approximately 10.6% when compared to more conservative state legislatures (set at one standard deviation below the mean on the ideological scale). Taken together, these findings show the important role political actors play in determining how Medicaid dollars will be spent.

Note: Standard errors are in parentheses. To simulate different levels of institutional ideology, ideology was set at one standard deviation below the mean, mean, and one standard deviation above the mean. Value for percent women in the state legislature, percent of the population over 25 with a high school degree, percent increase in population 65+, citizen ideology, recession recovery and state funded Medicaid expenditures were set at their mean. Values for governor's power, Medicaid expansion and legislative oversight were set at their median. Estimations were produced using Clarify: Software for Interpreting and Presenting Statistical Results, by Michael Tomz, Jason Wittenberg, and Gary King (2000).

IMPACT OF INTEREST GROUP STRENGTH AND THE INCREASE IN POPULATION AGE 65+

Table 4 presents the predicted percentages of Medicaid long term care spending allocated to community home health and personal care with varying levels of interest group strength and percent increase in population age 65+ (from 2003 to 2013). Increase in population 65+ was set at one standard deviation above the mean, the mean, and one standard deviation below the mean while interest group strength was set at its four categories ranging from complementary/ subordinate to dominant. The remaining control variables were set at their mean if they are continuous variables and categorical variables were set at their median. The probability estimates show in states where the population is aging and interest groups strength relative to other actors (including political parties) is stronger, state allocation of Medicaid long-term spending to community home health and personal care is more likely to be higher. As with Table 3, the percent of funds allocated to home health and personal care increased by roughly 17% when comparing states where interest groups are dominant to those where interest groups are complementary/ subordinate. Similarly, in states where the percentage increase of citizens 65+ is high (set at one standard deviation above the mean on the ideological scale), the percent of funds dedicated to home health and personal care increases by approximately 24% when the percent increase of citizens 65+ is low (set at one

Table 4. Impact of interest group strength and increase in population 65+ on the predicted percentage of Medicaid long-term care spending on community home health and personal care (2014)

Interest Group Strength/ Increase in Percent of Population Over Age 65	Complementary/ Subordinate	Complementary	Dominant/ Complementary	Dominant
High	43.0% (7.21)	48.6% (5.43)	54.2% (4.91)	59.8% (5.98)
Mean	30.9% (6.59)	36.5% (4.82)	42.1% (4.49)	47.7% (5.85)
Low	18.9% (7.16)	24.5% (5.78)	30.1% (5.71)	35.7% (7.00)
Difference (high-low)	24.1%	24.1%	24.1%	24.1%

Note: Standard errors are in parentheses. To simulate different levels of increase in population 65+, the population increase was set at one standard deviation below the mean, mean, and one standard deviation above the mean. Value for percent women in the state legislature, percent of the population over 25 with a high school degree, institutional ideology, citizen ideology, recession recovery and state funded Medicaid expenditures were set at their mean. Values for governor's power, Medicaid expansion and legislative oversight were set at their median. Estimations were produced using Clarify: Software for Interpreting and Presenting Statistical Results, by Michael Tomz, Jason Wittenberg, and Gary King (2000).

standard deviation below the mean on the ideological scale). Similar to Table 3, these findings show the important role political actors (interest groups) play in the allocation of long-term care Medicaid funds.

SOLUTIONS AND RECOMMENDATIONS

In 1965, Congress passes Medicaid at the urging of President Lyndon B. Johnson. Although this joint federal-state public assistance program helped bring needed healthcare to the aged poor, children and those living with disabilities, one provision soon came under fire. Both state officials and citizens raised concern about the lack of long-term care alternatives. By the 1970's, state officials found the payments to nursing facilities (nursing homes) continued to inflate their contributions to the Medicaid program. In addition, a series of scandals on the poor quality of care in nursing facilities had citizens demanding alternatives for long-term care. In 1981, the federal government began permitting states to use long-term care Medicaid funds for home and community-based services (HCBS) as an alternative to facilities. Overtime, many states have begun allocating more of their long-term care Medicaid funds to HCBS. How do we further increase the use of the nursing facility alternative across the states? One solution is for the federal government to give states greater financial incentive to move aged enrollees from costly nursing facilities back into the community for long-term care services. This recommendation is not supported by the findings of this study that shows federal incentives are unrelated to how Medicaid long-term care monies are allocated at the state-level. This might be a function of how federal incentives were measured in this study. Another answer is the continued interest group advocacy. A number of interests ranging from persons living with disabilities to average citizens concerned about nursing home quality have been instrumental in changing long-term Medicaid funding. Also, similar to other redistributive policies, this research found political actors to play a leading role in policy implementation. A final suggestion is to build public education. Often, long-term healthcare decisions are made by family abruptly following a medical event of a member, not in a position to carefully evaluate alternative long-term care options. Government agencies representing the aged are in a visible position to prepare the public for future long-term care needs of family, educating the public on care options.

FUTURE RESEARCH DIRECTIONS

What explains the difference in how states have responded to the federal government's encouragement to expand home and community-based services? Does the 2010 Patient Protection and Affordable Care Act (ACA) play an important role in this difference? This research represents an initial attempt at exploring these questions. The findings suggest that this policy area has responded like a classic redistributive policy in that political factors, more so than other factors, have determined how states allocate long-term care Medicaid healthcare dollars. This further suggests that federal inducements under ACA are not what is motivating state action in this policy area. It should be understood that these findings are preliminary.

This chapter used a fairly blunt instrument to measure federal inducements to states. It was coded 1 if a state had expanded Medicaid long-term care services under the ACA and 0 otherwise. This measure of federal inducement did not indicate how much additional monies a state received following the decision to expand Medicaid HCBS. In addition, there are other federal grants that encourage the expansion of HCBS, such as Real Choice System Change grants. This study focused on the impact of ACA on the states, but future research may consider the impact of other federal programs encouraging alternative options to traditional nursing home facilities. Furthermore, the Communication Model (Goggin et al., 1990) is designed to depict state-level policy implementation over time. This study only explores the impact of the ACA on long-term care options for the year 2014. Future research can improve upon this initial study by using a time-series approach. Finally, recent U.S. elections have brought in a new presidential administration (Donald Trump), where discussions are underway to make changes to ACA and Medicaid. The extent to which these changes will affect HCBS will require an evaluation.

CONCLUSION

Citizens are living longer, and meeting the care demands of an aging population is a fiscal challenge. This research explores one policy solution used in the United States to meet the demands of the aged: home and community-based services. Initially, Medicaid as the U.S. healthcare system for the poor limited public long-term care funding to nursing facilities. Within a few years of the 1965 Medicaid policy adoption, demands for an alternative to nursing facilities developed coming from citizen and public officials alike. Since 1981, the federal government has permitted states to use Medicaid long-term care dollars for both costly nursing facilities and alternative settings such as home and community-based services. Since community based care is often less costly and preferred by citizens, it would be expected that Medicaid funding for nursing facilities would soon dwindle. This has not happened; in some states community-based care is replacing the facilities, while in other states the nursing home facilities still receive the lion share of Medicaid long-term care dollars. Since Medicaid is a form of public assistance considered a redistributive policy, it was expected that the answer would be dominated by political factors (Lowi, 1964). The findings supported this prediction to an extent; greater funding of community-based care in the states was primarily explained by political factors and increased fiscal demands on the state. On the other hand, state resources and demand factors best explained which states continued to heavily fund nursing facilities. In addition, the findings did not suggest that federal grants such as those available through the Americans with Disability Act of 1990 impacted state decision on this policy question. The finding that political factors were important to the expansion of expenditures for home and community-based services and not nursing home facilities suggests that the facilities have become the default option. It is the option adopted by the states unless political actors force a change. Intrastate interest group advocacy efforts rather than federal level monetary inducements matter more in expanding home and community based long-term care services.

This study relied on the Communication Model to frame the exploration of why some states continue to spend more revenue on traditional nursing facility care while other states are spending more on HCBS. Over the years a number of studies have used this model as a guide for exploring intergovernmental policies. While Goggin et. al. (1990) had hoped that use of their Communication Model would ultimately lead to a generalizable theory of implementation, it hasn't happened. Instead, individual studies have resulted in findings that point to variables distinctive to each policy area (Winters, 2006). The same is true for this study; the findings from this study are unique to the area of government sponsored healthcare insurance. That does not lessen the usability of the Communication Model. Even though its subsequent use has not resulted in a generalizable theory of implementation, it is a useful heuristic for exploring intergovernmental policy.

REFERENCES

Berry, W., Ringquist, E., Fording, R., & Hanson, R. (1998). Measuring citizen and government ideology in the American states, 19601993. *American Journal of Political Science*, *42*(1), 327–348. doi:10.2307/2991759

Bratton, K., & Haynie, K. (1999). Agenda setting and legislative success in state legislatures: The effects of gender and race. *The Journal of Politics*, *61*(3), 658–679. doi:10.2307/2647822

Center for American Women and Politics. (2014). *Women in state legislatures*. Retrieved July 15, 2014, from http://www.cawp.rutgers.edu

Centers for Medicare & Medicaid Services, Office of the Actuary. (2014). *Report to congress. 2014 actuarial report on the financial outlook for Medicaid.* Retrieved July 5, 2016, from http://www.medicaid.gov/medicaid-chip-program-information/by-topics/financing-and-reimbursement/downloads/medicaid-actuarial-report-2014.pdf

Centers for Medicare and Medicaid Services. (2015). *Brief summaries of Medicare & Medicaid Title XVIII and Title XIX of the Social Security Act.* Retrieved July 5, 2016, from http://www.cms.gov/Research-Statistics-Data-and-Systems/Statistics-Trends-and-Reports/MedicareProgramRatesStats/Downloads/MedicareMedicaidSummaries2015.pdf

Cline, K. (2003). Influences on intergovernmental implementation: The states and the superfund. *State Politics & Policy Quarterly*, *3*(1), 66–83.

Donovan, T., Mooney, C., & Smith, D. (2013). *State and local politics: Institutions and Reforms* (3rd ed.). Stamford, CT: Cengage Learning.

Dotterweich-Bryan, L., & McNeal, R. (2004). *No child left behind: the report card—why are some states successfully implementing new law and others not?* Paper at the meeting of the Fourth Annual State Politics and Policy Conference, Cuyahoga Falls, OH.

Fording, R. (2012). *State ideology data*. Retrieved June 15, 2014, from http://rcfording.wordpress.com/state-ideology-data/

Gerber, B., Maestas, C., & Dometrius, N. (2005). State legislative influence over agency rulemaking: The utility of ex ante review. *State Politics & Policy Quarterly*, *5*(1), 24–46. doi:10.1177/153244000500500102

Goggin, M. (1999). The use of administration discretion in implementing the State Childrens Health Insurance Program. *Publius*, *29*(2), 35–51. doi:10.1093/oxfordjournals.pubjof.a030025

Goggin, M., Bowman, A., Lester, J., & O'Toole, L. (1990). *Implementation theory and practice: toward a third generation*. New York, N.Y.: Harper Collins Publishers.

Gray, V. (1973). Innovations in the states: A diffusion study. *The American Political Science Review*, *67*(4), 1174–1185. doi:10.2307/1956539

Hwang, S., & Gray, V. (1991). External limits and internal determinants of state public policy. *The Western Political Quarterly*, *44*(2), 277–299. doi:10.2307/448779

Kaiser Family Foundation. (2013). *Cumulative percentage change in Medicaid fees, by type of service timeframe: 2008-2012*. Retrieved June 10, 2016, from http://kff.org/medicaid/state-indicator/change-in-medicaid-fees/

Kaiser Family Foundation. (2013). *Cumulative percentage change in Medicaid fees, by type of service timeframe: 2008-2012*. Retrieved June 10, 2016, from http://kff.org/medicaid/state-indicator/change-in-medicaid-fees/

Kaiser Family Foundation. (2015a). *Distribution of Medicaid spending on long-term care*. Retrieved June 10, 2016, from http://kff.org/medicaid/state-indicator/spending-on-long-term-care/

Kaiser Family Foundation. (2015b). *State action on Medicaid expansion as of April 2015*. Retrieved June 10, 2016, from http://kff.org/health-reform/state-indicator/state-activity-around-expanding-medicaid-under-the-affordable-care-act/

Kaiser Family Foundation. (2015c). *Medicaid financing: how does it work and what are the implications?* Retrieved June 10, 2016, from http://kff.org/medicaid/issue-brief/medicaid-financing-how-does-it-work-and-what-are-the-implications/

Kaiser Family Foundation. (2015d). *Long-term care in the United States: a timeline*. Retrieved June 10, 2016, from http:// kff.org/medicaid/timeline/long-term-care-in-the-united-states-a-timeline/

Kaiser Family Foundation. (2015e). *Medicaid enrollment & spending growth: FY 2015 & 2016*. Retrieved June 10, 2016, from http:// kff.org/medicaid/issue-brief/medicaid-enrollment-spending-growth-fy-2015-2016/

Kaiser Family Foundation. (2015f). *Putting Medicaid in the larger budget context: an in-depth look at three states in FY 2015 and 2016, Alaska*. Retrieved June 10, 2016, from http://kff.org/report-section/putting-medicaid-in-the-larger-budget-context-an-in-depth-look-at-three-states-in-fy-2015-and-2016-alaska/

Kaiser Family Foundation. (2015g). *Putting Medicaid in the larger budget context: an in-depth look at three states in FY 2015 and 2016, California*. Retrieved June 10, 2016, from http://kff.org/report-section/putting-medicaid-in-the-larger-budget-context-an-in-depth-look-at-three-states-in-fy-2015-and-2016-california/

Kaiser Family Foundation. (2015h). *Medicaid and long-term services and supports: a primer.* Retrieved June 10, 2016, from http:// kff.org/medicaid/report/medicaid-and-long-term-services-and-supports-a-primer/

Kane, R. A. (2012). Thirty years of home- and community-based services: Getting closer and closer to home. *Generations (San Francisco, Calif.)*, *36*(1), 6–13.

King, G., Tomz, M., & Wittenberg, J. (2000). Making the most of statistical analysis: Improving interpretation and presentation. *American Journal of Political Science*, *44*(2), 347–361. doi:10.2307/2669316

Lowi, T. (1964). American business, public policy, case studies, and political theory. *World Politics*, *16*(4), 667–715. doi:10.2307/2009452

Lowi, T. (1979). *The end of liberalism: the second republic of the United States*. New York: W.W. Norton & Company, Inc.

Markell, D. (1993). The federal superfund program: Proposals for strengthening the federal/state relationship. *William and Mary Journal of Environmental Law*, *18*, 1–82.

Mathematica Policy Research. (2014). *The changing medical and long-term care expenditures of people who transition from institutional care to home- and community-based services*. Retrieved July 5, 2016, from https://www.mathematica-mpr.com/our-publications-and-findings/publications/the-changing-medical-and-long-term-care-expenditures-of-people-who-transition

McNeal, R. (2012). State response to Obama's broadband access policy: a study in policy implementation. In V. Weerakkody & C. Reddick (Eds.), *Public sector transformation through e-government: experiences from Europe and North America*. Routledge.

Medicaid and CHIP Payment and Access Commission (MACPAC). (2014). *Report to Congress on Medicaid and CHIP*. Retrieved July 14, 2016, from http://www.macpac.gov/reports

Meier, K. (1994). *The politics of sin: drugs, alcohol and public policy*. New York: Sharpe.

Mooney, C., & Lee, M. (1995). Legislating morality in the American states: The case of pre-Roe abortion regulation reform. *American Journal of Political Science*, *39*(3), 599–627. doi:10.2307/2111646

National Conference of State Legislatures. (2011). *Long-term care provisions in health reform*. Retrieved June 10, 2016, from http://www.ncsl.org/research/health/long-term-care-provisions-in-health-reform.aspx

National Conference of State Legislatures. (2017). *Children's health insurance program overview*. Retrieved February 15, 2017, from http://www.ncsl.org/research/health/childrens-insurance-program-overview.aspx

Nownes, A., Thomas, C., & Hrebenar, R. (2008). Interest groups in the states. In V. Grey & R. Hanson (Eds.), *Politics in the American states: A comparative analysis* (9th ed.; pp. 98–126). Washington, DC: CQ Press.

Olmstead v. L.C. (98-537) 527 U.S. 581 (1999)

Pew Charitable Trusts. (2014). *State health care spending on Medicaid: a 50-state study of trends and drivers of cost.* Retrieved June 12, 2016, from http://www.pewtrusts.org/en/Multimedia/Data-Visualizations/2014/Medicaid-Spending-Growth

Pew Charitable Trusts. (2015). *For first time, tax revenue has recovered in majority of states.* Retrieved June 12, 2016, from http:// www.pewtrusts.org/en/research-and-analysis/analysis/2015/12/10/for-first-time-tax-revenue-has-recovered-in-majority-of-states

Pew Charitable Trusts. (2016a). *Reserves remain short of pre-recession levels in most states.* Retrieved June 12, 2016, from http://www.pewtrusts.org/en/research-and-analysis/analysis/2016/01/05/reserves-remain-short-of-pre-recession-levels-in-most-states

Pew Charitable Trusts. (2016b). *Is Medicaid expansion near a tipping point?* Retrieved June 12, 2016, from http://www.pewtrusts.org/en/research-and-analysis/blogs/stateline/2016/01/26/is-medicaid-expansion-near-a-tipping-point

Pew Charitable Trusts. (2016c). *Revenue is up in most states; but weak forecasts prompt caution.* Retrieved June 12, 2016, from http://www.pewtrusts.org/en/research-and-analysis/blogs/stateline/2016/01/27/revenue-is-up-in-most-states-but-weak-forecasts-prompt-caution

Pew Charitable Trusts. (2016d). *Fiscal 50.* Retrieved June 12, 2016, from http:// www.pewtrusts.org/en/multimedia/data-visualizations/2014/fiscal-50

Public Law 101-336. (1990). *Americans with Disability Act of 1990.*

Public Law 105-33. (1997). *The Children's Health Insurance Program.*

Public Law 109-171. (2005). *Deficit Reduction Act of 2005.*

Public Law 111–148. (2010). *Patient Protection and Affordable Care Act.*

Public Law 111-5. (2009). *American Recovery and Reinvestment Act of 2009.*

Public Law 74-271. (1935). *Social Security Act of 1935.*

Public Law 89-97. (1965). *Social Security Amendments of 1965.*

Ripley, R., & Franklin, G. (1980). *Congress, the bureaucracy, and public policy.* Homewood, IL: The Dorsey Press.

Rockefeller Institute of Government. (2016). *State revenue report no. 102. softening third-quarter growth in state taxes, weak forecasts for fiscal 2016 and 2017.* Retrieved July 1, 2016, from http://www.rockinst.org

Schmeida, M. (2005). *Telehealth innovation in the American states.* Ann Arbor, MI: ProQuest.

Schmeida, M., & McNeal, R. (2015). Online health information: home caregiver population driving cyberspace searches in the United States. In M. Khosrow-Pour (Ed.), *Public affairs and administration: concepts, methodologies, tools, and applications* (pp. 1664–1683). Hershey, PA: Information Science Reference. doi:10.4018/978-1-4666-8358-7.ch085

Squire, P. (1992). Legislative professionalism and membership diversity in state legislatures. *Legislative Studies Quarterly*, *17*(1), 69–79. doi:10.2307/440081

United States Census Bureau. (2012a). *2010 Census urban and rural classification and urban area criteria*. Retrieved November 7, 2013, from http://www.census.gov/geo/reference/ua/urban-rural-2010.html

United States Census Bureau. (2012b). *2012 statistical abstract*. Retrieved December 9, 2013, from http://www.census.gov/compendia/statab/

United States Census Bureau. (2014). *Statistical abstracts in the United States*. Washington, DC: U.S. Government Printing Office.

United States Department of Commerce, Bureau of Economic Analysis. (2015). *GSP missions of current 2014 dollars*. Retrieved June 1, 2016, from http://www.bea.gov

United States Department of Health and Human Services, Administration of Aging. (2014). *A profile of older Americans: 2014*. Retrieved June 12, 2016, from http://www.aoa.acl.gov/aging_statistics/profile/2014/docs/2014-profile.pdf

United States Government Accountability Office. (2011). *Medicaid improving responsiveness of federal assistance to states during economic downturns. Report GAO-11-395*. Retrieved June 12, 2016, from http:// www.gao.gov/assets/320/317275.pdf

United States Government Accountability Office. (2015a). *Medicaid key issues facing the program. report to congressional addressees. Report GAO-15-677*. Retrieved June 12, 2016, from http:// www.gao.gov/assets/680/671761.pdf

United States Government Accountability Office. (2015b). *Medicaid managed care trends in federal spending and state oversight of costs and enrollment. Report GAO-16-77*. Retrieved June 12, 2016, from http://gao.gov/assets/680/674307.pdf

Urban Institute. (2014). *Reversing the Medicaid fee bump: how much could Medicaid physician fees for primary care fall in 2015?* Retrieved July 5, 2016, from http://www.urban.org/sites/default/files/alfresco/publication-pdfs/2000025-Reversing-the-Medicaid-Fee-Bump.pdf

Walker, J. (1969). The diffusion of innovation among the American states. *The American Political Science Review*, *63*(3), 880–899. doi:10.2307/1954434

Winters, S. (2006). Implementation. In B. Peters & J. Pierre (Eds.), *The SAGE handbook of public policy* (pp. 151–166). London: Sage. doi:10.4135/9781848608054.n9

World Health Organization. (2014). *"Ageing well" must be a global priority*. Retrieved July 5, 2016, from http://www.who.int/mediacentre/news/releases/2014/lancet-ageing-series/en/

ADDITIONAL READING

Degenholtz, H. B., Park, M., Kang, Y., & Nadash, P. (2016). Variations among Medicare beneficiaries living in different settings. *Research on Aging, 38*(5), 602–616. doi:10.1177/0164027515598557 PMID:26269562

Doty, P., Liu, K., & Wiener, J. (1985). Special report: An overview of long-term care. *Health Care Financing Review, 6*(3). PMID:10311163

Duckett, M., & Guy, M. (2000). Home and community-based services waivers. *Health Care Financing Review, 22*(1), 123–125. PMID:25372343

Kaiser Family Foundation. (2012). *The cost and coverage implications of the ACA Medicaid expansion: national and state-by-state analysis*. Retrieved June 10, 2016, from http://kaiserfamilyfoundation.files.wordpress.com/2013/01/8384.pdf

Kaiser Family Foundation. (November 25, 2013). *The role of Medicaid in state economies: a look at the research.* Retrieved June 10, 2016, from http://kff.org/medicaid/issue-brief/the-role-of-medicaid-in-state-economies-and-the-aca/

Kaiser Family Foundation. (October 15, 2015). *The Affordable Care Act drove record annual increases in enrollment and total Medicaid spending nationally in FY 2015, as newly eligible adults gained coverage in expansion states.* Retrieved June 10, 2016, from http://kff.org/medicaid/press-release/the-affordable-care-act-drove-record-annual-increases-in-enrollment-and-total-medicaid-spending-nationally-in-fy-2015-as-newly-eligible-adults-gained-coverage-in-expansion-states/

Kaiser Family Foundation. (October 15, 2015). *Putting Medicaid in the larger budget context: an in-depth look at three states in FY 2015 and 2016, Tennessee.* Retrieved June 10, 2016, from http://kff.org/report-section/putting-medicaid-in-the-larger-budget-context-an-in-depth-look-at-three-states-in-fy-2015-and-2016-tennessee/

Kaiser Family Foundation. (2016). *State health facts, federal medical assistance percentage (FMAP) for Medicaid and multiplier.* Retrieved June 10, 2016, from http://kff.org/medicaid/state-indicator/federal-matching-rate-and-multiplier/

Kaiser Family Foundation. (January, 2016). *Americans' views on the U.S. role in global health.* Retrieved June 10, 2016, from http://kff.org/global-health-policy/poll-finding/americans-views-on-the-u-s-role-in-global-health/

Kane, R. L. (2015). A new long-term care manifesto. *The Gerontologist, 55*(2), 296–301. doi:10.1093/geront/gnv010 PMID:26035606

Kane, R. L., & Kane, R. A. (2015). The long view of long-term care: Our personal take on progress, pitfalls, and possibilities. *Journal of the American Geriatrics Society, 63*(11), 2400–2406. doi:10.1111/jgs.13659 PMID:26515277

Kennedy, M. (2013). Community-based health plans take the (complex) path to integrated care. *Generations (San Francisco, Calif.), 37*(2), 30–32.

Mahoney, K. J., Sciegaj, M., & Mahoney, E. K. (2014). The future of participant direction in aging services. *Generations (San Francisco, Calif.)*, *38*(2), 85–93.

Miller, E. A., & Rudder, C. (2013). Engaging consumers in Medicaid nursing home reimbursement policy: Lessons from New York and Minnesota. *The Gerontologist*, *53*(4), 627–640. doi:10.1093/geront/gns141 PMID:23125075

Miller, S. C., Cohen, N., Lima, J. C., & Mor, V. (2014). Medicaid capital reimbursement policy and environmental artifacts of nursing home culture change. *The Gerontologist*, *54*(Supplement 1), S76–S86. doi:10.1093/geront/gnt141 PMID:24443609

National Association of Medicaid Directors. (November, 2015). *State Medicaid operations survey: fourth annual survey of Medicaid directors*. Retrieved July 5, 2016, from http://www.statecoverage.org/files/NAMD_Medicaid_Survey_Report_2015.pdf

National Health Policy Forum. (October 17, 2013). *The commission on long-term care: background behind the mission*. Retrieved July 5, 2016, from http://www.nhpf.org

Organisation for Economic Co-operation and Development (OECD). (2009). *The long-term care workforce: overview and strategies to adapt supply to a growing demand*. Paris: OCED. Retrieved July 5, 2016, from http://www.oecd.org/officialdocuments/publicdisplaydocumentpdf/?doclanguage=en&cote=delsa/elsa/wp2/hea (2009)1

Pew Charitable Trusts. (July 29, 2015). *State spending on Medicaid*. Retrieved June 12, 2016, from http://www.pewtrusts.org/en/research-and-analysis/analysis/2015/07/29/state-spending-on-medicaid

Pew Charitable Trusts. (December, 2015). *Why states save using evidence to inform how large rainy day funds should grow*. Retrieved June 12, 2016, from http://www.pewtrusts.org/~/media/assets/2015/12/whystatessavereport.pdf /

Pew Charitable Trusts. (February, 2016). *Insights from fiscal 50's key measures of state fiscal health*. Retrieved June 12, 2016, from http://www.pewtrusts.org/en/research-and-analysis/analysis/2015/11/11/insights-from-fiscal-50s-key-measures-of-state-fiscal-health

Pew Charitable Trusts. (May 17, 2016). *Long-term obligations vary as a share of state resources*. Retrieved June 12, 2016, from http://www.pewtrusts.org/en/research-and-analysis/analysis/2016/05/17/long-term-obligations-vary-as-a-share-of-state-resources

Popejoy, L. L. (2015). Comparing aging in place to home health care: Impact of nurse care coordination on utilization and costs. *Nursing Economics*, *33*(6), 306–313. PMID:26845818

Public Law 110-246. (2008). *The Older Americans Act*.

Public Law 89-73. (1965). *Older Americans Act*.

Reinhard, S. C. (2013). What do older adults want from integrated care? *Generations (San Francisco, Calif.)*, *37*(2), 68–71.

Rockefeller Institute of Government. (November, 2015). *State revenue report no. 101. another strong tax quarter for the states, but less promising forecasts for fiscal 2016.* Retrieved July 1, 2016, from http://www.rockinst.org

Rockefeller Institute of Government. (April, 2016). *Will April income tax returns surprise states*? Retrieved July 1, 2016, from http://www.rockinst.org

Salganicoff, A. (2015). Women and Medicare: An unfinished agenda. *Generations (San Francisco, Calif.), 39*(2), 43–50.

Stevens, A. B., Hochhalter, A. K., Basu, R., Smith, E. R., Thorud, J. L., Jo, C., & McGhee, R. (2015). A model program of community-based supports for older adults at risk of nursing facility placement. *Journal of the American Geriatrics Society, 63*(12), 2601–2609. doi:10.1111/jgs.13831 PMID:26663134

United States Census Bureau. (May, 2010). *The next four decades, the older population in the United States: 2010 to 2050.* Retrieved June 12, 2016 from http://www.census.gov/prod/2010pubs/p25-1138.pdf

United States Department of Commerce. Census Bureau. (November, 2011). *The older population: 2010.* Retrieved June 12, 2016, from http://www.census.gov/prod/cen2010/briefs/c2010br-09.pdf

United States Department of Health and Human Services. (2014). *2014 actuarial report on the financial outlook for Medicaid.* Retrieved June 12, 2016, from http://www.medicaid.gov/medicaid-chip-program-information/by-topics/financing-and-reimbursement/downloads/medicaid-actuarial-report-2014.pdf

United States Government Accountability Office. (July 29, 2014). *MEDICAID: completed and preliminary work indicate that transparency around state financing methods and payments to providers is still needed for oversight. Report GAO-14-817T.* Retrieved June 12, 2016, from http://www.gao.gov/assets/670/665069.pdf

Vestal, C. (2012). *Medicaid: a year of excruciating decisions.* Retrieved May 16, 2016, from http://www.stateline.org/live/prntable/story?contentId=624072

Williams, A., Straker, J. K., & Applebaum, R. (2016). The nursing home five star rating: How does it compare to resident and family views of care? *The Gerontologist, 56*(2), 234–242. doi:10.1093/geront/gnu043 PMID:24847846

Wysocki, A., Kane, R. L., Dowd, B., Golberstein, E., Lum, T., & Shippee, T. (2014). Hospitalization of elderly Medicaid long-term care users who transition from nursing homes. *Journal of the American Geriatrics Society, 62*(1), 71–78. doi:10.1111/jgs.12614 PMID:24383662

KEY TERMS AND DEFINITIONS

Assisted Living Industry: Community-based centers for persons requiring assistance with activities of daily living and/or personal care.

Expansion State: State choosing to expand their Medicaid program services in response to the 2010 Patient Protection and Affordable Care Act (ACA).

Family Home Caregiver: An individual who provides nursing care and/ or companionship, assistance for another person, such as parent, spouse, child with a disability or chronically ill.

Federal Fiscal Year: October 1 of previous year through September 30th.

Home Health and Personal Care: Services provided by Medicaid, including standard home health services, personal care, home and community-based care for the functionally disabled elderly, and services provided under home and community-based services waivers.

Medicaid: The second largest U.S. public health insurance program for the impoverished of all age groups, the blind, disabled, and medically needy considered impoverished.

Medicaid Enrollees: Persons enrolled in the Medicaid program in a fiscal year.

Medicare: The largest U.S. public health insurance program for persons under 65 years of age with a disability, age 65 or older, and all age groups with End-Stage Renal Disease.

State Fiscal Year: July 1st of previous year through June 30th for the majority of the 50 states.

Chapter 4
The Continuum of Care: A Case Study of a Senior Service Centre for Geriatric Care in Toronto, Canada

Kwong Yuen Liu
Yee Hong Centre for Geriatric Care, Canada

Maria Chu
Yee Hong Centre for Geriatric Care, Canada

Bonnie H. Y. Wong
Yee Hong Centre for Geriatric Care, Canada

William Y. W. Leung
Yee Hong Centre for Geriatric Care, Canada

ABSTRACT

This chapter examines the continuum of care in use at the Yee Hong Centre for Geriatric Care in Toronto, Ontario, Canada. The service continuum is a response to the needs of a diverse Chinese Canadian population, where services in the appropriate language and culture are limited. Within the funding context, service coordination for seniors within Ontario can be characterized as fragmented, with over-use of acute care hospitalization and long-term care institutionalization. Community agencies must find a way to adapt to changing systems as the Ontario government moves away from institutionalization and toward community care. This chapter explores challenges that are faced by a socially-minded organization within a medically-minded funding system. It also addresses ways to cope with the constraints.

INTRODUCTION

Evashwick (1989) defined the continuum of care as a "concept involving an integrated system of care that guides and tracks patients over time through a comprehensive array of health services spanning all levels of intensity of care" (p. 30). By Evashwick's definition, the continuum of care focuses on an individual's biomedical needs, ignoring a more holistic view of human needs. This chapter reviews different models of the continuum of care within the literature, explores each model's benefits and limitations, and presents the continuum of care model for senior service used at the Yee Hong Centre for Geriatric Care (Yee Hong).

Yee Hong began operation in 1994 as part of Dr. Joseph Wong's vision to serve Chinese seniors in Toronto. As a physician working in mainstream long-term care homes in the 1980s, Dr. Wong identified

DOI: 10.4018/978-1-5225-2633-9.ch004

unmet needs of many Chinese seniors. Dr. Wong mobilized a group of volunteers to advocate for a long-term care home that would provide culturally and linguistically appropriate services for Chinese seniors. With support from the University of Toronto, the Chinese Community Nursing Home for Greater Toronto (1989) completed a needs study to assess demographic data and conducted surveys and interviews with Chinese seniors, caregivers, and community members. The results highlighted that seniors' needs could not be met with a long-term care home alone. The first Yee Hong location was established in 1994. In addition to a small long-term care home, service space included a social housing complex, a community centre, and a medical centre. An expansion of the available community services was projected as part of Yee Hong's first strategic plan.

The Yee Hong (2016) mission states,

With strong roots in the Chinese Canadian community and our respect for seniors, we enable seniors of different backgrounds and needs to live their lives to the fullest—in the healthiest, most independent, and dignified way.

[The Centre] provide[s] a continuum of culturally and linguistically appropriate care to seniors of Chinese origin. Further, we provide culturally and linguistically appropriate long-term care services to seniors of other cultural backgrounds within the capacity of the centre.

Four elements in the mission statement underpin Yee Hong's approach to serving seniors in the community:

1. Focus is placed on client wellness and quality of life rather than just on physical care. The ultimate goal is to enable clients to live their lives to the fullest.
2. Yee Hong adopts an empowerment model to help seniors lead healthy, independent, and dignified lives.
3. With the above in mind, Yee Hong focuses on client needs. Special attention is paid to the need for appropriate culture and language rather than on services already available.
4. A continuum of service for seniors at different stages of the aging process addresses client needs and achieves the goal of living lives to the fullest.

With the mission in mind, Yee Hong expanded its continuum of services by serving approximately 20,000 seniors in the community annually, as well as providing 805 long-term care beds and services. This is a wellness model of care that moves away from the traditional North American biomedical model of health care. The Yee Hong model is client focused rather than focused on only biomedical needs. This chapter will present the philosophical underpinning for the continuum of care and services available at Yee Hong. In addition, it will discuss the challenges associated with implementing a wellness model in a medically minded funding structure.

CONTINUUM OF CARE MODELS IN THE LITERATURE

The term *continuum of care* does not capture the different care delivery models in the literature. Béland and Hollander (2011) used terms such as *integrated (health) care* and *continuing care* to elicit models of integrated care delivery. Gulliford, Naithani, and Morgan (2006) described *continuity of care* as a seamless transition between services through the coordination, integration, and sharing of information.

Béland and Hollander (2011) described integrated models as a way "to provide a continuum of care for frail elderly persons within a system of care with a broad range of services matched to their needs" (p. 138). Béland and Hollander (2011) defined two models of integrated care delivery. The first was a smaller community-based model, and the second was a national- or state-level model. Integration could be horizontal or vertical. While the former referred to improved care coordination across different settings, the latter referred to the delivery and coordination of services through a single organization (MacAdam, 2008). As the Yee Hong continuum of care focuses on community care within one agency, this chapter will explore the community-based continuum of care models. Current continuity of care models provided at the smaller community level identified by Béland and Hollander (2011) and MacAdam (2008) include the program of all-inclusive care for the elderly (PACE), the system of integrated care for older persons model (SIPA), and the program of research to integrate the services for the maintenance of autonomy model (PRISMA). It should be noted that currently Canada is still traditionally based in institutional care, and as of yet there is no formal state or national strategy that has been adopted – rather it is still in development. To address this, Yee Hong has adopted a continuum of care model to approach existing gaps in services that are not sufficiently meeting the needs of seniors in Canada.

The PACE Model

The United States of America's Centers for Medicare & Medicaid Services (2011) describe PACE as a way to improve the quality of life by maximizing participant autonomy and continued community residence. This targeted approach allows a single, local organization to provide seniors with chronic care needs to be met through a range of available community services. Service users are provided with multidisciplinary team case management, supplemented with services such as an adult day health centre, medical care, home and personal care, and other social services (National PACE Association, 2016). The continuum of care within PACE moves from "preventive, primary, acute, rehabilitative [toward] long-term care services" (Hirth, Baskins, & Dever-Bumba, 2009, p. 156). Research shows that PACE participants have an improved quality of life and health status, lower mortality rates, and greater confidence in managing late-life issues (Chatterji, Burstein, Kidder, & White, 1998; Mui, 2002).

However, eligibility for PACE services is limited. Participants must be eligible for long-term care services and live in a PACE service area. As a result, the program is only available to frail seniors. This limits services to a large number of seniors who may otherwise benefit from the range of services. Although PACE is effective in cutting costs and improving participant quality of life, implementation of PACE can be difficult (e.g., establishing a program requires a primary care specialist who is willing to work exclusively with a frail population) (Hirth et al., 2009). Critics note that the PACE model has limited service choices (based on available resources) and relies on adult day care (Hirth et al., 2009).

The SIPA Model

The SIPA model is an integrated service delivery model created through intensive research development in collaboration with stakeholders within the health and social services network of Quebec, Canada (Béland et al., 2006b). Coordinated services (e.g., intensive home care, 24-hour on-call services) are provided through a case manager and a multidisciplinary team with the involvement of a general practitioner (MacAdam, 2008). Older adults involved in the SIPA program are active participants in the decision-making process (Béland et al., 2006b).

SIPA lowered the risk of long-term care placement from acute care hospitals. It was able to coordinate care without additional funding as well as increase quality of care (Béland et al., 2006b). In addition, it increased the satisfaction of both participants and caregivers (Béland et al., 2006a). SIPA program eligibility requires that the participant be severely disabled in one of the following areas or mild to moderately disabled in two of the following areas: activities of daily living, instrumental activities of daily living, mobility, mental status, or continence (Bergman et al., 1997). It should also be noted that SIPA did not affect all participants in the same manner. It is effective for at-risk seniors and the frailest of seniors (Béland et al., 2006b).

One of the major challenges within SIPA was family physician involvement. Not all physicians were willing or able to fulfill the case manager's requests because there were limited incentives for their involvement (Béland et al., 2006a, 2006b).

The PRISMA Model

The PRISMA model of coordinated care spans three systems of governance: the strategic level, the tactical level, and the clinical level (MacAdam, 2015). This multilevel system allows PRISMA to include six necessary elements for integrated care: (1) single entry point, (2) case management, (3) individualized service plan, (4) single assessment instruction, (5) computerized clinical chart, and (6) coordination between partner organizations at regional and local levels (PRISMA, 2016). PRISMA focuses on meeting the physical needs of the frail elderly and aims to provide psychological and social support (Hébert, Durand, Dubuc, & Tourigny, 2003). Services are needs based instead of resource based (Hébert et al., 2003). The case manager is responsible for evaluating client needs and for planning and arranging the required services while the individualized service plan is shared among the multidisciplinary team (Hébert et al., 2003). Program participants were significantly more satisfied and empowered, had fewer cases of functional decline (Stewart, Georgiou, & Westbrook, 2013), and had a lower number of hospitalizations and emergency room visits than comparable groups (Hébert et al., 2009).

An eligibility criterion for joining PRISMA coordinated care requires that the participant needs two or more healthcare or social services. This reduces the misuse of resources. However, participants must also meet the standardized criteria of being moderately to severely disabled (Hébert et al., 2003). This may limit individuals with chronic diseases who require more services but whose functional decline has not yet met the disability criteria. Challenges to this model include reduction in unmet need related to case management and home care services and the need to increase physician involvement (MacAdam, 2015). It requires coordination at all levels of healthcare and social services systems as well as adoption at the policy level.

Comparing Continuity of Care Models

Kodner (2006) compared these three service integration models and found that four conditions must be met for the success of service integration models:

1. A multilevel organizational structure that encourages and supports operations, with accountability of service quality and costs

2. An interdisciplinary team with case management that will assess and plan client care based on individual needs
3. A closed network of service providers that have standardized referral processes and service agreements
4. Established financial incentives to promote prevention and rehabilitation, allowing for service integration and efficiency

Veras et al. (2014) reiterated that care plans and case management are essential to the continuity of services. Similarly, CARP (2013) advocated for the creation of a "navigator" role to ensure that individuals and their families are able to easily navigate and access the healthcare system.

Beyond system integration, an individual's needs must be addressed in order to improve quality of care. The previously discussed models are current standards for continuum of care. However, it should be noted that not all of these models address the emotional, mental, and social components of healthcare needs. Some address only the physical care needs of the aging population. The need for physician involvement within all three models limits the establishment and availability of these models. Given the reliance on physician involvement, the models can be viewed as placing less emphasis on aspects that affect an individual's health and well-being.

CARP (2013) advocated for an attitude change in healthcare delivery, which places the individual's needs and wishes at the forefront. This requires a care continuum in which different components within the healthcare system work together toward a more efficient and seamless quality of health care and that services are available "when and where they are needed" (CARP, 2013, p. 1). Yee Hong is a non-profit community service and long-term care organization. Therefore, without the support of funders and policymakers, constraints exist for Yee Hong. The organization prides itself on providing high-quality care and advocates for a more holistic continuum of care. It aims to address both the physical and the psychosocial needs of clients and caregivers.

CONTINUUM OF CARE AT YEE HONG CENTRE

Aging as a Process

The medical approach to health is dominant in North America. Within this model, it presumes that all illnesses can be classified and treated in an objective way (Taylor & Hawley, 2010). Older adults are viewed as a homogenous group that can be treated in a standardized manner. As a result, the focus of aging within this paradigm is on the deficiencies and absence of disease. To manage physical deficiencies, service provisions are standardized in the sense that services can be "prescribed" to "treat" the condition at hand. In reality, health status ranges greatly within the older population. The aging process differs on physical, cognitive, mental, and psychosocial levels, and standardized services are unable to meet the changing needs of this population.

Rather than view aging as a stagnant life stage, Yee Hong views it as a dynamic process with many transitions. A study commissioned by Yee Hong in conjunction with the University of Toronto (Tsang et al., 2013) found that, during the aging process, individuals are faced with many circumstantial changes:

- **Retirement:** Whether the transition to retirement is gradual or abrupt, an individual faces the following changes: role, economic status, friends, affiliation, daily routine, and (possibly) control over one's life.
- **Children Leaving the Home:** Aging parents can face depression and/or anxiety, a change of family dynamics, a loss of affection and intimacy, and a loss of purpose when children leave the home.
- **Caregiving:** Becoming a caregiver may be a gradual or an abrupt transition, creating a new identity as an individual takes on responsibilities to care for a spouse, parent, and/or other relatives.
- **Deterioration of Health:** Deteriorating health may lead to a change in economic status and a diminished ability to provide care for oneself, influencing self-esteem, self-confidence, independence, and the need for control.
- **Death of a Partner:** When a significant other passes away, an individual also loses the affection and intimacy that was once part of the relationship. Individuals face changing roles, economic status, and daily routines and may lose their meaning in life.
- **Change in Living Arrangements:** Seniors may need to change homes (whether temporarily or permanently). The loss of familiarity could be substantial, especially if there is also a change in social circles. If the move is into an institutional setting, then an individual may feel a loss of independence, autonomy, and control.

Given all of these transitions, seniors are faced with multiple levels of loss. Individuals react and cope differently to loss and change. For some, grief may have a larger effect. In this regard, the focus of care shifts away from biomedical needs. Instead, it focuses on a more holistic view of the aging process and overall wellness. A client's biopsychosocial needs can be appreciated as a specific and unique "journey." As the Yee Hong model is built on this premise, service provision is targeted at assisting the aging adult in achieving developmental tasks (adjusting and coping with the many changes in the aging process). By completing these developmental tasks, seniors—regardless of age—are able to make improvements to their quality of life and are capable of change.

Understanding Client Needs

The medical approach views aging as a physical health issue. It ignores the fact that aging affects an individual on cognitive, emotional, and social levels. Yee Hong recognized that long-term care homes alone could not meet the needs of older adults experiencing the aging process. Yee Hong realized that senior needs may change when interacting with provided services and will continue to change during the process of transition (Tsang et al., 2013).

Further exploring how culture shapes and creates the context by which individuals identify with the world around them is also a crucial element when understanding client needs. Yee Hong recognizes that culture plays a different role in each individual's life, and in turn, influences the way a person self-identifies. Thus, focusing on a wellness and holistic approach (which should encompass cultural sensitivity) is an effective way to understand and address the subjective identity-based needs of the service user – a component that is extremely relevant to an individual's aging process, but often overlooked and not accounted for in the medical approach.

In an effort to evolve with the changing needs of seniors and the community, the Social Services division of Yee Hong adopted a framework of practice based on the Strategies & Skills Learning & Development (SSLD) system. Professor Ka Tat Tsang from the Factor-Inwentash Faculty of Social

Figure 1. Comparing continuity of care models

Continuity of Care Model:	Characteristics	Challenges
The PACE Model	▪ allows for single, local organization to provide services ▪ multidisciplinary team case management, supplemented with range of health, personal care, and social services	▪ eligibility for PACE requires participants to first be eligible for long-term care services and must live in a PACE service area ▪ only available to frail seniors ▪ limited service choices based on available resources
The SIPA Model	▪ coordinated services by case manager, multidisciplinary team, and a general practitioner ▪ service users can be active participants in the decision-making process	▪ eligibility for SIPA requires that participant be severely disabled in one criteria or mild to moderately disabled in two areas ▪ seems effective for only at-risk seniors and the frailest of seniors
The PRISMA Model	▪ has multilevel systems of governance in forming its integrated approach ▪ single entry point for services ▪ services are needs based instead of resource based	▪ eligibility for PRISMA requires participants to have two or more healthcare or social services ▪ participants must meet standardized criteria of being moderately to severely disabled
Continuum of Care at Yee Hong Centre	▪ looks at aging as a process rather than criteria for services ▪ has multiple entry points for services depending on need of user ▪ empowers participants and caregivers to have choice in their service utilization ▪ services are needs based, culturally appropriate, and fluid – developed as the population needs change overtime	▪ resources are limited within the current biomedical minded funding model ▪ participation in certain programs are still governed by requirements of the funders which often times set eligibility (or exclusion) criterion based on biomedical conditions

Work at the University of Toronto founded the SSLD system. It is "an intervention system for bringing about change in human life, including our thinking, action, motivation, emotion, and body, as well as our environment" (SSLD, 2014, para. 1). When needs are unmet, the exhibited behaviours, which may or may not be deemed appropriate by others, are aimed to meet that need. The SSLD system seeks to identify these needs and aims to help the individual formulate better strategies to address the issues at hand. On a macro level, the versatility of SSLD allows for its application in analysing communities, as well as organisational cultures and practices, to identify needs within larger systems and plan for better strategies in embracing change.

The SSLD model looks at the individual, organizational, and community needs, circumstances, characteristics, and capacity (Tsang, 2013). For example, the dominant medical model focuses on the notion that aging is a problem and that physical deterioration is the main contributor. SSLD translates this view that aging is a problem to that of "aging as a process," which improves understanding of seniors' needs. In addition, the SSLD framework is premised on multiple contingency thinking (Tsang, 2013), where all factors that may affect the senior must be considered to determine needs. Yee Hong's capacity for understanding is expanded in order to work on strategies and skills to meet the changing needs of both the individual and the community. By using the SSLD system as a guiding framework, Yee Hong assesses the needs of clients, caregivers, and the community to determine service provision. Services provided based on this framework can be seen as strategies and skills for clients and caregivers to address their individual needs. SSLD consequently empowers the organization and its clients as it provides more options and choices (Tsang, 2013). Therefore, the objective is to assist clients, caregivers, and the organization to express their needs through the use and engagement of services provided by Yee Hong.

Shifting the Paradigm Toward a Wellness Model

Yee Hong defines wellness as a philosophy that involves a positive and proactive attitude toward life. Achieving a high level of wellness is a lifelong process in which a person makes conscious choices and decisions in an effort to reach his or her highest potential (Dunn, 1959). It encompasses a whole and balanced perspective on the individual and his or her relationships with others, the community, and the environment. Wellness is a dynamic process of maximizing one's potential. Yee Hong's mission statement places an emphasis on empowering seniors to live their lives to the fullest while focusing on overall wellness. As Yee Hong focuses on client well-being and quality of life, the individual is seen as an agent of change rather than as a patient requiring a health expert's supervision.

Services developed through the medical model of health care can be construed as preplanned or prepackaged programs because they are standardized models that can be structured, manualized, easily learned, and replicated (Tsang, 2013). On the other hand, services based on client needs can be viewed as contingency-based interventions, where emphasis is placed on meeting an individual's needs and characteristics. To assist clients in making changes to effectively meet their needs, the organization must explore how and what kind of services will best help clients. This is a significant shift from the medical model of health care in which the individual is seen as a passive participant in his or her own health. The Yee Hong model places emphasis on empowerment, where the individual takes charge of his or her health management and condition. The senior does not need to depend on the healthcare provider, as the professional is just a part of the support system to provide knowledge and advice. The individual has the right to make his or her own decisions. As a result, services must empower the senior to develop effective strategies and skills to cope with the decline in health.

The Yee Hong continuum, with client well-being and wellness in mind, places an emphasis on client strength rather than on illness. Therefore, its services assist clients to remain independent by encouraging the use, development, and improvement of strength. Every individual, regardless of age, has the capacity to change and improve his or her quality of life. Yee Hong's services support a client in revealing his or her capacity and self-efficacy in individual healthcare management in order to achieve physical and mental wellness. A few services utilize individualised care plans along the continuum, with ongoing input and review from the client and caregivers.

Quality indicators used along the Yee Hong continuum determine if a client's wellness needs are being met. The number of falls, which is a medically minded quality indicator, is monitored in the long-term care home as mandated by the Ontario government. However, other quality indicators used by Yee Hong are geared toward monitoring client well-being. For example, at the adult day programs, clients without dementia are regularly assessed using the Geriatric Depression Scale (Short Form), while dementia clients are regularly assessed using the Mini Mental State Examination. Other examples include the use of a goal attainment scale to determine change in confidence levels after participating in Yee Hong's caregiver education or chronic disease self-management programs.

Data currently collected from Yee Hong's day programs suggest that the programs may have a positive effect on clients' Geriatric Depression Scale (GDS) scores. For Chinese seniors living in Hong Kong, researchers found the mean GDS score to be 3.9 (Lee, Chiu, Kwok, & Leung, 1993). Chinese senior immigrants living in Canada showed a mean of 3.15 (Lai, 2000). Mean scores collected during 2014 from Yee Hong's day programs ranged from 2.2 to 3.77 (this falls within the earlier range). This finding is significant because day program clients generally suffer from various chronic illnesses. It is likely that day program clients report more depressive symptoms. However, it does not appear to be reflected in the mean scores of Yee Hong's day program clients. The statistics used above are not to be interpreted as comparisons between Chinese seniors living in Hong Kong and Chinese senior immigrants living in Canada, but rather an internal benchmark for Yee Hong to monitor clients' well-being. By meeting individual needs through contingency-based programming and individualized care plans, it appears that the day program services are enhancing client well-being.

The choice of quality indicators deployed by Yee Hong is reflective of its desire to shift from the current biomedical paradigm towards a wellness model. As mentioned previously, the use of goal attainment scale is used to determine change in the clients' confidence levels which attributes to self-esteem – an underlying need that is known to have significant impact on ones well-being. The Geriatric Depression Scale (Short Form) can help monitor the mood of clients which ultimately is as an indicator of psychosocial well-being. Finally, the use of N3C (Needs, Circumstances, Characteristics, Capacity) assessments from the SSLD framework allows for evaluation of programs and participants to assess whether needs, potential, and capacity have been met. Yee Hong has conscientiously selected indicators that are driven by client needs and aims to assess clients from a wellness and holistic framework.

Service Continuum at Yee Hong

The Yee Hong service continuum and support services have evolved as part of the organization's responsiveness to individual and community needs. Yee Hong started by developing services along the process of transition, from an active and healthy retiree to an older individual who moves into a long-term care home. Yee Hong meetings and focus groups provide platforms for client and caregiver feedback. Yee Hong recently completed a study on the "Changing Needs of Chinese Seniors in the Greater Toronto Area" (Tsang et al., 2013) as a way to inform the organization on program development and future service planning. Because many of Yee Hong's service users are immigrants to Canada, the services are provided in a culturally and linguistically appropriate manner.

Figure 2 presents the current continuum of care services available at Yee Hong. It provides a broad range of services to enable seniors to live independently and with dignity. The model delivers services at different levels of care, from the most independent to the most dependent seniors, with seamless transition between services. The programs do not focus solely on physical health. Instead, they centre on well-being as a whole. The services available on the continuum include:

- **Active Senior Program:** This program provides a spectrum of social, recreational, and educational activities for seniors 55 years and older. It aims to enhance the client's physical, emotional, and mental well-being. The program targets seniors who are considering retirement, those who are taking steps toward retirement, and those who are already retired. Retirement is a life-changing transition for these clients. The program provides an opportunity for them to develop a healthy lifestyle to face this life transition, create new friendships, cultivate new hobbies, and establish

Figure 2. Continuum of services available at Yee Hong

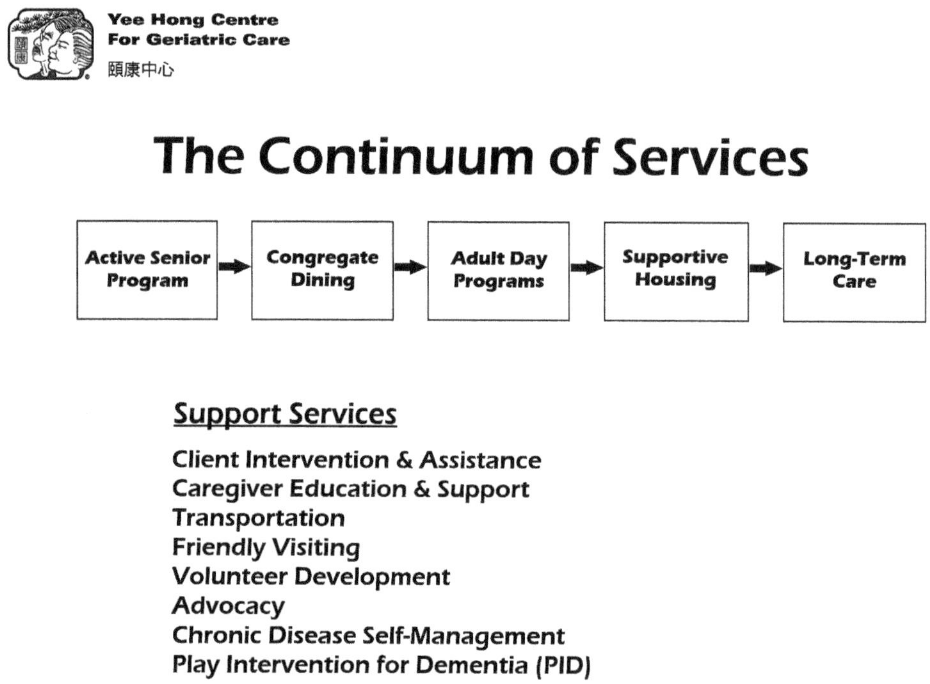

new routines and life patterns to adapt to a new stage of life. Yee Hong has four Active Senior Programs across different locations in the Greater Toronto Area, serving approximately 3,000 clients each year. There is also a self-programming seniors' social group called Macrobian Club, which has its own board of directors. With professional support from an Active Senior Program social worker, Macrobian Club members are encouraged to manage, contribute to, and organize their own affairs. Despite the need for such service in this developmental stage of retirement, the government has not provided any funds to support this program since its establishment. Yee Hong fundraising currently supports this program.

- **Congregate Dining:** This is a funded program to provide seniors a hot, nutritious meal once a week. This is a typical prescription program under the medical funding model. Yee Hong uses congregate dining to bridge the gap between the Active Senior Program and the adult day program, targeting seniors who are not active and independent enough to join the Active Senior Program but who are not frail enough to join the adult day programs. Eligible members are typically those who have retired, new immigrants, individuals with limited English proficiency, individuals with limited transportation means, and/or those living alone. Typically, this group of clients is socially and physically isolated. Yee Hong made use of the funded meal and expanded the program into a half-day service, which included different activities and transportation for eligible clients. Apart from a nutritious meal, the program provides a space for isolated seniors to participate in social, recreational, and educational activities. It aims to promote the client's health and mental well-being. The program not only satisfies the physical need for food but also aims to satisfy the clients' need for stimulation, affiliation, self-efficacy, and self-esteem and helps integrate clients into the community. Unfortunately, within a medical paradigm, the funder only sees the need to provide a healthy meal for eligible seniors, and the funding provided is only enough to cover this portion of the program. Yee Hong has to support the monetary deficiency via fundraising.

- **Adult Day Programs:** These programs target seniors who are very frail with different physical challenges and conditions. The average age of the current clientele is over 80 years. At present, Yee Hong operates six different adult day programs in different parts of the Greater Toronto Area. Under the medical paradigm, the funder sees adult day programs as a prescription to senior frailty and takes a one-size-fits-all approach. From a needs/social paradigm, Yee Hong recognizes that clients have different challenges and needs and require different strategies and services to meet those challenges and needs. Yee Hong thus developed subprograms under the umbrella of the adult day programs.
    - **Program for Frail Seniors:** This program is designed for seniors who have mobility issues and require support from others for daily living activities. Currently, the average age of attendance is over 85 years. The strategy focus for this group is to provide physical care, offer different opportunities to combat social isolation and alienation, develop capacity in self-management to improve self-efficacy, alleviate depressive symptoms common in community dwelling frail seniors (St. John, Tyas, & Montgomery, 2013), and develop a meaning of life.
    - **Program for Dementia Clients:** This program targets seniors diagnosed with mild to moderate dementia. The program's aim is, on the one hand, to provide respite for the family caregiver, and on the other hand, to provide social stimulation to the client in order to maintain current abilities and to slow the deterioration caused by dementia. Yee Hong uses the Mini Mental State Examination to assess clients' cognitive abilities. Statistics show that the majority of clients with dementia attending Yee Hong's day programs (88%) do not show decline in the exam's suggested annual decline rate of 3.3 after they have attended the program (Han, Cole, Bellavance, McCusker, & Primeau, 2000). Almost half of the clients (44%) have shown improvement. Geriatricians and caregivers support these findings. This spurred interest from the Factor-Inwentash Faculty of Social Work of the University of Toronto and resulted in the co-development of the Play Intervention for Dementia program.
    - **Program for Young Stroke Survivors:** The program targets a growing population of stroke survivors under the age of 65. The needs and subjective well-being of younger stroke survivors differ from older stroke survivors (Wyller, Holmen, Laake, & Laake, 1998). The program's aim is to help clients cope with the physical and social losses as a result of the stroke, manage their changing roles, adapt to a new self-identity, and regain and reclaim their independence. This program supplements the medical model of service to stroke survivors that stops after physical rehabilitation.
- **Supportive Housing:** Yee Hong's housing services do not stop at providing physical housing. Currently, Yee Hong supports five buildings, two are housing projects owned and managed by Yee Hong, another building is a private condominium where Yee Hong is the contracted service provider, and the last two buildings are supportive housings with Yee Hong as the service provider. All five buildings have support service programs that provide care coordination for the aging residents, including personal care, homemaking, medication reminders, and security checks. Of the two housing projects, Yee Hong owns and manages a social housing complex providing rental units on a rent geared to income basis. Additional support services provided at this complex include 24-hour emergency on-call assistance. The government stopped this kind of brick-and-mortar funding model in the early 1990s and no longer provides funding for new subsidized

housing buildings. As a result, Yee Hong explored other models of providing housing services, developing, building, owning, and managing a life-lease community project, where the tenant buys a lifetime lease hold to live in the housing complex. The life-lease project limits tenancy to those aged 55 and older. All units are equipped to ensure the safety of each resident and include an emergency medical response unit, a shower stall with grab bars and seating, and non-motion sensors. Support services are also offered 24 hours a day, and each resident is provided with up to two hours of free social activities per week. The overall objective of Yee Hong's supportive housing is to promote independent living, to keep seniors from early institutionalization, and to help them age at home by meeting their physical and psychosocial needs.

- **Long-Term Care:** Yee Hong operates four long-term care homes with a total of 805 beds. These residential facilities provide interdisciplinary care for individuals who are no longer able to live independently in their homes. The care provided focuses not only on the residents' physical needs but also on their psychosocial needs. As Yee Hong's services are linguistically and culturally appropriate, admission to the homes requires a long waiting period, and for some, can take up to 10 years. Currently, the four long-term care homes together have more than 4,000 people on their waiting lists.

Although many Chinese elderly prefer to age in their own homes, institutionalization may be their only option when community supports are not sufficient for safe and independent community living. Long-term care is an important part of the Yee Hong continuum. It should be noted that long-term care is not necessarily determined by the need for heavy care in a client's activities of daily living/functional abilities but the need for support in instrumental activities of daily living (Williams et al., 2009).

Emphasis has been placed on developing support services in order to delay institutionalization. Caregivers play a crucial role in supporting community living. Therefore, Yee Hong makes support services available to both the clients and their informal caregivers. A team of coordinators and social workers engages with clients and caregivers at different levels of service to determine an appropriate service plan. To better serve clientele, individual teams hold regular case review meetings to identify clients' changing needs in the programs. Teams hold regular case coordination meetings to determine additional support for clients who will remain in a particular program. In addition, they discuss ways to provide support when clients transition between services.

The service continuum and available support services have evolved as part of Yee Hong's responsiveness to community needs. Through ongoing dialogue, support services were enhanced to ensure a seamless transition between levels of the care continuum. The following support services are important to support the continuum of services:

- **Client Intervention and Assistance:** This program consists of a social worker providing professional case management for seniors and caregivers as a way to cope with the demands of independent community living. The social worker communicates, refers, and follows up with services both inside and outside the organization. This is an unfunded program and is grossly inadequate. Under the medical paradigm, the funder was unable to see the importance of this service and stopped its funding in the early 1990s. However, Yee Hong views this service as essential to assist clients and caregivers to navigate a fragmented healthcare system to ensure that their needs are met. Thus, Yee Hong supports this service through fundraising.

- **Caregiver Education and Support:** In order to enable seniors to age at home, it is important to support family caregivers who provide care for seniors 24 hours a day, 7 days a week. The government sees the importance of supporting family caregivers but focuses only on the provision of physical respite. The psychosocial needs of caregivers are ignored, even though they are more likely than non-caregivers to be stressed, have higher levels of depression, and have lower levels of subjective well-being (Pinquart & Sörensen, 2003). Yee Hong's caregiver education and support program consists of three pillars: (1) knowledge: to provide caregivers with the knowledge of the nature of health issues and challenges; (2) skills: to provide instruction on practical skills in caring for seniors, such as lifting and transfer, proper feeding techniques, and communication skills; and (3) wellness: to provide psychosocial support through improving relaxation techniques, helping caregivers discover their strengths, developing support networks, and participating in mutual support groups. To supplement face-to-face training workshops, Yee Hong has also developed an e-learning platform to allow caregivers to access training videos within the comfort of their homes as needed.
- **Transportation:** This service provides seniors with the ability to participate in Yee Hong's continuum of services and to attend medical appointments. Yee Hong operates a fleet of 10 vehicles, several of which are wheelchair accessible. This program enhances social and community involvement and promotes independence.
- **Friendly Visiting:** This program includes telephone reassurance, where volunteers visit or contact an isolated senior. These services provide community support and contact and ensure the senior's emotional and mental well-being.
- **Volunteer Development:** Yee Hong relies on volunteer support to ensure quality of care. Through ongoing development, about 1,200 volunteers support Yee Hong services annually, contributing approximately 100,000 hours of service. Yee Hong ensures that volunteers are well trained, dependable, and motivated.
- **Advocacy:** Yee Hong advocates for the implementation of new or increased services without compromising the quality of care.
- **Chronic Disease Self-Management:** Since 2006, Yee Hong has adopted the Stanford model of Chronic Disease Self-Management Program. This program helps individuals living with chronic diseases to translate their knowledge into action, allowing clients to be empowered to self-manage their conditions and to improve their quality of life. This aligns with Yee Hong's mission to empower seniors to live their lives to the fullest.
- **Play Intervention for Dementia:** With a wellness model and an empowerment model underpinning Yee Hong services, Yee Hong believes that everyone has the potential to continue to develop and improve. As mentioned earlier, Yee Hong developed the Play Intervention for Dementia program, providing an innovative approach to work with individuals living with dementia. The program is a short-term, targeted intervention using the play process to create stimulation through engagement and synchronization. These activities are developed based on the clients' needs profiles and strengths and aimed toward enhancing clients' functionality and emotional well-being. Changes and observations are not standardized for the group, but rather, individualized to be meaningful and relevant to the particular participant.

The Yee Hong continuum of care differs from other service providers by breaking away from medical professionals. With the exception of direct care provided by personal support workers or mandated assistance offered by regulated health professionals, services provided within the community are delivered by staff trained in social services, social work, gerontology, and/or activation. While care focuses on physical needs, it also concentrates on the psychosocial needs of the service users. The emphasis of care is placed on overall client wellness. The Yee Hong continuum also differs in the sense that services are designed according to client needs, not as a "prescription" provided by the funder. The price to pay for this approach is that the government will not fund some programs that do not fit into the medical paradigm, and Yee Hong must find alternative means to support these programs. Also, as this program was designed according to clients' life transitions, clients can move along this continuum as they age and their needs and abilities change.

Challenges

As the major funder of health services, the Ontario government uses an acute care medical model for health service provision. According to Spalding, Williams, and Watkins (2006), this model requires that service users rely on expert knowledge and skills to determine their needs and provide the appropriate services. Based on the medical model, government-funded services are nothing more than prescriptions to manage conditions identifiable through an objective lens.

In recent years, the Ontario government has promoted the concept of aging at home. But the medical model continues to push nonmedical community support, as there is no universal entitlement to homecare services (Williams et al., 2016). More funds have been injected for home and community care. However, there is no guarantee of free services. Services through publicly funded, regional Community Care Access Centres (CCAC) are free. However, they may not be accessible to many individuals due to eligibility criteria, funding constraints, and long wait lists (Williams et al., 2016). In turn, individuals in need of services will look toward community service agencies such as Yee Hong. However, as per the government service agreements, Yee Hong is mandated to charge user fees. Therefore, hospital and physician care covered by universal healthcare insurance appears to be the more viable economic solution (Williams et al., 2016).

The medical approach to health service provision ignores the social determinants of health as well as an individual's wishes and emotional and mental health needs. Funding is focused on hospital discharge, and through their Home First Program, Community Care Access Centres (2014) provide intensive homecare services for up to 60 days. However, this creates a cycle where hospitals rush patients home in order to keep costs low. After 60 days, the individual may not be able to live safely at home, leading to re-hospitalization or institutionalization. This results in inadequate funding for home and community care outside the discharge realm. Hence, Yee Hong must find alternative ways to support these services in order to keep the continuum intact and viable.

Although Yee Hong services fall outside the acute medical domain, they are important when empowering seniors to remain in their homes. To guarantee continued backing from a medically minded funder, Yee Hong must meet the requirements set by service provider accountability agreements. For example, parameters may include the number of clients served and time spent with each client. Funders do not focus on client and caregiver satisfaction and quality of life. As long as the requirements are not met (and regardless of client outcomes), funding can be pulled with limited notice.

SOLUTIONS AND RECOMMENDATIONS

According to Williams et al. (2016), planning for a continuum of community-based care is required in order to meet the growing needs of an aging population. However, the current Canadian system of integration—with its limited coordination—can only be described as links between service providers (Hébert et al., 2003). Leutz (1999) described three levels of service integration: linkage, coordination, and full integration. The linkage level of service integration views an organization's independent service providers with limited communication and coordination. At the other end of the integration spectrum, full integration means that care in all settings is controlled or provided through a specific agency. In this regard, Yee Hong sits between the linkage and coordination levels of service integration. Within the organization, there is coordination and transition between services. With limited government support, Yee Hong is unable to ensure smooth transition to and from all external agencies. To confirm partial coordination of services, partnerships have been established with community agencies. However, the financial decision to use external services falls on the client and caregiver.

Yee Hong continues to develop services according to client needs, foregoing the medical model lens. A realistic challenge for the organization is that the government will not fund all of the services. Yee Hong has met this challenge by fundraising and developing productive enterprises. This has ensured Yee Hong's sustainability within a medically minded model. This chapter recommends a multilevel system change, where services are fully integrated into the region to ensure the highest quality of care. Yee Hong's role will be to advocate for better service continuity and to lead by example to show how an agency can coordinate seamless client transitions among services. The Ontario government must explore continuum of care models. This will require major changes to its existing healthcare model.

FUTURE RESEARCH DIRECTIONS

Current healthcare delivery systems will no longer meet the changing needs of the population, according to the World Health Organization (2015), which has presented a global strategy to move toward person-centred care and integrated health services. To ensure that health and long-term care services are sustainable for an aging population, governments must explore integrated care delivery to meet an individual's needs. It is pertinent that the model of service delivery is both financially feasible and promotes quality community care. The development of these health delivery systems must be context specific, as the needs of each government and population will differ.

Caregivers' wishes and needs must also be taken into consideration. When preferences for institutionalized care are compared, elder adults were less likely than caregivers to prefer institutionalization (Chau et al., 2010). Caregivers play an important role in supporting older adults in successful aging in the home (Williams et al., 2009). Therefore, future research must explore how caregiver needs can be met to ensure a seamless transition among services.

The ultimate goal would be a context-specific continuum of care model that will meet healthcare quality and financial objectives while improving client and caregiver satisfaction. The healthcare delivery system focus would require shifting the paradigm away from medical care and toward a person-centred and integrated system. Global well-being can no longer spotlight physical health. It must have a more holistic understanding of the changing needs of an aging population. Research into the models in paradigm changes from a medical model to a socially minded, client-based model may be effective in addressing the barriers governments will face, as shifting away from the medical model would require changes in multiple policy levels. The research will also require governments at different levels to be willing to commit to the successful remoulding of healthcare services.

CONCLUSION

The current Ontario model of service funding focuses on the medical needs of the population. The focus is aimed at reducing hospitalization and delaying institutionalization. As the major stakeholders of care address the lack of institutional and community-based resources available to the aging population, they have yet to fully recognize that moving away from the biomedical model will be a necessary step towards providing sufficient care. Yee Hong is thus advocating change in this process and believes there is a need to transition from this medical model, moving away from acute care toward a socially minded, person-centred model of integrated care delivery. The Yee Hong Centre for Geriatric Care, through its mission statement and service provision, highlights the importance of client-centred care. Client needs must be met in order to allow seniors to live at their optimal level of well-being. Despite the challenges of being a socially minded organization within a medically minded funding model, Yee Hong has developed a continuum of care model that is client focused. In its model, client, caregiver, and community needs are taken into consideration to improve program quality and service development.

Every service provider talks about client-centred care and claims to be client centred. However, to be a truly client-centred provider, it is necessary to design services according to clients' individual needs and not according to how and what part of the program is funded. Clients should not be expected to "fit" into the services that are made available through funding but should be part of the dialogue in developing services that meet their needs. Yee Hong has conducted two needs studies, one in the 1980s and the other in the 2010s, with ongoing communication with clients and caregivers to ensure that their needs are met. As a result, Yee Hong has tried to form service strategies according to the feedback, developed a continuum of care based on client needs, and made a commitment to these programs by bearing the cost of services not funded by the government.

REFERENCES

Béland, F., Bergman, H., Lebel, P., Clarfield, A. M., Tousignant, P., Contandriopoulos, A. P., & Dallaire, L. (2006a). A system of integrated care for older persons with disabilities in Canada: Results from a randomized controlled trial. *The Journals of Gerontology. Series A, Biological Sciences and Medical Sciences*, *61*(4), 367–373. doi:10.1093/gerona/61.4.367 PMID:16611703

Béland, F., Bergman, H., Lebel, P., Dallaire, L., Fletcher, J., Tousignant, P., & Contandriopoulos, A. P. (2006b). Integrated services for frail elders (SIPA): A trial of a model for Canada. *Canadian Journal on Aging*, *25*(1), 25–42. doi:10.1353/cja.2006.0019 PMID:16770746

Béland, F., & Hollander, M. J. (2011). Integrated models of care delivery for the frail elderly: International perspectives. *Gaceta Sanitaria, 25*, 138–146. doi:10.1016/j.gaceta.2011.09.003 PMID:22088903

Bergman, H., Béland, F., Lebel, P., Contandriopoulos, A. P., Tousignant, P., Brunelle, Y., & Clarfield, M. et al. (1997). Care for Canada's frail elderly population: Fragmentation or integration? *Canadian Medical Association Journal, 157*(8), 1116–1121. PMID:9347783

CARP. (2013). *One patient: CARP's care continuum.* Retrieved from http://www.carp.ca/wp-content/uploads/2013/12/One-Patient-Paper-Dec-2013.pdf

Centers for Medicare & Medicaid Services. (2011). *Programs of all-inclusive care for the elderly (PACE).* Retrieved from https://www.cms.gov/Regulations-and-Guidance/Guidance/Manuals/downloads/pace111c01.pdf

Chatterji, P., Burstein, N. R., Kidder, D., & White, A. (1998). *Evaluation of the program of all-inclusive care for the elderly demonstration. The Impact of PACE on participant outcomes.* Retrieved from https://www.cms.gov/Medicare/Demonstration-Projects/DemoProjectsEvalRpts/downloads/PACE_Outcomes.pdf

Chau, P. H., Kwok, T., Woo, J., Chan, F., Hui, E., & Chan, K. C. (2010). Disagreement in preference for residential care between family caregivers and elders is greater among cognitively impaired elders group than cognitively intact elders group. *International Journal of Geriatric Psychiatry, 25*(1), 46–54. PMID:19551703

Chinese Community Nursing Home for Greater Toronto. (1989). *Health care needs of the Chinese elderly population: A needs assessment.* Toronto, ON: Author.

Community Care Access Centre. (2014). *Home first.* Retrieved from http://healthcareathome.ca/central/en/Getting-care/Getting-Care-at-Home/home-first

Dunn, H. L. (1959). What high-level wellness means. *Canadian Journal of Public Health, 50*(11), 447–457. PMID:13818678

Evashwick, C. J. (1989). Creating a continuum. The goal is to provide an integrated system of care. *Health Progress (Saint Louis, Mo.), 70*(5), 36–39, 56. PMID:10293328

Gulliford, M., Naithani, S., & Morgan, M. (2006). What is continuity of care? *Journal of Health Services Research & Policy, 11*(4), 248–250. doi:10.1258/135581906778476490 PMID:17018200

Han, L., Cole, M., Bellavance, F., McCusker, J., & Primeau, F. (2000). Tracking cognitive decline in Alzheimers disease using the mini-mental state examination: A meta-analysis. *International Psychogeriatrics, 12*(2), 231–247. doi:10.1017/S1041610200006359 PMID:10937543

Hébert, R., Durand, P. J., Dubuc, N., & Tourigny, A. (2003). PRISMA: A new model of integrated service delivery for the frail older people in Canada. *International Journal of Integrated Care, 3*(1). Retrieved from http://www.ijic.org/articles/10.5334/ijic.73/ doi:10.5334/ijic.73 PMID:16896376

Hébert, R., Raîche, M., Dubois, M. F., NDeye, R. G., Dubuc, N., & Tousignant, M. (2009). Impact of PRISMA, a coordination-type integrated service delivery system for frail older people in Quebec (Canada): A quasi-experimental study. *The Journals of Gerontology. Series B, Psychological Sciences and Social Sciences*, *65B*(1), 107–118. doi:10.1093/geronb/gbp027 PMID:19414866

Hirth, V., Baskins, J., & Dever-Bumba, M. (2009). Program of all-inclusive care (PACE): Past, present, and future. *Journal of the American Medical Directors Association*, *10*(3), 155–160. doi:10.1016/j.jamda.2008.12.002 PMID:19233054

Kodner, D. L. (2006). Whole-system approaches to health and social care partnerships for the frail elderly: An exploration of North American models and lessons. *Health & Social Care in the Community*, *14*(5), 384–390. doi:10.1111/j.1365-2524.2006.00655.x PMID:16918830

Lai, D. W. (2000). Depression among the elderly Chinese in Canada. *Canadian Journal on Aging*, *19*(3), 409–429. doi:10.1017/S0714980800015063 PMID:10765589

Lee, H. C. B., Chiu, H. F., Kowk, W. Y., & Leung, C. M. (1993). Chinese elderly and the GDS short form: A preliminary study. *Clinical Gerontologist: The Journal of Aging and Mental Health*, *14*(2), 37–42.

Leutz, W. N. (1999). Five laws for integrating medical and social services: Lessons from the United States and the United Kingdom. *The Milbank Quarterly*, *77*(1), 77–110. doi:10.1111/1468-0009.00125 PMID:10197028

MacAdam, M. (2008). *Frameworks of integrated care for the elderly: A systematic review*. Toronto, ON: Canadian Policy Research Networks.

MacAdam, M. (2015). PRISMA: Program of research to integrate the services for the maintenance of autonomy. A system-level integration model in Quebec. *International Journal of Integrated Care*, *15*(6). doi:10.5334/ijic.2246 PMID:26417212

Mui, A. C. (2002). The program of all-inclusive care for the elderly (PACE): An innovative long-term care model in the United States. *Journal of Aging & Social Policy*, *13*(2–3), 53–67. doi:10.1300/J031v13n02_05 PMID:12216362

National PACE Association. (2016). *PACE services*. Retrieved from http://www.npaonline.org/pace-you/pace-services

Pinquart, M., & Sörensen, S. (2003). Differences between caregivers and noncaregivers in psychological health and physical health: A meta-analysis. *Psychology and Aging*, *18*(2), 250–267. doi:10.1037/0882-7974.18.2.250 PMID:12825775

PRISMA. (2016). *Overview*. Retrieved from http://www.prisma-qc.ca/cgi-cs/cs.waframe.content?topic=5796&lang=2

Spalding, K. L., Williams, A. P., & Watkins, J. R. (2006). *Self managed care programs in Canada: A report to Health Canada*. Retrieved from http://healthycanadians.gc.ca/publications/health-system-systeme-sante/2006-self-managed-soins-autogeres/index-eng.php#a1

St. John, P. D., Tyas, S. L., & Montgomery, P. R. (2013). Depressive symptoms and frailty. *International Journal of Geriatric Psychiatry*, *28*(6), 607–614. doi:10.1002/gps.3866 PMID:22961757

Stewart, M. J., Georgiou, A., & Westbrook, J. I. (2013). Successfully integrating aged care services: A review of the evidence and tools emerging from a long-term care program. *International Journal of Integrated Care, 13*(1), e003. doi:10.5334/ijic.963 PMID:23687475

Strategies & Skills Learning & Development. (2014). *Background.* Retrieved from http://ssld.kttsang.com/html/introduction/background.html

Taylor, G., & Hawley, H. (2010). *Health and society: Key debates in health care.* New York, NY: Open University Press.

Tsang, A. K. T. (2013). *Learning to change lives: The strategies and skills learning and development system.* Toronto, ON: University of Toronto Press.

Tsang, A. K. T., Choi, C., Liu, K. Y., Chu, M., Wong, C., & Fung, K. K. (2013). *The changing needs of Chinese seniors in the Greater Toronto area.* Toronto, ON: Yee Hong Centre for Geriatric Care.

Veras, R. P., Caldas, C. P., Motta, L. B. D., Lima, K. C. D., Siqueira, R. C., Rodrigues, R. T., & Guerra, A. C. et al. (2014). Integration and continuity of care in health care network models for frail older adults. *Revista de Saude Publica, 48*(2), 357–365. doi:10.1590/S0034-8910.2014048004941 PMID:24897058

Williams, A. P., Challis, D., Deber, R., Watkins, J., Kuluski, K., Lum, J. M., & Daub, S. (2009). Balancing institutional and community-based care: Why some older persons can age successfully at home while others require residential long-term care. *Healthcare Quarterly, 12*(2), 95–105. doi:10.12927/hcq.2009.3974 PMID:19369817

Williams, A. P., Lum, J., Morton-Chang, F., Kuluski, K., Peckham, A., Warrick, N., & Ying, A. (2016). *Integrating long-term care into a community-based continuum.* Montreal, QB: Institute for Research on Public Policy.

World Health Organization. (2015). *WHO global strategy on people-centred and integrated health services: Interim report.* Geneva, CH: Author.

Wyller, T. B., Holmen, J., Laake, P., & Laake, K. (1998). Correlates of subjective well-being in stroke patients. *Stroke, 29*(2), 363–367. doi:10.1161/01.STR.29.2.363 PMID:9472875

Yee Hong Centre for Geriatric Care. (2016). *Mission & vision.* Retrieved from http://www.yeehong.com/centre/mission.php

KEY TERMS AND DEFINITIONS

Biomedical Model: A model of health where illness and disease are presupposed; therefore, healthcare services emphasize diagnosis and medical treatment of the illness and its symptoms.

Client-Centred Care: An approach to health service provision that is focused on the individual's needs and wishes, where the client is an active participant in decision making.

Continuum of Care: A model of care provision that allows seamless transition for a client between different health and community care services.

Needs-Based Care: An approach to health service provision that is grounded in the individual's physical, emotional, mental, and social needs.

Service Integration: A model of service provision where acute, primary, and community care are systematically coordinated.

Strategies and Skills Learning and Development System (SSLD): An intervention model to enable individuals to address their needs.

Wellness Model: A model of health where the biopsychosocial aspects are taken into consideration; therefore, healthcare services encompass physical, emotional, and psychosocial care.

Chapter 5
United Kingdom Health Promotion Initiatives for Healthy Aging

Susan Dawkes
Edinburgh Napier University, UK

Simon T. Cheung
The Hong Kong Polytechnic University, Hong Kong

ABSTRACT

People are living longer but not, unfortunately, living longer healthy lives as there is an increasing number of years spent in ill-health from the age of 65 years onwards. Rates of chronic non-communicable diseases are increasing. This purpose of this chapter is to describe how modern healthcare aims to involve patients more in their care (so called self-management) to reduce the incidence of complications linked to chronic disease while attempting to promote healthy ageing. Support for patients' self-management is multifaceted but patients require support from healthcare professionals and this will be discussed as well as the educational requirements of the healthcare professionals who support those patients. How well nurses are prepared for giving patients health promotion advice will be described using an example of research from the United Kingdom. The chapter will conclude with an outline of how healthcare professionals are considered as role models for healthy living.

INTRODUCTION

Although one of the greatest achievements of the last century is that people are living longer, that has resulted in us now facing one of the greatest challenges in this century: a rapidly growing ageing population. The world population is rising and the fastest growing group is the over 60 years age group. It is predicted in the United Kingdom (UK) that between 2013 and 2039 the number of people aged 60 years and older will rise by 7 million to almost 22 million people and that will account for 70% of the whole UK population growth (Harper et al., 2016). While people are living longer they are not, unfortunately, living longer healthy lives as there is an increasing number of years spent in ill-health from the age of 65

DOI: 10.4018/978-1-5225-2633-9.ch005

years onwards in the UK (Harper et al., 2016). The rates of non-communicable diseases are increasing with chronic non-communicable diseases such as cardiovascular disease, cancer, respiratory disease and diabetes becoming a growing burden.

A recent cross-sectional study found that over 42% of Scots living in the United Kingdom had one or more co-morbidity with almost a quarter of those studied being classed as 'multi-morbid' (>2 co-morbidities) (Barnett et al., 2012). Around 70% of healthcare expenditure in the United Kingdom and Australia is spent on providing care for people with chronic non-communicable conditions and the elderly population account for a significant proportion of this (College of Medicine, 2013).

Scotland has much lower life expectancy rates than the rest of the UK with an average lifespan for men of 77.1 years and 81.1 years for females, but there is wide variation between the different areas of Scotland and between remote / rural and urban living (National Records for Scotland, 2015). Although life expectancy has been very slowly improving in Scotland, the rates remain significantly lower than the rest of the United Kingdom, and despite efforts to improve this, the gap between Scotland and the rest of the United Kingdom is in fact widening. The health of Scottish people when compared with others in Western European countries is poor. Life expectancy rates of males living in Scotland are low and are only surpassed by those of Portugal. Scottish females have the lowest life expectancy rate in Western Europe (Scottish Government, 2015).

Healthcare in Scotland, as in the rest of the United Kingdom through the National Health Service, is free at the point of use. This free healthcare system is available to all British citizens and yet life expectancy has remained relatively static for Scotland over the last decade with only slight improvement. Consequently, health care support for promoting population health has had to change and the effect of that has not yet been measured. The changes necessitated the need for healthcare professionals to be educated in effective methods of promoting and supporting healthy ageing.

This chapter will focus on two main themes; how people are supported to live healthily in their older years, and how healthcare professionals are educated and prepared to support that healthy ageing. Examples of how healthcare has changed over recent years to cope with the ageing population will be discussed with a focus on the changing landscape of the healthcare system in the UK as this aligns with much of the developed world. Additionally, how healthcare professionals are educated to be more effective in their health promotion will be highlighted with specific focus on how this happens in the UK and North America and the effectiveness of this education / preparation will be highlighted using an example from a UK study. Role modeling of health promoting behaviours by healthcare professionals can also impact on people's likelihood to adopt more healthy behaviours as they age and this will be mentioned in the latter part of the chapter.

CHANGES TO HEALTHCARE SUPPORT FOR HEALTHY AGEING

Care of patients with acute diseases was the focus of the majority of healthcare providers in Scotland but a shift around the 1950s was necessary to concentrate more on the promotion of health and the management of increasingly prevalent chronic conditions, particularly in the elderly population (Holman & Lorig, 2004). This was not unique to Scotland as many other countries also reformed health care services to enhance effectiveness. Modern healthcare aims to involve patients more in their care to reduce the incidence of complications linked to chronic disease and the number of readmissions to hospital, while also attempting to improve patients' health, quality of life and well-being (Mead et al.,

2010; Munir et al., 2009). It was necessary, therefore, for healthcare to move away from the paternalistic style of care, where patients were relatively passive recipients of care provided by healthcare experts, to a more shared responsibility model, wherein patients are central to the approach but are supported by healthcare practitioners to together, strive for the best possible outcomes (Du and Yuan, 2010; Self Management UK, 2013). So called self-management.

Self-Management

Self-management (or self-care as it is often termed) is what individuals do for themselves to maintain or enhance their health and wellbeing, to preserve their physical function and to prevent further illness (Conn, 2011). Its aim is for the person to be able to live independently with a good quality of life and have positive, healthy ageing (Holman and Lorig, 2000). Healthcare providers should support and educate patients to enable them to solve any problems they have, make decisions regarding their lifestyle choices and disease management and take appropriate action if or where required (Clark et al., 2010; Gibson et al., 2009; Self-Management UK, 2013).

The ability of the person to engage in self-management improves their chronic disease management. While some research has found self-management to be effective (Gibson et al., 2009; Lau-Walker and Thompson, 2009; Ricci-Cabello et al., 2014), other studies have had more ambiguous findings (Jonsdottir, 2013; Khunti et al., 2012; Oliveira et al., 2012) but the reasons for that are not known. Ultimately, the responsibility for self-management of chronic conditions and modification of lifestyle factors to prevent or minimize disease progression lies with patients or individuals. It is known though that about 90% of the time, patients manage their chronic conditions alone with little in the way of support and education from healthcare providers (The Heath Foundation, 2011).

Healthcare Support for Self-Management

It has been documented that when patients are not supported in their chronic disease self-management, they have difficulty in modifying unhealthy behaviours or risk factors. The study from Chow et al. (2010) illustrates this phenomenon as they found that where support and advice was given initially after an acute coronary syndrome, any behaviour change made by patients in the first four weeks was not sustained beyond six months. Even where some support is given, issues arise in relation to the provision of ongoing assistance to patients for behaviour change. Cole et al. (2013) found that general practitioners stopped giving patients support when their health promotion advice had not been acted on. Newer technologies, such as telehealth, may be beneficial in that they can be accessible to patients who would not normally join rehabilitation programs or seek support from community care healthcare providers but evidence suggests that this type of support may not be valued or used effectively by patients and resultantly, behaviour change and risk factor reduction is often not attempted or not maintained beyond just a few weeks (Dalleck, Schmidt and Lueker, 2011; Kerr et al., 2010). This is unfortunate given that lifestyle factors can be extremely challenging to modify.

As indicated in the chapter providing information on the eating habits of students in Hong Kong, behaviours often originate in childhood or adolescence and the long-standing nature of them, coupled with potential pressure from the patients' social environment, hinder their modification (Joint Task Force of the European Society of Cardiology and Other Societies on Cardiovascular Disease Prevention in Clinical Practice, 2012). It seems that despite clinical guidelines advocating that patients are supported in their chronic disease self-management, ongoing assistance from healthcare professionals is not given, newer methods of providing support may not be valued by patients, particularly the elderly, and the result is that any initial gains in lifestyle modification are not sustained. Patients consequently, are left to self-manage alone and evidence shows that this may not be effective (Department of Health, Social Services and Public Safety, 2011). The notion of a shared responsibility model where patients are supported by healthcare professionals to, together, effectively self-manage their chronic condition is not apparent. Resultantly, poor self-management is common (Conn, 2011) and this can be evidenced through greater use of unscheduled care services and failure to meet outcomes associated with health (Purdy, 2010).

Support for patients' self-management is multifaceted but patients require support from healthcare professionals to alter lifestyles for healthy ageing as well as manage their long-term condition. Clinical guidelines have been published that recommend patients are supported by healthcare professionals and given information about topics related to their long-term condition, how to manage any symptoms they may have, as well as the benefits and purpose of any pharmacological treatment they receive (National Institute for Health and Care Excellence (NICE), 2011). For the majority of patients modifying lifestyle factors or behaviours known to contribute to ill health it is often advisable to reduce their risk of disease progression and enhance their health for older age. The clinical guidelines were informed by findings from randomized controlled trials that provided strong evidence that supporting and giving information and health promotion advice to the elderly and those with chronic diseases results in a reduction in unhealthy behaviours and improves their quality of life but the support needs to be structured and ongoing (Murchie et al., 2003).

In light of the evidence, some healthcare providers in the United Kingdom established Managed Clinical Networks in an attempt to integrate services more to improve the care and support for all patients with chronic conditions (Hamilton et al., 2005). Also General Practitioners were incentivized in the United Kingdom to identify elderly patients and those who had chronic conditions and support them more in their self-management (Vidal-Alaball, 2011). Despite these initiatives, however, it was found that support from healthcare professionals was still lacking (Buckley, Byrne and Smith, 2010) and this was not unique to the United Kingdom (Batic-Mujanovic, Zildzic and Beganlic, 2006).

Rehabilitation Support for Self-Management

Support may also be provided through comprehensive rehabilitation where patients receive help with lifestyle modification (NICE, 2013; British Association for Cardiovascular Prevention and Rehabilitation, 2012). Globally though, rehabilitation programs are often under resourced and, consequently, struggle to meet the needs of the patients. Despite being of proven benefit to patients, attendance at such programs is known to be poor (Zetta et al., 2011). The lack of resourcing, combined with the number of patients with chronic conditions who should be rehabilitated, leads to significant waiting times and so many patients often miss out on that support and are subsequently left to manage their condition and adopt more healthy behaviours alone. To meet patient needs and ensure the optimal support for patients to enhance their health through lifestyle modification it is essential that healthcare professionals are adequately knowledgeable and skilled. The preparation of these healthcare professionals is key and that should begin in the undergraduate educational programmes that these professionals undertake. There is however, a need for continuing professional education to ensure professionals remain up-to-date with current practices and guidelines related to supporting patients' adoption of healthier lifestyles and self-managing long-term conditions or non-communicable diseases.

EDUCATIONAL PREPARATION OF NURSES AND DOCTORS

Globally, professional governing bodies for nursing, medicine and other healthcare professionals set out the minimum standards that practitioners should achieve prior to their entry on to professional registers. These standards often give specific information regarding what healthcare professionals should be taught in relation to promoting health and supporting people with healthy ageing.

Educating Nurses to Support Healthy Ageing

Within the United Kingdom, the Nursing and Midwifery Council (2010) state in the standards that they set out for the preparation and education of pre-registration nurse education that nurses should take every opportunity available to them to promote healthy ageing to their patients. They indicate that nurses along with all other health care professionals require an understanding of health, causes of ill-health, the social determinants of health and causes of health inequalities in order to be adequately prepared to meet the health promotion needs of patients and fulfill their social responsibility to contribute to the health of the public. These standards ensure that every higher education institution that provides a nursing degree program in the United Kingdom incorporates all of these factors so that nurses, at the point of registration, have adequate knowledge and skills to support patients and enhance their health as they age. The Nursing and Midwifery Council goes no further than to stipulate the requirements for pre-registration nurses and so continuing professional development and the necessity to keep abreast of changes to the most effective approaches to promoting health and healthy ageing lies with the individual registered nurse. Resultantly, practices can vary in approach and success.

Guidance and standards from other countries is also helpful in informing the content of higher education programs used to prepare healthcare professionals. The standards set out for baccalaureate education for professional nursing practice from United States of America have a greater degree of specificity regarding what is expected of registered nurses during the completion of their program of study for professional registration. There is an expectation that nurses will have an awareness of health and its determinants but they must also be able to assess factors that contribute to or influence health such as the health or illness beliefs individuals have as well as determine their values and attitudes to health. Nurses must develop knowledge and skills of behavior change theories and techniques so that they can effectively assist individuals or patients in optimizing health. There is a strong indication from the guidance from the United States of America that nurses cannot be the sole provider of health promotion for patients or individuals but rather it should be a multi-disciplinary approach with each professional discipline contributing to the health of patients or individuals as well as their families, communities and populations. Although the detail of the minimum standards for nurse education is helpful in informing higher education providers of nursing programs, information about post-registration expectations is lacking.

As result of the proliferation of nursing programs in Canada, the Canadian Association of Schools of Nursing (2015) have helpfully set out a framework detailing not only what expectations of the nurses at the point of entry to the professional register would be in relation to promoting health and healthy ageing but also the standards for nurses being educated to Master's and doctoral level. This document is far reaching as it demonstrates the progression that is expected as nurses progress through their careers. Many of the same principles for educating student nurses about health promotion should be encompassed in the baccalaureate programs in Canada but there is also a requirement that the students would gain from the program a self-awareness of how their personal beliefs, attitudes and values could influence the health promotion advice they give to their patients.

These standards also provide guidance that general (or Adult) nurses should always advocate the notion of self-management to patients with long-term conditions and seek to educate the patients about how they can enhance their health and how best to approach lifestyle modification. This obviously relies on the nurses having that knowledge themselves and having the desire to foster a patient-centered approach to chronic disease management rather than adopt a more paternalistic approach.

Educating Doctors to Support Healthy Ageing

The General Medical Council (GMC) of the United Kingdom (GMC, 2015) expect more from the students studying medicine in that in addition to the expectations stated previously, medical students would be expected to have an awareness of the global factors that determine health and how diversity affects health as well as understand health risks and the principles of health and health economics. The standards also indicate that medical students need to develop specific knowledge and skills. For example, they require knowledge of how nutrition contributes to health and need to be able to apply that knowledge to their medical practice and have effective communication skills to allow them to raise health promotion issues with their patients and discuss it competently. Again, there is scant guidance on continuing professional development in relation to health promotion after registration with the medical governing body and so there is also a risk of varied and ineffective medical practices that may be sub-optimal in supporting patients in living and ageing healthily. Worryingly, research from Peckham, Hann and Boyce (2011) found that the majority of General Practitioners in the United Kingdom do not feel equipped with the necessary skills to discuss lifestyle modification and health ageing with their patients and so some doctors may not be keeping up to date with health promotion advice and effective approaches.

Although this is not an exhaustive list of standards set by professional governing bodies, it provides a notion that minimum standards should be relatively comparable across the developed world. Scott (2011) however, found that the translation of theory to healthcare practice was problematic. The ability to form collaborative partnerships with patients is poor and the notion that healthcare professionals are no longer the 'expert' but people who will work with patients and individuals to enhance healthy ageing seems difficult for some to comprehend and act upon.

SUCCESS OF HEALTH PROMOTION PREPARATION

A cross sectional, mixed methods study by Dawkes (2016, unpublished) aimed to explore registered nurses' experiences of giving health promotion advice to their patients. The four research questions for the study were:

1. What experience do registered nurses have in giving health promotion advice to patients / clients?
2. What approach to giving health promotion advice is used by the registered nurses?
3. How effective do the registered nurses perceive they are in giving health promotion advice?
4. How well prepared do the registered nurses think they are for giving their patients / clients health promotion advice?

Study Design and Methods

The study used a convergent parallel, mixed methods design and data were collected by two methods; a self-administered survey and a focus group. The survey tool was examined for face and content validity by experienced researchers prior to use with the study sample and was piloted with a small number of nurses to check for face validity and reliability. The sample was drawn from registered nurses studying a post-graduate nursing program. Participants for the focus groups (n=15) were taken from the original sample who completed the survey. As the study used a convergent parallel, mixed methods design, the quantitative and qualitative data were analyzed separately and then the findings brought together to gain a better understanding of the registered nurses' experience of giving health promotion advice.

Study Findings

The study recruited a convenience sample of sixty-four registered nurses from a possible 157 potential participants who met the inclusion criteria (enrolment on nursing program, ability to speak / read English, ability to provide written consent to participate). This gives a response rate of 41% which is reasonable. Just over two-thirds of the sample held a nursing diploma (n=46) and a quarter had been trained to advanced or specialist practitioner level. Over half the sample (n=38) were within four years of having trained and registered as a nurse and around 12% (n=8) had been registered for twenty years or more. The majority worked in government funded hospitals and were involved in the care of patients with a multitude of long-term conditions. Over half the sample (n=36) gave health promotion advice to patients every day or on a frequent basis. The vast majority of these nurses 84% (n=54) responded that they were confident in giving health promotion advice to the patients they encountered in their professional lives but fewer 69% (n=44) regarded the task of giving health promotion advice to patients as easy. Despite this 92% (n=56) were confident that they were adequately well prepared and knowledgeable to give effective health promotion advice. When asked though how many patients were likely to take their advice and modify unhealthy behaviours, 72% (n=46) participants perceived their advice to be successful in fostering behavior change. Although confidence levels were high among participants, all provided suggestions about what would help them give 'better' advice and this included more training in effective health promotion / behavior change techniques, contemporary literature that could be used as reference material and support from multidisciplinary colleagues.

Focus groups provided some greater understanding of the nurses' practices in giving health promotion advice. Many chose to resort to telling the patients what they should and should not do from a lifestyle behaviour perspective, despite having knowledge that this approach is rarely successful in fostering change. A theme that recurred was that the nurses 'blamed' the patients for not changing their behaviors, citing stubbornness, resistance to change and misunderstanding of what healthy living entailed. This seemed particularly problematic in older patients who were regarded 'difficult' and older age was considered a barrier to changing lifestyle. The participants seemed to have little awareness of how they could support and encourage their patients to maker lifestyle changes and appeared to have little comprehension that not all patients are at a stage where they are contemplating or in fact changing lifestyle factors.

Conclusion from the Study

The conclusions that can be drawn from the findings are therefore, that although registered nurses perceive themselves to be knowledgeable and skilled in giving health promotion advice, they lack awareness of how much their advice is likely to bring about lifestyle modification in patients and older individuals. Although giving health promotion advice was regarded as easy and participants had great confidence in providing it, the patients were blamed for not taking heed of that advice and being resistant to change rather than reflective on the approach used by the nurse. Although the conclusions from this study need to be viewed with caution given the limitations of the sampling method, they do provide some evidence that there may be a mismatch between the perceived success of health promotion advice by registered nurses and the reality. Further research would be required to support or refute this. With this and the previous discussion regarding standards in education and the difficulty healthcare professionals have in translating theory to practice in mind, new methods of preparing healthcare professionals to give health promotion advice and support to patients are required and further research is needed to determine the most effective pedagogical approach to achieve this.

ROLE MODELING

In addition to healthcare professionals having difficulty putting health promotion theory into practice, they are notoriously bad at having healthy lifestyles themselves and that echoes the Hong Kong perspective of university students highlighted earlier. Some professional governing bodies have stipulated in their standard statements related to the education that the professionals should act as role models in relation to lifestyle behaviours and one example of this comes from the Nursing and Midwifery Council in the United Kingdom. Underwood (1998) have suggested that role-modeling does play a role in healthy lifestyle practices that can allow nurses to be potentially more effective in health promoting interventions. This position statement is not unique to that particular country. Often healthcare professionals have a good understanding of what behaviours would enhance their health but all too many studies have found that the health of these professionals is often poor and subsequently, their example should not be advocated for patients.

One cross sectional study conducted by Dawkes (2016, unpublished) found that not one registered nurse of a group of 350 took the recommended amount of physical activity in one week. Although this study used a convenience sample of registered nurses attending classes for a program of educational study and the results are not generalizable, there is an indication that the health of the professionals who would be providing health promotion advice to patients to promote healthy ageing is sub-optimal due to their own lifestyle choices. This poses a potential risk that these professionals will not promote behaviours to patients and the public that they do not engage in themselves. The success of positive role modeling is therefore questionable. Role-modeling healthy lifestyles can be a challenge especially for nurses with stressful job duties although nursing is not a sedentary occupation. Nurses are not immune to unhealthy habits such as smoking, drinking, eating on the run, or skipping a regular exercise routine with only limited free time during the day. As Jackson et al. (1999) suggested that role-modeling by nurses is a choice, it is a challenge for nurses to do this. People learn from others not only through what they say but also by their actions. Knowledge of lifelong patterns of health promotion is the foundation of self-management, and nurses and other healthcare professionals play an important part as a role models and this would further serve to enhance their professional credibility while encouraging people to adopt healthy behaviours as they age (Borhcardt, 2000).

CONCLUSION

In this chapter, two main themes have been discussed. Firstly, how people are supported by healthcare professionals to adopt more healthy behaviours and self-manage their non-communicable, chronic diseases effectively was discussed with mention of the changes in modern healthcare to reflect the central role that the patient now has in looking after him / herself. Secondly, the role higher education institutions have in preparing healthcare professionals to promote healthy ageing and support people in doing this was outlined in relation to pedagogical content of educational programs. How effective such programs are in educating nurses to promote health and healthy ageing was discussed drawing an example from a study conducted in the UK. Also, healthcare professionals as role models and the importance of this on promoting health was summarized.

While this chapter has had somewhat of a focus on the UK, the alignment to the rest of the developed world is clear as similar challenges are faces by many countries. This chapter serves to provide an insight into how healthcare and healthcare education have had to change to cope with an ageing population so that not only people live longer but that they are also encouraged and supported to age healthily.

REFERENCES

American Association of Colleges of Nursing. (2008). *The Essentials of Baccalaureate Education for Professional Nursing Practice*. Washington, DC: American Association of Colleges of Nursing.

Barnett, K., Mercer, S., Norbury, M., Watt, G., Wyke, S., & Guthrie, B. (2012). Epidemiology of multimorbidity and implications for health care, research, and medical education: A cross-sectional study. *Lancet*, *380*, 37–43.

Batic-Mujanovic, O., Zildzic, M., & Beganlic, A. (2006). Secondary prevention of heart disease in primary health care. *Bosnian Journal of Basic Medical Sciences*, *6*(2), 37–41. PMID:16879111

Borchardt, G. (2000). Role Models for Health Promotion: The Challenge for Nurses. *Nursing Forum*, *35*(3), 29–32. doi:10.1111/j.1744-6198.2000.tb01002.x

Buckley, B., Byrne, M., & Smith, S. (2010). *Service organization for the secondary prevention of ischaemic heart disease in primary care.* Retrieved from: http://onlinelibrary.wiley.com/doi/10.1002/14651858.CD006772.pub2/full on 24.07.16

Canadian Association of Schools of Nursing. (2015). *National Nursing Education Framework*. Retrieved from: http://www.casn.ca/wp-content/uploads/2014/12/Framwork-FINAL-SB-Nov-30-20151.pdf

Clark, A., Davidson, P., Currie, K., Karimi, M., Duncan, A., & Thompson, D. (2010). Understanding and promoting self-care during heart failure. *Current Treatment Options in Cardiovascular Medicine*, *12*(1), 1–9. doi:10.1007/s11936-009-0053-1 PMID:20842477

Cole, J., Smith, S., Hart, N., & Cupples, M. (2013). Do practitioners and friends support patients with coronary heart disease in lifestyle change? *BMC Family Practice*, *14*(1), 126. doi:10.1186/1471-2296-14-126 PMID:23984815

College of Medicine. (2013). *The crisis in costs.* Retrieved from: http://www.collegeofmedicine.org.uk/crisis-costs

Conn, V. (2011). Helping patients help themselves: Chronic disease self-management interventions. *Western Journal of Nursing Research*, *33*(2), 159–160. doi:10.1177/0193945910386194 PMID:21252383

Dalleck, L., Schmidt, L., & Lueker, R. (2011). Cardiac rehabilitation outcomes in a conventional versus telemedicine-based programme. *Journal of Telemedicine in Healthcare*, *17*(5), 217–221. doi:10.1258/jtt.2010.100407 PMID:21508077

Du, S., & Yuan, C. (2010). Evaluations of patient self-management outcomes in healthcare: A systematic review. *International Nursing Review*, *57*(2), 159–167. doi:10.1111/j.1466-7657.2009.00794.x PMID:20579149

General Medical Council. (2015). *Outcomes for Graduates (Tomorrow's Doctors).* Manchester, UK: GMC.

Gibson, P., Powell, H., Wilson, A., Abramson, M., Haywood, P., Bauman, A., . . . Roberts, J. (2009). *Self-management education and regular practitioner review for adults with asthma.* Retrieved from: http://onlinelibrary.wiley.com/doi/10.1002/14651858.CD001117/pdf

Government Office for Science, UK Government. (2016). *Future of an ageing population.* Retrieved from: https://www.gov.uk/government/uploads/system/uploads/attachment_data/file/535187/gs-16-10-future-of-an-ageing-population.pdf

Hamilton, K., Sullivan, F., Donnan, P., Taylor, R., Ikenwilo, D., Scott, A., & Wyke, S. et al. (2005). A managed clinical network for cardiac services: Set-up, operation and impact on patient care. *International Journal of Integrated Care*, *5*(3), 1–13. doi:10.5334/ijic.135 PMID:16773161

Holman, H., & Lorig, K. (2000). Patients as partners in managing chronic disease. *British Medical Journal*, *320*(7234), 526–527. doi:10.1136/bmj.320.7234.526 PMID:10688539

Holman, H., & Lorig, K. (2004). Patient self-management: A key to effectiveness and efficiency in care of chronic disease. *Public Health Records*, *119*, 239–243. PMID:15158102

Jackson, B. S., Smith, S. P., Adams, R., Frank, B., & Mateo, M. A. (1999). Healthy life styles are a challenge for nurses. *Image*, *31*, 196.

Joint Task Force of the European Society of Cardiology and Other Societies on Cardiovascular Disease Prevention in Clinical Practice. (2012). European guidelines on cardiovascular disease prevention in clinical practice. *European Heart Journal*, *33*, 1635–1701. PMID:22555213

Jonsdottir, H. (2013). Self-management programmes for people living with chronic obstructive pulmonary disease. *Journal of Clinical Nursing*, *22*(5-6), 621–637. doi:10.1111/jocn.12100 PMID:23398312

Kerr, C., Murray, E., Noble, L., Morris, R., Bottomley, C., Stevenson, F., & Nazareth, I. et al. (2010). The potential of web-based interventions for heart disease self-management: A mixed methods investigation. *Journal of Medical Internet Research*, *12*(4), 56. doi:10.2196/jmir.1438 PMID:21156471

Khunti, K., Gray, L., Skinner, T., Carey, M., Realf, K., Dallosso, H., & Davies, M. et al. (2012). Effectiveness of a diabetes education and self-management programme (DESMOND) for people with newly diagnosed type 2 diabetes mellitus. *British Medical Journal*, *344*(apr26 2), 2333. doi:10.1136/bmj.e2333 PMID:22539172

Lau-Walker, M., & Thompson, D. (2009). Self-management in long-term health conditions. *Patient Education and Counseling*, *75*(2), 290–292. doi:10.1016/j.pec.2009.02.001 PMID:19272746

Long, V., Cates, S., Blitstein, J., Deehy, K., Williams, P., Morgan, R., & Hersey, J. (2013). *Supplemental Nutrition Assistance Program Education and Evaluation Study (Wave II)*. Ann Arbor, MI: Altarum Institute.

Mead, H., Andres, E., Ramos, C., Siegel, B., & Regenstein, M. (2010). Barriers to effective self-management in cardiac patients. *Patient Education and Counseling*, *79*(1), 69–76. doi:10.1016/j.pec.2009.08.003 PMID:19748205

Munir, F., Khan, H., Yarker, J., Haslam, C., Long, H., Bains, M., & Kalawsky, K. (2009). Self-management of health behaviours among older and younger workers with chronic illness. *Patient Education and Counseling*, *77*(1), 109–115. doi:10.1016/j.pec.2009.02.014 PMID:19356885

Murchie, P., Campbell, N., Ritchie, L., Simpson, J., & Thain, J. (2003). secondary prevention clinics for coronary heart disease: Four year follow up of a randomised controlled trial in primary care. *British Medical Journal*, *326*(7380), 84–87. doi:10.1136/bmj.326.7380.84 PMID:12521974

National Institute for Health and Care Excellence. (2011). *Management of stable angina*. Retrieved from: http://www.nice.org.uk/guidance/cg126/chapter/1-recommendations#information-and-support-for-people-with-stable-angina

National Institute for Health and Care Excellence. (2013). *Cardiac rehabilitation services*. Retrieved from: http://publications.nice.org.uk/cardiac-rehabilitation-services-cmg40/43-delivery-of-programme on 26.07.16

National Records of Scotland. (2015). *Life expectancy for areas within Scotland*. Retrieved from http://www.nrscotland.gov.uk/files//statistics/life-expectancy-areas-in-scotland/12-14/life-exp-in-scotland-2012-to-2014.pdf

Nursing and Midwifery Council. (2010). *Standards for Pre-Registration Nursing Education*. London: Nursing and Midwifery Council.

Oliveira, V., Ferreira, P., Maher, C., Pinto, R., Refshauge, K., & Ferreira, M. (2012). Effectiveness of self-management of low back pain. *Arthritis Care and Research*, *64*(11), 1739–1748. doi:10.1002/acr.21737 PMID:22623349

Peckham, S., Hann, A., & Boyce, T. (2011). Health promotion and ill-health prevention: The role of general practice. *Quality in Primary Care, 19*, 317–323. PMID:22186174

Purdy, S. (2010). Avoiding hospital admissions: what does the research evidence say? London: The King's Fund. Retrieved from https://www.kingsfund.org.uk/sites/files/kf/Avoiding-Hospital-Admissions-Sarah-Purdy-December2010.pdf

Ricci-Cabello, I., Ruiz-Perez, I., Rojas-Garcia, A., Pastor, G., Rodriguez-Barranco, M., & Goncalves, D. (2014). *Characteristics and effectiveness of diabetes self-management educational programmes targeted to racial / ethnic minority groups.* Retrieved from: http://www.biomedcentral.com/content/pdf/1472-6823-14-60.pdf

Scott, S. (2011). A tripartite learning partnership in health promotion. *Nursing Praxis in New Zealand Inc, 27*(2), 16–23. PMID:21957557

Scottish Government. (2015). *Long-term monitoring of health inequalities*. Retrieved from http://www.gov.scot/Publications/2015/10/6061

UK Self-Management. (2013). *What is self-management?* Retrieved from: http://www.selfmanagementuk.org/what-is-self-management

Vidal-Alaball, J. (2011). *Health services evaluation*. Academic Press.

Zetta, S., Smith, K., Jones, M., Allcoat, P., & Sullivan, F. (2011). Evaluating the Angina Plan in patients admitted to hospital with angina. [PubMed]. *Cardiovascular Therapeutics, 29*, 112–124.

Chapter 6
Public-Private Partnership in Health and Long-Term Care: The Hong Kong Experience

Wing Tung Ho
The Chinese University of Hong Kong, Hong Kong

Ben Yuk Fai Fong
The Hong Kong Polytechnic University, Hong Kong

ABSTRACT

An exponential growth in elderly population reflects a proportional increase in recourses that are unaffordable and unsustainable to the economy. This rapid demand for health services and long-term care not only leads to non-financial implication like shortage of manpower and long waiting time, but this also creates a large burden on health and related services in the public sector. Involving the private sector to provide better and more efficient facilities and services and to encourage innovation will enhance productivity, speed up project and service delivery, and increase opportunities for investment in health. This chapter examines existing problems within health care systems in aging populations such as Hong Kong, explores the advantages and challenges of Public Private Partnership (PPP), identifies successful factors in establishing PPPs models, reviews the PPP projects in Hong Kong and elsewhere and recommends methods in promoting PPP in health and long-term care as sustainable solutions.

INTRODUCTION

An exponential growth in elderly population reflects a proportional increase in recourses that are potentially unaffordable and unsustainable to the economy. This rapid demand for health services and long-term care not only leads to non-financial implication like shortage of manpower and long waiting time for services, but this also creates a large burden on health and related services in the public sector. Compared to around thirty years ago, most diseases of the aged are not acute nowadays, but rather, most of them are chronic, and thus demanding long-term care. The cost of treating chronic diseases is much

DOI: 10.4018/978-1-5225-2633-9.ch006

greater than acute diseases because of the non-episodic nature. Elderlies suffering from chronic diseases have to bear expensive medicines and treatment to stay alive and to prolong their life (Yuen, 2014).

Involving the private sector to provide better and more efficient facilities and services and to encourage innovation will enhance productivity, speed up project and service delivery, and increase opportunities for investment in health. Merits of such collaboration in the form of public private partnership (PPP) include utilizing the skills and experience, access to technology, and innovation of the private sector for better delivery of public services and enhancing unity of responsibilities for delivering services. Potential problems of PPP are unreliable levels of service and greater secrecy and lack of transparency resulting in benefits not being shared with the public agency (Lee, 2005).

The objectives of the chapter are (i) to examine existing problems within health care systems in aging populations such as Hong Kong, (ii) to explore the advantages and challenges of PPP, (iii) to identify successful factors in establishing PPPs models, (v) to reviewing the PPP projects in Hong Kong and elsewhere, (vi) to recommend methods in promoting PPP in health and long-term care.

BACKGROUND

Private Sector Involvement (PSI) is a strategy to involve the private sector in delivering infrastructure projects and services so as to improve public services. Government departments are encouraged to make good use of private sector resources if there is a chance to uphold the economic and fiscal objectives of maintaining an efficient government, promote employment opportunities, and involve the private organizations in civil services. There are two types of PSI, including outsourcing and public-private partnership (Efficiency Unit, 2015).

In PPP, the public and private sector join forces to provide public facilities or services. In this setting, both sectors are expected to contribute their resources and expertise to the project and share the risks involved. Nevertheless, the definition of PPP may defer in different objectives of projects. It depends on which part of the important arrangement is focused on. For instance, PPP can be defined as any agreement where both public and private sectors bring their skills to a project, with a high level of responsibility and involvement, and aim in providing public services or projects (Chan & Cheung, 2014).

In 2008, PPPs in healthcare was proposed by the Hong Kong Government as an agenda of, and a significant step in, the healthcare reform in Hong Kong. This proposal aims to provide more healthcare service choices to the individuals, to boost healthy competition within the private sector, to achieve better allocation of resources through the collaboration between the public and private sectors, as well as to facilitate cross-fertilization of healthcare expertise, and to benchmark the cost-effectiveness and efficiency of healthcare services. This proposal has gained a broad support from the community (Legislative Council, 2015b).

Public Private Partnership in healthcare is expected to redress the imbalance between the public and private sectors with the objectives of improvement in the quality of care, better use of the resources, enhanced training and sharing of experience and expertise, and ultimately helping to ensure the sustainability of the health care system. These aims will be achieved through savings, enhanced cost-effectiveness, optimal use of human resources, cross-fertilization of expertise and experience, and promotion of healthy competition and collaboration. In primary care, services are purchased from the private sector, allowing greater choice of services for individuals in the community. In secondary and tertiary care, again services are purchased from the private sector, and private doctors are employed on a part-time basis in public hospitals, particularly in tertiary and specialized services. There are also potentials in the development of hospital facilities and medical centers of excellence.

Although the current pilot PPP projects in Hong Kong have already benefited a number of patients, there are still rooms for the health care system to develop PPP more widely and effectively. As most of the patients accessing health services in the public sectors come from relatively low income group, it appears essential to reform the legal framework for PPP models in focusing on the needs of the low income groups and in facilitating them to access the health service under PPP.

PROBLEMS WITHIN THE HEALTH CARE SYSTEM WITH AN AGING POPULATION IN HONG KONG

There are currently around 1.12 million people aged 65 years or above in Hong Kong, about one sixth of the total population. It is estimated that this proportion will be rising to 30% in 2034, and further to 35.9% in 2064. The aging population may probably be resulting from the persistent improvement of life expectancy and low birth rate (Legislative Council, 2015a). Increasing number of aging population places a huge burden on the Hong Kong health care system. Yuen (2014) has found that the aged people are more susceptible to sickness and their hospitalized cases have been increasing at a much faster rate than that of the overall population. Hospitalization rate of the elderly is four times more than those aged below 65, and the ratio grows proportionally as the age increases. According to the Hong Kong Census and Statistic Department (2009b), 70.4% of the elderly population are suffering from chronic diseases and 41.1% of them have consulted a doctor in the previous month.

It has been shown that the government expenditure (37%) on improving the provision of healthcare service has more than five times outpaced the population growth (7%). Nevertheless, there is no significant improvement in the quality of the public hospital services like the long waiting time at Specialist Outpatient Clinic, shortage of healthcare workers and insufficient hospital beds. In order to quantify the challenge of aging, the Hong Kong Hospital Authority (HA) has estimated that an additional 8,800 hospital beds are needed to add in the public sector so as to fulfill the demand for and provision of the public health services in the next 20 years (Yuen, 2014). To cope with the needs of the increasing aging population, it becomes more important in developing a sustainable health care system. Thus, more and more resources will be needed in finding out the weaknesses in the existing system and solving the problems in a long-run measure (Lam, 2011).

Cost

Similar to other countries, Hong Kong has been making several reforms to the healthcare financing system to ensure its long-term sustainability in the past few decades. The "Towards Better Health" document in 1993 recommended increasing fees for public healthcare services. The "Harvard Report" in 1999 suggested the introduction of social health insurance, and the "Lifelong investment in Health" consultation document in 2000 raised the possibility of mandatory medical saving accounts (Ko, 2014; Yuen, 2014). However, The Food and Health Bureau (2008) projection has indicated that if the current health care system remains unchanged until 2033, by taking into account to both demographic changes and rising medical costs, the total health expenditures are expected to increase at an average annual rate 59% faster than the real GDP growth. This rise in the health expenditures would make the health care system, which is still predominantly funded by the Government through taxation, difficult to ensure its long run sustainability (Ko, 2014). These rapidly increasing needs of the healthcare services will also increase the share of public health expenditures and the financial burden on the future generations. By 2033, it has been estimated that the public health expenditures as a share of GDP and total public expenditures will be increased by 2.6% and 12.6% respectively, and will be increased by 148.8 billion and 16.7 thousand in terms of real dollars and per capita respectively. On the other hand, the proportion of working population will continually to decrease if the aging population persistently increase. This will lead to a decrease in the tax base, thus posing a great burden on the working population to support the government revenue through taxation (The Food and Health Bureau, 2008).

Manpower

Not only will there be a burden on public finance, but there are also other non-financial implications. A rapid rise in the demand of health services due to the progressive aging population will lead to a shortage of healthcare workers and qualified health professionals in Hong Kong, for example, general practitioners, nurses and healthcare assistants. This manpower shortage is probably not due to insufficient government funding in general. There has been a low intake of medical students by the two medical schools in Hong Kong all the years. Although the number of intake has already increased from 250 to 320 in 2009/10 and further to 420 in 2012/13, it needs 6 years to train a doctors and 13 years to qualify a specialist. Thus, as there was a reduction of the number of medical students due to economic downturn in 2003 to 2006, the number of well-trained doctors is not enough to satisfy the need of health services from the public nowadays (Yuen, 2014). On the other hand, the number of nursing graduates has dropped significantly when university nursing programs were introduced more than two decades ago, with the closure of all nursing schools in public hospitals, although some of the latter were "re-opened" in recent years. Furthermore, Hong Kong is still professional-led in medical and health services. Training programs for general healthcare workers have not been developed, or even discussed within the healthcare sector. School leavers can either get admitted to health professional courses or will not consider a career in health services at all, particularly in long-term care, community health and elderly services.

Facilities

In recent years, the utilization of acute medical wards is always over 100% capacity. It has been found that the beds are mostly occupied by the elderly patients who are suffering from chronic diseases and are more prone to weather change and influenza. In view of this, the aging problem seems to further aggravate the problem of insufficient hospital beds. Furthermore, as the natural resources are limited, land becomes a major concern in the hospital redevelopment and building programs. Thus, scarcity of land becomes a concern in dealing with the problem of aging population (Yuen, 2014).

For residential elderly care, there are 26,879 subsidized residential places against 7,089 community based places for the elderlies (Social Welfare Department, 2016). In financial terms, $2,549M are spent on residential places, compared to $381M spending on community-based places. There is also a high institutionalization rate of 6.8% of the population aged 60 and above. This figure is doubled that of Japan, and more than 3 times that of Singapore and Taiwan. 34,749 applicants appear in the Central Waiting List for subsidized residential care. The waiting time for a place in subsidized Care and Attention Homes is around 22 months, and for Nursing Homes 26 months (Social Welfare Department, 2016). Unfortunately, about 5,000 elderly persons die every year while waiting for a place in a subsidized nursing home (South China Morning Post 2014).

Compartmentalization in the Hong Kong Health Care System

The Hong Kong health care system is a dual track system. However, the involvement of the public and private sectors differs significantly. In term of total health expenditure, at around 5.2% of GDP, there is a comparable and equal share between the public and private services. The public sector shares about 2.5% of GDP while the private sector contributes to around 2.6% of GDP (Ko, 2014). Nonetheless, when referring to the provision of services, the Hong Kong system is a 90:10 dual track system. The public sector serves almost 90% of inpatient services whereas private hospitals only provide 10% of inpatient services. In outpatient clinics, the private sector delivers 70% and the public sector only serves 30% (EDB, 2016).

Compartmentalization is a structural deficiency in the Hong Kong health system, which is already over-stretched. Long-term residential care is under the jurisdiction of the Labor and Welfare Bureau, while all other health services are the responsibilities of the Food and Health Bureau. There is no flexibility for resources to be directed from acute care to long-term care. Such imbalance between residential LTC and community-based LTC has resulted in cost-ineffectiveness. Moreover, the lack of medical care in LTC institutions has resulted in frequent presentation to the Accident and Emergency Department and public hospital admissions. At the same time, it is difficult to recruit and retain healthcare professionals in LTC facilities because of the lack of a career structure in LTC and non-hospital services.

Health care systems in most developed societies continue to be a global concern due to the challenges arising from aging problems, population growth, increasing chronic and multiple morbidities, novel and chronic infectious diseases, increases in public health spending, incoherent healthcare, and rise in public expectations. Other factors are encountered in managing the health care system, such as manpower constraints, compartmentalization in health care systems, fragmentation among health professionals, and investment and advancement in medical technology. They will not only restrain the sustainability within the health care system, but will also put pressure on the financial capacity of the government and people in meeting the ever-escalating demands (Wong et al., 2015).

Hong Kong is ill-prepared to meet the serious challenges as the population continues to age, particularly in view of the fact that Hong Kong has been achieving the longest life expectancy in the world for both men and women. The current public sector has nearly stretched to its limits, but the private sector is not fully utilized as evident by the big difference in the waiting time. The use of public-private services in healthcare seems to be imbalanced. Persistent increase in the health services demand in the public sector may lead to a significant compromise in the quality of services and will further lengthen the waiting time of the largely subsidized services (Lam, 2011). To deal with these challenges, public-private partnership is suggested as a potentially feasible means in resolving issues arising from the aging population and growing demand for LTC.

ADVANTAGES OF PUBLIC PRIVATE PARTNERSHIP

PPP can bring together the expertise and resources from both the public and private sectors (The Food and Health Bureau, 2016). When compared to the services solely provided by the public sector, forming

PPP can reduce the burden of the public sector by involving the private sector in the project, and can be beneficial to the citizens, governments and even to the private sector itself. There is also a potential in increasing the efficiency and competition in the provision of services and in lowering the delivery costs while, at the same time, expanding the service coverage. PPPs can be more flexible in responding to market signals and market trends, and are more ready, as well as in an easy position, to purchase and adopt new technology than in the public sector. PPPs may help in addressing the imbalance between public and private healthcare subsystems, in improving the quality of care, making good use of the scarce available resources, enabling training of expertise, and ultimately ensuring the sustainability of the health care system (The Food and Health Bureau, 2016). PPPs are known to lead to improvements in innovation, efficiency and access to services (Mitchell, 2008), and is an effective way to help the Government to decrease public expenditure in the healthcare services by assuring an efficient resources allocation (Kirkpatrick, Clarke & Polidano, 2003; Cheng, 2009)

CHALLENGES OF PPP

According to Mitchell (2008), there are three challenges in adopting PPP in the health services, including equity, quality and cost, although PPP can bring better services to the community.

Equity

Equity is considered as one of the most important criteria and objective when providing health services (Bloom et al., 2000). Under the long-time policy "that no one is denied adequate medical treatment due to lack of means", the public sector in Hong Kong is generally viewed as a safety net in providing healthcare services to the poor and will take poverty and affordability as key elements in most and different policies, whereas the goal of private sector is to maximize the profit and thus the attention is almost solely on the wealthy people, who can afford and pay the high fees. Private providers are less interested in consumers who are unable to bear the full cost of health services. They only respond to the sector of the population that are most willing to pay for the expensive healthcare cost. This will increase the inequity in the access to healthcare services. As the poorer population have a lower willingness and ability to pay, private providers will decrease the supply of some socially desirable services like preventive care and health education, thus worsening the allocation efficiency in the health sector. They may even supply more unnecessary health services or provide low-quality services to the patients in order to drive up their profits. As the missions of public and private sectors are different, when adopting PPPs in the provision of healthcare services, equity poses a big challenge to both the policy makers and providers. The Government may form a partnership through the purchase of services from the private sector, but the private sector may try to provide lower quality of services to the poor so as to achieve profit maximization (Mitchell, 2008). This missing interlinkage between the goals of public and private sector, and pooling of risks will lead to equity and efficiency problems. As a result, the majority of the population cannot afford private health services, but the public sector cannot guarantee competitive services for all without the input from better-off and affordable contributors (Jütting, 2002).

Quality

The public sector services are traditionally known for its poor quality, affected by lack of motivation and training of the staff, little client-focus, waiting time, unmet demand and inadequate availability of services. As a contrary, private services are often praised for excellent quality in term of environments of hospitals and clinics that are catered for the wealthy, choice of professionals, friendly staff, timely arrangements, convenience and speedy services, etc. Nonetheless, they are primarily motivated by money and have no concern for equity, access or quality. Private healthcare is also known for the fraud, in which inappropriate and poor quality services are being provided to their patients, for example, the overuse of unnecessary medications and procedures in order to increase revenues. Five main problems are associated with private providers of health services. They are related to the use of illegitimate or unethical means to maximize profit, less concern towards public health goals, lack of interest in sharing clinical information, creating "brain drain" among public sector health staff, and lack of regulatory control over practices (Raman & Björkman, 2009). These issues place a challenge on improving the quality of both public and private sectors when adopting PPP projects. In order to strengthen the quality and to make the public much better informed about the partners, improvement is needed in two important areas and these are accountability and the regulatory environment (Mitchell, 2008).

Accountability

In terms of accountability, the collaborating partners are required to be accountable to each other, as well as to the consumers, in order to ensure a high standard of quality services they jointly offer to the community. In the private sector, unequal and incomplete information is always the case. Whereas in the public sector, quality indicators are often quoted, like re-admission rate for surgery, waiting time, and morbidity and mortality outcomes. In general, such statistics are not readily available in the private sector. Therefore, when a partnership is formed, it will be difficult for the consumers to make an informed choice about where to go for the healthcare services (Watson, 2003). To ensure this accountability, it is important to make the public better informed about the partners and the services they offer. People can be informed through publications, the media, internet, healthcare providers and insurance companies, etc., so that the public will better understand the providers they are choosing, and can select better quality of health services provided by providers who are competitors. The accountability in public sector is being more transparent in recent years. They are asked to report and provide information on some quality indicators like waiting time, facility-specific morbidity and mortality outcomes, as well as re-admission rate for surgery. When adopting PPP, it is essential on the one hand to make sure the public are informed about all data on quality indicators from the public sectors, and on the other hand to force the private providers to enhance their accountability so that all consumers can have a better informed choice (Mitchell, 2008).

Regulatory Environment

The regulatory environment and robust legal system are indispensable in maintaining and improving service quality. The essential objectives of these infrastructures in health service are to ensure access, to control costs, and to protect individual consumers. More importantly, they are useful in promoting public health activities such as cessation of smoking, healthy eating behavior, and the promotion of physical activity. Nevertheless, although enhanced regulatory environment is making apparent impacts in recent years, such as the government regulation on the safety of food production, toys products, construction of buildings, and cleaning materials, the changing patterns of diseases and mortality require the Government and policy makers to take a more active role in this area (Mitchell, 2008).

Unmet Demand in an Aging Population

In an aging population, changes in disease patterns, and technology advancement for treatment have resulted in a rapid increase in the need for healthcare, and thus costs in health services, particularly LTC. The health care system is no longer able to provide all the needed healthcare service to the entire population. The exponential growth in elderly population reflects a proportional increase in recourses that are unaffordable and unsustainable to the economy. This rapidly increasing demand for health services not only lead to non-financial implication like shortage of manpower and long waiting time, but also create a large burden on the public sectors (Yuen, 2014). Compared to around thirty years ago, most diseases are not acute nowadays, but rather, most of them are classified chronic such as diabetes, hypertension, coronary heart disease, and lung conditions. People suffering from acute disease are usually either cured or dead, but when they are suffering from chronic diseases, they have to bear the expensive long-term treatment and medicines to maintain their life, with the hope of improving living quality. The cost is much greater than acute disease. Therefore, even when the PPP is formed, this will not only create a huge burden to the public sector, but the private sector also has to share this service load. The tremendous increase in healthcare costs will offset the foreseeable and expectant efficiency gains from the partnership, in a magnitude larger than any savings that may be expected to have achieved.

High Transaction Cost and Lengthy Lead Time

Contracting a PPP project is practically very complex because it involves several parties' conflicting objectives and interests. This is understandable. PPP projects usually need an extensive expertise input and will take a long time in the negotiation. A PPP project often involves a high transaction cost than the traditional public sector procurement, including high legal and advisory fees, costs of private sector finance, and bidding costs. These financial and time costs may not be acceptable to the private consortium. Therefore, when the stakeholders believe that a project does not have a good value or an expected return, the contract may not have a good start at the beginning or may even fail in the end (Chan, Lam, Chan, & Cheung, 2008).

SUCCESSFUL FACTORS IN ESTABLISHED PPP MODELS

According to Cheung, Chan, and Kajewsk (2012), the most important factor affecting the development of PPP project in Hong Kong is the favorable legal framework, followed by commitment and responsibility of public and private sectors, strong and good private consortium, stable macroeconomic condition, and appropriate risk allocation and risk sharing. These factors are similar to the Malaysian study by Ismail in 2013, which had ranked eighteen critical successful factors for PPP, in which the top three were a good governance, commitment and responsibility, and a favorable legal framework. The National Treasury

Figure 1. Challenges of PPP

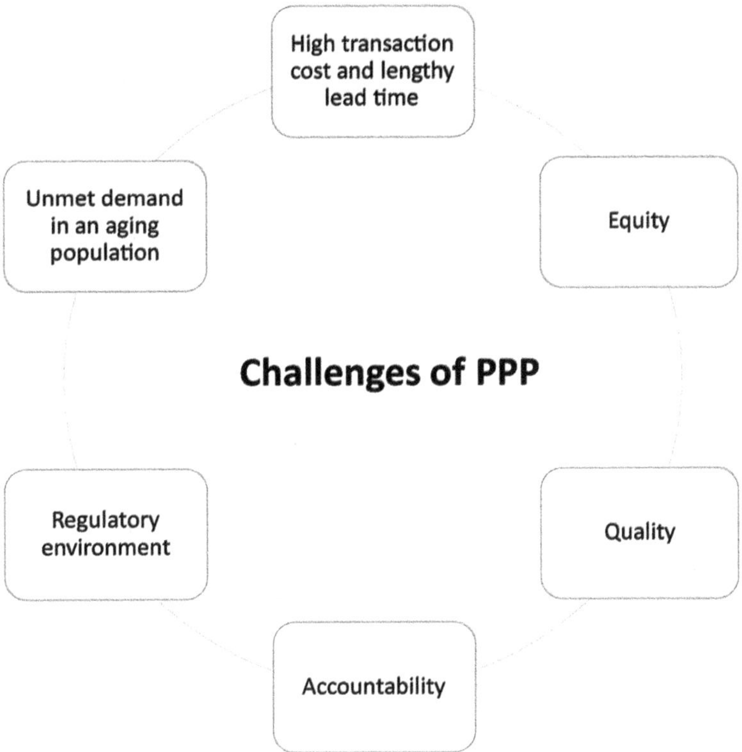

Figure 2. Successful factors in established PPP models

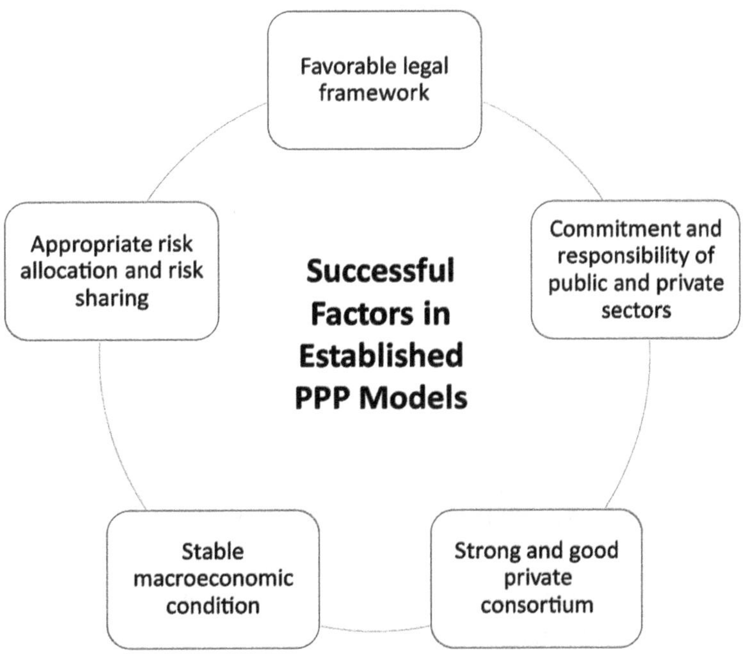

PPP Unit of South Africa (2007) has mentioned that an efficient, independent and fair legal framework is a key successful factor for PPPs.

However, in Australia and the United Kingdom (UK), where there has already been a long history of PPP models of more than 20 years, a favorable legal framework is only ranked medium, while the most important factors for a successful PPP model in these two countries are commitment and responsibility of public and private sectors, and strong and good private consortium respectively. This may imply that they have already had a well-developed legal framework that caters for PPP projects.

A well-established legal framework is also important for a country's economic development, mechanism for developing infrastructure and regeneration (Chan, Lam, Chan, Cheung, & Ke, 2009). Thus, a fair, independent and efficient legal framework is a key factor in PPP projects. Furthermore, appropriate governing regulations related to PPP should also be implemented in order to facilitate the application of PPP. Practically sufficient legal resources should be made available to deal with the complicated legal documentation required (Cheung, Chan, Lam, Chan, & Ke., 2012).

To implement PPP projects successfully, both public and private partners must be highly committed and be responsive to the projects. They should fully contribute their complementary skills and the best resources into the projects. In such way, a good relationship between both partners can be maintained and the projects can be implemented in an effective way (Cheung, Chan, & Kajewski, 2012). Choosing a strong and trustworthy private consortium is one of the skills for the public sectors when planning PPP projects. The government should ensure that the private consortia are competent and have sufficient resources, including financial, to take up the projects. Otherwise, PPP projects will be much more difficult to implement (Chan, Lam, Chan, Cheung, & Ke, 2009).

A predictable market in the stable macroeconomic environment is desirable for PPP projects. The financial risks in implementation can thus be lowered, in terms of interest rate, employment rate, exchange rate and inflation (Cheung, Chan, Lam, Chan, & Ke, 2012). As a result, the PPP projects can motivate private investors to join in view of a reasonable return for them. Apart from ensuring a reasonable return on investment, the public agencies and private consortium are expected to bear other risks due to political, social, environment, technical and economic factors. Appropriate and equitable risk allocation and sharing must be fully communicated and agreed upon, before a PPP project starts as there may be unforeseeable situations that go beyond the control and prediction of all concerned parties (Chan, Lam, Chan, & Cheung, 2008).

In Hong Kong,patients relying and using publicly-funded health services are mostly the low income group (LIG). Ndandiko and Ibanda (2016) have suggested three methods to reform the legal framework for PPP models that are focused on the needs of the LIG and to facilitate them to access the health service under PPP: (i) to strengthen and clarify the legal policy commits to the LIG under PPP models; (ii) segments of population constitute LIG and institution entity should have a common agreement in response to monitor patients from LIGs to access health services; (iii) consultation within LIG should be persistently performed so as to understand their needs, current service levels, preference and constraints.

HEALTHCARE PPP PROJECTS IN HONG KONG

Several PPPs projects have been adopted in HK, with apparent emphasis on elderly services and LTC. They include (i) Public-Private Interface Electronic Patient Record (PPI-ePR) Sharing Pilot Project, (ii)

Elderly Healthcare Voucher Pilot Scheme, (iii) Elderly Vaccination Subsidization Scheme, (iv) Patient Empowerment Project, (v) General Outpatient Clinic Public Private Partnership Program, (vi) Pilot Project on Enhancing Radiological Investigation Services through Collaboration with the Private Sector (Radi Collaboration), and (vii) Hemodialysis Shared Care Program.

Public-Private Interface Electronic Patient Record (PPI-ePR) Sharing Pilot Project

The PPI-ePR Sharing Pilot Project launched in 2005, now widely known as the Electronic Health Record Sharing System (eHRSS), was the earliest PPP healthcare project implemented in Hong Kong. The vision of this project is to develop a territory-wide Electronic Health Record (eHR) to underpin health transformation. The project does not aim at focusing on a specific treatment delivery, but rather it allows the patients' health information to be shared from the HA system to the private and non-government organizations through an IT platform, subject to the patients' consent and user authentication. Under this secure platform, registered private health professionals can have access to ePR of consenting individual patients. The information received can be used to assist in clinical decisions and treatments. As at January 2016, the project has enrolled over 48,500 patients, and 3,500 private healthcare professionals. Over 1,417,000 numbers of eHR have been accessed by the participating private and non-government sectors (Hospital Authority, 2016; Chan, & Choy, 2011)

Elderly Health Care Voucher Pilot Scheme

The purposes of the Elderly Health Care Voucher Pilot Scheme is to reduce the burden of existing public healthcare services by providing financial subsidies for elderly to choose private healthcare services, and to alleviate the burden of medical expenses on elderly persons and their families and to enhance health promotion and primary care services. This Scheme was launched on 1 January in 2009 initially for a period of three years. The scheme was then extended in 2012, based on the result of the Interim Review, and the annual voucher amount for each eligible elderly was increased from HK$250 to HK$500. There had been more positive feedbacks from the community. Hence, starting from 2014, the annual voucher amount was increased to HK$2,000, subject to an accumulated ceiling of HK$4,000. In 2017, the Government proposed to lower the eligibility age 70 to 65, so that about 400 000 more elderly persons will receive $2,000 a year to purchase private primary care services. (Health Care Voucher, 2016; Government of Hong Kong, 2017).

Elderly Vaccination Subsidization Scheme (EVSS)

The Scientific Committee on Vaccine Preventable Diseases of the Centre for Health Protection, Department of Health, has recommended a number of vaccinations for certain high risk groups so as to minimize the risk of infection and hospitalization (The Food and Health Bureau, 2010). EVSS was introduced in 2009/2010 by the Department of Health. The scheme continued in 2015/16 to encourage elderlies, aged 65 years or above, to receive seasonal influenza and pneumococcal vaccination. Under the EVSS 2015/2016, each eligible elder was subsidized HK$160 per dose of seasonal influenza vaccination and HK$190 per dose of 23-valent polysaccharide pneumococcal vaccination, for receiving vaccination given by enrolled private medical practitioners. Eligible elderlies are required to pay the difference after deducting the government subsidy from the fee charged by the private clinics (Centre for Health Protection, 2015).

Patient Empowerment Project

According to the National Council on Aging (2016), approximately 92% of older adults are suffering from at least one chronic disease, and 77% have at least two. In order to face this challenge, the Hospital Authority has implemented a Patient Empowerment Program which was launched in 2010 in all clusters of the HA in collaboration with non-government organizations (NGOs). The project aims at improving the medical knowledge of the patients on their chronic diseases so as to enhance their self-management skills. The HA multi-disciplinary team, which comprises different allied health professionals, is responsible in developing teaching materials for common chronic diseases and providing training for frontline staff of the collaborate NGOs (Hospital Authority, 2016; Chan, & Choy, 2011).

General Outpatient Clinic (GOPC) Public Private Partnership Program

Similar to the Patient Empowerment Project, this program has been implemented to deal with the increasing problems and demand for services of chronic diseases. The GOPC Public Private Partnership Program aims to increase the provision of primary care services by allowing an alternative choice for patients to receive primary care services from the private sector and to promote the concept of family doctors. The Program was first launched in mid-2014 in three pilot districts – Kwun Tong, Wong Tai Sin, and Tuen Mun (HA, 2016). In the first stage of implementation, clinically stable patients, who have hypertension, with or without hyperlipidemia, will be invited for voluntary participation. The program was then extended to include diabetes patients. Each participating patient is given a total of ten subsidized visits per year, including medical consultations for both chronic and acute care. Under this program, all participating patients only need to pay HKD$45 for each consultation, which is equivalent to the HA GOPC fee (Primary Care Office, 2016).

Pilot Project on Enhancing Radiological Investigation Services Through Collaboration With the Private Sector (Radi Collaboration)

This publicly-funded pilot project was launched in May 2012 in response to the overwhelming demand and workload for radiological imaging services in public hospitals over the years. It aimed to improve the radiological investigation services for cancer patients through the involvement of the private sector. In 2012, the project targeted at only four groups of cancer patients, but in 2014, the service was extended to another seven cancer groups (Legislative Council, 2015b). The eleven target cancer groups include prostate, breast, nasopharyngeal, cervix cancer, lymphoma, colorectal, stomach, corpus uteri, head and neck, sarcoma and germ cell tumor. Through the invitation from the Hospital Authority, patients can choose their private healthcare providers from five private partners, including private hospitals and diagnostic centers (Hospital Authority, 2010a). Until early March 2015, 18,730 patients have been served by the project. (Legislative Council, 2015b).

Figure 3. PPP pilot projects in Hong Kong

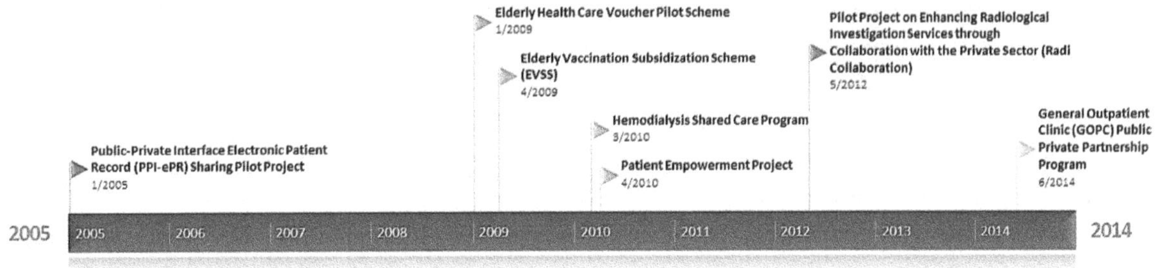

Hemodialysis Shared Care Program

This program was launched in March 2010 to provide better quality services to end-stage renal failure (ESRF) patients, to enhance collaboration between community hemodialysis centers and the HA, and to provide more choices for ESRF patients for hemodialysis. Eligible patients were invited by nephrologists of HA to join the program. Patients were only required to pay the same treatment fee as charged by HA to the private hemodialysis centers (Hospital Authority, 2010b). As at March 2015, there were 265 ESRF patients benefited from this program (Legislative Council, 2015b).

HEALTHCARE PPP PROJECTS IN SINGAPORE AND UNITED KINGDOM

There is a big difference between the approach of the application of PPP in healthcare in Hong Kong and other countries, say, Singapore and United Kingdom. In Hong Kong, the healthcare public sector only appoints some private healthcare organizations to co-operate with them in some designated PPP projects. PPP is not adopted in the whole health care system. In contrast, health care systems in Singapore and UK are actually PPP based. A series of healthcare programs, including long-term care, are being provided in these systems. They use PPP in the early stage of building and managing a hospital, instead of setting up individual PPP programs afterwards. The followings are the overview of PPPs in the Singapore and UK health care systems.

PPPs in Singapore

The Singaporean health care system is made up of three pillars: (i) promoting preventive care and healthy lifestyles, (ii) emphasizing citizens' healthy living responsibility through 3M (Medisave, Medishield, and Medifund), and (iii) controlling the healthcare cost and providing subsidies in public healthcare institutions. The philosophy behind is individual responsibility and affordable healthcare for all citizens. The Singapore government emphasizes that no medical service is provided free of charge, with the intention to reduce the over-use of healthcare services, and through regulating the doctor supply and salary as well. It also avoids over relying on national welfare or third-party health insurance, by establishing a sense of responsibility among individuals for their own health. (Lim, 2004)

In 1983, the Singapore government promoted the national health plan on the infrastructure of the health care system for the next 20 years with the idea of Medisave, giving a great protection for the long-term care for the citizens. Medisave is a kind of national savings scheme which allows members of the Central Provident Fund (CPF) to save part of their income into the Medisave Account for future or immediate personal or family's (including spouse, children, parents and grandparents) medical expenses, mainly after retirement. Medisave can be used for acute care, rehabilitative care, end-of-life care and outpatient treatment, at all public healthcare organizations, as well as approved private hospitals and medical parties under the PPP health care system (Central Provident Fund Board, 2016).

The Singaporean government recognizes the role of the private sector in meeting national healthcare needs. The Community Health Assist Scheme (CHAS) was introduced in 2012 to strengthen partnerships with General Practitioners (GPs) and dental clinics in providing subsidized primary care for Pioneers and Singaporean households. In 2015, 650,000 Singaporeans benefited from CHAS. In addition, Family Medicine Clinics are being established under CHAS, with a focus on chronic disease management (Ministry of Health Singapore, 2015).

In hospital care, the Emergency Care Collaboration with Raffles Hospital was introduced in 2015 for Singaporean Citizens and Permanent Residents to attend this private hospital for emergency care, inpatient or specialist outpatient care, but on charges similar to what they would pay at our public hospitals. Similar collaboration is made with Parkway Hospitals, another local private hospital group.

Public acute hospitals have close partnership with community hospitals run by Voluntary Welfare Organizations (VWOs) in intermediate residential care. They jointly develop clinical governance standards, care pathways, manpower capacity and capability to facilitate the transfer of patients between the institutions.

For long-term care, the Ministry has been working with the private sector to meet the needs of the aging population, via a portable subsidy scheme with up to 75% subsidy at participating private nursing homes. Through PPP, palliative care services are also being enhanced with expansion of capacity for inpatient, home and day hospice services in order to benefit more end of life patients.

In addition, the Pioneer Generation Package (PGP) provides several forms of healthcare supports to eligible elderly pioneers. PGP co-operates with private clinics enrolled in CHAS. People will be subsidized in some services and treatments provided in these private clinics, which share the burden and workload of elderly care services. PGP is an effective strategy to manage the imbalanced health care system, and financial sustainability in long term (Singapore Government, 2016).

PPP Infrastructure Projects by the Government of United Kingdom

UK is well known for its expertise in developing PPPs as it is the first country to apply this concept for public services projects. UK is also the leader in the healthcare PPPs around the world, with excellent public and private sector skills and innovation for the healthcare facilities so that the health care system can meet the complex health demand of a large population.

The UK Government mainly use PPP for the infrastructure projects in healthcare. They usually apply Private Finance Initiative in adopting PPP projects by inviting the private sector to finance the projects' capitals and design, build and operate specific facilities (GOV.UK, 2013). Since 1991, they have successfully built more than 130 healthcare PPP programs for acute, primary, community and mental health facilities. The UK government has managed to collaborate with a range of private commercial healthcare companies and academia to set up integrated, high-quality and cost-effective systems of care. Examples include Barts and the Royal London new hospitals program, Alder Hey Children's NHS Foundation Trust Hospital redevelopment and The Health Services Renewal Program for Grand Turk and Providenciales.

Barts and the Royal London New Hospitals Program

In 2006, the St. Bartholomew's and Royal London project was set up. It was the largest private finance initiative hospital scheme in the UK, with and investment of £1.1 billion. The successful bidding private consortium is Skanska-Innisfree, who was required to advise on the development control plans for the two hospitals and detailed planning of clinical departments (UK Trade & Investment, 2013). This project involved re-configuration and re-provision of hospital equipment, enhancement of the operational effectiveness and improvement of the provision of the hospital services in the two major acute hospital sites in London (European Investment Bank, 2016).

Alder Hey Children's NHS Foundation Trust Hospital Redevelopment

In this project, the Acorn consortium, comprising John Laing, Laing O'Rourke and Interserve, is the private party. John Liang and Laing O'Rourke each hold 40% of the total investment equity, whereas Interserve holds 20%. John Liang and Laing O'Rourke are required to design and build the new hospital and Interserve is responsible to maintain the hospital infrastructure (UK Trade & Investment, 2013). This hospital is built entirely in a park and is a specialist teaching hospital that provides a range of services for the children (NHS Foundation Trust, 2014).

The Health Services Renewal Program for Grand Turk and Providenciales

This program mainly focused on promoting healthy lifestyle and wellness initiatives by renewing the public health services and facilities. Private finance initiative was used to construct two new local general hospitals. The idea was developed by the expertise from UK advisors. The hospitals provide services to the population of seven islands. The private consortium in this project is required to provide a diverse range of health services for the 25 years of the contract. The hospital was constructed completely and successfully in 2009 and was opened as planned in April 2010 (UK Trade & Investment, 2013).

SOLUTIONS AND RECOMMENDATIONS

In 2012, the Audit Commission of the Hong Kong Government was giving some suggestions to the PPP programs organized by HA, and some of the suggestions are listed below (Food and Health Bureau, 2012).

Broadening the Patient Base of PPP Programs

When launching a pilot PPP program, the HA has only invited a part of eligible patients to participate. Take the Shared Care Program as an example, the HA has only invited about 60% of the potential participants. HA has tried to extend the invitation, but the invitation process is slow. It is recommended the HA should approach a larger number of potential participants to extend its patient base. Broadening the patient base one hand can help HA to test more deeply about the effectiveness and operations of the PPP program, and on the other hand, it could also benefit more eligible patients.

Improving Healthcare Providers' Take-Up Rate of PPP Program

In reviewing the take-up rate of three invitation exercise conducted between 2009 and 2010, the private healthcare providers taking up the HA's invitation to join the Programs were 11%, 15% and 29% respectively. This low take-up rate was not sufficient to enrich the patients' choices of health services. As private providers aim at earning profit, some of the PPP program did not appear to be attractive for them to join. It may also due to resource constraints, and uncontrollable recruitment procedures. Some suggestions are given to increase this take-up rate. HA should ensure the information of private medical practitioners in relevant district up to date, enhance the transparency of PPP program, and enhance the attractiveness of the programs.

Stepping Up Promotional Efforts

Using the PPI-ePR as an example, the patients and medical practitioners had a low satisfaction with the promotional material of the PPI-ePR. PPI-ePR was mainly promoted to the public through the HA's website, posters and leaflets at hospital and clinic, but it is rarely seen to be promoted through advertising on the public area like transport and the media. Implementing the PPI-ePR signature label is also a good method to help the patients to locate the private medical practitioners who are using electronic patient record. It was found that the private medical practitioners were welcome to use the PPI-ePR signature label that posted at the clinic or the name card of the practitioners.

Social Benefit Bonds

To deal with the unmet demand of aging population and to maximize the involvement and commercial opportunities of the private sector in the PPPs policy, the Hong Kong Government is suggested to take on the aging strategy by the Government of New South Wales as a reference, by setting up an open platform with the private sector to initiate a social investment partnership forum with the aims to develop action plans from specific industries and to explore opportunities for social investment. Social outcomes will be improved by such PPP social benefit bonds (NSW Government, 2012).

FUTURE RESEARCH DIRECTIONS

Future research will focus on innovation and sustainable solutions on long-term care that are relevant to both policy makers and managers of healthcare organizations in the planning and developing long-term care for an aging population with contemporary knowledge for an aging population. Studies of the service gap of the existing system through input from various stakeholders, and of the customer expectations, are also important, particularly with the view of establishing a client-oriented and community-based system in LTC. Data collected from existing PPPs in Hong Kong, though mostly being pilot projects, will provide important insights for the improvement of in-service development of knowledge and skills for service providers in long-term care, and will help in the development of relevant training programs in higher education institutions in order to meet the needs of the aging population.

CONCLUSION

PPP brings together the expertise, complementary skills, and resources from both the public and private sectors and thus can potentially bring better healthcare services to the public. PPPs can reduce the burden of the public sector and allow public facilities to focus more on the high priority services, for instance, acute cases and complex diseases. Promoting PPPs will result in a better allocation of resources, reduce the cost spent in the human resources and training of healthcare professionals, through improvements in innovation, and efficiency and access to services. PPPs models are beneficial to patients particularly when there is excess demand of services and insufficient manpower in the public sectors, as in the case of long-term care arising from a progressive aging population.

The success of PPP projects is highly dependent on a few factors, including favorable legal framework, commitment and responsibility of public and private sectors, strong and good private consortium, stable macro-economic condition, and appropriate risk allocation and risk sharing. More importantly, government policy and initiatives are crucial to PPPs, which may help in addressing the imbalance between the public and private sector as in the case of Hong Kong, improving the quality of care, making good use of the scarce available resources, enabling training of expertise, and ultimately ensuring the sustainability of the health care system.

However, issues of equity, quality, accountability, regulatory environment, unmet demand in an aging population, and high transaction cost and lengthy lead time are mainly concerned with the private partners and must be addressed in great details by the government, in conjunction with the private service providers. Ideally practical solutions and guidelines should be implemented before the introduction of PPP programs in order to maximize the benefits to the community. Furthermore, both public and private partners must be fully committed and be responsive to the needs and expectations of the users.

Involving the private sector in PPPs has been shown to benefit the government, the public and private healthcare service providers, as well as the community at large. Well developed and effectively operating PPPs in long-term care have great potentials to prepare the entire society in meeting the projected increasing needs of long-term healthcare arising from the aging population in terms of efficiency in utilization of resources and sustainability of the health care system.

REFERENCES

Bloom, D. E., Craig, P., & Mitchell, M. (2000). *Public and private roles in providing and financing social services: Health and education. In Public-Private Partnerships in the Social Sector: Issues and Country Experiences in Asia and the Pacific*. Tokyo: ADBI Publishing.

Central Provident Fund Board. (2016). *Medisave*. Retrieved 1 July 2016, from https://www.cpf.gov.sg/Members/Schemes/schemes/healthcare/medisave

Centre for Health Protection. (2015). *Elderly vaccination subsidy scheme*. Retrieved 10 August 2016, from http://www.chp.gov.hk/en/view_content/21863.html

Chan, A., & Cheung, E. (2014). *Public-private partnerships in international construction*. Routledge.

Chan, A. P., Lam, P. T., Chan, D. W., & Cheung, E. (2008). Application of public private partnership (PPP) in Hong Kong special administrative region – the critics' perspectives. *Proceedings of the First International Conference on Construction in Developing Countries,* 302-11.

Chan, A. P., Lam, P. T., Chan, D. W., Cheung, E., & Ke, Y. (2009). Potential obstacles to successful implementation of public-private partnerships in Beijing and the Hong Kong special administrative region. *Journal of Management Engineering*, *26*(1), 30–40. doi:10.1061/(ASCE)0742-597X(2010)26:1(30)

Chan, S. Y., & Choy, K. M. (2011). Fostering PPP in the Hong Kong healthcare system. *The Quarterly.* Retrieved 8 August 2016, from http://racma.edu.au/index.php?option=com_content&view=article&id=352:fostering-ppp-in-the-hong-kong-healthcare-system&catid=146:the-quarterly-2011&Itemid=61

Cheng, P. F. (2009). *An analysis of public private partnership in Hong Kong: a study of West Kowloon Cultural District. HKU Theses Online.* HKUTO. doi:10.5353/th_b4676044

Cheung, E., Chan, A. P., & Kajewski, S. (2012). Factors contributing to successful public private partnership projects: Comparing Hong Kong with Australia and the United Kingdom. *Journal of Facilities Management, 10*(1), 45–58. doi:10.1108/14725961211200397

Cheung, E., Chan, A. P., Lam, P. T., Chan, D. W., & Ke, Y. (2012). A comparative study of critical success factors for public private partnerships (PPP) between Mainland China and the Hong Kong Special Administrative Region. *Facilities, 30*(13/14), 647–666. doi:10.1108/02632771211273132

Education Bureau (EDB). (2016). *Economic analysis and evaluation of government policies: Health and healthcare in Hong Kong*. Retrieved 22 March 2016, from http://www.edb.gov.hk/attachment/en/curriculum-development/kla/pshe/references-and-resources/economics/health_eng.pdf

Emanuel, E. J., & Emanuel, L. L. (1996). What is accountability in health care? *Annals of Internal Medicine, 124*(2), 229–239. doi:10.7326/0003-4819-124-2-199601150-00007 PMID:8533999

European Investment Bank. (2016). Royal London and Barts Hospital PPP Project. *The EU bank.* Retrieved from http://www.eib.org/projects/pipeline/2003/20030038.htm

Food and Health Bureau. (2012). *Hospital Authority: Public-private prartnership (PPP) programmes.* Retrieved 26 Feb 2017, from http://www.aud.gov.hk/pdf_e/e58ch03.pdf

Food and Health Bureau. (2016). *Executive Summary for Improving Hong Kong Health Care System.* Healthcare Planning and Development Office. Retrieved 25 Feb 2017, from http://www.hpdo.gov.hk/en/doc/improving_hk_healtcare_system_summary_eng.pdf

GPnotebook. (2016). *Lead Time Bias.* General Practice Notebook-a UK medical reference. Retrieved 25 Feb 2017, from http://www.gpnotebook.co.uk/simplepage.cfm?ID=577437764

Health Care Voucher. (2016). *Background of elderly health care voucher scheme.* Retrieved 24 March 2016, from http://www.hcv.gov.hk/eng/pub_background.htm

Hospital Authority. (2010a). *Pilot project on enhancing radiological investigation services through collaboration with the private sector (Radi Collaboration).* Retrieved 25 March 2016, from https://www3.ha.org.hk/ppp/radi.aspx

Hospital Authority. (2010b). *Haemodialysis public private partnership programme (HD PPP)*. Retrieved 23 March 2016, from https://www3.ha.org.hk/ppp/hdscp.aspx?lang=eng

Hospital Authority. (2016a). *PPI-ePR sharing pilot project & eHR sharing system*. Retrieved 10 August 2016, from http://www3.ha.org.hk/ppp/ppiepr_a.aspx

Hospital Authority. (2016b). *General Outpatient Clinic Public Private Partnership Programme (GOPC PPP)*. Retrieved 12 Feb 2017, from http://www3.ha.org.hk/ppp/gopcppp.aspx?lang=eng

Ismail, S. (2013). Critical success factors of public private partnership (PPP) implementation in Malaysia. *Asia-Pacific Journal of Business Administration*, *5*(1), 6–19. doi:10.1108/17574321311304503

Jütting, J. (2002). *Public-private partnerships in the health sector: experiences from developing countries. Social Security Policy and Development Branch*. International Labour Office.

Kirkpatrick, C., Clarke, R., & Polidano, C. (2003). *Handbook on development policy and management*. Cheltenham, UK: Edward Elgar.

Ko, W. M. (2014). *Steps address aging population, rising costs*. Hong Kong Information Services Department. Retrieved 10 June 2016, from http://www.news.gov.hk/en/record/html/2014/08/20140815_162410.shtml

Lam, A. C. Y. (2011). Quality healthcare for an aging population. *Improving Hong Kong*, *8*, 7–9.

Lee, V. (2005). *Public Private Partnerships*. Research and Library Services Division. Legislative Council Secretariat. Retrieved 12 Feb 2017, from http://www.legco.gov.hk/yr04-05/english/sec/library/0405rp03e.pdf

Legislative Council. (2015a). *Challenges of population ageing*. Research Brief, 1. Retrieved 25 Feb 2017, from http://www.legco.gov.hk/research-publications/english/1516rb01-challenges-of-population-ageing-20151215-e.pdf

Legislative Council. (2015b). *Proposed $10 billion endowment fund to the Hospital Authority for public-private partnership initiatives*. Panel on Health Services. Retrieved 22 March 2016, from http://www.legco.gov.hk/yr15-16/english/panels/hs/papers/hs20151116cb2-235-7-e.pdf

Lim, M. K. (2004). Shifting the burden of healthcare finance: A case study of public-private partnership in Singapore. *Health Policy (Amsterdam)*, *69*(1), 83–92. doi:10.1016/j.healthpol.2003.12.009 PMID:15484609

Ministry of Health, Singapore. (2015). *Public-private partnerships*. Retrieved 3 July 2016, from https://www.moh.gov.sg/content/moh_web/home/pressRoom/Parliamentary_QA/2016/public-private-partnerships-.html

Mitchell, M. (2008). *An overview of public private partnerships in health. International Health Systems Program Publication*. Harvard School of Public Health.

National Council on Aging. (2016). *Facts about healthy aging*. Retrieved 8 August 2016, from https://www.ncoa.org/news/resources-for-reporters/get-the-facts/healthy-aging-facts/

National Treasury PPP Unite of South Africa. (2007). *Public private partnership manual*. Retrieved 24 March 2016, from http://www.treasury.gov.za/organisation/ppp/default.htm

Ndandiko, C., & Ibanda, S. (2016). *Public private partnerships guidelines for local governments*. United Nation Development Programme. Retrieved 27 May 2016, from http://www.undp.org/content/dam/uganda/img/Research%20and%20Publications/PPP%20Guidelines%20Final.pdf

NHS Foundation Trust, United Kingdom. (2014). *Strategic plan document for 2014-19 Alder Hey Children's NHS Foundation Trust*. Retrieved 27 May 2016, from https://www.gov.uk/government/uploads/system/uploads/attachment_data/file/389689/Alderhey_Publishable_Summary_Strategic_Plan_1415.pdf

Primary Care Office, Hong Kong. (2016). *Primary care initiatives*. Retrieved 8 August 2016, from http://www.pco.gov.hk/english/initiatives/projects.html

Raman, A. V., & Björkman, J. W. (2009). *Public/Private partnership in healthcare services in India*. Research study funded by the Indo-Dutch Programme on Alternatives in Development (project 5.3.96). Retrieved 27 May 2016, http://www.pppinharyana.gov.in/ppp/sector/health/report-healthcare.pdf

Singapore Government. (2016). *Pioneer generation package: Know the benefits*. Retrieved 20 May 2016, from https://www.ecitizen.gov.sg/Topics/Pages/Pioneer-Generation-Package-Know-the-benefits.aspx

Social Welfare Department. (2005). *Care and Attention Homes for the Elderly. Residential Care Services for the Elderly*. Retrieved 25 Feb 2017, from http://www.swd.gov.hk/en/index/site_pubsvc/page_elderly/sub_residentia/id_careandatt/

Social Welfare Department. (2016). *Overview on residential care services for elders*. Retrieved 6 August 2016, from http://www.swd.gov.hk/en/index/site_pubsvc/page_elderly/sub_residentia/id_overviewon/

South China Morning Post. (2014). *Hong Kong faces challenge ensuring the elderly feel right at home*. Retrieved 10 August 2016, from http://www.scmp.com/news/hong-kong/article/1433787/hong-kong-faces-challenge-ensuring-elderly-feel-right-home

The Food and Health Bureau. (2008). The need for Change. *Your Health Your Life*. Retrieved from http://www.fhb.gov.hk/beStrong/files/consultation/chapter1_eng.pdf

The Food and Health Bureau. (2010). Healthcare Reform- Progress to Date. *My Health My Choice*. Retrieved 11 August 2016, from http://www.myhealthmychoice.gov.hk/pdf/chapter2_eng.pdf

The Food and Health Bureau. (2016). Promote Public Private Partnership in Healthcare. *Your Health, Your Life*. Retrieved 22 March 2016, from http://www.fhb.gov.hk/beStrong/files/consultation/chapter3_eng.pdf

The Government of Hong Kong. (2017). *2017 Policy Address*. Retrieved 1 March 2017, from http://www.policyaddress.gov.hk/2017/eng/p195.html

The Government of United Kingdom. (2013). *Healthcare: Public Private Partnerships. Promotional material*. Retrieved 3 July 2016, from https://www.gov.uk/government/publications/public-private-partnerships/public-private-partnerships

The Hong Kong Census and Statistics Department. (2009b). *Thematic household survey* report - Report No. 40. Retrieved 12 July, 2016, from http://www.censtatd.gov.hk/products_and_services/products/publications/statis tical_report/social_data/index_cd_B1130240_dt_latest.jsp

UK Trade & Investment. (2013). *Public private partnership*. HealthcareUK. Retrieved from https://www.gov.uk/government/uploads/system/uploads/attachment_data/file/266818/07_PPP_28.11.13.pdf

Unit, E. (2015). *Private sector involvement: Management consultancy*. Retrieved 20 March 2016, from http://www.eu.gov.hk/en/our-work/management-consultancy/private-sector-involvement.html

Watson, D. (2003). The rise and rise of public private partnerships: Challenges for public accountability. *Australian Accounting Review*, *13*(31), 2–14. doi:10.1111/j.1835-2561.2001.tb00167.x

Wong, E. L., Yeoh, E. K., Chau, P. Y., Yam, C. H., Cheung, A. W., & Fung, H. (2015). How shall we examine and learn about public-private partnerships (PPPs) in the health sector? Realist evaluation of PPPs in Hong Kong. *Social Science & Medicine*, *147*, 261–269. doi:10.1016/j.socscimed.2015.11.012 PMID:26605970

World Bank Group. (2015). *What are Public Private Partnership*. About PPPs. Retrieved 25 Feb 2017, from http://ppp.worldbank.org/public-private-partnership/overview/what-are-public-private-partnerships

World Health Organization. (2017). *Equity*. Health Systems. Retrieved 25 Feb 2017, from http://www.who.int/healthsystems/topics/equity/en/

Yuen, R. M. F. (2014). The challenges of an ageing society from a health care perspective. *Public Policy and Administration*, *17*(1), 1–14.

KEY TERMS AND DEFINITIONS

Accountability: Accountability means the parties justify and take responsibility for the procedures and processes of all its activities or actions. In healthcare, accountability is usually held in the area of professional competence, legal and ethical conduct, financial performance, adequacy of access, public health promotion, and community benefit (Emanuel & Emanuel, 1996).

Care and Attention Homes: Care and Attention Homes provide residential care, meals, personal care and limited nursing care for those who suffer from poor health condition in activities of daily living but are mentally suitable for communal living, and are assessed to be of moderate impairment level under the Standardized Care Need Assessment Mechanism (Social Welfare Department, 2005).

Compartmentalization: In health care, compartmentalization refers to the splitting of the health care system into different smaller parts (Food and Health Bureau, 2016).

Equity: Equity is the absence of avoidable or remediable differences among groups of people, whether those groups are defined socially, economically, demographically, or geographically. Health inequities therefore involve more than inequality with respect to health determinants, access to the resources needed to improve and maintain health or health outcomes. They also entail a failure to avoid or overcome inequalities that infringe on fairness and human rights norms (WHO, 2017).

Lead Time: Lead time refers to the period between early detection of a disease and its usual clinical presentation and diagnosis (GPnotebook, 2016).

Public Private Partnership: In health care, PPP is the long -term contract between a government entity and a private party, for providing a public healthcare service, in which the private party has the responsibility to bear significant risk and take the management role, and the remuneration is linked to the performance (World Bank Group, 2015).

Section 2
Management and Solutions

Chapter 7
Development of Accreditation Approach of Elderly Care Service Providers:
Experience from East and West

Artie W. Ng
The Hong Kong Polytechnic University, Hong Kong

Tiffany C. H. Leung
The Hong Kong Polytechnic University, Hong Kong

Jacky C. K. Ho
City University of Macau, Macau

ABSTRACT

The purpose of this book chapter is to explore the similarities and differences in the development of performance measures and accreditation systems for the quality assurance of elderly care service providers of Asian and Western origins, focusing on Hong Kong, Macau, Australia and Canada. Building on a proposed theoretical framework, this study utilizes a multiple-case study method to examine the influencing factors for the accreditation approach adopted by a jurisdiction. The findings suggest that the quality assurance of the elderly care service operators of the Asian origins as selected appears to lag behind those of the Western countries and undergo their own peculiar paths of development. Thus, Hong Kong and Macau could learn from the practical experience of Australia and Canada in terms of their concerted approaches for funding, accreditation and assessments under an increasingly market-driven service sector in which the well-being of the end-users needs to be adequately protected.

INTRODUCTION

The worldwide aging population has increasingly become one of the most transnational social issues to be addressed by policy makers in different countries and the global research agenda. As the elderly population is increasing rapidly (OECD, 2016), the demand for institutional elderly care and residential care for senior citizens is experiencing exponential growth (Bernoth et al., 2014). Policy makers, health

DOI: 10.4018/978-1-5225-2633-9.ch007

care professionals and care service providers for the elderly around the world need to take measures to address the growing demand of the aging society. Prior health care studies have paid relatively little attention to comparing various management perspectives in elderly care settings in various jurisdictions (KPMG, 2013). The purpose of this book chapter is to explore and examine the similarities and differences in the development of performance measures and accreditation systems for the quality assurance of care service providers of Asian and Western origins, focusing on Hong Kong, Macau, Australia and Canada.

This chapter is structured as follows. The next section provides general background information on the aging population and the elderly care service providers. A brief literature review of operational models and funding sources, performance measure systems and accreditation systems is then provided, followed by the proposed theoretical framework of the accreditation approach and research design. Then, multiple-case studies from four different jurisdictions are presented. Conclusions and future research directions are provided at the end.

BACKGROUND

The Aging Population and the Elderly Care Service Providers

The aging population has become one of the major transnational social issues to be addressed by policy makers. The global aging indicator shows that the number of people aged 60 or above is approximately 901 million, and this number is expected to grow to 2.1 billion by 2050, as the life expectancy rate will gradually increase from 70 years in 2015 to 77 years in 2050 (The United Nations Population Fund, 2015). The gap between older people and children under 15 will be 1.6 billion people, and approximately 48% of the retirement-age population does not receive any pension fund (The United Nations Population Fund, 2015). The aging of the Western population is mainly due to declining fertility rates, the aging of the baby boom generation born in the post-World War II era, and increased longevity in general (De Meijer et al., 2013).

Policy makers and health care planners have conducted various health-related and population-based studies to address issues pertinent to the aging population. These contemporary health issues could be viewed as social concerns that require insights from multiple disciplines, including political, economic, religious, legal, technological and medical perspectives (Lewis, 2002). Other factors that have also been taken into account include national income growth, new health and medical technologies for the elderly, and the social costs of health care to maintain the quality of life and sustain the lifespan of the local population (De Meijer et al., 2013). As such, substantial public and health expenditures could be required for allocation to resources pertinent to an economy with an aging population.

The sector of global healthcare service providers grew by 4.6% to reach a total revenue of US$ 7,142 billion in 2013, presenting a compound annual growth rate (CAGR) of 4.8% between 2009 and 2013, and this sector is predicted to grow at a rate of 6.1% in the period between 2013 and 2018 (MarketLine, 2014). The Americas, Europe and Asia-Pacific accounted for 49%, 28.6% and 20.7% of the global healthcare provider sector in 2013, respectively, (MarketLine, 2014). The average health expenditures increased significantly from 5% of the GDP in 1970 to almost 10% in 2015 in OECD countries (OECD, 2015). The Asia-Pacific and European sectors grew with compound annual growth rates (CAGRs) of 8.4 and 2.6% in 2013 to reach US$ 1,477 billion and US$ 2,039 billion, respectively (MarketLine, 2014).

The substantial growth of the health care provider sector is a boom for the aging business (medical and health) and related and supporting industries, such as insurance, finance and recreation. Health care will become more connected to daily life via mobile phones and social media (Ernst and Young, 2015).

LITERATURE REVIEW

Operational Models and Funding Sources

Caring for the elderly has shifted from home- and community-based care to institution-based care deliverable by both not-for-profit organizations and for-profit organizations (Bernoth et al., 2014). There is no single operational model of health care services that can meet the demands of all individuals across countries. A myriad of elderly home service operators could provide services up to 24 hours a day and up to 7 days a week, but these are highly dependent on patient needs (Lewis, 2002). The World Health Organization (WHO) suggests that governments should take greater responsibility for funding home-based care through a combination of NGOs and public and private agencies (WHO, 2000).

Based on the extant literature, the current elderly home services providers and residential care homes for the elderly (RCHEs) could be broadly divided into three main types: (i) non-governmental organizations (NGOs) partially or fully supported and funded by government subvention; (ii) NGOs operated by qualified charitable organizations or religious groups that may receive some subsidies from the local government; and (iii) private or for-profit operators with a self-financing model (See Lewis, 2002; KPMG, 2013).

Elderly people need to receive more formal care, either in an institution or at home (KPMG, 2013). Institution-based care is provided by three main types of facility: (i) nursing homes offer medical care and select therapies along with room and board and may be certified to provide medical care; (ii) sub-acute care facilities provide skilled nursing services and a higher level of medical supervision, although not to the level of a hospital or an acute care facility; and (iii) assisted living facilities provide basic care for chronic illnesses and varying degrees of help with daily living, typically in a home-like environment enabling a high degree of independence and autonomy (KPMG, 2013, p. 13). This may involve home healthcare services, for example, nursing care, care management, and day care (KPMG, 2013).

The sources of funding for elderly home service providers are similar to those of health care providers. The funding models could be broadly divided into four main types: (i) those for which the government provides full funding; (ii) those for which the government provides a partial subsidy; (iii) those without any government subsidy and (iv) those paid for by co-payments (KMPG, 2013).

The first type includes schemes that are funded or subsidized by federal, state or local governments, mainly from tax revenues. This financing model is suitable for countries that have the economic capacity to raise tax revenues and is commonly found in developed countries, such as Australia, Canada, Finland, Norway, the UK, the US, Japan and Hong Kong (KPMG, 2013; OECD, 2016). This funding model highly relies on high-income groups for tax contributions and is an unstable source of funding due to its vulnerability to economic turndowns, political pressure and inefficiency in elderly home services providers (KPMG, 2013).

The second type includes schemes that are partially or fully subsidized by the government and executed by NGOs, religious groups or charitable organizations. This financing model is commonly found in Australia and Hong Kong (KPMG, 2013). The government or the state partially or fully supports NGOs operated by qualified religious groups or charitable organizations that provide elderly home services and monitors and evaluates the efficiency, quality and performance in the elderly home service delivery.

The third type includes schemes that operate without government subsidies. The elderly home services providers are private or for-profit operators with a self-financing model. This type is an out-of-pocket payment model and is mostly found in developed countries, such as Australia, Canada, the US, Hong Kong, and China (KPMG, 2013; OECD, 2016). International and domestic healthcare companies have started to enter the emerging market to provide high-end home care services and facilities (Deloitte, 2014). This funding model is supported mainly by the significant population who are likely to be willing to pay for individual elderly home services. This model tends not to have the moral hazard problem but is likely to exclude the poor elderly who cannot afford to pay for private elderly home services.

The fourth type is based on co-payments that are funded by a mix of employer contributions, individual payments based on income-based insurance contributions, and/or central taxes (KPMG, 2013). This funding model is often used in developed countries, such as Canada, France, Germany, Netherlands, Japan, and Singapore. Individuals could share the financial burden with the government.

Despite the various operational models that exist to address the aging population, the quality standards and performance among these different types of elderly home service providers need to be carefully measured, examined and evaluated.

Performance Measurement Systems

Performance measurement systems embrace a range of indicators to assess how well an organization performs from financial and non-financial perspectives efficiently and effectively (Hilton and Platt, 2015). The commonly used operational performance measures for the modern production environment are broadly classified into seven types: raw material and scrap, inventory, machinery, product and service quality, production and delivery, productivity, and innovation and learning (Hilton and Platt, 2015).

Contemporary performance measurement systems (CPMS), for example, the balanced scorecard, provide an effective means of management to examine a range of financial and non-financial performance measures by typically examining four important areas: financial, internal business process, customer, and learning and growth (Franco-Santosa et al., 2012; Hilton and Platt, 2015). CPMS could be viewed as a system that translates business strategies into measurable results for targeting pre-set goals, thereby helping senior management review and adjust the organizational plans. Effective CPMS is regarded as an important management control system (MCS) that could seek to provide managers with more extensive feedback about the organization's operations and thereby unveil areas for enhancing performance (Hall, 2011). The balanced scorecard, for example, provides a fair range of measures linked with strategy to help facilitate the learning and development process (Hilton and Platt, 2015).

The effectiveness of CPMS in public sector organizations depends both on contractibility and on how the system is being used by managers. These findings have important implications, both for practitioners and for public policy makers (Spekléa and Verbeeten, 2014). Yuen and Ng's (2012) study shows that a balanced performance measurement system would also be relevant to elderly homes, and this result supports the operation of a proper governance system to monitor the quality performance beyond a minimal degree of compliance, with accountability to public funding providers.

Accreditation Systems

Quality assurance in nursing homes is achieved through a set of procedures within an accreditation scheme that aims to promote excellence in the provision of care in a given care facility. The specific performance standards act as levels of achievement to be maintained, referred to as the 'quality', and the process of verifying that the 'quality' is achieved is referred to as 'assurance' (Pallassana & Patchner, 1987). Efforts to contain operating costs while achieving an optimal number of residents (clients) have introduced competition among care providers. Means of measuring the care quality and comparing providers against a set of performance indicators were first developed in the 1960s, using structural measures to examine both the 'process' and 'outcome' of care (Mor et al., 2003).

Following the experience in developed nations, such as Australia, Canada, the U.K. and the U.S., Hong Kong started to adopt an accreditation scheme through a 2-year trial program beginning in 2002. The Hong Kong Association of Gerontology obtained recognition from the International Society for Quality Assurance in Health Care (ISQua) in 2008 and was acknowledged as an 'Accredited Certification Body of Certification of Residential Care Homes (Elderly Persons) Service Providers' Management System' by the Hong Kong Accreditation Service of the Innovation and Technology Commission in 2014. Hong Kong has now developed its own systematic quality assurance process. On the other hand, Macau has just initiated a movement to accredit nursing homes under the government subsidiary program, with few providers having obtained an accreditation certificate thus far.

Based on a literature review of operational models and funding sources, performance measurement systems and accreditation systems, the purpose of this study is to explore and examine the similarities and differences in the development of performance measures and accreditation systems for the quality assurance of care service providers in four different jurisdictions of the world. Prior health care studies have paid relatively little attention to comparing various management perspectives in elderly care settings in various jurisdictions (KPMG, 2013). This study could deepen the understanding of performance management in the context of elderly home care services. The next section will present a proposed framework to evaluate the accreditation approach.

PROPOSED THEORETICAL FRAMEWORK

This proposed theoretical framework suggests that the accreditation approach of a jurisdiction could be influenced by three main sets of factors, namely, Social and cultural background, Operational model and Externalities (See Figure 1). The social and cultural background is influenced by the historical development and country system and thereby the particular expectations of the local stakeholders for an acceptable model for developing elderly care service providers. The operational model is largely related to the type and range of financial resources that support the operations of an elderly home. Externalities would be dominated by the regulators' consideration of the need to strengthen regulatory controls as well as demands by the end-users for quality performance. These three main forces would ultimately determine the accreditation approach, compulsory or otherwise, for strengthening the elderly care service providers.

Figure 1.

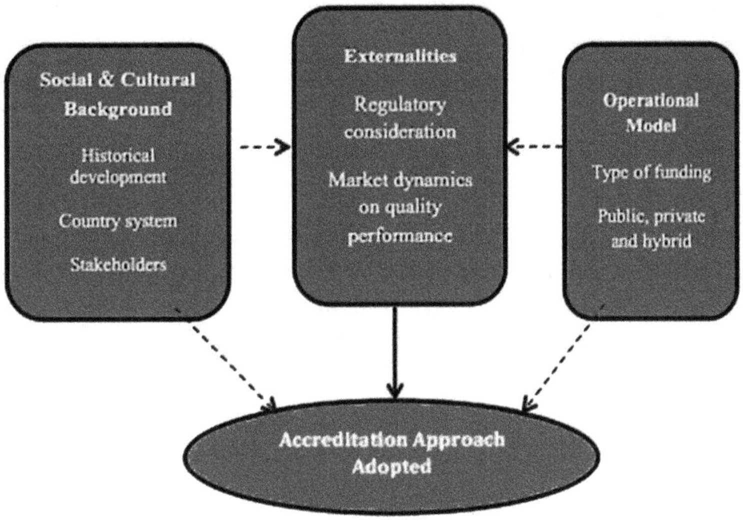

RESEARCH DESIGN

This book chapter will employ a multiple case study approach (Yin, 2003) to explore and examine the similarities and differences in the development of performance measurement systems and accreditation processes of health care service providers in four different jurisdictions of the world, Hong Kong and Macau in Asia and Australia and Canada in the West. Hong Kong and Macau have been selected for their British and Portuguese colonial backgrounds, so that they face an increasing rate of aging population growth with limited government support in providing elderly home care services under the mixture of a Western administrative system and traditional Chinese culture. Australia and Canada have been selected for both being Commonwealth nations that have long-term care systems for the elderly, supportive programs, and proper governance.

The elderly home service operators will be the embedded unit of analysis in the four different research contexts (See Yin, 2003). Evidence from multiple cases is often regarded as more compelling and robust than that from a single case study (Yin, 2003). This approach could allow researchers to compare and contrast the findings from various case studies (Bryman and Bell, 2007). Such an approach could in turn encourage researchers to consider the similarities and differences among multiple cases and promote theoretical reflection on the findings (Bryman and Bell, 2007). The secondary data were obtained from government official reports, consultancy reports and academic papers via websites to ensure data triangulation (Yin, 2003).

COMPARATIVE CASE STUDIES

Looking into the policies for regulating elderly care service providers in four different jurisdictions, comparative case studies are adopted to study the commonalities as well as contrasts among them. For instance, the common Euro-colonial backgrounds of Hong Kong and Macau and the development of their elderly care services under the influence of Western administrative systems within traditional Chinese cultures are characterized in comparison with the highlighted Commonwealth nations of Australia and Canada. Hong Kong, in particular, has been perceived as largely embracing a "laissez-faire" approach that allows the market to evolve and provide services as needed through profit-oriented and non-profit, charitable organizations, a mostly self-financing mechanism. Accreditation in Hong Kong is so far largely done on a voluntary basis by individual entities, aiming to differentiate oneself as a quality service provider as part of a marketing strategy with a competitive advantage for attracting premier customers and funding support. Under a seemingly more democratic process influenced by the stakeholders, the provinces of Canada have passed regulations to strengthen the accountability for quality performance, resulting in more public resources for accredited elderly care institutions. Top-down funding models for subvented entities continue to exist among the cases. It is worthwhile to highlight that each of these selected jurisdictions is considered a research context for these comparative case studies. This study approach enables us to understand the spectrum of performance measurements and accreditation approaches for elderly care service providers being adopted by governments in different parts of the world.

The Post-Colonial Cities

Hong Kong

The Hong Kong Social Welfare Department has implemented the 'Standardized Care Need Assessment Mechanism for Elderly Services' in 2000. This is an internationally recognized assessment tool to ascertain the type of care needed for each individual elderly person, including assignment to a nursing home under the government's subsidized scheme (Hong Kong Social Welfare Department, 2001). Services ranging from low to high levels of care (residential care services, hostels, homes for the aged, care and attention homes, nursing homes and infirmary units) are available to each eligible elderly person subject to the assessment. The purpose of this assessment is to provide appropriate care services to the elderly who cannot be adequately taken care of at home. Generally, the policy direction of the Hong Kong SAR Government has recognized the importance of 'aging in place' by which the majority of the elderly can age at their own homes; however, with a high institutionalization rate (6.8%) and a projected rise in the elderly population to close to 21.9% by 2026 accompanied by decreased fertility and increased longevity (Chui et al., 2009), Hong Kong will face an unprecedented challenge in meeting the long-term care demands.

Historically, NGOs mainly provided two different types of residential care services, 'care and attention homes' and 'nursing homes', but these settings may not be equipped with facilities or needed components for long-term care services. The government then introduced a conversion program in 2005 to incorporate long-term care components and upgraded facilities into these settings without relocating the residents as a continuum of the care strategy. 37% of the residential care services are provided through a subsidized scheme, while the majority of 63% are provided either by self-financed contract homes or private homes (Social Welfare Department, 2016). These services are largely funded through a tax-based model, which would pose a tremendous fiscal burden on public finance in the foreseeable future simultaneously with fast-growing demands on residential care services. To reduce the waiting time for residential care services for the elderly, the government recently launched "The Pilot Scheme on Community Care Service Vouchers for the Elderly" in 2013, and this new funding mode allowed eligible elderly persons to select community care services (CCS) for their individual needs (Social Welfare Department, 2017).

At present, the government does not provide long-term care services directly within its administrative structure but rather (i) provides subvention to service providers (NGOs) while the Social Welfare Department monitors the quality of their services delivered, (ii) provides subsidies for elderly placement at private residential care homes through the Nursing Home Place Purchase Scheme (NHPPS), and (iii) provides subsidies to selected service providers as Residential Care Homes for the Elder (RCHEs) through a competitive bidding program for contracts of operation under a specific termed subsidy scheme (Social Welfare Department, 2016). This is a mixed public-private service model where plans and management are devised by the central government but the specific operative functions are decentralized to a lower level of government office and the service providers are independently operated while being closely monitored by the government.

Though the Hong Kong Association of Gerontology is a recognized accredited body for the quality assurance and accreditation of elderly homes, the participation in such a quality assessment is on a voluntary basis, and there is not yet a locally agreed upon assurance system employed for all RCHEs. The Social Welfare Department is responsible to assure the quality of the operating RCHEs with its licensing control system, but this is only to ensure the basic quality of service and not a formal quality assessment process. A recent incident involving a breach of privacy and care in private nursing homes caused the general public to raise concerns about their quality, and this highlighted the importance of the proper regulation and promotion of healthy aging in homes for the elderly. However, the current mechanism of voluntary accreditation raised a number of practical concerns in the following (Chui et al., 2009):

1. A lack of standardization of an accreditation system that can be mandatorily employed for all RCHEs
2. The cost of accreditation is considerable, especially for private operators or self-financing RCHEs.
3. The time and cost for the training of staff required for the preparation for such an accreditation process are high and may not be aligned with the timeframe of the government's policy agenda.

Many large-scale NGOs are unlikely to develop new or large-scale self-financing residential care services as it was not the agency's vision or long-term strategy to start up 'market-oriented' services. Their services would mainly be 'need-driven'. If the NGOs were to maintain the same high level of service quality, it would be impossible for them to compete at a relatively low price (Social Welfare Department, 2001).

Macau

Macau has just initiated an accreditation movement for residential care facilities. With a total population of 588,000 and 14.8% of the population over 60, Macau is considered an aging society (The United Nations Population Fund, 2015). Residential care services are mainly provided by NGOs, with 11 not-for-profit service operators (10 under the government's subsidized scheme) and nine private operators. Similar to Hong Kong, social services in Macau are largely funded through a tax-based model, with the administrative government providing financial support while the service quality is monitored by the

Macau Social Welfare Bureau. This can also be considered a 'contemporary mixed economy' social service delivery approach with a heavy influence from the regional government, where the market occupancy has shrunk for the private sector due to resource shortages and quality concerns.

The quality assurance process has not been firmly established, and it is not a statutory requirement for residential care service operators to attain certification in Macau. At present, the service quality is mainly monitored by the Macau Social Welfare Bureau through a licensing system. Until 2010, NGO service operators were assessed against criteria partly extracted from the accreditation system adopted by the Hong Kong Association of Gerontology mentioned above, but this was without official certification. Service operators are encouraged to participate in a complete accreditation assessment as a self-initiated process. It is under the government policy agenda to increase the number of residential placements to 2,300 beds by 2018 (Government, 2016), so a proper accredited quality assurance system is greatly needed to promote continuing quality improvement in long-term care facilities.

As for private service operators, their market occupancy still remains low; they are not required to participate in the quality assurance process, and there is no incentive for it. There are concerns regarding the discrepancies in quality and service fees between private- and NGO- operated services; most elderly people and their family members prefer to reside in government-subsidized residential care services and are willing to be on their waiting lists given their higher service quality and being better equipped with professional personnel.

With the increase in the aging population and frailty of elderly people, the waiting lists for residential care services will continue to grow, and the waiting time will correspondingly increase, so the level of care to be provided in residential care settings would also be increased substantially. Government authorities need to formulate ways to promote quality homes for the elderly in addition to licensing requirements. A mandatory accredited quality assurance scheme will be necessary in the foreseeable future given the high expectations upheld by the service users and their family members, either from a practical or moral perspective. A low tax model in these two special administrative regions would support the current publicly funded industry; the heavily subsidized long-term care delivery model may not be sustainable in the long run.

However, the changing socio-economic profile of the future elderly cohort would imply that they would be better positioned financially to pursue a long-term retirement strategy. Thus, it is important to provide preventive health care and rehabilitation services to reduce their dependence and need for long-term care so that they can live independently with dignity.

Table 1. Comparison between Hong Kong and Macau regarding service delivery models and quality assurance systems for residential care services for elderly

	Hong Kong SAR	**Macau SAR**
Similarities	• A number of government-subsidized NGOs operations through subvention arrangement • Funding supported by low tax-based model • Accredited quality assurance is NOT mandatory • No standardization of the quality assurance system for all service operators • Basic quality checks are done by a government office through a licensing system • Assessment to referral through government office assessment unit	
Differences	Private operators have become major contributors to residential care services	NGO operators have become major contributors to residential care services

The New World Experiences

As part of the Commonwealth system, Australia and Canada represent New World examples in the development of their elderly care services. Both of them have developed legislations for regulating elderly care services and institutionalization of elderly care where public funding plays a key part for their source of financing. A non-profit provider accreditation system has become critical to ensure that public funding is utilized for quality service while safeguarding public interests under a democratic system: a model for accountability.

Australia

In Australia, standardized care measurements were first introduced in 1987. At a time when the assessment of the residential care quality had been poorly addressed, the government appointed 'Standards Monitoring Teams' for assessing residential care facilities' compliance with the Standards (Gibson, 1998). Then, the Australian government formalized the 'Quality of Care Principles' on the 1st of July, 2014 under the Aged Care Act 1997. The general goal of this principle is to ensure that aged care providers are operated in accordance with legislative requirements to provide the highest quality and safety of care under the framework of continuous quality improvement strategies (Australian Government Aged Care Financing Authority, 2015). Residential aged care homes are required to be accredited through an accreditation program to receive subsidies from the Australian Government. The accreditation process consists of self-assessment, review or assessment of performance, and monitoring of ongoing performance against predetermined standards by an external independent assessment body. This process comprises four standards with 44 outcome measures as the accreditation standards, including (i) management systems, staffing and organizational development; (ii) health and personal care; (iii) residents' lifestyle and (iv) physical environment and safe systems. The accreditation system is thus intended to provide a systematic approach to the management of care quality with sets of expected outcomes.

It is compulsory for all residential aged care providers to abide by this standard of care, despite the financial status of the residents, service fees and amount of residential care subsidy received. Thus, government funding is tied to the achievement of national benchmarks of quality for the care provided (CEPAR, 2014). Despite the Australian residential aged care system being highly regulated and subject to multiple assessments, there is still a gap in terms of determining the quality of care practices being utilized, especially in the clinical outcomes (Australian Government Aged Care Financing Authority, 2015).

The aged care industry is undergoing a significant change as it adjusts to a more consumer-driven market and demographic challenges. An annual report issued by the Aged Care Financing Authority estimated that the residential care sector will need to build approximately 76,000 additional places over the next decade based on the Government's service provision targets, which involve an investment of AUS $31 billion (Australian Government Aged Care Financing Authority, 2015). There are 1,024 providers in the residential care sector currently operating, with 66.7% of the services provided considered 'high-care' service but only 4.2% classified as 'low-care' service. 652 (63.7%) are considered either 'not-for-profit' or 'government'-owned services. This over-representation of not-for-profit and government providers is alarming for the financial sustainability of the government budget, since they are operated with either full or partial subsidy from the government (state and federal) or may rely on their communities' donations or past surpluses (which may not be stable over time). Since Australia ranked 10th in the world for life expectancy with a high standard of living GDP per capital estimated at US$ 42,400, population aging is expected to result in increased demand for long-term care services, in particular at a high level of care (Hibbert, Hannaford, Long, Plumb, & Braithwaite, 2013). The ARC Centre of Excellence in Population Ageing Research (CEPAR) reported that the aged care expenditure is projected to rise to 1.8-2.2% in 2050, while funding is channeled to care providers (home care and residential care) based on each individual's assessed care complexity and needs (CEPAR, 2014).

The OECD has classified aged care funding models into three types, including single universal, mixed and safety net systems. Mixed systems have three sub-types: parallel universal, means-tested and a fragmented mix of these. Australia has adopted the means-tested scheme under the mixed model type, where benefits are withdrawn based on an individual's level of income or wealth. Such benefits are traditionally related to in-kind services, where a provider delivers care to a needs- and means-assessed individual and is paid by the government. 93% of the aged care expenditure is contributed by the taxpayer through a relatively high tax scheme compared to regions mentions above. Though the Australian government attempted to transfer the funding responsibility for aged care from the states to the Commonwealth to ensure national standardization, there is still difficulty in estimating the societal 'actual' demand, since the demand may potentially outweigh our current supply (Australian Government Aged Care Financing Authority, 2015). It is also unclear whether the increased life expectancy will be accompanied by increased years in poor health, since evidence is mixed suggesting that the disability-free life expectancy has increased with the increased number of expected years with a disability and with severe functional limitations between 1998 and 2009 in Australia (CEPAR, 2014). In addition, the number of people with dementia is projected to increase significantly, which implies additional investment in specialist care in any format of long-term care services.

There is a complex interaction between the population aging and development in chronic disease trends, performance limitations and disability. The demands for formal aged care services depend on policy investment and the availability of service types and their functionality. Therefore, an accreditation system and an recognized accreditation body become critical to ensure that public funding is utilized for quality service while safeguarding public interests under a democratic system: a model for accountability.

Canada

As a country that respects human rights, Canada's Health Act imposes "criteria that guarantee all Canadians access to medically necessary physician and hospital services free of financial or other barriers within a system publicly administered on a non-profit basis" (Madore, 2004, p. 20). However, as Canada's constitution delegates health care responsibilities to its provincial jurisdictions, its health policy is developed through a range of interrelated federal–provincial relationships. There are 10 provinces and 3 northern territories in Canada, which vary in terms of size, fiscal budget and extent of economic and social developments. It is challenging to meet their various expectations and requirements of health care services with standardized financial arrangements and homogeneous efforts. While the federal government provides funding for particular health programs, such as public health, hospital construction, and training health personnel, the individual provinces are responsible for most of their operating expenses and capital expenditures.

Financing the Canadian health care system is strategized within individual provinces as they need to address market failure with a series of cost-sharing programs within the provinces (Deber, 2003). In 1957, the Hospital Insurance and Diagnostic Services Act was passed to support approximately half of the cost of provincial insurance plans for hospital-based care subject to specified national conditions.

In 1966, the Medical Care Act cost-shared provincial insurance plans for physician services were introduced under similar provisions. All provinces by 1971 developed plans to insure their populations for hospital and physician services. Since provinces have their own jurisdictions, there are still considerable variations among the Canadian provinces. While the financing arrangements were changed in 1977 to a combination of cash- and tax-based arrangements, through the Canada Health Act in 1984, the federal government ensured that the provinces and territories comply with certain requirements, such as free and universal access to publicly insured health care. Under such an arrangement, provincial plans are required to offer insured health services based on unified terms and conditions (Madore, 2004).

Under this background, elderly care services are currently stipulated at the provincial level. For instance, in Ontario, the Long-Term Care Act was legislated in 1994 to bring nursing homes, homes for the aged and charitable homes under the purview of the Ministry of Health and Long-term Care (MHLTC). Such regulations were passed in response to the "scandals" and poor evaluations of long-term care facilities with the objective of improving long-term care services while strengthening accountability under Residents' Bills of Rights (Banerjee, 2007). Each province in Canada tends to develop its own regulations emphasizing compliance with the expected quality of services for elderly care. To provide an economic incentive to participate in the process, Ontario elderly care services providers with accreditation status are reimbursed at a higher rate (per bed day) by the MHLTC (McDonald et al., 2015).

From a Market-Based Approach to a Public-Private Partnership Model

The proposed theoretical framework used three main factors, namely, social and cultural background, operational model and externalities, to examine the development of performance and accredited quality assurance of care service providers in four jurisdictions of the world, including Hong Kong, Macau, Australia and Canada (See Table 2). In the comparison between the 'Post-Colonial' and the 'New World' models based on the proposed framework of the analysis, it appears that the New World system has looked to accreditation as either mandatory or a necessary hurdle for economic incentives for the adoption of quality assurance.

Social and Cultural Background

All of the selected countries were previously British or Portuguese colonies. Hong Kong and Macau became a Special Administrative Regions (SARs) within the People's Republic of China (PRC) in 1997 and 1999, respectively, and have the obligation to abide by its Basic Law at a high degree of autonomy for 50 years. Hong Kong still continues to adopt the British common law system, while Macau adopts the Portuguese civil law system. In stark contrast, however, Australia and Canada declared independence in 1904 and 1867, respectively, as Commonwealth nations and continue to adopt the common law system and the democratic political system.

Across these countries, the estimated percentage of the population aged 60 or above in 2015 is 20%. However, the projected percentage of the population aged 60 or above in 2050 shows an alarming trend for Hong Kong (40.9%), Macau (34.5%), Australia (28.5%) and Canada (32.4%) (United Nations Population Fund, 2015). Elderly care services of the selected regions in Asia initiated performance measurement systems and accreditation systems in the 2000s. However, the quality assurance systems of the Asian countries tend to lag behind those of the Western countries. The accreditation of the elderly care

Table 2. Comparison of multiple cases based on the proposed theoretical framework

	Hong Kong	Macau	Australia	Canada
Part I – Social and Cultural Background				
Historical background	Previously a British colony	Previously a Portuguese colony	Previously a British colony	Previously a British colony
Country system	• Became a Special Administrative Region of China in 1997 • Continues to adopt Common Law while abiding to its Basic Law • High degree of autonomy for 50 years	• Became a Special Administrative Region of China in 1999 • Continues to adopt the Portuguese civil law system while abiding to its Basic Law • High degree of autonomy for 50 years	• Declared independence in 1904 (a Commonwealth nation) • Continues to adopt Common Law • Democratic political system • Federation of States and Territories	• Declared independence in 1867 (a Commonwealth nation) • Continues to adopt Common Law • Democratic political system
Population (2015)[1]	7,288 thousands	588 thousands	23,969 thousands	35,940 thousands
Aging Population (2015)[2]	1,581 thousands	87 thousands	4,887 thousands	8,021 thousands
Part II – Operational Model				
Operational model	NGOs and government-owned services; private operations	NGOs and private operators	NGOs and government-owned services	NGOs and government-owned services; private operations
Sources of funding	Tax-based model for subsidized operations; direct support by government; fees-based self-financing model	Tax-based model for subsidized operations; fees-based self-financing model	Tax-based model for subsidized operations; means-tested scheme under the mixed model; fees-based self-financing model	Tax-based model for subsidized operations; out-of-pocket payment model and co-payment model; fees-based self-financing model
Part III – Externalities				
Regulation on quality assurance system	Voluntary; licensing system	Voluntary; licensing system	Accreditation is mandatory for subsidies from government	Accreditation is voluntary to achieve better quality services, with economic incentives for accredited facilities
Market dynamics	Market-driven service > Need-driven market	Need-driven market > Market-driven service	Moving towards market-driven service from need-driven market	Moving towards market-driven service from need-driven market

[1] The information is based on the United Nations (2015)

[2] Aging Population in 2015 is referred to population aged 60 or over (The United Nations Population Fund, 2015)

services offered by the government with a combination of different operators could affect the expectations of local stakeholders.

The cultural factor could provide some thoughtful insights into why the elderly care services in Asian countries were commenced slower than those in the selected Western countries. Due to the traditional Chinese culture, 'home care' by their children, rather than home care or residential home care, could be the ideal choice for most of the elderly. Filial piety could be viewed as a core value in Chinese traditional culture but has been increasingly diluted due to the economic development, demographic change, and social migration over the past few decades (WHO, 2015). Over 60% of the Chinese elderly seek institutional care when their children could not provide health care at home or would be a financial burden for their children (Wong and Leung, 2012). Furthermore, more women work for a living rather than devoting their time to take care of their parents. In the absence of an adequate elderly care system and care management system, this is expected to have an adverse impact on family relationships and social harmony (WHO, 2015). Thus, home- and community-based care is seen as a cost-effective way to provide a better quality of life and a cultural preference, particularly in Asian countries (KPMG, 2013; WHO, 2015).

In the Western culture, the concepts of wellness and holism are the notion of self-care (Lewis, 2002). Self-care refers to individuals arranging meaningful and effective activities by themselves to maintain healthy lifestyles, and individuals are expected to be responsible for their life choices, such as in nutrition, exercise, and stress-management programs, to result in good health (Lewis, 2002). With decreasing fertility rates, higher divorce rates, and more children living away from their parents in the Western culture, elderly people tend not to receive traditional family-based care from their families (KPMG, 2013). Therefore, home care or residential home care could be regarded as the best options.

Both Australia and Canada under their existing political systems have managed to pass legislations to enforce more stringent measures for monitoring and inspecting quality performance among subsidized elderly home service providers. Such regulations are linked to the allocation of public funding for subsidizing the operations of accredited elderly homes.

Operational Model

The operational models of elderly care service operators in the Asian countries are somewhat similar to those in the Western countries. The governments of the selected countries tend to take greater responsibility for funding residential care services with a semi-systematic combination of NGOs and public and private operators. However, the Hong Kong SAR Government and the Macau SAR Government seemingly provide rather short-term solutions for elderly care services with subvention and subsidies to both private and non-profit service providers rather than long-term care services as provided by the Australian government and the Canadian government.

The sources of funding for elderly home service providers in Hong Kong and Macau are mainly a tax-based model from the local government for subsidized operation and a fees-based self-financing model. This financing model would be unsustainable in the future (Yuen, 2014), when a gradual increase in the aging population will be coupled with a decrease in the labor force participation rate, so that the government tax revenue will be expected to decline (Yuen, 2014).

On the other hand, the sources of funding for elderly home service providers in Australia include full or partial subsidy from the government (state and federal) or may rely on their communities' donations or past surpluses (which may not be stable over time). Therefore, the Australian government tends to employ a means-tested scheme under the mixed model. This scheme is based on an individual's level of income or wealth. Such benefits were traditionally related to in-kind services, where a provider delivers care to a needs- and means-assessed individual and is paid by the government. The Australian government attempted to allocate the funding to the Commonwealth to ensure the national standardization of aged care. Canadian provinces have attempted a similar approach as well. However, some provinces levy particular health premiums, and individuals are expected to contribute via co-payments, out-of-pocket payment models and fees-based self-financing models that vary by province, service and income level (KPMG, 2013).

Externalities

The performance measurement and accredited quality assurance of elderly care service operators in Hong Kong and Macau are completely different from those in Australia and Canada. Under these two jurisdictions in Asia, the performance measurement and accredited quality assurance are neither a statutory requirement by the Hong Kong government and the Macau government or mandatory from the health care industry. There is no standardization of the quality assurance systems for all service operators in Hong Kong and Macau. The current accreditation scheme tends to be on a voluntary basis due to the high cost of accreditation for private operators and time-consuming process of training staffs to prepare for the accreditation process. Thus, both the Social Welfare Department of the Hong Kong SAR Government and the Macau Social Welfare Bureau of the Macau SAR Government are responsible for accessing the basic quality check of elderly services provided by NGOs and public and private operators with its licensing control system.

By contrast, the Australian government has established the 'Quality of Care Principles' under the Aged Care Act 1997. This principle is to ensure that aged care providers are operated in accordance with legislative requirements to provide the highest quality and safety of care. Residential aged care homes are required to be accredited by an external independent assessment agency. Similar to Canada, the Australian government subsidy and financial funding is associated with the achievement of national benchmarks of quality assurance for elderly care service operators.

Several developed countries, such as Canada, Australia, and the UK, have adopted 'global budgeting' that creates a central funding pool for both institutional care and home-based and community-based services rather than separating these two budgets (KPMG, 2013). This innovative funding model has not only enhanced the flexibility in the elderly healthcare services but also better monitored them with a single administrative authority (KPMG, 2013).

Based on this observation, the market dynamics of the quality performance in Hong Kong are 'market-driven' markets rather than 'need-driven' markets due to over 60% of the elderly home care services being provided by private or self-financed operators. However, the aging population is still increasing in the future. Macau is primarily based on a 'need-driven' market from the government policy of 5 Year Development Plans between 2016 and 2020 (Macau SAR Government, 2016). The market dynamics of Australia and Canada could be shifted from 'need-driven' markets to 'market-driven' ones, as there are more demands on such services. The quality of unregulated and unaccredited profit-oriented service providers rushing to the market could remain a significant concern among the aging societies in the years to come.

CONCLUSION

This study is intended to explore and examine the similarities and differences in the development of performance measures and accreditation systems for the quality assurance of care service providers in four selected jurisdictions. This study is based on a multiple-case study approach with secondary data. According to the proposed theoretical framework, the selected case studies show the social and cultural background, operational model, and externalities of elderly service providers.

The findings suggest that the governments of the selected countries tend to take greater responsibility for funding residential care services with a semi-systematic combination of NGOs and public and private operators. The findings also indicate that the main source of funding for elderly home service providers in four selected countries is a tax-based model from the government for subsidized operation and a fees-based self-financing model. In addition, the overall performance measurement and accredited quality assurance of elderly care service operators in both Hong Kong and Macau operate largely on a voluntary basis. They appear to lag behind those of the Western countries and undergo their own peculiar paths of development. Thus, Hong Kong and Macau should look into practical experience from Australia and Canada in terms of the system of their funding, accredited quality assurance and assessment tools under an increasingly market-driven service sector in which the well-being of the end-users needs to be adequately protected.

Elderly care service operators in Hong Kong and Macau could obtain practical experience from Australia and Canada in a number of potential areas. First, the source of funding for elderly home service providers could shift from a tax-based model from the local government to a co-payment model that is funded by a mix of employer contribution, individual payment and central taxes. This model could share the fiscal burden on the public health expenditure on a long-term basis. Second, the accredited quality assurance of elderly care services is not mandatory in either Hong Kong or Macau. The government could appoint an external and independent assessment body or an international accreditation agency within the long-term care system to monitor the quality of elderly care service providers. With the accreditation standards and the benchmarks, the government could allocate resources effectively and efficiently. Third, the government should consider adopting elderly care standardized assessment tools and a rigorous performance measurement system to evaluate the long-term elder care services and care packages to cope with the increasing aging population. Such a system enables the effective monitoring of performance while providing adequate transparency over the services delivered to such a vulnerable group in society. Further, the active engagement of the stakeholders, particularly the family members, would bring in new opportunities for identifying areas for performance improvement while enhancing the overall quality of the elderly care services.

This book chapter is primarily based on a multiple-case study approach using secondary data. Future studies could be positioned in several research directions. First, future studies could draw on primary data, such as interviews, focus groups and participation observation. An in-depth case study approach could explore the possible challenges of performance measurement and accreditation systems. Second, future research is needed to examine which integrated operational models and funding sources could be the appropriate, effective and efficient to deliver the services of elderly care services. Third, future studies could investigate the relationship between elderly care service providers and users and other related stakeholder groups in particular cultural and institutional contexts.

REFERENCES

Australian Government Aged Care Financing Authority. (2015). *Factors Influencing the Financial Performance of Residential Aged Care Providers*. Canberra: Australian Government Aged Care Financing Authority.

Banerjee, A. (2007). *An Overview of Long-Term Care in Canada in Selected Provinces and Territories, Women and Health Care Reform Group*. Toronto: York University.

Bernoth, M., Dietsch, E., Burmeister, O. K., & Schwartz, M. (2014). Information Management in Aged Care: Cases of Confidentiality and Elder Abuse. *Journal of Business Ethics*, *122*(3), 453–460. doi:10.100710551-013-1770-7

Bryman, A., & Bell, E. (2007). *Business Research Method*. Oxford, UK: Oxford University Press.

Chui, W. T., Chan, K. S., Chong, M. L., Ko, S. F., Law, C. K., Law, C. K., ... Ng, Y. T. (2009). *Elderly Commission's Study on Residential Care Services for the Elderly*. Hong Kong: The University of Hong Kong.

De Meijer, C., Wouterse, B., Polder, J., & Koopmanschap, K. (2013). The effect of population aging on health expenditure growth: A critical review. *European Journal of Ageing*, *10*(4), 353–361. doi:10.100710433-013-0280-x

Deber, R. B. (2003). Health Care Reform: Lessons from Canada. *American Journal of Public Health*, *93*(1), 20–24. doi:10.2105/AJPH.93.1.20 PMID:12511378

Deloitte. (2014). *Fortune Favors the Bold Shifting to Private Health*. Deloitte.

Ernst and Young. (2015). *Megatrends 2015: Making sense of a world motion*. Ernst and Young.

Franco-Santosa, M., Lucianetti, L., & Bourne, M. (2012). Contemporary performance measurement systems: A review of their consequences and a framework for research. *Management Accounting Research*, *23*(2), 79–119. doi:10.1016/j.mar.2012.04.001

Gibson, D. (1998). *Aged care: Old policies, new problems*. Melbourne: Cambridge University Press.

Hall, M. (2011). Do comprehensive performance measurement systems help or hinder managers mental model development? *Management Accounting Research*, *22*(2), 68–83. doi:10.1016/j.mar.2010.10.002

Hibbert, P., Hannaford, N., Long, J., Plumb, J., & Braithwaite, J. (2013). *Final Report: Performance indicators used internationally to report publicly on healthcare organisations and local health systems*. Australian Institute of Health Innovation.

Hilton, R. W. & Platt, E. W. (2015). *Managerial Accounting: Creating Value in a Dynamic Business Environment*. Singapore: McGraw Hill Education.

KPMG (2013). *An uncertain age: Reimaging long term care in the 21st century*. KPMG International.

Lewis, C. B. (2002). *Aging: The Health-Care Challenge*. Philadelphia: F. A. Davis Company.

Madore, O. (2004). *The Canada Health Act: Overview and Options*. Parliamentary Information and Research Service.

MarketLine. (2014). *MarketLine Industry Profile: Healthcare Providers in Asia-Pacific*. London: MarketLine.

McDonald, S.M., Wagner, L.M., & Gruneir, A. (2015). Accreditation and Resident Safety in Ontario Long-Term Care Homes. *Healthcare quarterly (Toronto, Ont.)*, *18*(1), 54-9.

Mission of the Statistics and Census Service (DSEC). (2016). *Population Statistics 2016 1st Quarter Report*. Macau: Statistics and Census Service.

Mor, V., Berg, K., Angelelli, J., Gifford, D., Morris, J., & Moore, T. (2003). The Quality of Quality Measurement in U.S. Nursing Homes. *The Gerontologist*, *43*(2Supplement 2), 37–46. doi:10.1093/geront/43.suppl_2.37 PMID:12711723

OECD. (2015). *Health at a glance 2015: OCED indicators*. Paris: OECD Publishing.

OECD. (2016). *OECD Health Statistics 2015*. Retrieved May 14, 2016, from http://stats.oecd.org/index.aspx?DataSetCode=HEALTH_STAT

Pallassana, R. B., & Patchner, M. A. (1987). *Quality Assurance in Nursing Homes: Jane Addams School of Social Work*. Urbana, IL: Illinois University.

Spekléa, R. F., & Verbeeten, F. H. M. (2014). The use of performance measurement systems in the public sector: Effects on performance. *Management Accounting Research*, *25*(2), 131–146. doi:10.1016/j.mar.2013.07.004

The ARC Centre of Excellence in Population Ageing Research (CEPAR). (2014). *Aged care in Australia: Part I - policy, demand and funding*. Australian Research Council.

The Hong Kong Social Welfare Department. (2001). *Legislative Council Panel On Welfare Services - Allocation of New Social Welfare Service Units, Provision of Residential Care Home Services for the Elders through Open Tender*. Hong Kong: Social Welfare Department.

The Hong Kong Social Welfare Department. (2016). *Provision of Residential Care Services for Elders (Subsidised versus Non-subsidised Places)*. Hong Kong: Social Welfare Department.

The Macau SAR Government. (2016). *Consultative Paper on the 5 Year Development Plans (2016-2020)*. Macau: The Macau SAR Government.

The Social Welfare Department. (2017). *First Phase of the Pilot Scheme on Community Care Service Voucher for the Elderly (Pilot Scheme)*. Retrieved 11 Feb 2017, from http://www.swd.gov.hk/en/index/site_pubsvc/page_elderly/sub_csselderly/id_firstphase/

The United Nations. (2015). *World Population Prospects: The 2015 Revision, Key Findings & Advance Table*. New York: The United Nations.

The United Nations Population Fund. (2015). *World Population Ageing in 2015*. New York: The United Nations.

The World Health Organization (WHO). (2000). Health Systems: Improving Performance. Geneva: The World Health Organization.

The World Health Organization (WHO). (2015). China country assessment report on ageing and health. Geneva: Department of Ageing and Life Course, The World Health Organization.

Wong, Y. C., & Leung, J. (2012). Long-term care in China: Issues and Prospects. *Journal of Gerontological Social Work*, *55*(7), 570–586. doi:10.1080/01634372.2011.650319 PMID:22963116

Yin, R. K. (2003). *Case Study Research: Design and Methods*. SAGE Publication. Inc.

Yuen, P. P. (2014). Financing health care and long-term care in a rapidly ageing context: Assessing Hong Kong's readiness. *Public Policy and Administration*, *17*(1), 56–64.

Yuen, P. P., & Ng, A. W. (2012). Towards a balanced performance measurement system in a public health care organization. *International Journal of Health Care Quality Assurance*, *25*(5), 421–430. doi:10.1108/09526861211235919 PMID:22946241

KEY TERMS AND DEFINITIONS

Accreditation System: A system where operators are accredited by an independent agency to attain a certain level of service quality.

Ageing Population: A social phenomenon in which the median age of population in a country increases substantially due to decreasing fertility rates and increasing life expectancy.

Elderly Care: A long-term care composed of different types of services for the special needs of senior citizens.

Funding Sources: The act of providing financial resources to support a project, program or recurring operations.

Multiple-Case Study: A research design that involves the detailed analysis of multiple cases for comparative purposes.

Operational Model: A model of operations adopted by an organization to deliver services to its customers. It takes into consideration the type of legal and ownership structure at formation.

Performance Measurement System: A system that embraces a range of indicators to assess how well an organization performs in financial and non-financial perspectives efficiently and effectively.

Quality Assurance: A series of systematic activities to ensure the quality of products and services in conformance with certain standards in a quality system.

Chapter 8
Integrated Care as a Strategic Solution for Active Aging in the Community:
Tools and Models

Eman Leung
City University of Hong Kong, Hong Kong

Alison Lee
City University of Hong Kong, Hong Kong

Cheuk Wing Chau
City University of Hong Kong, Hong Kong

Youhua (Frank) Chen
City University of Hong Kong, Hong Kong

Diana T. F. Lee
The Chinese University of Hong Kong, Hong Kong

ABSTRACT

A rapidly aging population is an international challenge. Although much has been done, senior citizens today are not experiencing better health than our ancestors (WHO, 2016). This chapter reviews evidence on the current international good practices, the positive clinical and economic impact of integrated care, and how Operations Research/Management Science (OR/MS) methodologies add value to the implementation of integrated care. In the second half of the chapter, three enablers of implementing integrated care are reviewed: 1) a common technological platform, 2) service-restructuring with the introduction of new job roles and recruitment, and 3) creation of a financial model that incentivizes integrated care. In conclusion, while research has shown that integrated care is effective in fostering aging in place, challenges remain as to how it could be implemented given that population aging has increased the demands on healthcare resources. This chapter reviews how OR/MS methodologies can facilitate the implementation of integrated care.

DOI: 10.4018/978-1-5225-2633-9.ch008

BACKGROUND

With the cost of medical and social care skyrocketing in relation to population aging, countries like the UK, Canada, Australia, New Zealand and those in the European Union have shifted their care strategies away from institution-based acute and long-term care (LTC) toward community-based preventive and proactive care, with the goal of maintaining the independence of the elderly.

Achieving this will require care integration that ensures that the right mix of services are available in the right place at the right time, where care is coordinated around the full spectrum of an individual's needs (rather than on single diseases), and prevention of diseases and support for maintaining functional independence of the elderly are prioritized. Successful integrative care employs comprehensive geriatric assessment at the proper time, and offers effective provision of coordinated primary, community and social care services close to home.

It has become clear to the above countries that, while the individual health or care facilities across the care continuum provide high quality services, the previously fragmented services are not meeting the needs of the aging population. Sectorization is seen as a major obstacle to the management of better health, especially for healthcare professionals treating patients with chronic conditions (Busse and Stahl, 2014). It has been shown that the elderly is a group that is most likely to suffer from the challenges in the coordination of care and the transitions between services, and integrated care is therefore a solution to enhance the quality and cost-effectiveness of care for an aging population.

Integrated care has many definitions. Armitage et.al (2009) in a review of the literature concluded that there are 175 definitions and concepts. Most of the definitions are referred to as a continuity of care within the healthcare system, and one expanded that scope to include social services (e.g. housing and meals). Evidence suggests that the integration between medical and social care improves subjective experience, care outcomes, and efficiency. In terms of care outcomes, Ouwens, Wollersheim, Hermens, Hulscher and Grol (2005) conducted a systematic review of integrated care programs for chronically ill patients, and found that functional health status has a positive trend. In one of two studies that performed meta-analyses, the result is found to be significant. There is also a decreasing trend in hospital readmission and length of stay in the three reviews. The authors concluded that integrated care programs have positive effects on care quality. While people of all ages require acute care, post-acute rehabilitation and enablement services, the majority of these resources are currently being allocated to the care of older people. This is true around the world, and particularly in Asia. Hence, an effective integrated elderly care program that improves the cost-effectiveness of elderly care and shortens acute lengths of stay for older people would release poorly utilized resources and make the healthcare system efficient for everyone.

THE HEALTH ECONOMICS OF INTEGRATED CARE AND WAYS OPERATIONS RESEARCH/MANAGEMENT SCIENCES (OR/MS) CAN ADD FURTHER VALUE

In addition to clinical research that demonstrates the impact of integrated care on clinical outcomes, health economists and researchers in the discipline of OR/MS have also demonstrated the health economic values of integrated care, and how healthcare resources could be optimized to deliver integrated care cost-effectively and sustainably in order for the population to age in place. Research has found that hospital admission and cost associated with acute care and long-term care could be reduced if preventive or follow-up care could be provided adequately at the community beyond the walls of hospitals or long-term care institutions.

Care Beyond Acute Care

In the following, studies from Canada, the United States and Hong Kong are reviewed to illustrate how integrated care enhances the cost-effectiveness of the healthcare system.

When the cost and cost-drivers for acute myocardial infarction (AMI) were studied in Canada (Cohen, Manuel, Tugwell, Sanmartin, & Ramsay, 2014), it was found that the cost could be divided into three phases: pre-event state, event state and post-event state, with 25% of the cost associated with pre- and post-event states, which reflect the substantial economic impact of AMI beyond acute care.

The results above resonate with findings indicating that investment in such post-event care is not only good clinical practice but also makes perfect economic sense. Trybou, Spaepen, Vermeulen, Porrez, and Annemans (2013) found that the estimated total financial burden of 1 month and 3 months readmissions across Belgian acute hospitals is around €2.8 billion. If such readmission rate could be reduced to 75 percentile, around €14 million would be saved.

In the United States, Carey and Stefos (2015) found that hospitals could expect to save $2,140 for the average 30-day readmission that had been avoided by care provided beyond the walls of the acute care hospitals. In fact, using sophisticated data mining techniques, Golmohammadi and Radnia (2016) can specify with 80% accuracy a trade-off between taking preventive action such as post-discharge community care, AND planning required resources in advance to care for patients who will be readmitted to the hospital but whose readmissions are avoidable. The author concluded that "the investment will produce a quick payback in eliminating unnecessary claims and achieving a better level on metric that will be an important indicator of the quality of care in ranking health care units in the future".

In the context of Hong Kong, Yam et al. (2010) analyzed all public medical specialty admissions in the year of 2007, and found that around 40.8% of unplanned readmissions could be avoided by an effective discharge planning system, which included improving discharge decision, enhancing patient education on self-management, and better community care. In light of Yam et al.'s insight, a program titled "Integrated Care and Discharge Support for elderly patients" (ICDS) was developed by the Hong Kong Health Authorities (HA) and was implemented in one Hong Kong hospital between 2013 and 2014 as pilot. Patients 60 years of age or older who were identified as high risk by a home-grown clinical risk assessment tool were recruited in this program. A nurse would first assess the needs of the elderly prior to discharge, and those who were at an elevated risk would receive community services coordinated by the hospital's post-discharge multidisciplinary team. The range of services the discharged patients received from the ICDS team included home healthcare and health assessment, telephone support, home assessment and modification, and other social care services such as meal delivery, and household cleaning. Preliminary evaluation (Lin, Luk, Chan, Mok, & Chan, 2015) showed that within a 6-month period, the program had reduced acute hospital admission by 47%, reduced emergency department attendance by 40%, and decreased hospital bed days by 31%. It was estimated that a total of HKD$22.5 million could potentially be saved 1 year after the implementation of the program.

It is clear that care beyond acute care is effective in terms of economics and quality of life, and care coordination has thus become the trend.

OPTIMIZING INTEGRATED CARE PRACTICES WITH OR/MS

While the above research has highlighted the cost-effectiveness of integrating acute care and community care, challenges remains as to how to implement such integrated care given the increasing demands on the scarce healthcare resources. The following review studies employed OR/MS methodologies to further improve the integrated care model in terms of reducing readmission to acute care hospitals, improving access to primary care, improving the care quality across different levels of community care, and optimizing resource planning across the broader care continuum.

Optimizing Access to Community Care and Primary Care

Kucukyazici, Verter, and Mayo (2011) developed an analytical framework for community-based care for chronic diseases utilizing the Markov model to forecast the outcome of stroke survivors in Canada. Their framework has taken into consideration the case-mix biases and care-provider level clustering of the patients. The result suggests that, scheduling a planned visit for post-stroke patients to consult a primary-care provider (PCP) at the point of hospital discharge could reduce the total number of Emergency Room (ER) visits by 13%, re-hospitalizations by 12%, and mortality by 8%; and if the planned visits were with a specialist, ER visits and re-hospitalizations could be reduced by 17% and 11% respectively. However, the average cost per patient is reduced by 10% if the planned visit was with a PCP, versus 7% reduction for a visit with a specialist. Hence this study recommends post-discharge planned visit to a PCP rather than a specialist, in view of the same efficiency that is achieved with lower cost.

Along the same vein, Li, Kong, Chen, and Zheng (2016) suggested that access to care was an essential factor for delivering integrated care in a cost effective manner. They studied travel costs and developed an optimization model for chronic mental diseases. In their study, they criticized the poor access to outpatient care and called for changes in the delivery mode, while exploring ways to optimize multi-site integrated care networks. The team tackled physician assignment and patient demand allocation in the US, and provided solutions for better patient access to outpatient chronic mental care by scheduling appointments.

Kucukyazici and Verter (2013) examined the management of community-based care (CBC) for chronic diseases with different quantitative approaches. For instance, they applied a discrete time finite horizon discounted Markov Decision Process (MDP) in examining capacity allocation in CBC, which comprised of patients with different health states during limited appointment slots in each period. After calibrating their models with operation parameters and disease transitions using historical data, it was shown that CBC could improve the health gains of the community by up to 15% over the current policy.

Minimizing Readmission

In addition to optimizing services in the community and primary care, studies showed that the hospital readmission rate could also be reduced. According to Foster and Harkness (2010), patient readmission accounted for more than $15 billion dollars per year in the U.S., and $12 billion out of this $15 billion was associated with potentially preventable readmission through better post-discharge management. Integrated care beyond acute care is critical to reducing readmission by 40% at least according to 1 study reviewed above, which is not only imperative to the performance of the healthcare system but is also beneficial to the health outcomes of the entire population. In their seminal paper, Helm and colleagues (2016) demonstrated that by integrating methods in big data such as statistical machine learning and OR/

MS techniques, it would be possible to optimize the priority and schedules of post-discharge follow-up based on individualized profile in readmission risk. Helm and colleagues (2016) also showed that 40% to 70% of 28-days readmission could be mitigated through this methodology.

Optimizing Resource Allocation Across the Care Continuum

With a simulation model based on mathematical programming, Cardoso, Oliveira, Barbosa-Póvoa, and Nicke (2015) were able to reduce the number of alternate level of care patients who use expensive acute care services (on average €403 per patient) by optimizing the provisioning of convalescence care, rehabilitation care, long-term and maintenance care, and palliative care that were of lower cost (on average €82 per patient). The model aims at improving the delivery of non-acute care to achieve access equity, geographical equity and socioeconomic equity. The results provided information on the identification of different types of long-term care, the distribution of capacity, and the changes needed.

In sum, given the challenges in implementing integrated care in an aging population with overstretched healthcare resources, OR/MS methodologies is proposed above as a means to minimize the cost of healthcare delivery and maximize the health outcomes of elderly. In addition to applying OR/MS methodologies for optimizing the implementation of integrated care, research has also shown that information technology, human capital cultivation and innovation in financing and commissioning models can enable integrated care. In the following, enablers of integrated care will be reviewed.

ENABLERS OF INTEGRATED CARE

There isn't a single model for integrated care. The right approach varies according to the local context and is likely to involve actions at multiple levels.

At the local system level, successful integrated care requires leaders to set shared strategies and enable resources to be pooled across organizations. In operational terms, the setting of shared strategies requires an underlying strategic alignment of incentives and payoffs of all relevant stakeholders. On the other hand, pooling resources across organizations requires the identification of the optimal level of resources assignments across the care continuum given the demands.

Research has shown that these multi-level processes could be facilitated by innovations in 1) information technology, 2) new service construction in an organization with human resources implications and 3) financing & commissioning models. At the clinical or care team level, it will require shared information and new ways of working such as single assessment processes and shared care plans. This operationally will require an information technology platform that is conducive to communication, and that will provide a common language for the client/patient. In the following, three enablers identified above will be reviewed.

Enabler One: Information Technology

A common platform that allows quality information to share effectively will enable integrated care. This section will highlight the role of technology, how it has been used, what the key driver is, and under what circumstances the utilization of information could be optimized; new developments in information technology such as Data Lake in enhancing big-data analytics will also be reviewed.

Lluch and Abadie (2013) suggested that Information and Communication Technology (ICT) is crucial to integrated care delivery in ensuring continuity and coordination of care by multidisciplinary teams. They studied the role of tele-healthcare across eight European countries: Denmark, Estonia, Germany, France, Italy, Netherlands, Spain and the UK, and found that aligned incentives, sound governance and evidence consolidation are essential factors for successful delivery of integrated care with support from ICT, where innovative organizational redesign also plays a major role.

They also found that countries with outcome-based incentives (e.g. France, Italy, Spain and the UK) could positively promote ICT applications and chronic care delivery, whilst fee-for-service scheme (e.g. Germany) tends to have a negative effect. In the study, they quoted the outcome of Whole System Demonstrator (WSD) program in UK, a tele-health and tele-care program for patients with any of the three chronic conditions: Diabetes, Heart Failure and Chronic Obstructive Pulmonary Disease. Early headline findings of 12 months implementation of WSD suggested 15% reduction in ER visits, 20% reduction in emergency admissions, 14% reduction in elective admissions, 14% reduction in bed days, 8% reduction in tariff costs, and most importantly, 45% reduction in mortality rates.

A joint report published by King's Fund and Nuffield Trust (Goodwin, Smith, Davies, Perry, Rosen, Dixon, and Ham, 2012) identified that the major barrier to effective integrated care is the lack of information sharing, such as shared clinical records. Currently in the UK, all patient records are stored in computerized form, yet information is not integrated and patient record is not shared in any National Health Service (NHS) information sharing platforms between public and private providers.

Nevertheless, NHS has started to take initiatives to enhance information sharing through Patient Online (NHS England, 2016), a NHS England program designed to support General Practitioner (GP) practices to offer and promote online services to patients, including online booking of appointments, ordering repeat prescriptions and, by the 31st of March 2016, access to detailed coded information held in patients' records.

One of the system supplier specific webinars is The Phoenix Partnership (TPP). They developed the system called SystemOne launched in 2011, which is holding 40 million patient records with one fifth of GP records and two fifths of community and child health records across England. The system has different modules for every healthcare setting from primary care to hospitals, social care and mental health, providing clinicians and health professionals with a single shared Electronic Health Record (EHR) available in real time at the point of care. This information sharing system allows ER physicians to gain access to patient's medical and pharmaceutical records from GP to aid their clinical decisions (Torjesen, 2012).

In contrast to NHS' Patient Online, which was built with the intention of bring together medical and social care, the Electronic Health Record Sharing System (eHRSS) was developed by the Hong Kong Hospital Authority for hospitals, with community care providers are mere end-users of the system.

Data Lake

The importance of ICT does not limit to information sharing. With a well-designed data structure, it can also serve as a building block for evaluation and even forecasting. More recently, large enterprises and research institutes such as the University of California Irvine Medical Center, Google, Facebook have accepted and made use of the new concept of Data Lake, which is a repository and management engine for big data. It stores different types of data in large quantities, and possesses great data management power and immense capacity to manage the exponential growth of tasks.

The term Data Lake was first coined by James Dixon, chief technology officer of Pentaho, based on the idea of data mart. Data mart is a smaller repository of attributes extracted from raw data. Dixon once said if data mart is the bottled water in a store, filtered, packaged and categorized for consumption, Data Lake is the immense body of water under natural conditions. Data from the data lake come from an array of sources, from which users can extract the needed information. Dixon holds that data mart can only provide the basic solution, while Data Lake can provide the optimal solution to users. Roski, Bo-Linn and Andrews (2014) recognized the value of Data Lake in healthcare, and suggested that relevant policies such as data use, access, sharing, privacy and stewardship should be revised so as to maximize the success of big-data analytics.

Enabler Two: Innovations in Human Services and Human Capital

The implementation of integrated care involves restructuring the existing service and associate workforce. Studies had focused on two directions: new job role and the sustainability of the workforce.

Oliver, Foot and Humphries (2014) outlined the 10 components of care for older adults that contribute to a continuum of care: 1) Healthy active aging and support of independence, 2) Helping people live well with simple or stable long-term conditions, 3) Helping people live with complex co-morbidities, including dementia and frailty, 4) Providing rapid support close to home in times of crisis, 5) Providing acute hospital care, 6) Discharge planning and post-discharge support, 7) Rehabilitation and re-ablement (outside acute hospitals) after acute illness or injury, 8) Long-term nursing residential care, 9) Choice, control, care and support towards the end of life, and 10) Integrated care to support older people and their families and bring the other 9 components toward a patient-centred path.

Among the components, the final and overarching component, which is the integrated services to provide person-centered care, binds the other components together. The focus on social and health care integration, together with the shift of care from acute care and long-term care to community care and primary care, create a demand for integrated care coordination services.

In many countries, case manager exists to deliver continuity and quality care to client. Studies showed that case management could reduce readmission to hospitals. Popejoy, Stetzer, Hicks, Rantz, Galambos, Popescu, and Marek (2015) compared care coordination managed by registered nurses and routine care through home health care in terms of utilization and cost outcomes. While the differences between care coordination managed by nurses and routine care through home health are not statistically significant, care coordination managed by nurses exhibits positive influence on the outcomes (functional and cognitive) and health care utilization for the frail elderly. The nurse-coordinated AIP program was found to reduce both hospitalization and emergency department visits (0.44 and 0.2 events per year respectively). Both AIP and HHC programs resulted in 80% decrease of re-hospitalization, and over 40% of elderly in both programs had no emergency visits in a year. Hence it was concluded that care coordination managed by a nurse was more cost-effective; and reimbursement models are needed that allow independent care coordination practices by nurses to function. Althaus et al. (2011) reviewed the intervention methods that reduce the number of visits to Emergency Department (ED). Out of all the studies, case management was the most described intervention. The author concluded that case management not only could reduce cost but could also enhance some clinical and social outcomes.

Current public social and health services for the elderly and existing personnel in Hong Kong are reviewed respectively with the reference to the ten components of care for older people. As indicated above, comprehensive social and health care services are identified from components 1 to 9. It is found that the services are generally bound to a few components of care in which component 10 is not adequately fulfilled. The concept of integrated care coordination in relation to component 10 has been well developed and implemented in the U.S. It is essential to smooth the transition between different care services for older adults who interact frequently with social and health care systems (AARP Public Policy Institute, 2015). Currently, the concept is supported by the Government of Hong Kong. Pilot integration programs named Integrated Discharged Support Programme for Elderly Patients (IDSP) and Integrated Care and Discharge Support for Elderly Patients (ICDS) are implemented, targeting mainly older adults who attended acute care in hospitals. The preliminary findings have shown that these programs have successfully reduced emergency attendance, hospital readmission, length of hospitalization and potentially healthcare expenditure (Lin, et al., 2015; Ng, Sha & Tong, 2011). However, these programs are limited to hospital-based setting. The full-scale care coordination services target not only those who are discharged from hospitals but also those at-risk elderly in the community. With appropriate models, effective integrated care services in Hong Kong could be transferrable from acute to community care settings in full scale.

In addition to current services, major types of personnel working in elderly care services have been identified: 1) generic skilled healthcare professionals: doctors, nurses and allied healthcare professionals, 2) generic skilled social care professionals: social workers, 3) specially trained healthcare paraprofessionals: health workers and personal care workers; and 4) non-formally trained paraprofessional as well as informal care providers such family and volunteers.

The existing job roles highlight the insufficient employment opportunities to attract young adults into the field of elderly services. The roles also fail to address the full-spectrum of needs of the elderly from community care to the coordination of health and social care. Therefore, there is a pressing need to prepare specialized and skilled personnel to fill the integrated care coordination roles in a continuum of elderly care.

Labour shortage in elderly care not withstanding, in recent years, the number of jobless youth (under age 25) in Hong Kong, especially male, has drastically increased. The International Labour Organisation estimates Hong Kong's male youth unemployment rate at over 20%. To ensure sufficient employable opportunities to attract young school leavers into elderly care services, this new community-recognized job role should be created with support from formal vocational training. Our preliminary study on local formal training programs related to elderly care and services found that: 1) A small number of programs offer a comprehensive curriculum covering a wide spectrum of elderly care, and 2) For programs covering wider topics in relation to the elderly care curriculum, none of them covers topics of integrated care coordination in depth.

Another group that will serve a crucial role is the volunteers. Given that a large percentage of human capital in the community are familial caregivers and volunteers, a supply of manpower in elderly care can be strengthened with structured training designed to accommodate different groups. Indeed, volunteer training on elderly care can sustainably maximize the impacts on the community. Training for young-adult volunteers serves as service learning experience to prepare these young adults to transition from school to work and facilitate life-learning practices. It is also the policy objective of the Hong Kong Government to promote a sense of worthiness among older adults by engaging them in elderly care support networks. It is therefore critical and appropriate that a flexible curriculum is designed so as to create a new elderly care job role, mobilize existing human capital, and strengthen the capability of informal caregivers and volunteers.

In short, with formal vocational training, these two groups could play an important part in integrated care.

Enabler Three: Innovation in Financing Models

There is a great difference between the American healthcare system and the universal healthcare systems found in Europe, Canada, Australia and New Zealand. The variability among universal healthcare systems offered by different countries is also substantial. Hence, the nature and outcome of the financing models which different countries utilize to incentivize and sustain integrated care within the context of their own systems are likely to be different, though there may be minor similarities between the American healthcare system and the national health insurance systems in countries like Austria, Germany and Netherlands.

The Quality and Outcomes Framework (QOF) in England, Gesundes Kinzigtal Integrated Care initiative in Germany, Team Care Arrangements in Australia, and Family Health Teams (FHT) in Ontario Canada are examples of how different counties adopt financing models to incentivize the coordination among primary care, acute care and community care within the context of their unique healthcare systems (for reviews, see Hernandez-Quevedo, Llano and Mossialos, 2013). In the following, different financing models for incentivizing integrated care will be reviewed within the context of the healthcare systems that adopt them.

Pay-For-Performance

Outcomes-Based Commissioning

Pay-for-performance in health care is defined as 'physicians receive differential payments for meeting or missing performance benchmarks' (Tsiachristas et al., 2013). In a single-payer public healthcare system like UK's NHS, it takes the form of outcomes-based commissioning (OBC). In outcomes-based commissioning the payer provides a fixed budget for the care of a particular population in order to incentivizes different care providers to work together with more coordination to deliver services that are cost-effective and high quality.

An example of this model is the Oxfordshire Clinical Commissioning Group for mental health. Oxford Health NHS Foundation Trust is contracted by NHS to serve as the lead provider in the area. Oxford Health NHS Foundation Trust then subcontracted the services out in 5-year terms, where 80% of contract value is paid as block (£28m) and 20% (£7m) paid according to the achievement of outcomes. It has been shown that NHS' OBC has reduced service cost and increased revenue (Corrigan and Hocks, 2012).

Despite a reduction of annual spending by 20%, it was revealed that the Oxfordshire group was £6.1M in debt. Hence, additional research is required to evaluate the viability and effectiveness of the OBC model.

Kotitori Model: Extending OBC With a Penalty Add-On

The Kotitori model is similar to OBC, but instead of incentivize service integration through cost-saving, service integration is paid on a capitation basis under the Kotitori model. Payment methods to different integrator services vary from full subsidies to co-payment to out-of-pocket plans. Bonuses are rewarded if the integrator services are able to meet 3 targets: Transfers to sheltered housing, use of hospital wards and utilization of A&E services. On the other hand, penalty is inflicted if the integrator services cannot meet the targets (Tynkkynen et al., 2012).

Despite having a universal healthcare system, the Finns have a strong tradition of utilizing the private sector in care services. With the shift in the Finnish elderly care policy in the past two decades, from institutional care to promoting home-based care, there is an effort to incentivize public-private partnerships in delivery care at the home of the elderly. It has been reported that the city had approximately saved €2-3 million with this public-private partnership under the Kotitori model. €290,000 were paid to the service integrators as bonus from 2009-2011.

Gesundes Kinzigtal

The Kinzigtal region of Germany has adopted a population-based integrated care system that involves all health sectors. The "Gesundes Kinzigtal" model finances integrated care initiative based on a shared compensation structure. With a shared savings contract, the management company and two "sickness funds" share profit generated from the difference of realized savings compared to the average costs of care (Llano, 2013). The compensation mechanism is managed by a governmental agency, the Federal Insurance Authority, which provides the financial incentives for the management group to improve the margin by US$203 per person per year (Busse and Stahl, 2014). Busse and Stahl (2014) found that the initiative has significant decreased length of stay and mortality (1.76% compared with 3.74% two and a half year later), though admissions have increased.

Pay-For-Coordination

Similar to Pay-for-Performance, Pay-for-coordination is characterized by 'payments to providers providing care coordination services that integrate care between providers' (Tsiachristas et al., 2013).

Lead Provider in Outcomes-Based Commissioning for Pay-for-Coordination

Within the context of NHS, Pay-for-Coordination is also achieved through the outcomes-based commissioning. By improving the market power of the lead provider, who is responsible for managing and supporting the care pathway through incentivizing other providers to better coordinate with each other in the care delivery, it is believed that outcomes-based commissioning can achieve integrated care that addresses patient needs with reduced transaction cost and increased efficiency (Billings & Weger, 2015). Corrigan and Laitner (2012) suggested that the pay-for-coordination framework can be the solution for acute care providers to adapt the new healthcare business model for integrated care without destabilizing existing local NHS providers. Especially in the case of the accountable lead provider model, where the lead provider does not only serve as the integrator but it also provides the major treatment, the different aspects of social and medical care can be brought together in a coherent patient journey and improved the coordination of the patient pathway (Corrigan & Laitner, 2012).

For example, the Clinical Commissioning Groups of the NHS has a contract with a single organization to take care of the day-to-day management of other providers (Addicott, 2014). The prime contractor acts as an integrator to manage supply of services through its sub-contracts different providers (Addicott, 2014).

The effectiveness of the outcome-based commissioning of the pay-for-coordination model lies in the fact that, as the lead provider gains increased direct control across the pathway, it has an incentive to reduce the administrative costs and enhance opportunities for innovative service delivery to achieve economies of scale (O'Flynn et al., 2014; Billings & Weger, 2015). This in turn enables money to move within the pathway.

Disease Management Programs

There are different pay-for-coordination models other than the one UK has adopted. In Germany and Australia, where its health insurance scheme is statutory and jointly supported by the central government and the employers, Disease Management Programs (DMP) are implemented to 'coordinate treatment and care of patients during the entire duration of a disease across boundaries between providers and on basis of scientific and up-to-date evidence'. (Nolte et al., 2012).

In Germany, primary care physicians who registered in DMP act as the principal coordinator of care. Patients voluntarily enroll in DMPs. The quality of care is assured by putting in place clinical guidelines and regulations to ensure proper documentation by the physicians (Nagel et al., 2008). On the other hand, DMP-registered GPs will receive additional remuneration for courses they attend and proper documentation (Tsiachristas et al., 2013). In Austria, regional SHI and federal state combine funds to create a financial pool at the state level. This financial pool funds projects in integrated care, including DMPs. The incentives for DMP physicians include patient sign-up, quarterly fees for treatment and documentation (Nolte et al., 2012).

In terms of evidence, there is a significant cost reduction in terms of overall drug and hospital cost, as well as decrease in hospitalization and the average length of hospital stay associated with the implementation of DMPs; in addition, there is a (Stock et al., 2010). Research has also revealed a significant difference in mortality rate between patients associated DMP and patients who do not. Nagel et al. (2008) reported that 12.3 per 1000 patients died in the non-disease management program compared to 9.5 per 1000 patients in DMP.

De Bruin, Baan and Struijs (2011) conducted a systematic review to evaluate the effects of disease management programs on healthcare quality and healthcare costs. In addition to the general positive effect on the quality of care delivery, the effect is most prominent in incentivizing an improvement in the quality of diabetes care management, as reflected in an increase of HbA1c test being ordered.

Bundled Payment

Bundled Payment is characterized by bundling payment for services delivered during an episode of care related to a specific medical condition or procedure that involves multiple providers across different care settings. Despite the apparent differences between Netherlands and US' healthcare systems, both adopt the bundled payment method to incentivize integrated care. The bundled payment in Netherlands has an upstream focus on specific chronic diseases and outpatient care, while the bundled payment in US has a downstream focus on inpatient and post-acute care (Bakker et al., 2012).

Bundled Payment in the Netherlands

Similar to Germany and Austria, Netherlands' healthcare system is financed through the Bismarckian model of Statutory Health Insurance (SHI), where the insurance scheme is statutory and jointly supported by the central government and the employers. But unlike DMP in Germany and Austria, whose bundle payment is contracted through individual provider, Netherlands' disease-focused bundled payment scheme is contracted through a care group – health insurers who provide packages of care according to national standards (Nolte et al., 2012).

As the health insurers pay a single fee to the care groups for all healthcare services with respect to a particular disease, this scheme provides incentive for care groups which are clinically and financially responsible to the clients enrolled, and for insurers to negotiate a lower price for the care chain (Llano, 2013). This means that the insurer has incentive to sign care contracts with the lowest price, whereas the care group has incentive to reduce payment to the subcontractor (Tsiachristas et al., 2013). The care group can provide care itself or sign subcontracts with other healthcare providers. Although the care group bears full financial risk of care (Struijs and Baan, 2011). At the end, it reduces transaction cost and increases cost-effectiveness. This also increases the efficiency of subcontractors to attract care groups to cooperate with them.

Since 2007, a pilot scheme of applying bundled payment model to incentivize integrated care out-patient care was launched. The initial focus of the pilot scheme was only diabetes care, and was subsequently expanded to chronic obstructive pulmonary disease and vascular risk management (Llano, 2013). At this point, the cost reduction of the bundled payment method in Netherlands remains inconclusive (Struijs et al. 2010, cited in Nolte et al., 2012).

In the case of diabetes-focused programs, Busse and Stahl (2014) argued that, despite the savings of US$47 per patient per year (amount to a 25% decrease of diabetes specialist care in hospital), there was however an increase of US$189 per patient per year for specialist care in total.

Bundled Payment in the U.S.

While the U.S. has a predominantly private healthcare system, those who meet the inclusion criteria can receive publicly funded insurance via Medicare and Medicaid. The Shared Saving Program (SSP) for Medicare reimbursement is an incentive program tied to the Accountable Care Organizations (ACOs) to promote their formation and use (Billings & Weger, 2015). The SSP is an outcome-focused model that is applied in the U.S. under the Affordable Care Act (ACA).

When a physician treats a Medicare patient, he bills the government as fee-for-service. A fee-for-service provider can choose to register as Accountable Care Organizations. The shared saving program is an outcome-focused model for Medicare reimbursement to incentivize the formation and quality of ACO.

What is unique about SSP ACO is that the Centers for Medicare and Medicaid Services develops a benchmark for each ACO through several processes: 1) Medicare will first develop a savings plan for the ACO after reviewing its records of how much it charges for treating patients and 2) When the ACOs meet the quality and savings requirements, Medicare then share a percentage of the savings with them. There are four criteria for assessing if the ACOs are meeting the requirements according to SSP: patient experience, care coordination/patient safety, preventive health, and at-risk population.

Hence, SSP provides ACOs with a financial incentive to provide quality services to individual patients and employ preventive measures to maintain and improve the health of the population. In addition, as the revue increases with the number of patients utilizing the ACO, enhancing patient experience will strengthen the ACO's market position.

In terms of effectiveness, Center for Medicare & Medicare Services (CMS) reported that in 2014, ACOs generated more than $411 million in total savings. Despite the benefits of this model, one of the critiques is the high startup cost - most ACOs will require a $1.8 million investment to get started (Bennett, 2012).

CONCLUDING REMARKS: SOLUTIONS AND RECOMMENDATIONS

Research has shown that integrated care is the solution to foster aging in place, but globally countries face tremendous challenges in implementing integrated care in an aging population with overstretched healthcare resources. OR/MS methodologies is proposed above as a means to minimize the cost of healthcare delivery and maximize the health outcomes of elderly. In addition to applying OR/MS methodologies for optimizing the implementation of integrated care, research has also shown that information technology, human capital cultivation and innovation in financing and commissioning models can enable integrated care. In the following, enablers of integrated care will be reviewed.

Integrated care is better care. Three enablers are found to be significant to deliver better integrated care at the local system level and at the clinical level. This review served as a foundation for health professionals, Operations Research/Management Sciences scholars and policy makers for further study with focus on the following objectives using the three enablers: 1) shared key performance standards whereby all organizations can aspire to achieve in the care of the elderly, 2) evaluation of current practices with respect to good practices and their effectiveness in bringing positive changes, 3) identification of priorities for change according to cost-effectiveness, 4) shared data on the unmet needs and service gaps of the elderly to inform the service redesign, the progress and the performance of the programs.

REFERENCES

AARP Public Policy Institute. (2015). *Caregiving - Public Policy Institute*. Retrieved April 14, 2016, from http://www.aarp.org/ppi/issues/caregiving/

Addicott, R. (2014). *Commissioning and contracting for integrated care*. London: The Kings Fund.

Althaus, F., Paroz, S., Hugli, O., Ghali, W. A., Daeppen, J. B., Peytremann-Bridevaux, I., & Bodenmann, P. (2011). Effectiveness of interventions targeting frequent users of emergency departments: A systematic review. *Annals of Emergency Medicine*, *58*(1), 41–52. doi:10.1016/j.annemergmed.2011.03.007 PMID:21689565

Armitage, G. D., Suter, E., Oelke, N. D., & Adair, C. (2009). Health systems integration: State of the evidence. *International Journal of Integrated Care*, *9*(17), 1–11. PMID:19590762

Bennett, A. R. (2012). Accountable care organizations: Principles and implications for hospital administrators. *Journal of Healthcare Management*, *57*(4), 244–254. PMID:22905603

Billings, J., & Weger, E. (2015). Contracting for integrated health and social care: A critical review of four models. *Journal of Integrated Care*, *23*(3), 153–175. doi:10.1108/JICA-03-2015-0015

Busse, R., & Stahl, J. (2014). Integrated care experiences and outcomes in Germany, the Netherlands, and England. *Health Affairs*, *33*(9), 1549–1558. doi:10.1377/hlthaff.2014.0419 PMID:25201659

Cardoso, T., Oliveira, M. D., Barbosa-Póvoa, A., & Nickel, S. (2016). Moving towards an equitable long-term care network: A multi-objective and multi-period planning approach. *Omega*, *58*, 69–85. doi:10.1016/j.omega.2015.04.005

Carey, K., & Stefos, T. (2015). The cost of hospital readmissions: Evidence from the VA. *Health Care Management Science*, 1–8. PMID:25576391

Cohen, D., Manuel, D. G., Tugwell, P., Sanmartin, C., & Ramsay, T. (2014). Direct healthcare costs of acute myocardial infarction in Canadas elderly across the continuum of care. *The Journal of the Economics of Ageing*, *3*, 44–49. doi:10.1016/j.jeoa.2014.05.002

Corrigan, P., & Hicks, N. (2012). *What organisation is necessary for commissioners to develop outcomes based contracts? The COBIC case study*. Right Care Casebook Series. London: NHS. Retrieved from: http://www.rightcare.nhs.uk/downloads/RC_Casebook_cobic_final.pdf

de Bakker, D. H., Struijs, J. N., Baan, C. A., Raams, J., de Wildt, J. E., Vrijhoef, H. J., & Schut, F. T. (2012). Early results from adoption of bundled payment for diabetes care in the Netherlands show improvement in care coordination. *Health Affairs*, *31*(2), 426–433. doi:10.1377/hlthaff.2011.0912 PMID:22323174

De Bruin, S., Heijink, R., Lemmens, L. C., Struijs, J. N., & Baan, C. A. (2011). Impact of disease management programs on healthcare expenditures for patients with diabetes, depression, heart failure or chronic obstructive pulmonary disease: A systematic review of the literature. *Health Policy (Amsterdam)*, *101*(2), 105–121. doi:10.1016/j.healthpol.2011.03.006 PMID:21592607

eHealth HKSAR. (2016). *About eHR*. Retrieved 12 April, 2016, from http://www.ehealth.gov.hk/en/about_ehrss/index.html

Foster, D., & Harkness, G. (2010). *Healthcare reform: pending changes to reimbursement for 30-day readmissions*. Healthcare reform: reimbursement. Thomson Reuters.

Glied, S., & Smith, P. (2011). *The Oxford handbook of health economics*. Oxford, UK: Oxford University Press. doi:10.1093/oxfordhb/9780199238828.001.0001

Golmohammadi, D., & Radnia, N. (2016). Prediction modeling and pattern recognition for patient readmission. *International Journal of Production Economics*, *171*(Part 1), 151–161. doi:10.1016/j.ijpe.2015.09.027

Goodwin, N., Smith, J., Davies, A., Perry, C., Rosen, R., Dixon, A., & Ham, C. (2012). *Integrated care for patients and populations: Improving outcomes by working together*. London: King's Fund.

Helm, J. E., Alaeddini, A., Stauffer, J. M., Bretthauer, K. M., & Skolarus, T. A. (2016). Reducing Hospital Readmissions by Integrating Empirical Prediction with Resource Optimization. *Production and Operations Management*, *25*(2), 233–257. doi:10.1111/poms.12377

Hernández-Quevedo, C., Llano, R., & Mossialos, E. (2013). Paying for integrated care: an overview. *Euro Health Incorporating Euro Observer, 19*(2), 3-6.

Kucukyazici, B., & Verter, V. (2013). Managing Community-based Care for Chronic Diseases: The Quantitative Approach. In G. S. Zaric (Ed.), Operations Research and Health Care Policy, (pp. 71–90). New York: Springer.

Kucukyazici, B., Verter, V., & Mayo, N. E. (2011). An Analytical Framework for Designing Community-Based Care for Chronic Diseases. *Production and Operations Management*, *20*(3), 474–488. doi:10.1111/j.1937-5956.2011.01224.x

Li, Y., Kong, N., Chen, M., & Zheng, Q. P. (2016). Optimal physician assignment and patient demand allocation in an outpatient care network. *Computers & Operations Research*, *72*, 107–117. doi:10.1016/j.cor.2016.02.013

Lin, F. O. Y., Luk, J. K. H., Chan, T. C., Mok, W. W. Y., & Chan, F. H. W. (2015). Effectiveness of a discharge planning and community support programme in preventing readmission of high-risk older patients. *Hong Kong Medical Journal*, *21*(3), 208–216. PMID:25904292

Llano, R. (2013). Bundled payments for integrated care in the Netherlands. In Incentivising 2013 Integrated Care (pp. 15-16). Quarterly of the European Observatory on Health Systems and Policies.

Lluch, M., & Abadie, F. (2013). Exploring the role of ICT in the provision of integrated care—evidence from eight countries. *Health Policy (Amsterdam)*, *111*(1), 1–13. doi:10.1016/j.healthpol.2013.03.005 PMID:23587547

Nagel, H., Baehring, T., & Scherbaum, W. A. (2008). Disease management programmes for diabetes in Germany. *Diabetes Voice*, *53*(3), 17–19.

Ng, M., Sha, K., & Tong, B. (2011). *Bridging the Gap: Win-win from Integrated Discharge Support for Elderly Patients*. Presentation, HA Convention 2011.

NHS England. (2016). *NHS England Patient Online*. Retrieved 11 April 2016, from https://www.england.nhs.uk/ourwork/pe/patient-online/

Nolte, E., Knai, C., Hofmarcher, M., Conklin, A., Erler, A., Elissen, A., Vrijhoef, H. J. M. (2012). Overcoming fragmentation in health care: chronic care in Austria, Germany and the Netherlands. *Health Economics, Policy and Law, 7*(S1), 125–146.

O'Flynn, J., Dickinson, H., O'Sullivan, S., Gallet, W., Currie, K., Pettit, M., . . . Robinson, T. (2014), *The Prime Provider Model. An Opportunity for Better Public Service Delivery?* Social Policy Working Paper No. 18, published report. Melbourne: University of Melbourne and Brotherhood of St Laurence.

Oliver, D., Foot, C., & Humphries, R. (2014). *Making our health and care systems fit for an ageing population*. London: The King's Fund.

Ouwens, M., Wollersheim, H., Hermens, R., Hulscher, M., & Grol, R. (2005). Integrated care programmes for chronically ill patients: A review of systematic reviews. *International Journal for Quality in Health Care*, *17*(2), 141–146. doi:10.1093/intqhc/mzi016 PMID:15665066

Popejoy, L. L., Stetzer, F., Hicks, L., Rantz, M. J., Galambos, C., Popescu, M., & Marek, K. D. (2015). Comparing Aging in Place to Home Health Care: Impact of Nurse Care Coordination on Utilization and Costs. *Nursing Economics*, *33*(6), 306–313. PMID:26845818

Roski, J., Bo-Linn, G. W., & Andrews, T. A. (2014). Creating value in health care through big data: Opportunities and policy implications. *Health Affairs*, *33*(7), 1115–1122. doi:10.1377/hlthaff.2014.0147 PMID:25006136

Stock, S., Drabik, A., Büscher, G., Graf, C., Ullrich, W., Gerber, A., & Lüngen, M. (2010). German Diabetes Management Programs Improve Quality Of Care And Curb Costs. *Health Affairs*, *29*(12), 2197–2205. doi:10.1377/hlthaff.2009.0799 PMID:21134920

Struijs, J. N., & Baan, C. A. (2011). Integrating care through bundled payments—lessons from the Netherlands. *The New England Journal of Medicine*, *364*(11), 990–991. doi:10.1056/NEJMp1011849 PMID:21410368

Torjesen, I. (2012). Go with the flow. *The Health Service Journal*, *122*(6303), 2–3. PMID:22741355

Trybou, J., Spaepen, E., Vermeulen, B., Porrez, L., & Annemans, L. (2013). Hospital-acquired infections in Belgian acute-care hospitals: Financial burden of disease and potential cost savings. *Acta Clinica Belgica*, *68*(3), 199–205. doi:10.2143/ACB.3258 PMID:24156220

Tsiachristas, A., Dikkers, C., Boland, M. R. S., & Rutten-van Mölken, M. P. M. H. (2013). Exploring payment schemes used to promote integrated chronic care in Europe. *Health Policy (Amsterdam)*, *113*(3), 296–304. doi:10.1016/j.healthpol.2013.07.007 PMID:23937868

Tynkkynen, L. K., Hakari, K., Koistinen, T., Lehto, J., & Miettinen, S. (2012). Integrating public and private home care services: The Kotitori model in Tampere, Finland. *Journal of Integrated Care*, *20*(5), 284–295. doi:10.1108/14769011211270738

World Health Organization. (2016). *Ageing and health*. Retrieved August 23, 2016, from http://www.who.int/mediacentre/factsheets/fs404/en/

Yam, C. H., Wong, E. L., Chan, F. W., Leung, M. C., Wong, F. Y., Cheung, A. W., & Yeoh, E. K. (2010). Avoidable readmission in Hong Kong-system, clinician, patient or social factor? *BMC Health Services Research*, *10*(1), 1. doi:10.1186/1472-6963-10-311 PMID:21080970

Chapter 9
Knowledge Management for Health Care and Long-Term Care in the Technology-Organization-Environment Context

Man Fung Lo
The Hong Kong Polytechnic University, Hong Kong

Peggy Mei Lan Ng
The Hong Kong Polytechnic University, Hong Kong

ABSTRACT

The objective of this chapter is to propose a framework examining the impacts of technological, organizational and environmental factors on the innovation adoption of knowledge management (KM) in long-term care context. This chapter begins with the definition, rationale and importance of KM. Secondly, KM stories, KM in long-term care, prior frameworks in long-term care and knowledge barriers in health care settings will be reviewed. Furthermore, the KM for long-term care in Technology-Organization-Environment (TOE) framework is discussed and proposed. The technology dimension includes security, complexity and costs. Besides, organizational dimension is composed of top management support, firm size, nursing leadership and the readiness. For environmental dimensions, this chapter will focus on competitive pressure and vendor support. As KM is proven to understand performance in long-term care organizations, the proposed framework provides insight to health care organization leaders on how to enhance the effectiveness of KM system.

DOI: 10.4018/978-1-5225-2633-9.ch009

INTRODUCTION

Over the past ten years, more studies have shown that effective Knowledge Management (KM) improve the overall business performance (Choi et al., Fugate et al., 2009; Ho, 2008; 2008; Lee et al., 2012; Liao and Wu, 2009; Noruzy et al., 2013; Zack et al., 2009). Survival of any healthcare organizations heavily depends on KM, such as implementing evidence-based medicine in daily healthcare activities, retrieving evidence-based reports, and providing quality of care to patients by exchanging the knowledge among several partners of healthcare organizations. In fact, public health decision is evidence-based, which is mainly data-driven, and healthcare sector can be advantageous through the implementation of KM. KM in long-term care has focused exclusively on improving processes by incorporating KM practices. For example, employing digital dashboard can support touch-points in long-term care work flow by consolidating real-time information for users to view key performance indicators, making data much more useful for users. As mentioned by Pan & Jang (2008), Technology-Organization-Environment (TOE) framework was developed to study the adoption of technological innovations. This framework was widely adopted in many industries: information technology (Low, Chen, Wu, 2011), government (Pudjianto, Zo, Ciganek & Rho, 2011), auditing (Rosli, Yeow & Siew, 2012) and hospitality (Racherla & Hu, 2008). This chapter will overview KM, discuss the importance of KM in long-term care, KM stories and prior frameworks in long-term care, knowledge barriers and examine critical factors that enhance KM in long-term care using the TOE framework.

WHAT IS KNOWLEDGE MANAGEMENT?

KM aims to make the right knowledge available to the right people at the right time so that the best possible strategies and outcomes can be delivered. The purpose of KM is to identify, create, transfer and apply knowledge to achieve better strategic objectives, resulting in enhancing organizational performance (Choi et al., 2008, López-Nicolás and Meroño-Cerdán, 2011). KM is concerned with innovation and sharing behaviors and improvement of capabilities through learning (Moustaghfir and Schiuma, 2013). In addition, KM assists in managing complexity and ambiguity through knowledge networks and connections, exploring smart processes and deploying appropriate tools and technologies (Bharati et al., 2015). There are several sub-strategies discussed in the literature within the domain of KM. Firstly, the concepts of exploitation and exploration are introduced by March (1991). Secondly, Hansen et al. (1999) compare and contrast two KM sub-strategies for a classic study in managing knowledge - codification and personalization. The former one is concerned about how knowledge is codified, stored and accessed through computerized databases; whereas the latter one refers to how knowledge is shared through direct contact among organizational members and/or with technology support (Hansen et al., 1999). Pourhamidi (2013) further contends that the characteristics of codification are similar to those defined in exploitation whilst those attributes in personalization are consistent with the concept of exploration. A broader perspective has been adopted by Choi and Lee (2003), who argue that there are system-oriented and human-oriented KM sub-strategies. The adoption of different KM strategies in recent literature is summarized in Table 1.

Apart from the above-mentioned sub-strategies, there are several key models in KM domains. This section aims to provide an overview on these models. Firstly, Nonaka and Takeuchi (1995) have developed the knowledge spiral model which is composed of four quadrants: (1) socialization; (2) externalization; (3)

Table 1. KM in recent literature

Author(s) and Year	KM Strategy		
	Codification/ Personalization	Exploitation/ Exploration	System-Oriented/ Human-Oriented
Ju, Li, and Lee (2006)			X
Ajith Kumar and Ganesh (2011)	X		
Durcikova, Fadel, Butler, and Galletta (2011)		X	
López-Nicolás and Meroño-Cerdán (2011)	X		
Martín-de Castro, López-Sáez, Delgado-Verde, Donate, and Guadamillas (2011)	X		
Canzano and Grimaldi (2012)	X	X	
Chai and Nebus (2012)	X		
Jahn and Nielsen (2012)	X		
Liu, Chai, and F. Nebus (2013)	X		
Pourhamidi (2013)	X		
Shahzad, Zia, Aslam, Syed, and Bajwa (2013)			X
Yousif Al-Hakim and Hassan (2013)	X		
AL-Hakim and Hassan (2014)	X		
Arvanitis and Woerter (2014)		X	
Daraei and Vahidi (2014)	X		
Shamah (2014)	X		

Source: Lo and Ng (2015).

combination; and (4) internalization (SECI). This model demonstrates how different forms of knowledge conversion occur. First, socialization refers to the tacit-to-tacit conversion. Moreover, combination takes place when pieces of explicit knowledge are synthesized or combined. Thirdly, tacit knowledge from one's mind is converted to explicit form through externalization. When explicit knowledge is converted to tacit form, it is called internalization. Nonaka and Takeuchi (1995) have further pointed out that the sharing and conversion of knowledge is a continuous process and the knowledge spiral is developed. The second key model is the European Foundation for Quality Management (EFQM) KM Model. According to Dalkir and Liebowitz (2011), this model illustrates how KM is used to achieve organizational goals. Enablers in EFQM model include leadership, people, policy and strategy, partnerships and resources, and processes. These crucial factors have significant impact on the key performance result in the EFQM KM model. Lastly, Girard (2005) has built the inukshuk KM Model for the Canadian government. This model is derived from SECI components. In addition, leadership, technology, culture, measurement and the types of knowledge (tacit and explicit) are incorporated.

WHY IS KNOWLEDGE MANAGEMENT SO IMPORTANT IN HEALTHCARE?

Due to the generation of massive amounts of data, such as clinical trial data, electronic medical records, hospital records and administrative reports (Abidi, 2001), healthcare becomes a highly complex, evidence-based environment and a knowledge intensive industry (Ferlie et al., 2015). It is necessary to transform the "data rich" into a strategic decision-support system, so that the integration of knowledge and knowledge sharing can be better achieved among healthcare stakeholders. Bordoloi and Islam (2012, p.110) states that "healthcare delivery is a knowledge driven process and knowledge management provides an opportunity for improvement in process performance". Effective KM helps to develop a culture of learning among healthcare stakeholders with the following benefits:

- Sharing information and methodology on healthcare initiatives;
- Providing more accurate and accessible information and knowledge resources;
- Increasing speed of response as a direct result of better knowledge access and application;
- Improving efficiency and quality of work;
- Developing capability and clinical competency of staff;
- Enhancing the collaboration with partners and relevant strategic stakeholders.

In addition, "*knowledge translation*" has been widely discussed in healthcare studies (Boström, 2012; Kitson, 2009; Scott et al., 2012; Straus et al., 2009). In a recent study by Straus et al. (2011, p.6), knowledge translation is defined as "*the use of knowledge in practice and decision making*". Effective knowledge translation results in better decision making, and ultimately enhance productivity and improve health and quality of life (Straus et al., 2011). In the same vein, Metaxiotis (2011) points out that KM has the role to translate research results into policies and practices and finally lengthen survival and improve the quality of life.

Other than knowledge translation, "*knowledge transfer*" and "*knowledge exchange*" are the emerging strategies which aim to facilitate the accessibility, applicability and production of evidence to healthcare settings by an interactive interchange of knowledge between research users and researcher producers (Motten et al., 2007; Pentland et al., 2011). With the increased demands on healthcare resources, generating knowledge by means of knowledge transfer and exchange may have significant impacts on the management of large healthcare organizations. Pentland et al. (2011) points out the key characteristics of knowledge transfer and knowledge exchange in healthcare settings (Table 2).

With the proper design and implementation of knowledge transfer and exchange mechanisms in place, research knowledge can be communicated to clinical practitioners, thereby improving evidence-based practice and facilitating decision making by healthcare professionals in relevant large organizations and institutions. From these studies, it is observed that a close relationship exists among KM, knowledge translation, knowledge transfer and knowledge exchange, and quality healthcare. To sum up, KM plays an important role in achieving knowledge translation, knowledge transfer and knowledge exchange, which in turn achieves quality healthcare ultimately.

KNOWLEDGE MANAGEMENT SUCCESS STORIES IN HEALTHCARE

This section aims to share three KM stories in the healthcare sector. To illustrate the importance of KM at different levels, stories from Hong Kong (regional level), England (country level) and World Health Organization (international level) were discussed. A comparison table with respect to the responsible KM unit, objectives and key contributions in these stories are presented.

Table 2. Key characteristics of knowledge transfer and knowledge exchange

Key characteristics of knowledge transfer – *Sharing knowledge*	Relevance • Ensuring the relevance of research information or findings when sharing them with knowledge users
	Accessibility • Making research evidence information accessible to potential users • Tailoring the findings of research for specific audiences and ensuring its relevance
	Format and method • Clear and precise presentation is vital in improving probability of use • Knowledge sharing methods should be flexible enough to provide users with access to research evidence in various formats
Key characteristics of knowledge exchange – *Generating knowledge*	Collaborative research formulation • Collaboration and communication between researchers and health professionals during research formulation can generate new research knowledge
	Collaborative research production • Collaboration between those using research evidence and its producers in influencing clinical, planning and policy decisions • Establishing and maintaining quality relationships during collaborative research in knowledge exchange initiatives
	Collaborative dissemination • Collaboration during research makes action from knowledge more probable as it allows stakeholders the opportunity to inform implementation strategies by bringing local and context-specific knowledge to the process • Improving researchers' understanding and appreciation of clinical environments

Source: Pentland et al. (2011).

Hong Kong: E-Knowledge Gateway at Hospital Authority

Established in 1990, the Hospital Authority (HA) is a statutory body in Hong Kong which is responsible for the public hospitals and institutes management. By reviewing its vision, mission, values and strategic priorities, it can be ascertained that high quality medical services, staff learning and continuous improvement are advocated. Within the organization structure of the Hospital Authority, KM Unit was established under the Strategy and Planning Division of the HA Head Office. This establishment aims at "providing convenient, timely and easy access to expert-selected and best available information resources, and an environment conducive to research and knowledge sharing" (Hospital Authority, 2003, p.4). One of the key achievements is the "e-Knowledge Gateway". According to KM Unit (2016), e-Knowledge Gateway is a KM tool designed for Hospital Authority professional staff. With Internet connection, healthcare professionals can access this KM platform to obtain "comprehensive and quality" medical knowledge. In 2000, KM unit started the e-Knowledge Gateway pilot project which aimed at facilitating the knowledge sharing among healthcare professionals. At that moment, e-Knowledge Gateway acted as a resource platform sharing medical information in four specialties (Hospital Authority, 2003). With the experience gained from pilot project, e-Knowledge Gateway was then migrated to the HA intranet in 2002, and finally moved to Internet in 2004. As a result, physicians, nurses and other healthcare staff can access the platform from anywhere and at any time. The number of specialties was increased from four to thirty-four. For instance, Chinese medicine and nursing specialty were incorporated into the e-Knowledge Gateway in 2005 and 2007 respectively (Hospital Authority, 2005; Hospital Authority, 2007). With their slogan as stated in the website – "*knowledge · anytime · anywhere*", healthcare professionals are now able to access a variety of resources, electronic healthcare journals, e-books, and databases, hence the knowledge sharing objective is undoubtedly achieved with overwhelming success.

England: *Do Once and Share* a National Health Service

In England, National Health Service (NHS) is a publicly-funded healthcare system established in 1948. In order to reduce the medical errors occurrences and to improve the quality of patient care, National Health Service has been actively launching different KM initiatives since 2003 (De Brún, 2007). Plaice & Kitch (2003) have reviewed that the practical drivers for KM development in National Health Service include patient-centered healthcare, evidence-based healthcare, workforce development, merger of trusts, information technology and clinical education. One of the projects was called "*Do Once and Share*". In this project, different communities of practice were developed to facilitate healthcare professionals sharing their experience and practices in 50 clinical topics, like asthma and child health. As a result, commonly-agreed patient management approaches could be developed. According to NHS (2010), the "Do Once and Share" project has led to a win-win-win situation, namely:

- Patients can receive agreed and consistent treatment approaches;
- Healthcare professional are equipped with best medical knowledge at national standards; and
- National Health Service can save costs as inconsistencies are being reduced.

Apart from the "*Do Once and Share*" project, the National Health Service has also adopted the use of lesson cards Eurekas (a KM platform). When healthcare professionals learn a lesson, they externalize their experience in a form of document concisely and it will be shared via the platform. Other innovative KM initiatives include the use of Protocols and Care Pathways database and Map of Medicine. Recently, McCracken and Edwards (2015) conduct a qualitative study to examine key factors affecting the implementation of knowledge management systems at a National Health Service hospital. Seven factors are identified in this study and they are (1) business strategy; (2) fluid approach; (3) communication plan; (4) process mapping; (5) silo thinking and organizational structure; and (6) demand for knowledge. First, KM projects should be aligned with the organizational strategies which aim to solve business problems. Secondly, fluid approach refers to an adaptable and flexible way for KM systems implementation under the dynamic environment. Moreover, authors posit that both structured and unstructured communications should be incorporated in the communication plan. By winning their hearts and minds, healthcare professionals will be more eager to voice their opinions and barriers can be removed in an earlier stage. With the use of process map, clinical operations can be visualized. The effectiveness of KM projects can be enhanced by mapping appropriate initiatives with medical procedures. Furthermore, more knowledge can be shared across different units or specialties if silo thinking can be broken. Lastly, the study has developed the proposition that "KMS designed around patient care pathways are more effective than those organized by department" (McCracken and Edwards, 2015, p.9) – which emphasizes that understanding the knowledge needs is crucial to KM implementation.

World Health Organization

The World Health Organization (WHO) has been established as a specialized group under the United Nations since 1948 and it focuses on global public health issues. Aligned with the strategic review in 2003, WHO sets up its Department of KM and Sharing with the aim of utilizing "technology to enable people to create, capture, store, retrieve, use and share knowledge" (World Health Organization. 2016a). WHO has identified that the "know-do" gap exists in healthcare sector. A "know-do" gap is the disconnection between "what is known" and "what is done in practice" (World Health Organization, 2005a). Working closely with the region offices in Zimbabwe, India, Egypt, USA, Denmark and Philippines and some external parties, the Department of KM and Sharing has implemented different KM initiatives which aim at bridging this gap. The overview of the KM strategy can be illustrated with the slogan stated in their leaflet – "Innovation in sharing and applying knowledge for global health equity" (World Health Organization, 2005b). WHO's global KM strategy attempts to:

- Strengthen country health systems through KM;
- Establishing KM in public health; and
- Enable WHO to become a better learning organization

In order to achieve the above-mentioned strategies, WHO puts the focus on five areas: (1) improving access to the world's health information; (2) translating knowledge into policy and action; (3) sharing and reapplying experiential knowledge; (4) leveraging e-Health in countries; (5) fostering an enabling environment. Some countries have difficulties in accessing high-quality healthcare information while information overload exist in some regions. WHO has developed several measures to disseminate quality information and knowledge to healthcare professional located in different parts of the world. For instance, both print and electronic health-related multi-lingual journals and reports are available to be accessed through the network of libraries. Through the establishment of communities of practice, the best practice and lessons learned in public health are shared among healthcare professionals. Moreover, e-Health framework and its components are incorporated into existing health systems. In addition, the Department of KM and Sharing is also responsible to create and maintain the KM culture, to develop and deliver KM training workshops and to support the KM implementations in different regions and countries. Details of KM implementation are presented in Table 3.

Table 3. KM implementation in World Health Organization

Focus Area	Actions
Improving access to the world's health information	• Support for WHO publications • WHO flagship publications • WHO network of libraries • WHO Web communications
Translating knowledge into policy and action	• Good practice and guidance on knowledge translation and scale-up • Building capability in KM methods in public health practice • Promote evidence for policy and decision making
Sharing and reapplying experiential knowledge	• Improve ability to share knowledge in public health • WHO and Global Health Histories • WHO Collaborating Centres
Leveraging e-Health in countries	• E-Health frameworks, guidelines and tools • E-Health services in countries • Country capacity building via ICT • Public-private partnerships in ICT
Fostering an enabling environment	• Foster a knowledge management culture • Develop and deliver KM training programmes • Support countries, technical programmes and partners

Source: World Health Organization (2016b).

Although the sizes of the KM implementation and development in the Hospital Authority in Hong Kong, the National Health Service in England and the World Health Organization of United Nations differ substantially, KM still plays an important role in improving the healthcare service quality (Table 4).

KNOWLEDGE MANAGEMENT FOR LONG-TERM CARE

KM can be used as a powerful tool to facilitate the generation, utilization, assimilation, dissemination and exchange of knowledge and information in healthcare (Röling and Engel, 1990; Jadad et al., 2000). The value of KM is also paramount in long-term care organizations and KM helps nursing homes improve their performance so as to deliver quality care (Guptill, 2005; Surve and Natarajan, 2015). To make KM more effective in long-term care, nursing home administrators first need to know what features and attributes of KM that fits their long-term care services (Anderson et al., 2003). An article written by Kandasamy Pasupathy, the president and CEO of InforSys, Inc. in 2006 addressed that KM systems assist long-term care users to turn miscellaneous information intro practical knowledge by "extracting information form databases and other electronic sources, filtering information according to user profiles, presenting information in concert with user preferences, condensing information, retrieving evidence-based reports, holding current information in a single point of reference, routing relevant information in a timely manner, alerting users to changers, and informing decision making" (Pasupathy, 2016, p.3). A survey conducted by a consulting firm in 2008 indicated that more than 58% of home care agencies surveyed in that report had electronic medical records (EMR) in place and the figure is higher than the 32.1% of home care agencies reported in the 2000 National Center for Health Statistics (NCHS) report (Resnick and Alwan, 2010). The growing figure shows the important use of KM in home health and hospice (HHH) care, viewing KM as an essential tool for improving healthcare quality.

Table 4. A comparison of KM success stories

Criteria	Hospital Authority (Hong Kong)	National Health Service (England)	World Health Organization (United Nations)
Unit responsible for KM	KM Unit, Strategy and Planning Division, Head Office.	National Knowledge Service and The Knowledge & Intelligence team, NHS Improving Quality.	Department of Knowledge Management and Sharing.
Objective(s)	Provide convenient, timely and easy access to expert-selected and best available information resources, and an environment conducive to research and knowledge sharing.	Build knowledge sharing and learning capability, develop a repository storing success stories, form communities and adopt technology to share knowledge.	Improve the KM application through better information access, global collaborations, multilingual and quality publications and adoption of technologies.
Key contribution(s)	Developed a KM tool – e-Knowledge Gateway -which provides quality medical information to healthcare professionals.	Developed NHS Evidence (formerly called "National Electronic Library for Health") and communities of practices … etc.	Fostered KM culture, delivered KM training, developed e-Health framework and related services, translated knowledge into policy/action, published flagship products and provided network of libraries.

Source: Developed for this study.

By implementing KM system, the staff members of nursing homes have quality information to respond to situations in a timely manner. Moreover, KM helps improve decisions and facilitates communication within long-term care organizations (Jadad et al., 2000). For instance, a KM system can provide nurses real-time information regarding patient orders and other pertinent clinical care information, making long-term care organizations more accountable. In addition, use of paper-based forms by physicians and other professionals can be reduced with an effective KM system as they can use KM to get timely access to patients' information. Thus, physicians and other professionals are more encouraged to become involved in the care of nursing homes' residents. *"Almost all physicians and other professionals agreed that correct and complete patient information improves healthcare"* and long-term care delivery (Bordoloi and Islam, 2012, p.116). When the patient records and information can be accessed by physicians in a timely manner, patient care can be greatly improved so as to enhance quality of care. With KM systems in place, long-term care organizations are able to improve quality care on an ongoing basis.

PRIOR FRAMEWORKS IN LONG-TERM CARE

A framework about KM capabilities for healthcare management systems is adopted in the study by Bose (2003). In healthcare organizations, sources of knowledge include:

- **Documents:** Admission, billing, medical research and drug references.
- **Knowledge Warehouse:** Patient record, medical procedures and hospital operations.
- **Applications:** Clinical decision support, quality assurance and knowledge mining.
- **Best Practices:** Procedures, disease diagnosis, pharmacy, emergency and nursing practices.
- **Discussions:** Cost reduction, fraud prevention, performance measurement and coordination of care.

With the KM capabilities in Table 5, existing knowledge can be transformed to new knowledge through knowledge learning loops. Bose (2003) classified KM capabilities into presentation, personalization, collaboration, process, publishing and distribution, integrated search, categorization and integration. Shared new knowledge enables healthcare organizations to lower the administrative costs and enhance the healthcare quality.

In Japan, Miyagawa et al. (2014) have developed a framework for professionals who are responsible for long-term care services management. The framework is composed of six key components (four agents and two databases). The first component is user agent, which includes care provider, care recipient and care recipient's family. They can access information (e.g. aggregated case records) and submit requests to other agents. Secondly, the local information system access agent serves as the bridge between local information system and care community portal. Thirdly, the role of authentication/access control agent is to perform identity verification. After verification, sensitive information could be shared to care recipient. The last agent, namely priority control agent, is designed to determine / verify the priority of each update. Two databases include user database and care record index database. With this multi-agent framework, sensitive information can be shared / monitored with privacy and priority control.

Table 5. KM capabilities in healthcare organizations

KM Capabilities	Main Function	Illustrative Items
Presentation	Designed for user interaction	• Enterprise knowledge portal • Visualization
Personalization	Customize content and services	• Collaborative filtering • Intelligent agents
Collaboration	Staff connect together via communities of practice, discuss and work together	• Groupware • Discussion forums
Process	Variety of processes in healthcare organizations	• Clinical process • Administrative and financial processes
Publishing and Distribution	A platform for capture and distribute knowledge assets	• Authoring • Webcasting and notification
Integrated search	Reduce information overload	• Search agents and spiders • Data-mining and filtering
Categorization	Allow users to access and create knowledge categories	• Ontology • Semantic definitions
Integration	Seamless navigation across all functions	• Knowledge repository • Learning and document management

Source: Bose (2003).

KNOWLEDGE BARRIERS IN HEALTHCARE SETTINGS

Knowledge stickiness has been shown to be one of the main barriers of knowledge transfer in previous studies (Sheng et al., 2013; Law, 2014). Knowledge stickiness is the major reason for knowledge transfer failure due to the inability or unwillingness to transfer knowledge, keeping knowledge from flowing (Sheng et al., 2013). Szulanski et al. (2016) have investigated the factors that make knowledge sticky and how sticky knowledge impacts on the process of knowledge transfer. Four major gaps in knowledge stickiness are identified when transferring knowledge or best practice in healthcare settings (Table 6).

Table 6. Knowledge stickiness in transferring best practice in healthcare settings

Stages in Knowledge Transfer	Gaps	Remarks
Initiation stickiness	Difficulties in recognizing opportunities	Recognizing the opportunities for benchmarking best practice requires sufficient time and effort in delimiting and defining the best practice to be transferred.
Implementation stickiness	Technical and communication stickiness	Technical and communication gaps are developed during the phase when new knowledge is implemented. Thus, careful planning, establishing good relationship between the source and recipient of knowledge can minimize this gap.
Ramp-up stickiness	Casual ambiguity	Casual ambiguity means the basic ambiguity arising from the nature. This gap arises when precise reasons for success are not really understood during implementing the transferred knowledge. The bigger the casual ambiguity, the more likely the problems will be faced.
Integration stickiness	Obstacles when integrating new knowledge	When problems arise when implementing new knowledge or new practice, the new practice may be abandoned. Thus, success depends very much on the extent of removing obstacles and how to normalize new practice.

Source: Szulanski et al. (2016).

Apart from knowledge stickiness, an earlier study argues that both "knowledge source barriers" and "knowledge receiver barriers" hinder the flow of medical knowledge (Lin, Tan, & Chang, 2008). Healthcare professionals are busy and it may not be feasible for them to devote time in sharing or receiving knowledge. Other possible causes include the fear of losing ownership, not being adequately rewarded, lack of absorptive capacity and lack of retentive capacity (Lin, Wu, & Yen, 2012). Similarly, Khalifa (2013) has identified human barriers and financial barriers to KM implementation in health information systems and electronic medical records (EMR). Human barriers include lack of awareness of the importance and benefits of using KM as well as the lack of experience of KM systems (Manson and Pauleen, 2003). To reduce the human barriers, it is suggested that training on KM tools should be developed and implemented comprehensively as a course or a subject in medical education programmes. Dixon et al. (2013) point out that financial barriers is one of the major categories of barriers in the way of successful implementation of KM, including high initial cost of KM implementation, and high operations and maintenance cost of KM systems. In order to overcome such financial barriers, Khalifa (2013) suggests the followings:

- Allocating proper ongoing funding and adequate capital investments.
- Designing systems for the annual budgets of the healthcare organizations to accommodate the higher recurrent operation and maintenance costs.
- Proper planning of healthcare resources and logistics in the phases of KM implementation.
- Conducting feasibility studies regarding benefits vs costs of initiating / implementing KM.

To overcome knowledge barriers and foster knowledge transfer, healthcare organizations should focus and rely on factors regarding people, organization, technology and environment, i.e. the Technology-Organization-Environment (TOE) framework.

KNOWLEDGE MANAGEMENT FOR LONG-TERM CARE IN THE TOE FRAMEWORK

KM focuses on achieving a balance across people, organization and technology which helps connecting people with organizations through the use of technology (Bhatt, 2001). The optimum KM theoretically relies on the TOE framework (Lin, 2014; Kim et al., 2014). The TOE framework is an organization-level theory that explains three different elements of a firms' context influence adoption decision (Baker, 2012). TOE framework is a comprehensive tool for explaining the adoption of innovation, such as KM, in an organizational context (Ahmadi et al., 2015). Different contextual factors affecting KM effectiveness for long-term care can be closely examined in the TOE context.

Dimension of Technology

Technology plays a crucial role in innovative KM adoption among healthcare professionals. The results in the study by Yun (2013) have revealed that at the hospital level, the capacity for IT-based innovation positively influences the usage of KM systems among nurses in Seoul, Korea. A number of technologies are implemented in hospitals and healthcare organizations. First, cloud applications are frequently adopted in the healthcare industry (Li, Zheng, Ren & Lou, 2013; Lian, Yen & Wang, 2014; Sultan, 2014). Lai, Tam

& Chan (2012) have developed a model of knowledge cloud system (known as knowledge-as-a-service (KaaS) framework), which facilitates the information sharing and collaboration among professionals in Chinese medical service industry. Secondly, the adoption of radio frequency identification (RFID) is increasing significantly in healthcare sector (Chong & Chan, 2012; Lu, Lin, & Tzeng, 2013; Yao, Chu & Li, 2012). Yao et al. (2012) point out that the barriers of RFID implementation include technological limitations, costs (including hardware, software, training and maintenance) and privacy issue.

The Application of Technologies in Long-Term Care Organizations

Blaschke et al. (2009) argue that both assistive technologies and information and communication technologies can help long-term care patients or the elderlies to improve their quality of life, and physical and mental health status. Assistive technologies, including behaviour monitoring tools, smart homes, and telehealth tools, could tackle the safety and health issues. Recently, an integrated tracking with 3G smartwatch was designed for elderly. Without connecting to mobile phone, elderly or dementia patients just simply press the one-touch SOS button and the alert, with identification of the location, will be transmitted to family members (McGlaun, 2016). Moreover, The Hong Kong Polytechnic University (PolyU) and its licensee Rehab-Robotics Company Limited have designed a robotic technology, namely "*Hand of Hope*", to assist stroke patients in moving their paralyzed hands (PolyU, 2008). This device has been adopted by seven public hospitals and rehabilitation centres in Hong Kong. Moreover, it is now recognized by the European Commission, and has been exported to more than twenty countries (BIPAsia, 2016). According to Muoio (2015), one fifth of the population in Japan are elderlies, aged 65 or older. The current number of care-givers cannot meet the demand of elderly services. Therefore, several Japanese companies have designed "*Carebots*" to address this issue. "*Carebots*" are robots designed for the elderlies, long-term care patients, blind people and those in need. Based on the information provided by The International Organization for Standardization, robots can be classified into three groups: (1) person carrier robots; (2) physical assistant robots; and (3) mobile servant robots. ASIMO, a humanoid robot developed by Honda, is able to help the elderlies by feeding them food, by walking up and down steps with them in a house and by turning on and off the lights (Honda, 2004). Feedback from long-term care users and data collected from these devices can be analyzed for better clinical decision-making and better knowledge sharing.

Apart from the assistive technologies, there are a variety tools supporting clinical KM. In a healthcare KM study, Dwivedi (2007) has highlighted that KM technologies (including Internets, intranets and extranets) support a variety KM processes (identification, creation, collection, storage and access). Sittig et al. (2010) have identified four tools to support clinical KM. The first one is the web-based clinical content repository. The browse-able and searchable repository provides a platform for healthcare professionals to maintain, share and review clinical knowledge. Secondly, a web-based collaborative content management system definitely facilitates the knowledge sharing among doctors, nurses, pharmacists and other healthcare professionals. Through asynchronous discussion, opinions from different stakeholders can be voiced and consensus can be reached faster. The third and fourth tools are the enterprise-wide clinical terminology controlling tool and users' feedback tool respectively. Both positive and negative experience from patients can be shared among healthcare professionals and the top management. However, Sittig et al. (2010) point out that costs, user involvement (incentive issue), and regulatory reporting and compliance requirements are the barriers to effective clinical KM. More recently, Dixon et al. (2013) have conducted a pilot study to examine a cloud-based KM and clinical decision support system. Although the performance of this KM tool is satisfactory, several concerns (including governance, semantic interoperability and usability) have to be further explored and addressed. Particularly, security under the governance theme is considered as a critical issue. Both the healthcare and technology professionals should work closely in order to enhance the adoption of cloud-based KM systems.

Factors influencing the innovative KM adoption are widely discussed. Technology integration, technology competence and security concern are the criteria adopted in the study by Lu et al. (2013). Lian et al. (2014) have measured technology in terms of security, complexity, compatibility and costs. In a more recent study, relative advantage, compatibility, complexity and security are the variables used in technology dimension of the research framework (Ahmadi et al., 2015). Based on the discussion above, this chapter adopts three dimensions, namely: security, complexity, and costs for measuring the technological context in healthcare organizations.

Dimension of Organization

Several studies have supported that top management support is considered to be highly important in the KM process in the healthcare organizations (Lu et al., 2013; Yun, 2013; Ahamdi et al., 2015). Top management support is a key factor in overcoming resistance to changes caused by new technology adoption and diffusion, and providing vision and commitment to create a positive effect in the successful KM process (Lu et al., 2013). As the value of KM investments has been considered as an important issue for top management, a balanced scorecard approach may be appropriate to measure KM performance in long-term care organizations (Wu and Kuo, 2012). A suitable balanced scorecard structure was established by Voelker et al. (2001) for the healthcare sector (Figure 1).

Figure 1. The balanced scorecard structure for nonprofit organizations
Source: Voelker et al. (2002).

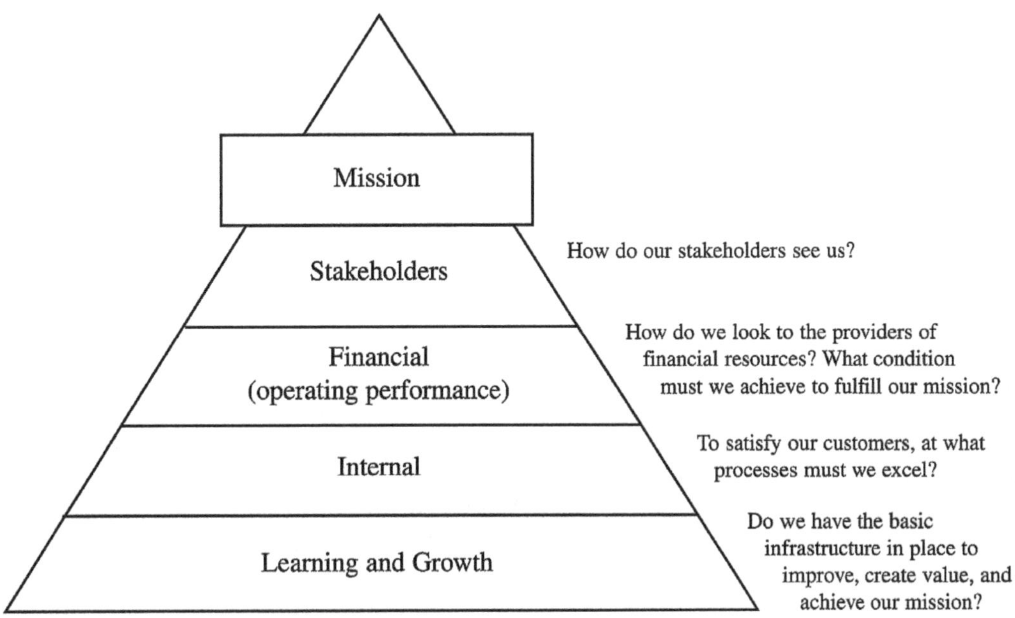

In order to effectively link mission, stakeholders, financial, internal process, and learning and growth in long-term care organizations, the balanced scorecard structure becomes an integrated as well as crucial tool for measuring them. Innovation process and information capital can be evaluated within the perspectives of internal process and learning and growth in order to measure the overall effectiveness of KM. The performance measures of innovation process and information capital are presented in the following table.

Organizational size has been regarded as important in the literature. Large firms, i.e. large healthcare institutes, typically have more resources necessary for implementing KM with the adoption of innovative technology. Thus, the size of healthcare organizations (Baker, 2012) has contributed a significant influence on the success factor of the KM process. Large healthcare organizations have resources dedicated to internal knowledge management efforts in support of the KM process so as to provide the best possible healthcare, achieving operational excellence while fostering innovation. Apart from the organizational size and in order to achieve better performance in long-term care, enhancing nursing leadership is a vital move. It is well recognized that nurses are essential in the improvement of the quality of care (Harvarth et al., 2008). Thus, enhancing nursing leadership in long-term care is absolutely necessary and is considered as "a must". According to McBride et al. (2006), leadership in nursing ties with personality characteristics or traits, such as responsiveness, commitment, vision, courage, innovation, etc. Other than the importance of personality traits, it is also imperative for nurses or nursing leaders to develop necessary skills and knowledge to motivate long-term care organizations to implement changes. Nursing leadership enhancement programmes can be delivered so as to provide comprehensive training for nurses or nursing leaders in order to strengthen their leadership skills. The dimensions of skills that nursing leaders should acquire include interpersonal skills, clinical skills, organizational skills and management skills (Harvarth et al., 2008). Table 8 shows the core content for nursing leadership enhancement programmes that can be implemented, especially in long-term care service organizations.

Healthcare professionals include medical doctors, nurses, caretakers, and other frontline staff. There are many prior studies discussing the critical role of nurse in long term care (Brazil, Brink, Kaasalainen, Kelly, & McAiney, 2012; Brühl, Luijendijk & Muller, 2007; Edwards, McClement, & Read, 2013); Hunter & Levett-Jones, 2010; Joy, Carter, & Smith, 2000) This study would put the emphasis on nursing leadership. Leadership training programmes for nurses in long-term care are needed in order to improve the quality of care in long-term care organizations. If nursing leaders are fully equipped with a set of leadership skills, the demand on ability to effect changes at all levels within an organization could be maximized.

Table 7. Balanced scorecard measures for KM

Perspectives	Objectives	Measures
Internal process	Innovation process	• Identify more innovative opportunities for long-term care • Develop innovative medical service • Design innovative administrative service
Learning and growth	Information capital	• Improve quality of information • Improve capabilities of KM • Improve accessibility of various information

Source: Wu and Kuo (2012).

Table 8. Contents for nursing leadership enhancement programmes

Dimensions	Beaulieu (1997)	Hollinger-Smith and Ortigara (2004)	Wilson (2005)	Huber (2013)
Interpersonal Skills				
Communication	X	X	X	X
Motivation				
Conflict resolution		X		X
Relationship building	X	X		X
Clinical Skills				
Use of best practices				X
Person-centered care		X		
Organizational Skills				
Vision				X
Team building	X	X	X	X
Change Theory		X	X	X
Management Skills				
HR policy and procedures			X	
Employee supervision & mentoring	X	X		X
Quality improvement	X		X	X

Source: Developed for this study.

Organizational readiness refers to the extent of readiness of healthcare sectors to get prepared for making business process changes. According to Weiner et al. (2008), the estimated success rates for businesses implementing changes range from 20% to 60% depending on the type of change. Hence, getting long-term care organizations prepared for change, e.g. adopting innovative KM technology, is significant. In fact, innovative cultures have been shown to link efficient organizational practice and high quality long-term care (Berta et al., 2005; Aylward et al., 2003). KM stimulates cultural change and innovative practices, while innovation cultures facilitate "the creation and implementation of new ideas and work methods" in long-term care (Nieboer & Strating, 2012, p.166). Scott et al. (2003) have also reported that organizational characteristics influence the innovation cultures in long-term care settings. Nieboer and Strating (2012) have conducted a study in Dutch long-term care service in order to investigate how organizational characteristics influence the innovative cultures in long-term care. Their findings have shown that formal external exchange of information, transformational leadership, commitment to quality and exploratory innovative strategy were all significantly linked to innovative cultures. Therefore, in order to develop and strengthen innovative cultures for making organizations change, efforts should be made to align organizational characteristics with organizational goals that foster innovation.

Al-Balushi et al. (2014) have determined that communication is the critical organizational readiness factor to healthcare organizations. The readiness factor assists organizational transformation by eliminating inhibitors or providing the required capabilities and knowledge in order to establish change for organizations, leading for success (Abdolvand et al., 2008; Shea et al., 2014). As several customer groups exist in long-term care setting, (such as patients, relatives of the patients, nursing home administrators, nurses, doctors, decision makers, etc., there is a need for each customer group to be communicated appropriately so as to prevent conflicts and reduce resistance to change. Thus, getting prepared for change or organizational shift, communication strategy is an essential contributor to the readiness factor (McKay et al., 2013).

Dimension of Environment

Long-term care organizations are increasingly aware of the dynamic change of the competitive environment. The influence of the external environment in an organization's decision to adopt an innovation is highlighted in the healthcare industry, especially in long-term care settings. Competitive pressure and vendor supports are regarded as the important external factors in previous studies (Baker, 2012; Bhattacharya et al., 2015; Lu et al., 2013). Competitive pressure refers to the extent to which an innovation is adopted in the firm's industry (Bhattacharya et al., 2015). The implementation of KM systems is an innovation adoption in the healthcare sector. If the healthcare organization perceives that the adoption of KM systems by other healthcare organizations is beneficial or successful, the healthcare organization faces high level of competitive pressure that triggers corresponding strategic move of similar innovation adoption (Ahmadi et al., 2015). According to Nieboer and Strating (2012), the extent of an organization's competitive environment influences the organization's innovative culture positively. In order to improve the development and implementation of innovations, a clear strategic vision should be set in response of changes in the environment.

The role of vendor has been discussed for a long period of time. One of the pitfalls that KM professionals should avoid is the "challenging software with poor vendor support" (Sharp, 2003). Ngai and Chan (2005) put forward that the successful KM systems installation and maintenance depended on the matching quality of vendor support. The study further classifies the vendor supports into five main categories: (1) vendor reputation; (2) training; (3) implementation partner; (4) KM consulting services; and (5) support, maintenance, upgrade and integration. First, vendor reputation includes their expertise and experience in KM industry. For example, an experienced KM system vendor can provide quality support services and more confidence to their clients. Secondly, both KM training and product-specific user training should be available to the clients. Moreover, successful implementation highly depends on a reliable and experienced implementation partner. Fourthly, consulting service is essential to those organizations without any KM experience. Similar to other information systems, organizations may need to improve and upgrade their KM systems so as to meet the changing needs. Ongoing vendor support should be available to the clients. In the same vein, Buyukozkan and Feyzioglu (2008) have advised organizations to evaluate vendor reputation, stability and service support when choosing KM tools or solutions. As mentioned by Bhattacharya et al. (2015), vendors are more willing to invest in larger healthcare organizations so as to maintain an innovation of the long-term care organizations. Vendor support has been identified as a determinant of innovation adoption. Thus, long-term care organizations which experience greater vendor support are more likely to adopt innovative KM systems as part of the initiatives for changes and long-term improvements.

By summarizing the factors affecting the adoption of KM, the conceptual framework for this study is proposed on the basis of the TOE framework which is shown in Figure 2.

Figure 2. A conceptual framework
Source: Developed by authors.

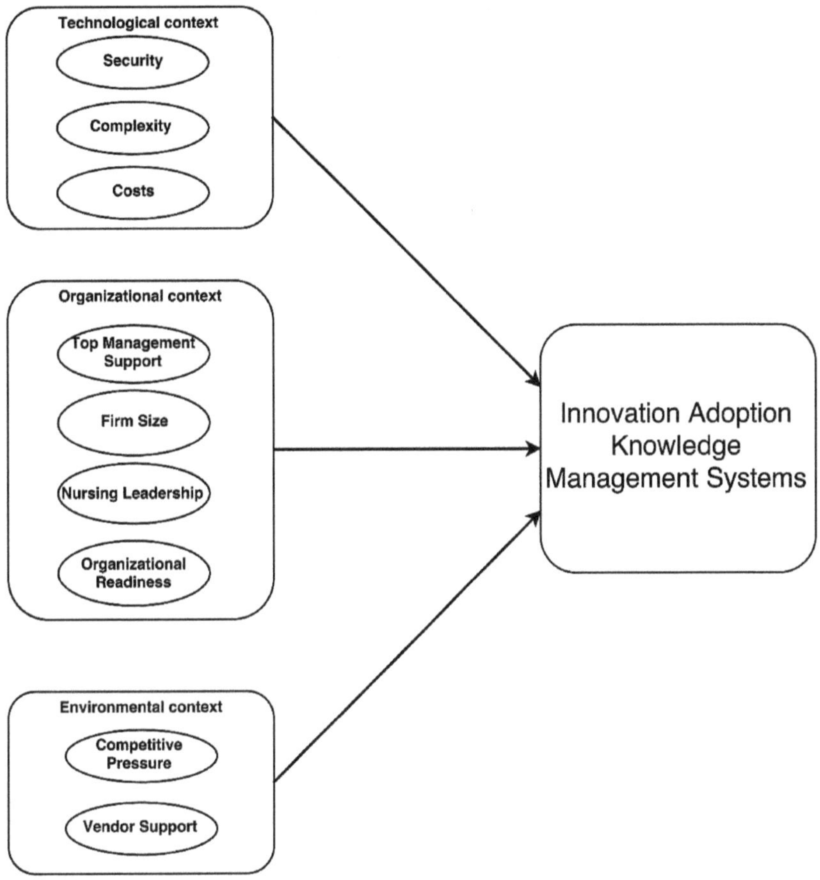

CONCLUSION AND FUTURE RESEARCH DIRECTION

KM in the long-term care service industry is progressing and the use of KM is promising to enhance the quality of care for patients by conducing evidence based practice with the best knowledge available. The delivery of healthcare service is knowledge-intensive and data-driven process, while KM and KM tools provide opportunities for improving the process performance in the long-term care industry. In addition, KM can be used to appraise performance in long-term care organizations and previous studies have noted that KM processes do have positive effect on organizational performance. The adoption of KM can impact the efficiency of healthcare delivery in terms of turning miscellaneous information into practical knowledge as a source of competitive advantage.

Through literature analysis and cases, this chapter seeks to develop a suitable framework to understand the effectiveness of KM in long-term care organizations. To overcome knowledge barriers and foster knowledge transfer, healthcare organizations should rely on a number of crucial factors such as people, organization, technology and environment. Moreover, to enhance the effectiveness of KM system, critical factors have been examined using the TOE framework. From prior studies, security, complexity, costs, top management support, firm size, leadership, organizational readiness, competitive pressure and vendor support have been proven as critical factors affecting the innovation adoption of KM systems in the context of technological, organizational and environmental dimensions.

In the future, researchers are encouraged to design a questionnaire and to collect primary data from healthcare organizations which are specialized in long term care. In the questionnaire, each construct in technological context, organizational context and environmental context is measured with multi-items. Partial Least Squares can be adopted to examine the relationships within the model in this study. From the result, the management from healthcare organizations is expected to gain insights in formulating appropriate KM strategy for performance excellence.

REFERENCES

Abdolvand, N., Albadvi, A., & Ferdowsi, Z. (2008). Assessing readiness for business process reengineering. *Business Process Management Journal*, *14*(4), 497–511. doi:10.1108/14637150810888046

Abidi, S. S. R. (2001). Knowledge management in healthcare: Towards knowledge-driven decision-support services. *International Journal of Medical Informatics*, *63*(1), 5–18. doi:10.1016/S1386-5056(01)00167-8 PMID:11518661

Ahmadi, H., Ibrahim, O., & Nilashi, M. (2015). Investigating a new framework for hospital information system adoption: A case on Malaysia. *Journal of Soft Computing and Decision Support Systems*, *2*(2), 26–33.

Al-Balushi, S., Sohal, A. S., Singh, P. J., Al Hajri, A., Al Farsi, Y. M., & Al Abri, R. (2014). Readiness factors for lean implementation in healthcare settings–a literature review. *Journal of Health Organization and Management*, *28*(2), 135–153. doi:10.1108/JHOM-04-2013-0083 PMID:25065107

Anderson, R. A., Issel, L. M., & McDaniel, R. R. Jr. (2003). Nursing homes as complex adaptive systems: Relationship between management practice and resident outcomes. *Nursing Research*, *52*(1), 12–21. doi:10.1097/00006199-200301000-00003 PMID:12552171

Aylward, S., Stolee, P., Keat, N., & Johncox, V. (2003). Effectiveness of continuing education in long-term care: A literature review. *The Gerontologist*, *43*(2), 259–271. doi:10.1093/geront/43.2.259 PMID:12677083

Beaulieu, R., Shamian, J., Donner, G., & Pringle, D. (1997). Empowerment and commitment of nurses in long-term care. *Nursing Economics*, *15*(1), 32–42. PMID:9087042

Berta, W., Teare, G. F., Gilbart, E., Ginsburg, L. S., Lemieux-Charles, L., Davis, D., & Rappolt, S. (2005). The contingencies of organizational learning in long-term care: Factors that affect innovation adoption. *Health Care Management Review*, *30*(4), 282–292. doi:10.1097/00004010-200510000-00002 PMID:16292005

Bharati, P., Zhang, W., & Chaudhury, A. (2015). Better knowledge with social media? Exploring the roles of social capital and organizational knowledge management. *Journal of Knowledge Management*, *19*(3), 456–475. doi:10.1108/JKM-11-2014-0467

Bhatt, G. D. (2001). Knowledge management in organizations: Examining the interaction between technologies, techniques, and people. *Journal of Knowledge Management*, *5*(1), 68–75. doi:10.1108/13673270110384419

Bhattacharya, M., & Wamba, S. F. (2015). A Conceptual Framework of RFID Adoption in Retail Using TOE Framework. *International Journal of Technology Diffusion*, *6*(1), 1–32. doi:10.4018/IJTD.2015010101

BIPAsia. (2016). *Actively Promoting Intellectual Property Trading HK PolyU's "Hand of Hope" gains international recognition*. Retrieved 20 July 2016, from http://bipasiaforum.com/en/success_stories/int_Actively_Promoting.html

Blaschke, C. M., Freddolino, P. P., & Mullen, E. E. (2009). Ageing and technology: A review of the research literature. *British Journal of Social Work*, *39*(4), 641–656. doi:10.1093/bjsw/bcp025

Bordoloi, P., & Islam, N. (2012). Knowledge management practices and health care delivery: A contingency framework. *Electronic Journal of Knowledge Management*, *10*(2), 110–120.

Bose, R. (2003). Knowledge management-enabled health care management systems: Capabilities, infrastructure, and decision-support. *Expert Systems with Applications*, *24*(1), 59–71. doi:10.1016/S0957-4174(02)00083-0

Boström, A. M., Slaughter, S. E., Chojecki, D., & Estabrooks, C. A. (2012). What do we know about knowledge translation in the care of older adults? A scoping review. *Journal of the American Medical Directors Association*, *13*(3), 210–219. doi:10.1016/j.jamda.2010.12.004 PMID:21450230

Brazil, K., Brink, P., Kaasalainen, S., Kelly, M. L., & McAiney, C. (2012). Knowledge and perceived competence among nurses caring for the dying in long-term care homes. *International Journal of Palliative Nursing*, *18*(2), 77–83. doi:10.12968/ijpn.2012.18.2.77 PMID:22399045

Brühl, K. G., Luijendijk, H. J., & Muller, M. T. (2007). Nurses and nursing assistants recognition of depression in elderly who depend on long-term care. *Journal of the American Medical Directors Association*, *8*(7), 441–445. doi:10.1016/j.jamda.2007.05.010 PMID:17845946

Buyukozkan, G., & Feyzioglu, O. (2008, July). A decision framework for the evaluation of the knowledge management tools. In *PICMET'08-2008 Portland International Conference on Management of Engineering & Technology* (pp. 1075-1084). IEEE. doi:10.1109/PICMET.2008.4599717

Choi, B., & Lee, H. (2003). An empirical investigation of KM styles and their effect on corporate performance. *Information & Management*, *40*(5), 403–417. doi:10.1016/S0378-7206(02)00060-5

Choi, B., Poon, S. K., & Davis, J. G. (2008). Effects of knowledge management strategy on organizational performance: A complementarity theory-based approach. *Omega*, *36*(2), 235–251. doi:10.1016/j.omega.2006.06.007

Chong, A. Y. L., & Chan, F. T. (2012). Structural equation modeling for multi-stage analysis on radio frequency identification (RFID) diffusion in the health care industry. *Expert Systems with Applications*, *39*(10), 8645–8654. doi:10.1016/j.eswa.2012.01.201

Dalkir, K., & Liebowitz, J. (2011). *Knowledge Management in Theory and Practice*. Cambridge, MA: MIT Press.

De Brún, C. (2007). Knowledge management and the national health service in England. In R. Bali & A. Dwivedi (Eds.), *Healthcare Knowledge Management* (pp. 179–188). New York, NY: Springer. doi:10.1007/978-0-387-49009-0_13

Dixon, B. E., Simonaitis, L., Goldberg, H. S., Paterno, M. D., Schaeffer, M., Hongsermeier, T., & Middleton, B. et al. (2013). A pilot study of distributed knowledge management and clinical decision support in the cloud. *Artificial Intelligence in Medicine*, *59*(1), 45–53. doi:10.1016/j.artmed.2013.03.004 PMID:23545327

Dwivedi, A. N., Bali, R. K., & Naguib, R. N. (2007). Building new healthcare management paradigms: A case for healthcare knowledge management. In R. Bali & A. Dwivedi (Eds.), *Healthcare Knowledge Management* (pp. 3–10). New York, NY: Springer. doi:10.1007/978-0-387-49009-0_1

Edwards, M. P., McClement, S. E., & Read, L. R. (2013). Nurses responses to initial moral distress in long-term care. *Journal of Bioethical Inquiry*, *10*(3), 325–336. doi:10.1007/s11673-013-9463-6 PMID:23793936

Ferlie, E., Crilly, T., Jashapara, A., Trenholm, S., Peckham, A., & Currie, G. (2015). Knowledge mobilization in healthcare organizations: A view from the resource-based view of the firm. *International Journal of Health Policy and Management*, *4*(3), 127–130. doi:10.15171/ijhpm.2015.35 PMID:25774369

Fugate, B. S., Stank, T. P., & Mentzer, J. T. (2009). Linking improved knowledge management to operational and organizational performance. *Journal of Operations Management*, *27*(3), 247–264. doi:10.1016/j.jom.2008.09.003

Girard, J. P. (2005). The Inukshuk: A Canadian knowledge management model. *KMPro Journal*, *2*(1), 9–19.

Guptill, J. (2005). Knowledge management in health care. *Journal of Health Care Finance*, *31*(3), 10–14. PMID:16080410

Hansen, M. T., Nohria, N., & Tierney, T. (1999). What's your strategy for managing knowledge? In J. A. Woods & J. Cortada (Eds.), *The Knowledge Management Yearbook 2000–2001* (pp. 55–69). Butterworth Heinemann.

Harvath, T. A., Swafford, K., Smith, K., Miller, L. L., Volpin, M., Sexson, K., & Young, H. A. et al. (2008). Enhancing nursing leadership in long-term care: A review of the literature. *Research in Gerontological Nursing*, *1*(3), 187–196. doi:10.3928/00220124-20091301-06 PMID:20077963

Ho, L. A. (2008). What affects organizational performance? The linking of learning and knowledge management. *Industrial Management & Data Systems*, *108*(9), 1234–1254. doi:10.1108/02635570810914919

Hollinger-Smith, L., & Ortigara, A. (2004). Changing Culture: Creating a Long-Term Impact for a Quality Long-Term Care Workforce. *Alzheimer's Care Today*, *5*(1), 60–70.

Honda. (2004). *The Bronx Says "Hello" to ASIMO*! Retrieved 20 July 2016, from http://asimo.honda.com/event-details.aspx?XML=Events/PostEvent_0026.xml

Hospital Authority. (2003). *HA and Clinical Research - Support, Output & Direction*. Retrieved 20 July 2016, from http://www.ha.org.hk/ho/research_ethics/msdc_p181.pdf

Hospital Authority. (2005). *Highlights of Hospital Authority Annual Plan 2005/06*. Retrieved 20 July 2016, from http://www.ha.org.hk/haho/ho/cad_bnc/126135e.pdf

Hospital Authority. (2007). *Chief Executive's Progress Report on Strategic Priorities*. Retrieved 20 July 2016, from http://www.ha.org.hk/haho/ho/cad_bnc/131443e.pdf

Hunter, S., & Levett-Jones, T. (2010). The practice of nurses working with older people in long term care: An Australian perspective. *Journal of Clinical Nursing*, *19*(3-4), 527–536. doi:10.1111/j.1365-2702.2009.02967.x PMID:20500289

Jadad, A. R., Haynes, R. B., Hunt, D., & Browman, G. P. (2000). The Internet and evidence-based decision-making: A needed synergy for efficient knowledge management in health care. *Canadian Medical Association Journal*, *162*(3), 362–365. PMID:10693595

Joy, J. P., Carter, D. E., & Smith, L. (2000). The evolving educational needs of nurses caring for the older adult: A literature review. *Journal of Advanced Nursing*, *31*(5), 1039–1045. doi:10.1046/j.1365-2648.2000.01392.x PMID:10840236

Khalifa, M. (2013). Barriers to health information systems and electronic medical records implementation. A field study of Saudi Arabian hospitals. *Procedia Computer Science*, *21*, 335–342. doi:10.1016/j.procs.2013.09.044

Kim, T. H., Lee, J. N., Chun, J. U., & Benbasat, I. (2014). Understanding the effect of knowledge management strategies on knowledge management performance: A contingency perspective. *Information & Management*, *51*(4), 398–416. doi:10.1016/j.im.2014.03.001

Kitson, A. L. (2009). The need for systems change: Reflections on knowledge translation and organizational change. *Journal of Advanced Nursing*, *65*(1), 217–228. doi:10.1111/j.1365-2648.2008.04864.x PMID:19032518

Lai, I. K., Tam, S. K., & Chan, M. F. (2012). Knowledge cloud system for network collaboration: A case study in medical service industry in China. *Expert Systems with Applications*, *39*(15), 12205–12212. doi:10.1016/j.eswa.2012.04.057

Law, K. K. (2014). The problem with knowledge ambiguity. *European Management Journal*, *32*(3), 444–450. doi:10.1016/j.emj.2013.07.010

Lee, S., Gon Kim, B., & Kim, H. (2012). An integrated view of knowledge management for performance. *Journal of Knowledge Management*, *16*(2), 183–203. doi:10.1108/13673271211218807

Li, M., Yu, S., Zheng, Y., Ren, K., & Lou, W. (2013). Scalable and secure sharing of personal health records in cloud computing using attribute-based encryption. *IEEE Transactions on Parallel and Distributed Systems*, *24*(1), 131–143. doi:10.1109/TPDS.2012.97

Lian, J. W., Yen, D. C., & Wang, Y. T. (2014). An exploratory study to understand the critical factors affecting the decision to adopt cloud computing in Taiwan hospital. *International Journal of Information Management*, *34*(1), 28–36. doi:10.1016/j.ijinfomgt.2013.09.004

Liao, S. H., & Wu, C. C. (2009). The relationship among knowledge management, organizational learning, and organizational performance. *International Journal of Business and Management, 4*(4), 64. doi:10.5539/ijbm.v4n4p64

Lin, C., Tan, B., & Chang, S. (2008). An exploratory model of knowledge flow barriers within healthcare organizations. *Information & Management, 45*(5), 331–339. doi:10.1016/j.im.2008.03.003

Lin, C., Wu, J. C., & Yen, D. C. (2012). Exploring barriers to knowledge flow at different knowledge management maturity stages. *Information & Management, 49*(1), 10–23. doi:10.1016/j.im.2011.11.001

Lin, H. F. (2014). A multi-stage analysis of antecedents and consequences of knowledge management evolution. *Journal of Knowledge Management, 18*(1), 52–74. doi:10.1108/JKM-07-2013-0278

Lo, M. F., & Ng, P. M. L. (2015). *Role of codification and personalization in organizational learning, innovation and performance: A conceptual framework and research propositions.* The 12th International Conference on Intellectual Capital, Knowledge Management & Organizational Learning, Bangkok, Thailand.

López-Nicolás, C., & Meroño-Cerdán, Á. L. (2011). Strategic knowledge management, innovation and performance. *International Journal of Information Management, 31*(6), 502–509. doi:10.1016/j.ijinfomgt.2011.02.003

Low, C., Chen, Y., & Wu, M. (2011). Understanding the determinants of cloud computing adoption. *Industrial Management & Data Systems, 111*(7), 1006–1023. doi:10.1108/02635571111161262

Lu, M. T., Lin, S. W., & Tzeng, G. H. (2013). Improving RFID adoption in Taiwans healthcare industry based on a DEMATEL technique with a hybrid MCDM model. *Decision Support Systems, 56*, 259–269. doi:10.1016/j.dss.2013.06.006

March, J. G. (1991). Exploration and exploitation in organizational learning. *Organization Science, 2*(1), 71–87. doi:10.1287/orsc.2.1.71

Mason, D., & Pauleen, D. J. (2003). Perceptions of knowledge management: A qualitative analysis. *Journal of Knowledge Management, 7*(4), 38–48. doi:10.1108/13673270310492930

McBride, A. B., Fagin, C. M., Franklin, P. D., Huba, G. J., & Quach, L. (2006). Developing geriatric nursing leaders via an annual leadership conference. *Nursing Outlook, 54*(4), 226–230. doi:10.1016/j.outlook.2006.05.003 PMID:16890042

McCracken, S. S., & Edwards, J. S. (2015). Implementing a knowledge management system within an NHS hospital: a case study exploring the roll-out of an electronic patient record (EPR). *Knowledge Management Research & Practice,* 1-11

McKay, K., Kuntz, J. R., & Naswall, K. (2013). The effect of affective commitment, communication and participation on resistance to change: The role of change readiness. *New Zealand Journal of Psychology, 42*(2), 29–40.

Metaxiotis, K. S. (2011). Healthcare Knowledge Management. In D. G. Schwartz (Ed.), *Encyclopedia of Knowledge Management* (pp. 204–210). London, UK: Idea Group Inc.

Mitton, C., Adair, C. E., McKenzie, E., Patten, S. B., & Perry, B. W. (2007). Knowledge transfer and exchange: Review and synthesis of the literature. *The Milbank Quarterly*, *85*(4), 729–768. doi:10.1111/j.1468-0009.2007.00506.x PMID:18070335

Miyagawa, S., Yamasaki, S., Uchiyama, E., & Amoroso, D. L. (2014). Framework for information sharing with privacy and priority control in long-term care in Japan. *International Journal of E-Health and Medical Communications*, *5*(1), 46–62. doi:10.4018/ijehmc.2014010103

Moustaghfir, K., & Schiuma, G. (2013). Knowledge, learning, and innovation: Research and perspectives. *Journal of Knowledge Management*, *17*(4), 495–510. doi:10.1108/JKM-04-2013-0141

Muoio, D. (2015). *Japan is running out of people to take care of the elderly, so it's making robots instead*. Retrieved 20 July 2016, from http://www.techinsider.io/japan-developing-carebots-for-elderly-care-2015-11

Ngai, E. W., & Chan, E. W. C. (2005). Evaluation of knowledge management tools using AHP. *Expert Systems with Applications*, *29*(4), 889–899. doi:10.1016/j.eswa.2005.06.025

NHS. (2010). *Do Once and Share Factsheet*. Retrieved 20 July 2016, from http://webarchive.nationalarchives.gov.uk/20130502102046/http://www.connectingforhealth.nhs.uk/resources/systserv/do-once-and

Nieboer, A. P., & Strating, M. M. (2012). Innovative culture in long-term care settings: The influence of organizational characteristics. *Health Care Management Review*, *37*(2), 165–174. doi:10.1097/HMR.0b013e318222416b PMID:21720249

Nonaka, I., & Takeuchi, H. (1995). *The knowledge-creating company: How Japanese companies create the dynamics of innovation*. Oxford University Press.

Noruzy, A., Dalfard, V. M., Azhdari, B., Nazari-Shirkouhi, S., & Rezazadeh, A. (2013). Relations between transformational leadership, organizational learning, knowledge management, organizational innovation, and organizational performance: An empirical investigation of manufacturing firms. *International Journal of Advanced Manufacturing Technology*, *64*(5-8), 1073–1085. doi:10.1007/s00170-012-4038-y

Pan, M. J., & Jang, W. Y. (2008). Determinants of the adoption of enterprise resource planning within the technology-organization-environment framework: Taiwan's communications industry. *Journal of Computer Information Systems*, *48*(3), 94–102.

Pasupathy, K. (2016). *Knowledge Management in Long-term Care: What You Need to Now*. Accessed at: http://www.ltlmagazine.com/article/knowledge-management-long-term-care-what-you-need-know

Pentland, D., Forsyth, K., Maciver, D., Walsh, M., Murray, R., Irvine, L., & Sikora, S. (2011). Key characteristics of knowledge transfer and exchange in healthcare: Integrative literature review. *Journal of Advanced Nursing*, *67*(7), 1408–1425. doi:10.1111/j.1365-2648.2011.05631.x PMID:21466576

Plaice, C., & Kitch, P. (2003). Embedding knowledge management in the NHS south-west: Pragmatic first steps for a practical concept. *Health Information and Libraries Journal*, *20*(2), 75–85. doi:10.1046/j.1471-1842.2003.00417.x PMID:12786906

Pourhamidi, M. (2013). Prioritisation of knowledge management strategies in the learning organisation: An integrated Shannons entropy-TOPSIS methodology. *International Journal of Learning and Intellectual Capital, 10*(3-4), 213–227. doi:10.1504/IJLIC.2013.057431

Pudjianto, B., Zo, H., Ciganek, A. P., & Rho, J. J. (2011). Determinants of e-government assimilation in Indonesia: An empirical investigation using a TOE framework. *Asia Pacific Journal of Information Systems, 21*(1), 49–80.

Racherla, P., & Hu, C. (2008). eCRM system adoption by hospitality organizations: A technology-organization-environment (TOE) framework. *Journal of Hospitality & Leisure Marketing, 17*(1-2), 30–58. doi:10.1080/10507050801978372

Resnick, H. E., & Alwan, M. (2010). Use of health information technology in home health and hospice agencies: United States, 2007. *Journal of the American Medical Informatics Association, 17*(4), 389–395. doi:10.1136/jamia.2010.005504 PMID:20595305

Röling, N. G., & Engel, P. G. (1990). Information technology from a knowledge system perspective: Concepts and issues. *Knowledge, Technology & Policy, 3*(3), 6–18.

Rosli, K., Yeow, P. H., & Siew, E. G. (2012). Factors influencing audit technology acceptance by audit firms: A new I-TOE adoption framework. *Journal of Accounting and Auditing, 2012*, 1–11.

Scott, S. D., Albrecht, L., OLeary, K., Ball, G. D., Hartling, L., Hofmeyer, A., & Thompson, D. (2012). Systematic review of knowledge translation strategies in the allied health professions. *Implementation Science; IS, 7*(1), 1–17. doi:10.1186/1748-5908-7-70 PMID:22831550

Scott, T., Mannion, R., Davies, H., & Marshall, M. (2003). The quantitative measurement of organizational culture in health care: A review of the available instruments. *Health Services Research, 38*(3), 923–945. doi:10.1111/1475-6773.00154 PMID:12822919

Sharp, D. (2003). Knowledge management today: Challenges and opportunities. *Information Systems Management, 20*(2), 32–37. doi:10.1201/1078/43204.20.2.20030301/41468.6

Shea, C. M., Jacobs, S. R., Esserman, D. A., Bruce, K., & Weiner, B. J. (2014). Organizational readiness for implementing change: A psychometric assessment of a new measure. *Implementation Science; IS, 9*(1), 1. doi:10.1186/1748-5908-9-7 PMID:24410955

Sheng, M. L., Chang, S. Y., Teo, T., & Lin, Y. F. (2013). Knowledge barriers, knowledge transfer, and innovation competitive advantage in healthcare settings. *Management Decision, 51*(3), 461–478. doi:10.1108/00251741311309607

Straus, S. E., Tetroe, J. M., & Graham, I. D. (2009). Defining knowledge translation. *Canadian Medical Association Journal, 181*(3-4), 165–168. doi:10.1503/cmaj.081229 PMID:19620273

Straus, S. E., Tetroe, J. M., & Graham, I. D. (2011). Knowledge translation is the use of knowledge in health care decision making. *Journal of Clinical Epidemiology, 64*(1), 6–10. doi:10.1016/j.jclinepi.2009.08.016 PMID:19926445

Sultan, N. (2014). Making use of cloud computing for healthcare provision: Opportunities and challenges. *International Journal of Information Management, 34*(2), 177–184. doi:10.1016/j.ijinfomgt.2013.12.011

Surve, M. B. A., & Natarajan, G. (2015). Knowledge Management Tools: Recognition for The Support To Healthcare Practitioners. *International Journal of Advanced Information and Communication Technology*, *1*(12), 923–927.

Szulanski, G., Ringov, D., & Jensen, R. J. (2016). Overcoming Stickiness: How the Timing of Knowledge Transfer Methods Affects Transfer Difficulty. *Organization Science*, *27*(2), 304–322. doi:10.1287/orsc.2016.1049

The Hong Kong Polytechnic University. (2008). *Robotic hand responds to intention signals.* Retrieved 20 July 2016, from https://www.polyu.edu.hk/ife/corp/upload/docs/8_publication/KT_Eng_2012/pdf/06_4.pdf

Tourangeau, A., Cranley, L., Spence Laschinger, H. K., & Pachis, J. (2010). Relationships among leadership practices, work environments, staff communication and outcomes in long-term care. *Journal of Nursing Management*, *18*(8), 1060–1072. doi:10.1111/j.1365-2834.2010.01125.x PMID:21073577

Unit, K. M. (2016). *eKG Home Page.* Retrieved 20 July 2016, from https://www.ekg.org.hk

Voelker, K. E., Rakich, J. S., & French, G. R. (2001). The balanced scorecard in healthcare organizations: A performance measurement and strategic planning methodology. *Hospital Topics*, *79*(3), 13–24. doi:10.1080/00185860109597908 PMID:11794940

Weiner, B., Amick, H., & Lee, S. Y. (2008). Conceptualization and measurement of organizational readiness for change: A review of the literature in health services research and other fields. *Medical Care Research and Review*, *65*(4), 379–436. doi:10.1177/1077558708317802 PMID:18511812

Wilson, A. A. (2005). Impact of management development on nurse retention. *Nursing Administration Quarterly*, *29*(2), 137–145. doi:10.1097/00006216-200504000-00008 PMID:15923977

World Health Organization. (2005a). *World Health Organization Knowledge Management Strategy.* Retrieved 20 July 2016, from http://www.who.int/kms/about/strategy/kms_strategy.pdf

World Health Organization. (2005b). *Knowledge Management in WHO: Bridging the Know–Do Gap.* Retrieved 20 July 2016, from http://www.who.int/kms/en/kms_leaflet.pdf

World Health Organization. (2016a). *Knowledge management and health.* Retrieved 20 July 2016, from http://www.who.int/kms/en/

World Health Organization. (2016b). *WHO knowledge management strategy.* Retrieved 20 July 2016, from http://www.who.int/kms/about/strategy/en/

Wu, L., & Kuo, Y. Z. (2012). A balanced scorecard approach in assessing IT value in healthcare sector: An empirical examination. *Journal of Medical Systems*, *36*(6), 3583–3596. doi:10.1007/s10916-012-9834-2 PMID:22366918

Yao, W., Chu, C. H., & Li, Z. (2012). The adoption and implementation of RFID technologies in healthcare: A literature review. *Journal of Medical Systems*, *36*(6), 3507–3525. doi:10.1007/s10916-011-9789-8 PMID:22009254

Yun, E. K. (2013). Predictors of attitude and intention to use knowledge management system among Korean nurses. *Nurse Education Today*, *33*(12), 1477–1481. doi:10.1016/j.nedt.2013.05.018 PMID:23806194

Zack, M., McKeen, J., & Singh, S. (2009). Knowledge management and organizational performance: An exploratory analysis. *Journal of Knowledge Management*, *13*(6), 392–409. doi:10.1108/13673270910997088

KEY TERMS AND DEFINITIONS:

Access Control: A procedure used to check if a user is permitted to enter a (computerized) system.

Assistive Technology: Specialized hardware and software designed to improve the performance of individuals with disabilities.

Best Practices: The best way to solve problems in organizations and be codified and stored in knowledge repositories.

Clinical Decision: An outcome of a disease or injury process of diagnosis based on evidence, professional examination and judgement.

Information Overload: When excessive amount of information are available, individuals may feel anxious as well as confused and have difficulty in absorbing them into proper workflow in managing related tasks.

Knowledge Management System: An organization-wide information system that can capture, store, share and manage knowledge existed at individual, group and organizational levels.

Knowledge Translation: A process to transform knowledge into practice or decision-making in workplace.

Chapter 10
Using Pervasive Computing for Sustainable Healthcare in an Aging Population

Adam Ka Lok Wong
The Hong Kong Polytechnic University, Hong Kong

Man Fung Lo
The Hong Kong Polytechnic University, Hong Kong

ABSTRACT

Statistics have shown that not only the proportion of elderly as part of the world's population is growing, but there also is a growing deficit of the working population compared to the retired population. Therefore, the provision for age-related medical conditions will put a heavy pressure on the healthcare system. This chapter discusses how pervasive computing can be used to help to achieve sustainability in healthcare for the elderly. Mobile devices can facilitate old adults to actively seek for health and nutrition information, beware of their vital signs, and follow an active life style in a safe manner. Light-weight wearable electronic devices can provide acute care and rehabilitation services to the elderly without causing a big impact to their quality of life. A model is suggested to integrate the use of pervasive computing in health education, health management, doctor support, and monitored rehabilitation at home.

INTRODUCTION

This chapter discusses the use of pervasive computing in health care at a time when the world is facing the challenge of an aging population and uncertain economic future. The world's population is expected to grow to 9.2 billion by 2050. Although the rate of growth is dropping, from approximately 1.2% per year at 2012 to less than 0.5% per year by 2050, this is a trend of population aging. The median age of the world's population was 28 in 2012, and it will be about 38 in 2050. Moreover, the problem of the population aging will be more serious in developed countries than in developing countries. By 2050, the median age will be 41 in North America and Asia, 45 in China, and 47 in Europe (Magnus, 2012).

DOI: 10.4018/978-1-5225-2633-9.ch010

As people grow old, their needs for health care increase. For example, old people may suffer from acute illness such as stroke or bone fracture due to falling, and chronic illnesses such as dementia, diabetes, or high blood pressure. The provision for age-related medical conditions will put a heavy pressure on the healthcare system. In China alone, it is estimated that the expense on age-related diseases will be more than 200 billion yuan by 2050 (Sun et al., 2016). Therefore, there is a real and urgent need to find ways to improve the quality of healthcare, while controlling the cost of diagnostics, treatment and rehabilitation. An important part of the solution to the problem is to change the focus of health care for the elderly from a reactive model to a preventive model. This means on one hand, old adults have to be encouraged and educated to actively seek for health and nutrition information, beware of their vital signs, and follow an active life style in a safe manner. On the other hand, another part of the solution is to use light-weight wearable electronic devices, in association with communication technologies, to provide acute care and rehabilitation services to the elderly without causing a big impact to their quality of life. As the elderly take a more active role in self-care, they can help to prevent injuries, minimize illness and reduce the cost on healthcare and rehabilitation.

BACKGROUND

The problem of the aging population can be measured by the Elderly Dependency Ratio (EDR). Basically, EDR is ratio of the number of people who have reached retirement age to the number of people of working age. An EDR of greater than 50% means there is a person at the working age has to support more than one elderly person. The specific definition depends on the designated retirement age of the society under study. For example, Athauda et al. (2015, p.97) defined EDR as "the ratio between the population over 65 years, and the population between 15-65 years of age". The Organization for Economic Co-operation and Development (OECD) defined EDR as the number of persons of working age (aged 15 to 64) per person aged 65 or over (Harper, 2014). The OECD estimated that by 2050, the EDR is expected to reach 51% for the European Union members, and 74% for Japan. An alternative measure is the difference in the number of people reaching the working age to the number of people reaching the retirement age. Based on this measure, there is a demographic deficit for the OECD members around 2016. In the foreseeable future, the world will see an EDR of greater than 51% and a demographic deficit. This implies that not only a working person has to support more than one elderly, but also that the trend will get worse as time goes by. Therefore, new and sustainable forms of health care will be crucial to meet the growing demand for more and more age-related spending, in the face of a declining portion of people of the working age.

Blowfield (2013, p.6) defined sustainability as "meeting the needs of the present generation without compromising the ability of future generations to meet their own needs". This definition has implications for governments and businesses. One of the implications is that it must meet the increased expectations of today's citizens and consumers. With today's advances in telecommunications network and high proliferation of technology, the elderly and their care-takers expect that they can get better healthcare without substantial increase in cost and causing excessive burden on future generations. The use of pervasive computing is a solution to achieve that sustainability.

Korhonen and Bardram (2004, p. 229) defined pervasive computing as "the integration of computing power (microprocessors) and sensing (sensors) into anything, including not only traditional computers, personal digital assistants (PDAs), printers, etc., but also everyday objects like white goods, toys, houses and furniture". The term pervasive computing is often used interchangeably with "personal technology". In fact, the word "pervasive" is used to define personal technology. For example, Weiss, Whiteley, Treviranus, and Fels (2001) defined personal technology as "ubiquitous, pervasive and/or mobile computing in entertainment, business or educational contexts". This means pervasive computing is an approach to computing in which advanced technologies are personalized to meet the unique educational, social and emotional needs of individual users (Weiss et al., 2001). According to the World Health Organisation (WHO), health is "a state of complete physical, mental and social well-being and not merely the absence of disease or infirmity". The definition remains unchanged since 1948. Therefore, this chapter reviews the use of information technologies not only on the physical well-being of people, but also on the social and mental well-being of them.

PERVASIVE COMPUTING AND HEALTH CARE

Pervasive computing is often called ubiquitous computing. It is a new field of research that leverages on the advanced developments in technologies such as wireless communications, mobile computing, wearable and handheld devices, embedded systems, sensors, RFID tags and the like. The goal of pervasive computing is to improve the human experience and quality of life by having intelligent sensors and network devices embedded in an environment so that unobtrusive connectivity and services are provided to the user without explicit knowledge of the underlying communication and computing technologies. In such an environment, the objects, such as computers, cars, houses, and even the human body, are interconnected. These objects communicate autonomously to collect, process and transport information in order to adapt to the relevant context and activity (Elsevier, 2009). One example of pervasive healthcare is the use of a sensor that can be worn around the wrist to measure and record the pulse rate of the wearer. The device has small LED lights that are in close contact with the skin, but invisible to the human eye. The LED lights detect the changes in the reflected light from the capillaries as the wearer's heart beats. A built-in algorithm converts the changes to heart rate so that it can be automatically and continuously (Fitbit, 2016).

Healthcare is one of the most important applications for pervasive computing. Uses of pervasive computing in healthcare include support for independent living, wellness and disease management. It is possible to access health-related information, such as measurement data or medical knowledge, from wearable or embedded sensors in both in-hospital and out-hospital conditions, without interfering with our daily lives. The advances in mobile telephone networks and wireless technologies make it possible to collect data and present information to users, from healthcare professionals to citizens. This kind of ubiquitous monitoring and transfer of biological data creates the notion of pervasive healthcare. There are three aspects of pervasive computing in healthcare. Firstly, pervasive computing enables relatives and peers of chronically ill persons to stay in touch with a patient via mobile phones and WIFI monitor cameras. Secondly, pervasive computing enables the patient or citizen to better manage his or her own illness. Finally, pervasive computer technologies can enhance communication and collaboration between patients and healthcare professionals, and among healthcare professionals themselves (Korhonen & Bardram, 2004).

Education for Medical Students

The current state of mobile computing and wireless communications make it feasible for doctors to make better decisions when they visit the wards and give consultation to patients. The doctors can have quick access to medical information and patient history using mobile devices such as mobile phones and tablets. While the benefits are obvious, there are studies which show that doctor may resist the use of such technologies (Sun et al., 2016). In order to make doctors and other medical professionals to better accept the use of technologies, it is important that the medical students start to learn to use the technologies at the university. They can use mobile-learning to study anywhere and anytime they want. This part discusses the uses of mobile-learning, virtual patients and student response systems.

Mobile-Learning

The technology will start with the medical students. They can use mobile-learning to study anywhere and anytime they want. Meanwhile, most medical schools offer the computer-assisted learning opportunities in the medical curricula and training. According to Ventola (2014), the role of mobile devices and apps in healthcare education will be more and more important. Mobile-learning has been adopted in medical education for more than ten years. With the wireless infrastructure, medical students were able to access drug reference and diagnostic reference resources with their Personal Digital Assistants in the University of British Columbia (Garrett and Jackson, 2006). Another application is the audio and video podcasts. Students can download lecture recordings and other multimedia resources in their portable devices and learn at their own pace. Aligned with the concept by Sandars (2009), Schreiber, Fukuta et al. (2010) conducted an empirical study at the Imperial College Medical School, London and those medical students pointed out that the control feature (stop and repeat) in video podcast helped them to consolidate their learning. Another study advocated the effective use of wikis, blogs and podcasts enhanced medical students' learning (Boulos, Maramba et al. 2006). Both Flu Wiki (http://flu.wikia.com/) and Ganfyd (http://www.ganfyd.org/) are the examples of wikis in healthcare education. Furthermore, the School of Medicine, University of California, conducted another mobile learning study and the project involved more than 100 third-year medical students. Apple iPad and several mobile apps were introduced and medical students used the devices during their clinical rotations, sharing that experience in the journal Clinical Teacher (Cerrato and Satish, 2015). There are three key benefits stated in the survey report: (1) ability to retrieve electronic medical records; (2) study during downtime; and (3) ability to provide "on the go" access to information. These applications were mainly used as electronic reference tools and the interactive feature was not fully utilized. This chapter will discuss two special applications of mobile-learning - virtual patients and student response systems in medicine schools (Ozdalga, Ozdalga et al. 2012; Wong, 2016).

Virtual Patients

In the past decade, virtual patient was widely discussed in medical education research and practice. Several recent papers adopted this virtual patient definition: "a specific type of computer program that simulates real-life clinical scenarios; learners emulate the roles of health care providers to obtain a history, conduct a physical exam, and make diagnostic and therapeutic decisions" (Cook and Triola, 2009; Albarrak, 2011; Cendan and Lok 2012; Papadopoulos, Stamati et al. 2013). By reviewing more than three hundreds papers, Kononowicz, Zary et al. (2015) further classify the virtual patient applications into different forms and the top three are: (1) interactive patient scenarios; (2) high fidelity software simulations; and (3) virtual standardized patients. According to Cendan and Lok (2012), virtual patient system was composed of inputs, simulation and outputs. Learners provide inputs through the virtual patient interface and the simulation engine inside then processes. Patient responses are generated and these outputs include verbal responses, facial expressions, gestures and the change of heart rate and blood pressure. There are several applications in medical schools. First, Wakefield (2012) reported an application of virtual patient on an interactive operating table at St Mary's Hospital, London. Such table is equipped with a huge touchscreen and can be connected to desktop PCs, USB drive and other devices. On this table, there is a virtual body, namely Melanie, and it is created by 3D computer graphics and CT scans pictures. Medical students can either use mouse or touch screen to interact the operating table and examine the internal organs of Melanie. With this virtual body and stored patient cases, students can put their studies into practice and are useful in studying anatomy and surgery.

Another application of virtual patient is Patrick at Drexel University and at the University of Florida. Patrick is composed of virtual patient software and a robotic butt. It was designed to enhance the performance of medical students when conducting intimate exams, for instance prostate exam. Weller (2013) reported that there were two purposes of this virtual patient project: personal/professional and functional. For the former one, medical students are trained to communicate with Patrick effectively so as to comfort the patients with fears. From the functional perspective, the sensors inside Patrick detect and provide feedbacks to medical students when they are too aggressive during the examination. Through this virtual patient application, medical students can improve their knowledge and skills in both communicative and technical aspects. However, many studies argue that such simulation is not a substitute to practicum, Saleh (2010) provided the pros and cons summary shown in Table 1 of utilizing virtual patients as a teaching aid.

Student Response Systems

Research of student response systems in medical or healthcare education has a long history. Miller, Ashar et al. (2003) argued that interaction between presenter and audience is crucial in healthcare continu-

Table 1.

Advantages	Disadvantages
• Decreased instructor workload • Easy accessibility • Efficacy • Efficiency • Exposure to rare but critical cases • Immediate and personalized instruction and feedback • Improvement of clinical skills in a non-threatening experimental environment • Interactivity • Links to the medical literature • Personalized learning • Standardization • Student autonomy	• Difficult to integrate into medical curricula • Difficult to edit and author • Expensive and resource intensive • Limited by technology • Poor at evaluating complex cognitive skills such as empathy, negotiation, and conveying bad news • Limited by lack of diversity (race, culture, and discipline)

Source: Advantages and Disadvantages of Virtual Patients (Saleh, 2010).

ing education. Their study revealed that the use of audience response system was favorably perceived by respondents in continuing education context. In recent studies, there were many medical or nursing schools adopting this kind of systems. First, the George Washington University adopted the blog and audience response system in "Introduction to Clinical Medicine" - one of core courses in the medical curriculum (Abate, Gomes et al. 2011). Both students and instructors had positive feedback on this and the study also found that students did not have much difficulty in using the response system. However, the study highlights that instructor has to spend more time on planning and preparation. Students will lose interest in submitting responses if questions are too easy. In contrast, students may have hesitations in answering the questions. Abate, Gomes et al. (2011) provide guidance to instructors that questions should be challenging enough but accessible within a couple of minutes. Secondly, a cross-sectional study was carried out in a hundred-student medical class. When the topic of asthma was delivered, the faculty designed a pre-test and post-test (each with ten multiple choice questions). Based on the survey result, students reported that the adoption of student response system helps them to:

- Increase their attention and participation in lecture;
- Voice their opinions and receive instant feedback; and
- Follow the learning materials in the module (Sharma, 2016).

A more comprehensive study was conducted by De Gagne (2011) who reviewed more than fifteen studies about the application of student response system in healthcare education. The study summarized the impacts of student response system into three areas: (1) interactivity and participation; (2) satisfaction and learning outcomes; and (3) formative assessment and contingent teaching. For the interactivity and participation, student response systems are proven to maintain healthcare students' motivation in class. Due to the anonymity, passive students could also be changed to an active one. Secondly, both students and instructors are satisfied with the student response system. Students obtain instant feedback while instructors can establish a pleasant and active learning environment (De Gagne, 2011). However, preparation time is still an obstacle in the implementation. Drawing on literature in this area, De Gagne (2011) has pointed out that student response system is an effective tool for formative assessment. Based on students' responses, instructors can adjust their teaching during the learning process.

To sum up, information technology has already transformed many aspects in different industries. Both advantages and challenges of using mobile technology in healthcare are widely discussed. But no matter what the discussion is, the use of mobile devices must increase in the future medical education and practice. As suggested by Wallace, Clark et al. (2012), medical school leaders should develop a plan on how to integrate educational technology in their curricula so as to maximize the benefits among medical students, faculty, practitioners and ultimate provide better medical care to patients.

Support to Doctors Using Mobile Devices

When doctors consult patients and visiting the wards, they can have quick access to medical information using mobile devices such as mobile phones and tablets. Within the clinical settings, healthcare professionals use the mobile devices and apps in eight key domains: (1) information management; (2) time management; (3) health record maintenance and access; (4) communications and consulting; (5) reference and information gathering; (6) clinical decision-making; (7) patient monitoring; and (8) medical education and training (West, 2012; Ventola, 2014). For instance, doctors and nurses can use Dynamed,

Micromedex, and Epocrates for reference and information gathering. In addition, medical knowledge can be shared among healthcare practitioners through Doximity – a social networking site. Furthermore, physicians can install medical calculator apps (such as Archimedes, MedCalc and Mediquations) for patient monitoring and management.

Benefits of using these apps include enhanced efficiency and productivity, better clinical decision-making and improved accuracy (Ventola, 2014). Aligned with the theme of long term care, West (2012) provided several examples on how mobile technology helps these patients. Firstly, "On-Cue Compliance" (a text messaging system) was developed to help doctors in South Africa. A daily message is sent to remind their patients taking Rifafol for tuberculosis treatment. Another mobile coaching app was designed to help chronic disease patients. This software is used to track patients' status, including weight and blood pressure, and medical advices are then provided. Ultimately, this can help to prevent and manage patients with diabetes, heart disease and obesity (Ventola, 2014). While the benefits are obvious, there are studies which show that doctors may resist the use of such technologies (Sun, Guo et al. 2016). Some older doctors may hesitate to use new technologies in their work (Ventola 2014). Both West (2012) and Ventola (2014) put forward that several stakeholders have a key concern on the privacy and security of these devices and mobile apps. Besides, senior management and doctors would also pay attention to other issues, like the reliability of clinical decisions, impact on doctor-patient relationship, the proper integration in workplace and the legal and regulation issues (West, 2012; Aungst, 2013; Ventola, 2014).

Health Knowledge Acquisition

The increase in older adults represents an increasing percentage of the whole population and number of persons living with one or more chronic health conditions. However, extant research has largely overlooked older adults when examining current Internet users and the potential for the Internet as a health management resource. A research has found that older adults, who use the computer less, are more likely to suffer from low mood (Thielke et al., 2014). It is important to investigate how old adults can be encouraged to use the Internet to gain health-related knowledge.

Cresci and Novak (2012) conducted focus groups with urban elders in Detroit to elicit, in their own words, 'their collective perceptions about their interest, current uses, and desired uses for health management via the Internet in tandem with their current abilities and needs for technological training and support'. The findings reveal that many urban elders access the Internet, or would like to, and they clearly articulate many ways that management tools on the Internet do/could empower and assist them in actively engaging in their health management and knowledgably interacting with their health care providers. The findings also support the premise that survey measurement instruments need to be developed in collaboration with those who will directly benefit from research findings and the practice applications. It has been found that among the elderlies who received training on how to find medical information, women are more willing than men to find medical information on the Internet to manage their chronic health problems (Campbell, 2004). This finding is aligned with other studies by Jung and Padman (2014), and Tennant et al. (2015), which report that female are more likely to seek healthcare information online for their health management.

Three hundred elderlies participated in another study to examine their health information seeking behaviors (Tennant et al. 2015). Two regression results were reported in the study. First, the predictors of eHealth Literacy include age, education, and total number of electronic devices owned by each elderly. Lower age predicts higher eHealth Literacy. Contrast to previous findings, this study reports that elderly with more education claimed to have higher self-reported eHealth literacy. Besides, the increased mobile devices ownership enhances the access of online health information, thus leading to greater eHealth Literacy. The second regression result exhibits that sex, education level at baccalaureate or postgraduate, use of one or more than one electronic device are the five predictors of Web 2.0 Use for Health Information (Facebook or Twitter). As discussed earlier, female are more likely than male to use online health information. Respondents who have used of one or more than one device are three times and seven times more likely to retrieve Web 2.0 healthcare information than non-users of electronic device respectively. In order to encourage elderly accessing online health information, Tennant et al. (2015) suggests that practitioners and experts can utilize these findings and customize training opportunities for them.

From the above studies, Internet is one of the popular sources to obtain health information. However, the level of perceived reliability of healthcare website is relatively low in an Australian study (Burns, Jones et al. 2013). This is consistent with the finding obtained by Yan (2010) in Hong Kong, showing that more than 40% respondents were not sure about the reliability of the online healthcare information obtained. The promotion of credible websites by doctors and nurses is crucial to the acquisition of health knowledge by elderly or chronic disease patients. Researchers can conduct more studies in the future so as to raise the perceived reliability of healthcare websites.

Health Management in Elder Care

To achieve sustainability in healthcare for the elderly, it is important to change the paradigm of reactive medical care to a preventive one. It implies a shift from physician-centric systems to individual-centric operational models, in which the individual becomes an active partner in the care process (Korhonen & Bardram, 2004). Patients, and their care-takers, must be enabled and encouraged to take more responsibility of their own health. If illnesses are effectively screened at an early stage, the cost of subsequent medical treatment will be greatly reduced, and the patient's quality of living will not be greatly affected. For example, the elderly can be encouraged to follow a more active life style by having more physical exercises while their health is continuously monitored. This will prevent cardiovascular diseases. Their sugar intake can be measured by mobile applications to reduce the occurrence of obesity and to prevent the development of type II diabetes. Certain light-weight wearable technologies have been designed to monitor the vital signs of the patients and provide accurate and up-to-date records that enable doctors to make a more accurate diagnosis (Rudner et al., 2016; Shennib, 2014).

When patients see the doctor for consultations, they often cannot provide vital records, such as blood pressure and pulse rate, except from their memory or poorly kept paper records. McArthur (2016) described a scenario in which an elderly, at the age of 73, went to see a doctor because he had been suffering dizzy spells. The doctor performed scans on his heart and found no abnormalities. However, the doctor took the extra step of reviewing the heart-monitoring data from the patient's FitBit, a bracelet-like device that can track movements and heart beats of the wearer. Then it was found that the patient's heart could jump to a life-threatening pace for a minute before returning to normal. The patient was sent for a more scientific examination on his heart. Eventually, the examination found that the patient had been suffering a ventricular tachycardia condition and was given an implanted defibrillator in case the condition striked again.

Mobile devices can also be used for early detection of possible mental problems like dementia. The World Alzheimer's Report of 2015 estimates that there are 9.9 million new cases of dementia each year, and that the global annual cost of the disease will reach US $818 billion this year. There is a strong need for better detection through cost-effective approaches to population screening (Prince et al, 2015). One of the early detection of the onset of dementia is Mild Cognitive Impairment (MCI). Ruggeri et al. (2016) have converted the traditional pen and paper screen examination for MCI and create a mobile application called the Cambridge University Pen to Digital Equivalence assessment (CUPDE). The CUPDE was piloted and compared to the traditional pen and paper version on sixty healthy participants aged between 50 and 79. Significant differences in the overall scores between the two testing versions as well as within individual items were observed. Although this study is not conclusive in itself, it represents a possible development towards a cost-effective screen method that may one day be carried out at home by everyone.

Pervasive Technology for Self-Care and Acute Care for Older Adults

With an aging population, there is a growing demand for more health services, which are not only becoming more effective, but are also more expensive. A feasible solution to meet the growing demand in health services is to move from managing illness to maintaining wellness. Pervasive computing is an effective way to "personalize and consumerize health and wellness technologies, pushing them into the home, where real-time prevention, diagnosis, and treatment can occur" (Korhonen & Bardram, 2004, p. 230). This means a change in the approach to healthcare from professional-operated technologies in the hospital to consumer-operated interoperable generic technologies at home. The use of technologies such as Bluetooth-enable measuring devices, mobile phones and home networks plays an important role in making this happen.

For monitoring the physical wellness of elders, there are wearable technologies such as Fitbit Jawbone UP, and Samsung Gear Fit. Millions of people are measuring and monitoring their own vital signs with the objective of having a healthy lifestyle. The children and friends of elders can use these devices to find out if they are fine (Schofield, 2014). These wearable technologies can measure things like heart rates, blood pressure, calorie intake, blood sugar levels, sleep quality, and the number of steps they take each day. Almost all of these devices can connect to a smartphone using Bluetooth. For example, the Fitbit Flex wristband uploads data to the Fitbit website via a PC with a wireless sync dongle or an Android or iPhone app. If the user chooses to "share with friends" for her data, then the user's friends and relatives can have a good indication that the user is fine. The unobtrusive and easy-to-use nature of the device will encourage the elder to use it on a daily basis (Schofield, 2014). The GPS function of the FitBit allows children, and grandchildren, of the users to monitor them while they live alone independently (McArthur, 2016). There are also mobile phone applications that can inform the relatives and children of an elderly person if he or she remains inactive for a pre-set time. One such application is ManDown. The application will send an alert if an Android or Apple phone is immobile for a pre-set time, up to 24 hours. It also includes an SOS button. For an elderly person living alone, the ManDown app turns their phone into a check-in device. Just set the timer for a once or twice per day movement (Schofield, 2014).

Wearable technology also helps rescue life by saving the precious time in providing emergency treatment. There are disposable programmable electrocardiogram (ECG) sensor patches for non-invasive detection of risk patterns according to programmed criteria. The patch can be programmed by a medical professional to select one or more monitoring parameters for detection and alarm indication (Shennib, 2014). For example, when a patient takes cardioactive drugs, the patch can be used to detect changes in the ECG. Another example is the triggering of an alarm for a cardiac patient during a stress condition. The programmable patch operates in conjunction with an external programming unit for selecting the detection monitoring parameters. Rudner et al. (2016) had reported a case in which a 42-year-old man was sent to the emergency department (ED) with a newly diagnosed atrial fibrillation of unknown duration. The medical staff retrieved data from the patient's wrist-worn activity tracker and smartphone application. It was then identified the onset of the arrhythmia as within the previous 3 hours, permitting electrocardioversion and subsequent discharge of the patient from the ED.

Rehabilitation for Elderlies

Rehabilitation is an integral part of healthcare, particularly in elderly care. If people need to do rehabilitation exercises, they often need to travel to a specific location. For old adults, they may require the care-takers to accompany them and it may involve the use of wheelchairs and special vehicles. These requirements often discourage the elderly to attend rehabilitation exercises, which in turn lengthen their recovery and adversely affect their quality of life. The use of pervasive technology will allow old adults who suffer from certain medical conditions to do their rehabilitation exercises at a location which is more convenient to them, or even at home.

When motion sensing technology and artificial intelligence, elderly patients can do some exercises at home and get instant feedback. Their exercise data will be sent to the doctor or therapist via IoT (Internet-of-Things) connections (Gonz'alez-Villanueva et al., 2013; Lim et al., 2011; Songyuan et al., 2015). The Internet-of-Things can be defined as "A global infrastructure for the information society, enabling advanced services by interconnecting (physical and virtual) things based on existing and evolving interoperable information and communication technologies" (Mulani & Pingle, 2016, p.1). Gonz'alez-Villanueva et al. (2013) have developed a wearable multi-sensor system for human motion monitoring for use in rehabilitation. The sensors have embedded high-precision accelerometers and wireless communications to transmit the information related to the body motion to near-by computer to capture and record the data. Although it is still a prototype, it has demonstrated its usefulness in human motion acquisition and tracking, as required, for example, in activity recognition, physical/athletic performance evaluation and rehabilitation.

Rehabilitation is not limited to physical injuries. Most sufferers with cognitive disorder need to perform mental exercise as a continual treatment after they are discharged from hospitals. However, they cannot regularly go to professional rehabilitation centers for rehabilitation therapy. Computer-aided training has become an effective means of cognitive rehabilitation. The Intelligent Therapy Assistant (ITA) is a cognitive tele-rehabilitation platform that provides neuropsychological services. The ITA automatically selects, configures and schedules rehabilitation tasks for patients with cognitive impairments (Solana et al., 2014). According to a clinical observation, over a period of 18 months, of 528 cases with cognitive disorder, ITA can improve the rehabilitation effect of patients with cognitive impairment. The results reveal that the rehabilitation treatment proposed by the ITA is as effective as the one performed manually by therapists. Although it is not meant for use by the patients themselves at home, the ITA is potentially a useful supporting tool for the therapists.

SOLUTIONS AND RECOMMENDATIONS

A framework is suggested to enable the major stakeholders in the healthcare industry to achieve sustainable operations in health education, health management, better doctor consultations, and monitored rehabilitation at home. The adoption of the framework allows the society to train better medical professionals, alert elderlies of their health situation, enable elderly patients to rehabilitate at home, and allow doctors to give more accurate diagnosis and better advice to elderlies at the lower cost, without creating much burden on manpower requirements for the medical professionals. The model is shown in Figure 1.

FUTURE RESEARCH DIRECTIONS

The application of pervasive computing technology for healthcare is, however, not without its own inherent challenges. "Pervasive computing technology" is in itself not a well-defined technology but more like a multidisciplinary research agenda involving technologically oriented research on things like hardware, communication technology, embedded hardware and software, software infrastructures, sensor technology, distributed computing, computer-supported cooperative work, human–computer interfaces, sociological studies of the use of technology, etc. Hence, pervasive technology is not some specific technology any consumers simply buy and use in a healthcare setting, but rather a new kind of a holistic concept of integrated and embedded application of modern technology in everyday settings. (Korhonen & Bardram, 2004)

The implementation of pervasive computing technology for healthcare will depend on a number of factors. These include advances in miniaturization of devices, penetration of wireless broadband networks, culture and a change in government's policy. One promising development is the invention of the high-performance magnetic memory chip on a flexible plastic surface. The technology can embed magnetic memory and data processing components on a flexible transparent piece of plastic. It is important for the creation of light-weight, flexible, wearable electronics in future (National University of Singapore, 2016).

Figure 1. A model of integrated use of pervasive computing for healthcare

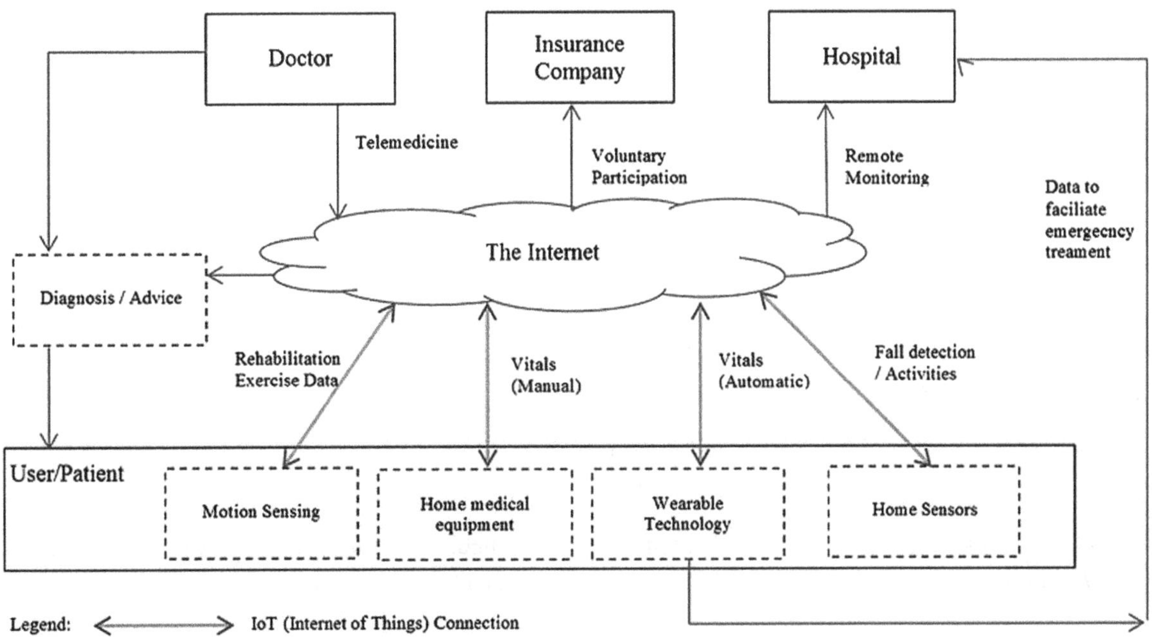

CONCLUSION

Pervasive Computing will have an important role in order to provide healthcare to the elderly in a sustainable manner. More research needs to be done, not only in the technologies themselves, but also in the acceptance of the technologies by the elderly, their care-takers and the medical staff. It is also important to bear in mind that pervasive computing should be seen as a tool that works as an integrated part of the established healthcare system. One of the concerns with using pervasive computing, especially in health monitoring, is the precision and accuracy of the devices. Therefore, most wearable medical devices should not be seen as a diagnosis tool; rather, it should be used as a tool for disease management. Wearable medical devices should focus on dynamic data acquisition, transmission of personal health data and the provision of real-time data to medical professionals, which will facilitate more timely and accurate medical decisions (Sun et al., 2016). Also, the government should also monitor and understand trends in health concerns among old adults, so as to facilitate the flow of data and information to prevent data captured by the devices from becoming islands of data, while protecting the privacy of the patient.

REFERENCES

Abate, L. E., Gomes, A., & Linton, A. (2011). Engaging students in active learning: Use of a blog and audience response system. *Medical Reference Services Quarterly*, *30*(1), 12–18. doi:10.1080/02763869.2011.540206 PMID:21271448

Albarrak, A. (2011). E-learning in Medical Education and Blended learning approach. *Learning*, *13*, 14-20.

Athauda, L. K., Wickremasinghe, A. R., Kumarendran, B., & Kasturiratne, A. (2015). An ecological study for Sri Lanka about health effects of coconut. *The Ceylon Medical Journal*, *60*(3), 97–99. doi:10.4038/cmj.v60i3.8188 PMID:26520863

Aungst, T. D. (2013). Medical applications for pharmacists using mobile devices. *The Annals of Pharmacotherapy*, *47*(7-8), 1088–1095. doi:10.1345/aph.1S035 PMID:23821609

Blowfield, M. (2013). *Business and sustainability*. Oxford, UK: Oxford University Press.

Boulos, M. N., Maramba, I., & Wheeler, S. (2006). Wikis, blogs and podcasts: A new generation of Web-based tools for virtual collaborative clinical practice and education. *BMC Medical Education*, *6*(1), 41. doi:10.1186/1472-6920-6-41 PMID:16911779

Burns, P., Jones, S. C., Iverson, D. C., & Caputi, P. (2013). Where do older Australians receive their health information? Health information sources and their perceived reliability. *Journal of Nursing Education and Practice*, *3*(12), 60. doi:10.5430/jnep.v3n12p60

Campbell, R. J. (2004). Older women and the Internet. *Journal of Women & Aging*, *16*(1-2), 161–174. doi:10.1300/J074v16n01_11 PMID:15149930

Cendan, J., & Lok, B. (2012). The use of virtual patients in medical school curricula. *Advances in Physiology Education*, *36*(1), 48–53. doi:10.1152/advan.00054.2011 PMID:22383412

Cerrato, P., & Satish, M. (2015). *Study describes the UC Irvine experience with use of the iPad in medical education.* Retrieved 4 March 2017, from http://www.imedicalapps.com/2015/08/uc-irvine-ipad-medical-education-study/

Cook, D. A., & Triola, M. M. (2009). Virtual patients: A critical literature review and proposed next steps. *Medical Education, 43*(4), 303–311. doi:10.1111/j.1365-2923.2008.03286.x PMID:19335571

Cresci, M. K., & Novak, J. M. (2012). Information Technologies as Health Management Tools: Urban Elders Interest and Ability in Usingthe Internet. *Educational Gerontology, 38*(7), 491–506. doi:10.1080/03601277.2011.567185

De Gagne, J. C. (2011). The impact of clickers in nursing education: A review of literature. *Nurse Education Today, 31*(8), e34–e40. doi:10.1016/j.nedt.2010.12.007 PMID:21232831

Fitbit. (2016). *Fitbit PurePulse Continuous Wrist-Based Heart Rate.* Retrieved 28 July 2016, https://www.fitbit.com/hk/purepulse

Garrett, B. M., & Jackson, C. (2006). A mobile clinical e-portfolio for nursing and medical students, using wireless personal digital assistants (PDAs). *Nurse Education Today, 26*(8), 647–654. doi:10.1016/j.nedt.2006.07.020 PMID:17011674

Gonzalez-Villanueva, L., Cagnoni, S., & Ascari, L. (2013). Design of a Wearable Sensing System for Human Motion Monitoring in Physical Rehabilitation. *Sensors (Basel, Switzerland), 13*(6), 7735–7755. doi:10.3390/s130607735 PMID:23774987

Harper, S. (2014). Economic and social implications of aging societies. *Science, 346*(6209), 587–591. doi:10.1126/science.1254405 PMID:25359967

Jung, C., & Padman, R. (2014). Virtualized healthcare delivery: Understanding users and their usage patterns of online medical consultations. *International Journal of Medical Informatics, 83*(12), 901–914. doi:10.1016/j.ijmedinf.2014.08.004 PMID:25193501

Kononowicz, A. A., Zary, N., Edelbring, S., Corral, J., & Hege, I. (2015). Virtual patients-what are we talking about? A framework to classify the meanings of the term in healthcare education. *BMC Medical Education, 15*(1), 1. doi:10.1186/s12909-015-0296-3 PMID:25638167

Korhonen, I., & Bardram, J. (2004). Guest editorial introduction to the special section on pervasive healthcare. *IEEE Transactions on Information Technology in Biomedicine, 8*(3), 229–234. doi:10.1109/TITB.2004.835337 PMID:15484426

Lim, C. K., Luo, Z., Chen, I. M., & Yeo, S. H. (2011). Wearable wireless sensing system for capturing human arm motion. *Sensors and Actuators. A, Physical, 166*(1), 125–132. doi:10.1016/j.sna.2010.10.015

Magnus, G. (2012). *The age of aging: How demographics are changing the global economy and our world.* John Wiley & Sons. doi:10.1002/9781119207702

McArthur, G. (2016). *Melbourne grandfather's life saved by FitBit.* Herarld Sun. Retrieved 4 March 2017, from http://www.heraldsun.com.au/news/victoria/melbourne-grandfathers-life-saved-by-fitbit/news-story/cfcd28310c938a4de2811b97adb417af

Miller, R. G., Ashar, B. H., & Getz, K. J. (2003). Evaluation of an audience response system for the continuing education of health professionals. *The Journal of Continuing Education in the Health Professions, 23*(2), 109–115. doi:10.1002/chp.1340230208 PMID:12866330

Mulani, T. T., & Pingle, S. V. (2016). Internet of Things. *International Research Journal of Multidisciplinary Studies, 2*(3).

National University of Singapore. (2016). *Research team led by NUS scientists develop plastic flexible magnetic memory device*. Singapore: National University of Singapore.

Ozdalga, E., Ozdalga, A., & Ahuja, N. (2012). The smartphone in medicine: A review of current and potential use among physicians and students. *Journal of Medical Internet Research, 14*(5), e128. doi:10.2196/jmir.1994 PMID:23017375

Papadopoulos, T., Stamati, T., & Nopparuch, P. (2013). Exploring the determinants of knowledge sharing via employee weblogs. *International Journal of Information Management, 33*(1), 133–146. doi:10.1016/j.ijinfomgt.2012.08.002

Prince, M., Wimo, A., Guerchet, M., Ali, G. C., Wu, Y. T., & Prina, M. (2015). World Alzheimer's Report. The Global Impact of Dementia: An Analysis of Prevalence, Incidence, Cost and Trends. London: Alzheimer's Disease International (ADI).

Rudner, J., McDougall, C., Sailam, V., Smith, M., & Sacchetti, A. (2016). Interrogation of Patient Smartphone Activity Tracker to Assist Arrhythmia Management. *Annals of Emergency Medicine, 68*(3), 292–294. doi:10.1016/j.annemergmed.2016.02.039 PMID:27045694

Ruggeri, K., Maguire, Á., Andrews, J. L., Martin, E., & Menon, S. (2016). Are We There Yet? Exploring the Impact of Translating Cognitive Tests for Dementia Using Mobile Technology in an Aging Population. *Frontiers in Aging Neuroscience, 8*, 21. doi:10.3389/fnagi.2016.00021 PMID:27014053

Saleh, N. (2010). The value of virtual patients in medical education. *Annals of Behavioral Science and Medical Education, 16*(2), 29–31. doi:10.1007/BF03355129

Sandars, J. (2009). Twelve tips for using podcasts in medical education. *Medical Teacher, 31*(5), 387–389. doi:10.1080/01421590802227958 PMID:19140038

Schofield, J. (2014, 3 July). What tech can I use to keep an eye on an ageing parent? *The Guardian*.

Schreiber, B. E., Fukuta, J., & Gordon, F. (2010). Live lecture versus video podcast in undergraduate medical education: A randomised controlled trial. *BMC Medical Education, 10*(1), 1. doi:10.1186/1472-6920-10-68 PMID:20932302

Sharma, A. (2016). Attitudes of medical students toward use of clickers for assessment in classrooms: A cross-sectional study. *International Journal (Toronto, Ont.), 2*(1), 60.

Shennib, A. (2014). *Programmable ECG sensor patch*. Google Patents.

Solana, J., Cáceres, C., García-Molina, A., Chausa, P., Opisso, E., Roig-Rovira, T., & Gómez, E. J. et al. (2014). Intelligent Therapy Assistant (ITA) for cognitive rehabilitation in patients with acquired brain injury. *BMC Medical Informatics and Decision Making*, *14*(1), 58. doi:10.1186/1472-6947-14-58 PMID:25038823

Songyuan, Z., Shuxiang, G., Baofeng, G., Hideyuki, H., & Hidenori, I. (2015). Design of a Novel Telerehabilitation System with a Force-Sensing Mechanism. *Sensors*, *15*(5), 11511-11527. doi:10.3390/s150511511

Sun, J., Guo, Y., Wang, X., & Zeng, Q. (2016). mHealth For Aging China: Opportunities and Challenges. *Aging and Disease*, *7*(1), 53. doi:10.14336/AD.2015.1011 PMID:26816664

Tennant, B., Stellefson, M., Dodd, V., Chaney, B., Chaney, D., Paige, S., & Alber, J. (2015). eHealth literacy and Web 2.0 health information seeking behaviors among baby boomers and older adults. *Journal of Medical Internet Research*, *17*(3), e70. doi:10.2196/jmir.3992 PMID:25783036

Thielke, S. M., Mattek, N. C., Hayes, T. L., Dodge, H. H., Quiñones, A. R., Austin, D., . . . Kaye, J. A. (2014). Associations Between Observed In-Home Behaviors and Self-Reported Low Mood in Community-Dwelling Older Adults. *Journal of the American Geriatrics Society*, *62*(4), 685-689 685. doi:10.1111/jgs.12744

Ventola, C. L. (2014). Mobile devices and apps for health care professionals: Uses and benefits. *Pharmacy and Therapeutics*, *39*(5), 356. PMID:24883008

Wakefield, J. (2012). Virtual patient under the knife on hi-tech operating table. *BBC*. Retrieved from http://www.bbc.com/news/technology-18088337

Wallace, S., Clark, M., & White, J. (2012). Its on my iPhone: Attitudes to the use of mobile computing devices in medical education, a mixed-methods study. *BMJ Open*, *2*(4), e001099. doi:10.1136/bmjopen-2012-001099 PMID:22923627

Weiss, P. L. T., Whiteley, C. P., Treviranus, J., & Fels, D. I. (2001). PEBBLES: A personal technology for meeting educational, social and emotional needs of hospitalised children. *Personal and Ubiquitous Computing*, *5*(3), 157–168. doi:10.1007/s007790170006

Weller, C. (2013). Robotic Butt Offers Prostate Exam Training For Medical Students: How "Patrick" Teaches Empathy, Proper Technique. *Medical Daily*. Retrieved 4 March 2017, from http://www.medicaldaily.com/robotic-butt-offers-prostate-exam-training-medical-students-how-patrick-teaches-empathy-proper

West, D. (2012). How mobile devices are transforming healthcare. *Issues in Technology Innovation*, *18*(1), 1-11.

Wong, A. (2016). *Innovations in Health Education-M-Learning Facilitated Multimodal Learning using Clickable Images and Virtual Patients*. Paper presented at the CPCE Health Conference 2016, Hong Kong.

Yan, Y. Y. (2010). Online health information seeking behavior in Hong Kong: An exploratory study. *Journal of Medical Systems*, *34*(2), 147–153. doi:10.1007/s10916-008-9226-9 PMID:20433053

KEY TERMS AND DEFINITIONS

Elderly Dependency Ratio (EDR): EDR is defined as "*the ratio between the population over 65 years, and the population between 15-65 years of age*" (Athauda et al. 2015, p.97). An EDR of greater than 50% means there is a person at the working age having to support more than one elderly person.

Intelligent Therapy Assistant (ITA): The cognitive evaluation system provides an automatic analysis of patients' cognitive status and arranges rehabilitation content.

Internet of Things (IoT): A global infrastructure for the information society, enabling advanced services by interconnecting (physical and virtual) things based on existing and evolving interoperable information and communication technologies.

Pervasive Computing: The integration of computing power (microprocessors) and sensing (sensors) into anything, including not only traditional computers, personal digital assistants (PDAs), printers, etc., but also everyday objects including toys, houses and furniture. The goal of pervasive computing is to improve the human experience and quality of life by having intelligent sensors and network devices embedded in an environment.

Virtual Patient: A specific type of computer program that simulates real-life clinical scenarios; learners emulate the roles of health care providers to obtain a history, conduct a physical exam, and make diagnostic and therapeutic decisions.

Chapter 11
Corporate Social Responsibility of Long-Term Care Service Enterprises

Vincent T. Law
The Hong Kong Polytechnic University, Hong Kong

Candace W. Ng
The Hong Kong Polytechnic University, Hong Kong

ABSTRACT

This chapter attempts to construct a framework for Long-Term Care (LTC) service providers to utilize Corporate Social Responsibility (CSR) concepts as the guiding principles for improving management and operations in a socially responsible manner. The framework adopts selected dimensions of the ISO 26000:2010 standard and the Triple Bottom Line framework in the economic, social, and ethical perspectives. LTC service providers need to understand CSR and can benefit from adopting best practices of CSR. Application of the proposed framework for LTC service providers are discussed. This chapter concludes by proposing future research directions on the relation between LTC and CSR.

INTRODUCTION

Many countries are facing serious problem of aging population in the recent decades. This opens opportunities to the private healthcare sector, in particular Long-Term Care (LTC) service providers. LTC services are complex and may vary with characteristics of customers, content of services, and the physical environments. Corporate social responsibility (CSR) is a popular but evolving concept. Based on the socioeconomic view, private enterprises should also serve public or social purposes; managers need to go beyond profits and improve the society's welfare. LTC service providers need to understand CSR frameworks and their application in the industry, as well as learning from best practices of CSR for sustainability.

This chapter aims at constructing a CSR framework for LTC service providers and providing recommendations to the government and LTC service enterprises in the CSR context.

DOI: 10.4018/978-1-5225-2633-9.ch011

LONG-TERM CARE SERVICES

What Are Long-Term Care Services?

From the individual perspective, long-term care (LTC) is associated with physical and/or mental deficits that limit the recipient's ability to do regular daily tasks (Singh, 2016). LTC serves the most vulnerable individuals in the society (Singh, 2016) and can be provided in a range of environments (Applebaum et al., 2013). With an increasing attention to quality of care in LTC and demographic change of LTC consumers (Pratt, 2010), best practices are established to help address ethical issues regarding LTC services (Hirst et al., 2015). Service delivery under the LTC system often incorporates competing values which share some similarities with CSR, such as autonomy, justice, beneficence, and nonmaleficence (Gamroth et al., 1995).

Components of Long-Term Care Services and Common Problems

Using Hong Kong as an example, it was found that service providers of LTC include public organizations, non-governmental organizations (NGOs), and private providers (Chung et al., 2009). Services cover community care and support (i.e. non-residential care) and residential care (Table 1).

Institutional care for LTC services in Hong Kong has traditionally been mostly provided by the public or non-profit sector, the latter being directly subvented by the former (Cheng & Chan, 2003; Chung et al., 2009). Residential facilities are preferred because they provide 24-hour care with multi-disciplinary professionals (Lou, 2014). The private sector also provides residential care services for the elderly on either self-financed basis or through Enhanced Bought Place Scheme (EBPS) of the government to provide the same on subsidized rates (Kwong & Kwan, 2002; Chan & Pang, 2007). However, the enormous

Table 1. Long-term care services for the elderly in Hong Kong

<table>
<tr><td rowspan="4">Community Care and Support Services</td><td>Community Care Services</td></tr>
<tr><td>• District Elderly Community Centre(s)
• Neighborhood Elderly Centre
• Social Centre for the Elderly
• Holiday Centre for the Elderly
• Day Care Centre/ Unit for the Elderly
• Enhanced Home and Community Care Services
• Integrated Home Care Services</td></tr>
<tr><td>Community Support Services</td></tr>
<tr><td>• Support Teams for the Elderly
• Carer Support Service
• Opportunities for the Elderly
• Home Help Service</td></tr>
<tr><td>Residential Care Services</td><td>• Hostels for the Elderly
• Homes for the Aged
• Care and Attention Homes for the Elderly
• Nursing Homes (and the Nursing Home Place Purchase Scheme)
• Contract Homes
• Private Homes (Bought Place Scheme and Enhanced Bought Place Scheme)</td></tr>
</table>

Source: Social Welfare Department (2016a).

demand for residential care services is unmet. Financing arrangements for the public, not-for-profit sector, and private (for profit) sector are also different (Chi, 2002). According to Yuen (2014), community LTC in Hong Kong is provided predominantly by non-governmental organizations (NGOs) which receive funding mostly from the government, supplemented by donations and user fees.

The LTC industry in Hong Kong faces the following common problems: (1) inadequate services to meet the demands, poor service matching, and no prioritization of service recipients (Chi, 2002; Kwong & Kwan, 2002; Lou, 2014); (2) poor service coordination; (3) no standardized assessment or referral criteria among providers (Leung, 2002); (4) poor integration among different service sectors; (5) no quality control over services (Leung, 2002; Chan & Pang, 2007); (6) limitations in funding sources and questionable affordability (Chi, 2002; Chou et al., 2005; Chan & Pang, 2007), including absence of LTC insurance coverage (Chi, 2002; Leung, 2002); and (7) weakening family care for the elderly (Leung, 2002). Overall speaking, there are opportunities for the LTC service providers to achieve better quality and socially responsible service delivery.

CORPORATE SOCIAL RESPONSIBILITY

Definitions of Corporate Social Responsibility (CSR)

Milton Friedman (1970) argues that managers' primary concern is to operate the business in the best interests of the stockholders primarily based on financial concerns. However, contemporary view argues that managers need to convert social problems into business opportunities so as to benefit and strengthen the companies or the industry (Drucker, 2008). Managers, other than making profits, need to protect and improve society's welfare (Robbins & Coulter, 2016).

Corporate social responsibility (CSR) is a popular concept among businesses, policymakers, and academics (Peterson, 2006). The term CSR is commonly understood but difficult to condense in a definition (Van Marrewijk, 2003; Brammer et al., 2012; Amaeshi et al., 2013). The nature and meaning of CSR are still evolving (Okapara & Idowu, 2013). In his classical work, Carroll (1979) views CSR as the social responsibility of business embraces the economic, legal, ethical, and discretionary expectations that society has of organizations at certain time. The European Commission on CSR defined CSR as "the responsibility of enterprises for their impacts on society" (European Commission, 2011). From a managerial perspective, Daft and Marcic (2017) defined CSR as the management's obligation to take actions for the welfare and interests of the society, not just the organization.

Private or non-governmental healthcare service enterprises can also be benefited from CSR activities. While implementation of CSR may be beneficial to the relationship between an enterprise and its external stakeholders (Firszt, 2015), LTC service providers in Hong Kong can benefit from adopting best practices of CSR in the future.

APPLICATION OF CSR FRAMEWORKS

Several CSR frameworks or standards can be applied to evaluate practices among the LTC service providers. The following sections first highlight the essential features of the Triple Bottom Line (TBL) framework and the ISO 26000:2010 standard, followed by application of their selected dimensions to LTC service providers in Hong Kong. The proposed framework on CSR practices for LTC service providers is depicted in Table 2.

Triple Bottom Line (TBL) Framework

The TBL framework measures CSR performance by integrating financial, social, and environmental aspects into measurement (Elkington, 1994). To ensure sustainability, companies have to take all three aspects into account and evaluate their performance against the TBL (Aras & Crowther, 2012). To report

Table 2. Proposed CSR framework for long-term care service providers

Aspects of Corporate Social Responsibility	Dimension	Content
Economic (Financial) Aspects	ISO 6.8.5 *(Employment creation and skills development)*	• Employment is regarded as an internationally recognized objective related to economic and social development • Skills development assists people to secure decent and productive jobs
	ISO 6.8.6 *(Technology development and access)*	Promotion of advancement of economic and social development through full and safe access to modern technology
	ISO 6.8.7 *(Wealth and income creation)*	• Creation of wealth in the community • Fair distribution of benefits of economic activities
	ISO 6.8.8 *(Health)*	Promotion of health of both customers and employees
	ISO 6.8.9 *(Social investment)*	Resources investment in initiatives and programs which aimed at improving social aspects of community life
Social Aspects	ISO 6.4.3 *(Employment and employment relationships)*	• Employment for human development • Improvement of living standards of employees through full and secure employment and decent work
	ISO 6.4.4 *(Conditions of work and social protection)*	Working conditions such as wages and different forms of compensation greatly affect both the quality of life of workers and social development
	ISO 6.4.5 *(Social dialogue)*	Exchange of ideas with major stakeholders (such as government, customers, employees, etc.)
	ISO 6.4.6 *(Health and safety at work)*	• Promotion and maintenance of the highest degree of physical, mental and social well-being of workers • Prevention of harm to health caused by working conditions
	ISO 6.4.7 *(Human development and training in the workplace)*	Improvement of employees' abilities through training and development
Ethical (or Human Rights) Aspects	ISO 4.4 *(Ethical behavior)*	Organizational behavior should be based on the values of honesty, equity, and integrity
	ISO 6.6 *(Fair operating practices)*	• Ethical conduct in dealings with other organizations such as partners, suppliers, contractors, customers, competitors, etc. • Respect for property rights of various groups (including the customers)
	ISO 6.7.1.2 *(Consumer issues and social responsibility)*	• Addressing fair marketing practices • Protection of health and safety • Dispute resolution and redress • Data and privacy protection • Addressing the needs of vulnerable and disadvantaged consumers

on CSR based on the TBL framework, Daft and Marcic (2017) set out four criteria to gauze corporate social performance, namely: (1) economic responsibility - be profitable; (2) legal responsibility - obey the law; (3) ethical responsibility - be ethical, do what is right, and avoid harm; (4) discretionary responsibility - contribute to the community and be a good corporate citizen.

ISO 26000:2010 Standard

ISO 26000:2010 is one of the well-known CSR reporting standards based on the TBL framework. It was published by the International Organization for Standardization (ISO) in 2010. It covers three dimensions of social development - economic, environmental, and societal. It provides companies with guidelines on how to operate responsibly and practice social responsibility effectively (ISO, 2014).

The most commonly used sustainability reporting standards include stakeholder involvement as one of the key components of CSR. For instance, ISO 26000:2010 provides a detailed guideline on various stakeholder engagement issues. It also states that "an organization should respect, consider, and respond to the interests of its stakeholders" (ISO, 2010). The Global Reporting Initiative Guidelines (GRI, n.d.) also introduce the principle of stakeholder inclusiveness by engaging them in the reporting process (ISO, 2014).

CSR PRACTICES IN LTC SERVICE ENTERPRISES

A framework for LTC service providers is constructed utilizing CSR concepts as the guiding principles for improving management and operations in a socially responsible manner (see Table 2). The framework is based on a combination of the ISO 26000:2010 standard and the TBL framework. The ISO 26000:2010 standard serves as the backbone since it is recognized worldwide and its content can be adapted to fit various industries. The financial and social aspects of the latter framework were selected on a complementary basis.

Overall Views on CSR

Private LTC service providers need to demonstrate CSR and are accountable to their stakeholders, such as the elderly and their family members. The following paragraphs discuss the utilization of CSR practices by LTC service providers in three selected aspects of the proposed CSR framework: economic (financial) aspects, social aspects, and ethical (human rights) aspects.

Economic (Financial) Aspects of CSR

The ISO 26000:2010 standard advocates various activities that promote the economic aspects of CSR. Economic (financial) aspects of CSR are one of the three elements of the TBL framework of CSR (Elkington, 1994). Previous studies link CSR with healthcare services. Longest and Lin (2005) find positive association between good corporate citizenship and financial performance in nonprofit hospitals. Healthcare organizations can do well financially and engage in corporate citizenship activities simultaneously. Ahn and Park (2016) find that sustainable CSR practices facilitate long-term survival. LTC service providers can enjoy positive impacts of the economic (financial) aspects of CSR. Good performance helps survival from market conditions. There is a positive link between corporate social actions and corporate financial performance (Henisz et al., 2013). Manos and Drori (2016) find a strong link between corporate social actions and the firm's core managerial policies and practices. Engagement in CSR activities enhances firm reputation (Stephenson, 2009; Carroll & Shabana, 2010; Eisenegger & Schranz, 2014) while CSR can be used as a strategy to increase profits (Doh & Quigley, 2014).

Based on the ISO 6.8.1 to 6.8.9 of the ISO 26000:2010 standard, LTC service providers need to perform certain activities to promote the economic aspect of CSR. First, the "employment creation and skills development" dimension (ISO 6.8.5) regards employment as an internationally recognized objective related to economic and social development while skills development assists people to secure decent and productive jobs (ISO, 2010). This dimension can be viewed together with the dimension of "human development and training in the workplace" (ISO 6.4.7) under the social aspects of CSR. As patient care delivery in LTC requires a multi-skilled team approach (Sullivan-Marx & Gray-Miceli, 2008), human resource is very important to LTC service providers. LTC service providers can offer flexi-time for citizens who need a job at the community levels. The "human development and training" dimension enlarges people's choices by expanding human capabilities and functioning, thus enabling workers to be knowledgeable and enjoy a decent standard of living. LTC service providers can strengthen in-house training and mentoring which focus on job-related skills in serving the elderly, as well as soft skills such as sympathy and a serving attitude. Skills of front-line staff also need regular evaluation and upgrading.

Second, the "technology development and access" dimension (ISO 6.8.6) promotes advancement of economic and social development through full and safe access to modern technology (ISO, 2010). LTC service providers can utilize suitable information and communications technology or equipment to enhance overall service delivery.

Third, the "wealth and income creation" dimension (ISO 6.8.7) emphasizes enterprises create wealth in the community and distribute benefits of economic activities fairly (ISO, 2010). LTC service providers can promote recruitment at the community level. This would relieve pressure of the family members, so that the latter can continue to go to work and retain economic productivity. This would be beneficial to the whole society.

Fourth, the "health" dimension (ISO 6.8.8) emphasizes promotion of health of both customers and employees. LTC service providers can place health issues in the first priority. They should be aware of the occupational health and safety of the employees via various activities on health promotion. Regular promotional activities on health can also be organized for customers as a value-adding service.

Lastly, the "social investment" dimension (ISO 6.8.9) encourages organizations to invest resources in initiatives and programs which aim at improving social aspects of community life (ISO, 2010). LTC service providers can participate in social investment indirectly by collaborating with the local district organizations when the latter organize social activities. Service providers can also co-organize social activities with NGOs and any other suitable organizations.

Social Aspects of CSR

Social aspects of CSR constitute the second element of the TBL framework of CSR (Elkington, 1994). ISO 26000:2010 (ISO 6.4.1 - 6.4.7) advocates various social activities that promote the economic aspects of CSR. Firszt (2015) argues that implementation of CSR may be beneficial to the relationship between an enterprise and its external stakeholders such as customers, suppliers, and other business partners. LTC service providers can build a positive impact of the social aspects of CSR with corporate image.

While elderly care services gradually become one of the foci of NGOs or service organizations, serving the elderly is viewed as a CSR.

First, the dimension of "employment and employment relationships" (ISO 6.4.3) emphasizes the importance of employment for human development and encourages employers to improve living standards of employees through full and secure employment and decent work (ISO, 2010). Promoting CSR is a key element in ensuring long-term employee and consumer trust (Sørensen & Brand, 2011). CSR programs enhance employee's organizational commitment, satisfaction, and identification with their employer (Rupp et al., 2013). LTC service providers can maintain employment with existing staff as long as financially feasible.

Second, the dimension of "conditions of work and social protection" (ISO 6.4.4) states that the conditions of work such as wages and different forms of compensation greatly affect the quality of life of workers and thus social development (ISO, 2010). Since residential facilities compete fiercely for the same pool of LTC workers, LTC service providers need to provide better working conditions after fulfilling mandatory legal requirements.

Third, the dimension of "social dialogue" (ISO 6.4.5) concerns with exchange of ideas with major stakeholders which include the government, customers, employees, and others. Other than fulfilling requirements, LTC service providers can communicate with the regulatory bodies for service improvement. Regular meetings with customers and their family members are needed to gauze opinion on service quality. To promote communication with internal stakeholders, annual or even seasonal meetings for staff at different levels are needed.

Fourth, the dimension of "health and safety at work" (ISO 6.4.6) concerns the promotion and maintenance of the highest degree of physical, mental and social well-being of workers, as well as prevention of harm to health caused by working conditions (ISO, 2010). By nature, LTC service providers concern about health and safety of their workers since they are operating in the healthcare industry. Different types of equipment should be in place to ensure occupational health and safety at various levels. Health of workers can be further protected by resident nurses and doctors.

Fifth, the dimension of "human development and training in the workplace" (ISO 6.4.7) concerns with the improvement of employees' abilities through training and development. For frontline staff, LTC service providers can provide regular job-specific training on rotary hold, feeding, and bathing techniques for the elderly. Skill levels of workers need regular reassessment. For supervisory staff, LTC service providers need to step up regular training on performance appraisal for better human resource management.

Ethical (or Human Rights) Aspects of CSR

Ethical aspects of CSR emphasize that an organization should behave ethically (ISO 4.4) while its behavior should be based on the values of honesty, equity, and integrity (ISO, 2010). Other than fulfilling service standard set by local authorities, LTC service providers can set additional requirements for frontline care-takers. Mutual scrutiny among workers also ensures enforcement of ethical standards.

On the other hand, "fair operating practices" (ISO 6.6) of the ISO 26000:2010 standard concerns ethical conduct in an organization's dealings with other organizations such as partners, suppliers, contractors, customers, competitors, and so on (ISO, 2010) and respect for property rights of various groups (including the customers)(ISO, 2010). Other than competition, LTC service providers can cooperate with their industrial counterparts or help one another in contingent situations. As operators in the service industry, LTC service providers endeavor to maintain good relation with their customers.

Regarding "consumer issues and social responsibility" (ISO 6.7.1.2), organizations need to address fair marketing practices, protection of health and safety, dispute resolution and redress, data and privacy protection, as well as the needs of vulnerable and disadvantaged consumers (ISO, 2010). Both the older person and his or her family caregivers should be treated as service targets (Lou, 2014). Riding on the locally required service standards, LTC service providers need to protect privacy of customers and their human rights in accordance with the laws.

RECOMMENDATIONS

Based on literature review on LTC and CSR, a few policy recommendations were made. First, the government should scan and review the business environment of the LTC industry. Government needs to identify key drivers of LTC spending and develop relevant policy interventions (Chung et al., 2009). The government needs to explore and introduce more government-funded places for subvented service providers so as to enhance the overall quality of service delivery. It is suggested that the government perform this at the land planning stage for every geographical district in Hong Kong. Borderline service providers should also be subsidized so that they can provide reasonable LTC services in the market.

Second, the government needs to review and improve the resource allocation mechanism for residential care homes. While monopolization by sizable operators should be avoided, the survival space for small-and-medium sized NGOs should be protected. It also affects the quality of services provided and the salary of employees working in contracted residential care homes. To ensure reasonable service delivery, it is suggested that allocation of contracts be based on both past experience and quality levels.

Third, the government should also review the training courses for healthcare service industry. Provision of training courses needs to strike a balance in maintaining the quality of trainees and fueling new labor forces for the LTC industry. This would train and develop human resources to sustain CSR practices of the industry.

FUTURE RESEARCH DIRECTIONS

There are few literature researches into the relationship between CSR and the LTC industry. Some studies focused on the service quality of existing caring facilities. For example, Cheng and Chan (2003) conducted a socio-ecological investigation into the quality of care of nursing homes in Hong Kong. Chi et al. (2011) examine ways to strengthen community care services for elders through diverse mode of service delivery. Some studies focused on the individual perception and characteristics of the elderly customers. For example, Chou et al. (2005) examined the retirement economic status of three groups of elderly based on financial dependency. Chan and Pang (2007) researched into the perceptions of elders, family members, as well as healthcare professionals. Some studies focused on the policy-related issues of the LTC industry. For example, Chi (2002) sees the opportunities for containing residential care and building a care system based on community services.

Previous studies on LTC did not particularly use a CSR framework or international standards (such as ISO 26000:2010 and GRI guidelines) as a basis for research into the healthcare services. More future research in the relationship between CSR and LTC are needed.

CONCLUSION

Based on the economic (financial), social, and ethical (or human rights) aspects of CSR under the ISO 26000:2010 standard, LTC service providers need to understand and fulfil CSR. However, LTC practitioners are not aware of the definitions, drivers, and framework of CSR in details.

In the economic (financial) perspective of CSR, LTC service providers need to view CSR initiatives as fulfilling financial objectives. To fulfil the "employment creation and skills development" (ISO 6.8.5) and "wealth and income creation" (ISO 6.8.7) dimensions, LTC services can strengthen the recruitment of local residents at the community level and provide job-specific training to both supervisory and frontline staff. Economic productivity of the society is facilitated since family members of the elderly living in residential care facilities can continue to work. Regarding the "technology development and access" dimension (ISO 6.8.6), LTC service providers can utilize service-related technology and hardware as basic requirements for operations. This echoed the efforts made by LTC service providers in promoting health of both customers and employees under the "health" dimension (ISO 6.8.8). Under the "social investment" dimension (ISO 6.8.9), LTC service providers can perform social investment indirectly by collaborating with the local district organizations, NGOs, and other parties in organizing social activities that engage the elderly and their family members.

In the social perspective of CSR, LTC service providers can visualize a positive relation between CSR activities and corporate image since serving the elderly is primarily viewed as a social responsibility. For the "employment and employment relationships" (ISO 6.4.3), "human development and training in the workplace" (ISO 6.4.7), and "conditions of work and social protection" (ISO 6.4.4) dimensions, LTC service providers should endeavor to maintain employment with existing staff as long as financially feasible amidst fierce industrial competition. Flexi-time, tailor-made in-house training, and mentoring for employees are needed. Regarding the "social dialogue" (ISO 6.4.5) dimension, LTC service providers should be aware of and actively communicate with major stakeholders of the industry which include licensing unit of the government, as well as elderly residing in their facilities and their family members. Regarding the "health and safety at work" dimension (ISO 6.4.6), LTC service providers need to concern about health and safety of their workers and customers with the support of equipment and resident healthcare professional such as nurses and doctors.

In the ethical (or human right) perspective of CSR, LTC service providers, other than fulfilling local service standards, can step up service quality via internal staff manual and various guidelines for different types of frontline staff. LTC service providers need to protect privacy of customers and their human rights in accordance with the local laws.

This chapter also identifies a future research gap for LTC services. More studies are needed on the relationship between LTC and CSR based on frameworks or international standards.

REFERENCES

Ahn, S. Y., & Park, D. J. (2016). Corporate Social Responsibility and Corporate Longevity: The Mediating Role of Social Capital and Moral Legitimacy in Korea. *Journal of Business Ethics*. doi:10.1007/s10551-016-3161-3

Amaeshi, K., Nnodim, P., & Osuji, O. (2013). *Corporate Social Responsibility, Entrepreneurship and Innovation*. New York: Routledge.

Applebaum, R., Bardo, A., & Robbins, E. (2013). International approaches to long-term services and supports. *Generations (San Francisco, Calif.)*, *37*(1), 59–65.

Aras, G., & Crowther, D. (2012). *Governance and social responsibility: international perspectives*. Hampshire, UK: Palgrave Macmillan.

Brammer, S., Jackson, G., & Matten, D. (2012). Corporate Social Responsibility and Institutional Theory: New Perspectives on Private Governance. *Socio-economic Review*, *10*(1), 3–28. doi:10.1093/ser/mwr030

Carroll, A. B. (1979). A Three-Dimensional Conceptual Model of Corporate Social Performance. *Academy of Management Review*, *4*(4), 497–505.

Carroll, A. B. (1991). The Pyramid of Corporate Social Responsibility: Toward the Moral Management of Organizational Stakeholders. *Business Horizons*, *34*(4), 39–48. doi:10.1016/0007-6813(91)90005-G

Carroll, A. B., & Shabana, K. M. (2010). The Business Case for Corporate Social Responsibility: A Review of Concepts, Research and Practice. *International Journal of Management Reviews*, *12*(1), 85–105. doi:10.1111/j.1468-2370.2009.00275.x

Census and Statistics Department. (2016a). *Press Release*. Hong Kong: Hong Kong Special Administrative Region Government. Retrieved March 2, 2017, from http://www.censtatd.gov.hk/press_release/pressReleaseDetail.jsp?charsetID=1&pressRID=3810

Census and Statistics Department. (2016b). *Hong Kong Population Projections 2015-2064*. Hong Kong: Hong Kong Special Administrative Region Government. Retrieved March 2, 2017, from http://www.statistics.gov.hk/pub/B1120015062015XXXXB0100.pdf

Census and Statistics Department. (2016c). *Demographics*. Hong Kong: Hong Kong Special Administrative Region Government. Retrieved March 2, 2017, from http://www.censtatd.gov.hk/hkstat/sub/so160.jsp

Chan, H. M., & Pang, S. (2007). Long-Term Care: Dignity, Autonomy, Family Integrity, and Social Sustainability: The Hong Kong Experience. *The Journal of Medicine and Philosophy*, *32*(5), 401–424. doi:10.1080/03605310701631661 PMID:17924269

Cheng, S. T., & Chan, A. C. M. (2003). Regulating quality of care in nursing homes in Hong Kong: A Social-ecological Investigation. *Law & Policy*, *25*(4), 403–423. doi:10.1111/j.0265-8240.2003.00156.x

Chi, I. (2002). Long-term care policy for elders in Hong Kong. *Journal of Aging & Social Policy*, *13*(2), 137–153. doi:10.1300/J031v13n02_10 PMID:12216352

Chi, I., Lam, Z., & Chan, P. (2011). *Consultancy Report on Community Support Services for the Elderly People in Hong Kong*. Hong Kong: The University of Hong Kong.

Chou, K. L., Chow, N. W. S., & Chi, I. (2005). A Proposal for a Voucher System for Long-Term Care in Hong Kong. *Journal of Aging & Social Policy*, *17*(2), 85–106. doi:10.1300/J031v17n02_06 PMID:15911519

Chung, R. Y., Tin, K. Y. K., Cowling, B. J., Chan, K. P., Chan, W. M., Lo, S. V., & Leung, G. M. (2009). Long-term care cost drivers and expenditure projection to 2036 in Hong Kong. *BMC Health Services Research*, *9*(172), 1–14. PMID:19775476

Daft, R. L., & Marcic, D. (2017). *Understanding Management* (10th ed.). Boston, MA: Cengage Learning.

Doh, J. P., & Quigley, N. R. (2014). Responsible Leadership and Stakeholder Management: Influence Pathways and Organizational Outcomes. *The Academy of Management Perspectives*, *28*(3), 255–274. doi:10.5465/amp.2014.0013

Drucker, P. F. (2008). *Management* (revised edition). New York: Harper Collins Publishers.

Eisenegger, M., & Schranz, M. (2014). Reputation Management and Corporate Social Responsibility. In Ø. Ihlen, J. L. Barlett, & S. May (Eds.), *The Handbook of Communication and Corporate Social Responsibility* (pp. 128–146). Malden, MA: Wiley-Blackwell.

Elkington, J. (1994). Towards the sustainable corporation: Win-win-win business strategies for sustainable development. *California Management Review*, *36*(2), 90–100. doi:10.2307/41165746

European Commission. (2011). *A renewed EU strategy 2011-14 for Corporate Social Responsibility*. Brussels, 25.10.2011, COM (2011) 681 final. Retrieved August 28, 2016, from http://eurlex.europa.eu/LexUriServ/LexUriServ.do?uri1/4COM:2011:0681:FIN:EN:PDF

Firszt, D. (2015). Innovations and Their Diffusion Versus CSR Practices. In L. O'Riodan, P. Zmuda, & S. Heinemann (Eds.), *New Perspectives on Corporate Social Responsibility: Locating the Missing Link* (pp. 109–125). Essen, Germany: Springer Gabler. doi:10.1007/978-3-658-06794-6_6

Friedman, M. (1970, September 13). The Social Responsibility of Business Is to Increase Profits. *New York Times Magazine*, p. 13.

Gamroth, L. N., Semradek, J., & Tornquist, E. M. (Eds.). (1995). *Enhancing Autonomy in Long-term Care*. New York: Springer Publishing.

Global Reporting Initiative. (n.d.). *GRI's History*. Retrieved July 7, 2016, from https://www.globalreporting.org/information/about-gri/gri-history/Pages/GRI's%20history.aspx

Henisz, W. J., Dorobantu, S., & Nartey, L. J. (2014). Spinning Gold: The Financial Returns to Stakeholder Engagement. *Strategic Management Journal*, *35*(12), 1727–1748. doi:10.1002/smj.2180

Hirst, S. P., Lane, A. M., & Miller, C. A. (2015). *Miller's Nursing for Wellness in Older Adults* (Canadian Edition). Philadelphia, PA: Wolters Kluwer.

ISO. (2010). *ISO 26000:2010 Guidelines on Social Responsibility*. Retrieved August 20, 2016, from http://www.iso.org/iso/catalogue_detail?csnumber=42546

ISO. (2014). *GRI G4 Guidelines and ISO 26000:2010 How to use the GRI G4 Guidelines and ISO 26000 in conjunction*. Retrieved July 7, 2016, from http://www.iso.org/iso/iso-gri-26000_2014-01-28.pdf

Kwong, E. W. Y., & Kwan, A. Y. H. (2002). A Review of Private Residential Care in Hong Kong. *Journal of Aging & Social Policy*, *13*(4), 73–89. doi:10.1300/J031v13n04_05 PMID:12418383

Leung, E. M. F. (2002). Changing Needs and Changing Service Delivery for Long-term Care in Hong Kong. *Journal of Aging & Social Policy*, *13*(2-3), 155–168. doi:10.1300/J031v13n02_11 PMID:12216353

Longest, B. B. Jr, & Lin, C. J. (2005). Can Nonprofit Hospitals Do Both Well and Good? *Health Care Management Review*, *30*(1), 62–68. doi:10.1097/00004010-200501000-00009 PMID:15773255

Lou, V. W. Q. (2014). Case Management in Community-based Long-term Care: Good Practices and Challenges in Hong Kong. In K. W. Tong & K. N. K. Fong (Eds.), *Community Care in Hong Kong: Current Practices, Practice-research Studies and Future Directions* (pp. 17–36). Hong Kong: City University of Hong Kong Press.

Manos, R., & Drori, I. (2016). *Corporate Responsibility: Social Action, Institutions and Governance*. Hampshire, UK: Palgrave Macmillan. doi:10.1057/9781137450722

OECD. (2016). *Corporate responsibility: Frequently asked questions.* Retrieved May 2, 2016, from http://www.oecd.org/corporate/mne/corporateresponsibilityfrequentlyaskedquestions.htm

Okapara, J. O., & Idowu, S. O. (Eds.). (2013). *Corporate Social Responsibility: Challenges, Opportunities and Strategies for 21st Century Leaders*. New York: Springer. doi:10.1007/978-3-642-40975-2

Peterson, E. R. (2006). *Between Hopes and Realities: Reflections on the Promises and Practices of Corporate Social Responsibility (CSR)*. PhD School of Technologies of Managing/Copenhagen Business School.

Pratt, J. R. (2010). *Long-term Care: Managing Across the Continuum* (3rd ed.). Sudbury, MA: Jones & Barlett Publishers.

Robbins, S. P., & Coulter, M. (2016). *Management* (13th ed.). Harlow, UK: Pearson.

Rupp, D. E., Shao, R., Thornton, M. A., & Skarlicki, D. P. (2013). Applicants and Employees Reactions to Corporate Social Responsibility: The Moderating Effect of First-party Justice Perceptions and Moral Identity. *Personnel Psychology*, *66*(4), 895–933. doi:10.1111/peps.12030

Singh, D. A. (2016). *Effective Management of Long-term Care Facilities* (3rd ed.). Burlington, MA: Jones & Bartlett Learning.

Social Welfare Department, Hong Kong: Hong Kong Special Administrative Region Government. (2016a). *Services for the Elderly.* Retrieved August 23, 2016, from http://www.swd.gov.hk/en/index/site_pubsvc/page_elderly/

Social Welfare Department, Hong Kong: Hong Kong Special Administrative Region Government. (2016b). *Service Quality Standards (SQSs) and Criteria*. Retrieved March 10, 2017, from http://www.swd.gov.hk/doc/ngo/_SQSs%20and%20Criteria%20(Dec%2001)(Eng).pdf

Sørensen, K., & Brand, H. (2011). Health Literacy - A Strategic Asset for Corporate Social Responsibility in Europe. *Journal of Health Communication, 16*(supp. 3), 322–327. doi:10.1080/10810730.2011.606072 PMID:21951261

Stephenson, A. K. (2009). The pursuit of CSR and business ethics policies: Is it a source of competitive advantage for organizations? *Journal of American Academy of Business, 14*(2), 251–262.

Sullivan-Marx, E. M., & Gray-Miceli, D. (Eds.). (2008). *Leadership and Management Skills for Long-term Care*. New York: Springer Publishing.

Van Marrewijk, M. (2003). Concept and Definitions of CSR and Corporate Sustainability: Between Agency and Communion. *Journal of Business Ethics, 44*(2-3), 95 & 105.

Yuen, P. P. (2014). Financing Health Care and Long-term Care in a Rapidly Ageing Context: Assessing Hong Kong's Readiness. *Public Policy and Administration, 17*(1), 56–64.

KEY TERMS AND DEFINITIONS

Aging in Place: A government policy which enables older people to remain living in familiar physical and social environments.

Social Responsibility: A business's intention to do the right things beyond its legal and economic obligations and act in ways that are good for society.

Sustainable Reporting: Organizations adopt codes and standards and publicly express over social issues towards greater transparency and accountability.

Chapter 12
Contributions of Volunteers in Long-Term Care in Hong Kong

Ting-leung Lau
Auxiliary Medical Service, Hong Kong

Kin-yee Chan
The Hong Kong Polytechnic University, Hong Kong

ABSTRACT

With the efforts of Social Welfare Department, voluntary works in Hong Kong become systemic and popular. Volunteers have been involved in developing local elderly services in many organisations in recent years. Contributions of volunteers related to elderly services in some organisations have been reviewed in this chapter, introducing the scope of services among the volunteers. Training and rewarding systems are also highlighted in order to examine the engagement of volunteers. The case of a local welfare organisation is used to discuss the operational issues encountered in Hong Kong. With a view to relieve the shortage of manpower and demand of the healthcare system, suggestions of further enhancing the ability of volunteers and extending their scope of services in the home of elderly people are proposed. Pertinent issues in sustaining trained volunteers in the voluntary long-term care work are also presented.

THE ORIGIN OF VOLUNTEERISM

Many years ago, the religious groups such as the Christianity have been playing an important role to take care of the poor by providing them with food and other necessities because of their spiritual values. Members of the church started practicing voluntary work to look after the sick in hospitals or in their homes. They believe that the negative emotions of the patients such as pain, anxiety and despair would be alleviated by peace and hope after they have visited them. Therefore, churches have been participating hospital visitations and voluntary work up to present day (Williams, n.d.).

DOI: 10.4018/978-1-5225-2633-9.ch012

Volunteers

Volunteers refer to people contributing their time and talent willingly for betterment of the society without financial gain. There are countless non-government and charity organisations involving more and more volunteers in their operations and services across the globe. Due to the aging population, the demand of healthcare service increases while the supply of labour force decreases. This group of passionate volunteers and people with potential can give a helping hand in long-term care services to the elderly people.

Volunteers are valued resources in providing services to many aspects in the community. It is believed that volunteers with appropriate training can offer more creditable assistance widely in many areas of long-term care and elderly services. They serve as an adjunct manpower to supplement the regular providers. Hence the contributions of volunteers, when organized and managed systematically, is a sustainable solution to providing the long-term care in an aging population.

Evolution of Volunteerism in Hong Kong

Under the funding of the Community Chest of Hong Kong, the Hong Kong Jockey Club Charities Trust and private donations, the Agency for Volunteer Service (AVS) was formed in 1970 to promote the voluntary work and dedicated to develop volunteerism in Hong Kong. AVS assists in referral services through a Central Membership System for people who are interested in voluntary works. Volunteers are matched and deployed according to their personal preference and talent with suitable services in a voluntary organisation. A development centre has been established to provide diversified training as well as enhancing the capacity of volunteers and voluntary organisations. More importantly, training can earn the trust and respect of both the service users and providers. It helps to build up a positive image of local volunteers. AVS is the pioneer in local volunteerism (Agency for Volunteer Service, n.d.).

In 1998, the Social Welfare Department (SWD) introduced the on-going cross-sectional scheme, "Volunteer Movement" to encourage the public to participate in voluntary work. The Steering Committee on Promotion of Volunteer Service was set up to formulate the strategy and direction of local voluntary development. Apart from offering the public a platform of multi-faceted opportunity of performing voluntary work, it gives volunteers recognition by developing a reward system. A volunteer information system has also been established (Social Welfare Department, 2005).

Moreover, four sub-committees were formed to devise action plans. Each of these sub-committees focuses on one of the following areas: students and youth, corporations, community organizations, promotion and publicity. With the division of work, resources can be utilised more efficiently without overlap. Besides, 11 district coordinating committees are organised under the SWD to co-ordinate service providers and to formulate proposals for the growth of volunteerism. The proposals have taken into consideration the characteristics of each district to give direction to the districts' strategies and the allocation of their resources so that a greater impact of volunteerism can be made. Within the SWD, the Central Office for Volunteer Service was formed for facilitating the development of volunteerism with a series of promotional activities. Through the co-operation, voluntary work is promoted widely and effectively in the society (Volunteer Movement, n.d.).

In recent years, voluntary organisations become more and more important in the society especially when it comes to the welfare of the underprivileged and vulnerable groups. With the increasing demand for long-term care, the government and society have realised that the volunteer workforce can give help in meeting the demand and can promote the well-being of long-term care recipients in the community.

Contribution of Volunteers

Volunteers often come from all walks of life. They all have their heart in serving people in need. They perform the voluntary works with passion and love. Volunteers give a big helping hand in many health orgnisations, hospital, welfare agencies, and government and Non-Government Organizations (NGOs).

In most programmes and services, volunteers emerge as the key supporting workforce of welfare agencies. In 2014, more than 1.23 million volunteers from 2,840 voluntary organisations have participated in the ''Volunteer Movement'' and served 22.4 million hours in Hong Kong (Volunteer Movement, 2016). Taking Yan Oi Tong as an example, there are more than 3,500 registered volunteers. The number is approximately three times that of their salaried staff (Yan Oi Tong Limited, 2016). The services provided by volunteers of this welfare agency operate in the same way as other welfare agencies.

It is noted that all the NGOs in the welfare service have introduced volunteers in their services because volunteers comprise the significant and main human resources of welfare agencies. Volunteers are accepted and regarded as a "regular and stable" workforce in healthcare and welfare services (Agency for Volunteer Service, 2009).

In the paper presented by Liu (2010) about the Contributions of Christian-based Volunteers in Taiwan, it has been proposed that health care policy makers should pay more attention to the services provided by religious volunteers since it has been proved that they can assist the qualified chaplains to comfort and contribute the long-term care residents. A study concerning the impact upon patients of volunteering from the United Kingdom NHS Foundation Trust suggests that volunteers are excellent resources in providing services to patients and that the patients also agree with this assessment of their important (Teasdale, 2007).

INCREASING DEMAND FOR VOLUNTEERS

Life expectancy of Hong Kong people is going up. According to the Centre for Health Protection (2016) in Hong Kong, the average life expectancy was 81.2 years for males and 87.3 years for females in 2015. Compared with the life expectancy a decade ago, the life expectancy of males and females have increased by 2.4 and 2.7 years respectively (Food and Health Bureau, 2016). In addition, citizens aged 65 years or above accounted for 15.4% of the population in 2015 and the percentage is estimated to double to 29% in 2036 (Census and Statistics Department, 2015). Thus, the demand of supportive and health care for senior citizens will definitely increase.

In view of chronic diseases and degenerative conditions of general health, majority of the aging population needs supportive care, especially in the final three to five years of their lives. Among all age groups, patients aged 85 years and above require inpatient-services under the Hospital Authority (HA) most frequently (Census and Statistics Department, 2015). Among those in the last phase of their life journeys, 30% stay in a long-term care setting for a long time, and nearly half of them passed away in hospitals and hospices (Perrels, et al., 2013). The demand for end-of-life services is rising and the demand for healthcare workers in the public health system will increase due to the aging population.

However, there is a shortage of health professionals and human resources to meet the need for the provision of such services. As such, how to acquire adequate manpower in providing service to the elderly people becomes a priority in future strategies for societies and countries with an aging population

(Morris, Wilmot, Hill, Ockenden, & Payne, 2013). This calls for active and higher volunteer engagement. The development of a sustainable volunteer workforce will certainly help to meet the shortfall of service providers in the long-term care for the elderlies.

Services Provided by Voluntary Agencies

A voluntary agency may provide one single service or multiple services. The Samaritan Befrienders Hong Kong is an example of agencies providing one single service. This organisation mainly focuses on offering psychological support to distressed and helpless people through counselling services in order to address their negative emotions. The agency provides a platform for those in need to ventilate their feelings, so that they can face the problems in a positive manner, and avoid committing suicide (The Samaritan Befrienders Hong Kong, 2016).

There are voluntary agencies that provide multiple services to the public. The Po Leung Kuk offers services in several areas, including medical and integrated health services, social, recreational, educational and cultural services. As the needs of everyone are different, various departments in Po Leung Kuk have introduced multi-faceted services to take care of those in need. Hence, more problems in the community can be solved (Po Leung Kuk, 2011).

Services Provided to Elderly People

General speaking, voluntary services currently provided to elderly people in Hong Kong are mainly focused on non-healthcare services. These services usually refer to repair of domestic electric equipment, minor household repair and maintenance works, etc. For example, the repair of home electrical apparatus is a well-known project regularly organised by the China Light Power Limited Voluntary Team. This is because social responsibility and caring the community are the core values of the China Light Power Limited, one of the two local electricity suppliers in Hong Kong.

On the other hand, some organizations are more focused on health related services. Through the scheme of Enhanced Home and Community Care Service, St. James' Settlement offers services to senior citizens in the Central and Western District, and Wan Chai in basic nursing, personal care and support, and rehabilitation exercise in their home with the aim to improve their quality of life (St. James' Settlement, n.d.). Nevertheless, such services are mainly provided by salaried staff.

Some voluntary agencies conduct regular visits, say, once in a month, to the elderly people, especially those living alone. The volunteers are led by a social worker or by an experienced volunteer. They are concerned about their living and health conditions. They remind the elderlies to take their medicine and to attend the scheduled medical appointment. In case of special needs, they will refer the clients to other agencies for follow-up.

In addition, there are health promotional activities provided to the elderlies, such as blood pressure monitoring, blood sugar levels, and body weight checking, carried out in elderly centres. Doctors and nurses, in their voluntary capacity, are invited to conduct the check-up, supported by lay volunteers. The duties of volunteers in these healthcare and check-up services require certain levels of health knowledge and skills.

Case Study (1): Woo Chung District Elderly Community Centre

Established in 1930, Yan Oi Tong was registered as a nonprofit charitable organisation in 1977. It has been providing different kinds of services in areas such as social, educational, medical, recreational and environmental. The objective of Yan Oi Tong is to enhance the quality of life of the under-privileged groups in the community.

The elderly service is remarkable among the various services of Yan Oi Tong and it benefits approximately 1.17 million elderly people annually. Members can enjoy the services in district centres such as the Woo Chung District Elderly Community Center (WCDECC), where senior citizens are helped to improve their quality of life by participating in different training courses, health talks and outings. Apart from the more traditional programmes such as singing and language courses, members can also learn how to use the computer to enrich their information technology (IT) knowledge and meet people with similar interests and habits. The elderly people are trained to have a close connection with the modern world.

WCDECC also utilises community resources efficiently to provide better support and to develop a broader network of voluntary programmes by co-operating with different district service units. For example, in the Tuen Mun East district, WCDECC has joined the Hong Kong Young Women's Christian Association to deliver care and services to those elderly people without adequate support in their daily living. For the elderly people who live alone and rarely connect the society, Yan Oi Tong also co-operates with district organisations to reach them and the less active old people, in order to assess and improve their isolated situation. Through such a collaboration, more elderly people in need can be reached and be helped.

The physical health conditions of the elderly people are also taken into consideration by WCDECC. For those who are frail, living alone, lacking supports or living in remote villages, regular visits and caring phone calls, as well as repairing and cleansing works, are offered by Yan Oi Tong. There are 30 volunteers in a team and they visit about 600 elderly people regularly to contribute the services. During the visits, appropriate psychosocial support and referral services will be made according to the needs of the elderlies.

As elderly people are susceptible to dementia, the centre offers some memory and recognition training, talks and games to control the conditions of dementia. In addition, it provides preventive measures to elderly people in dementia screening, such as questionnaires and smart phone applications. These help to raise the public awareness of Alzheimer's disease and to identify elderly people with symptoms of the disease in the early stage. Around 5 in 100 elderly people have been found to show symptoms of dementia in screening. They are referred to follow-up assessments and treatments.

On the other hand, carers attending to the elderly people are also supported considerably. The centre arranges relievers to let the carers take time off to attend to their personal business, and to ease their daily pressure through peer sharing, counseling and social activities. Meanwhile, relevant and appropriate training on the skills of caring for the elderly has helped the carers to perform their roles in a better way.

Daily Operations

There are 50 salaried staff and more than 260 volunteers in the voluntary programmes in WCDECC. Salaried staff are mainly responsible for the administrative work and liaison with other organisations. Each program is taken charge by a staff member who contacts the leader, an experienced volunteer, of a voluntary group assigned to the program. Then, the leader will contact his or her group members to give assistance to the services required. Sometimes, if there are adequate experienced volunteers, salaried staff can spare their time to take part in other programmes. Thus, resources can be allotted in a more flexible manner with the help of volunteers.

Keeping a volunteer group small can facilitate better management. It is also easier to achieve a closer relationship among members. Moreover, building up a strong connection between staff and volunteers can cultivate a strong sense of belonging, helping to sustain the partnership and their passion. Every organization has their own norms and regulations to follow, and volunteers are expected to behave in a more "self-disciplined" manner.

Case Study (2): Work Groups of Volunteers in Yan Oi Tong

The works of volunteers at Yan Oi Tong can be divided into five units.

1. **Caring Service:** Voluntary groups under this category mainly provide home visit and care phone call.
2. **Supporting Team of Centre Duty and Activities:** Volunteers in the group will be on duty at the reception counter in the centre.
3. **Performing Teams:** Volunteers are invited to share their talents by performing in public events. For example, the Lion Dance Team is always invited during Chinese New Year and in festive events. This group runs projects with other voluntary organisations such as the Red Cross and Road Safety Association.
4. **The Green Volunteer:** This group focuses on promoting green messages by delivering meals under the Food Rescue and Food Assistance Programme. Surplus food from other food suppliers will be collected and distributed to those in need.

To support these diversified services, volunteers play an irreplaceable role in Yan Oi Tong as they are the key service providers in most programmes.

Recruitment of Volunteers

In Yan Oi Tong, members who are interested in voluntary work are invited to meet the staff individually for assessing their suitability a set of diversified roles of volunteer work. In the process, better understanding of why people intend to get involved in voluntary work and the area they are interested in helps to retain and sustain their engagement. The understanding is important as people may have different expectations. If the goals and purposes of the voluntary work do not match those of the individual's expectation, conflicts may arise, and the applicants might quit prematurely. So, when applicants are found not to have a clear understanding of the work and duties involved, they will be arranged to attend a briefing session, in which concepts on voluntary work, responsibilities of volunteers, nature of elderly services will be explained to them.

To attract new volunteers, information of the voluntary works is included in the Yan Oi Tong Elderly Newsletter which is published monthly. People interested in the opportunities of voluntary work can contact the staff to obtain further information. Senior members are invited to participate in voluntary work although they may suffer from common chronic illnesses themselves. Encouraging senior members in the community to get involved in voluntary works has an implication to broaden their social engagement and networking. They make use of their experience and talents to serve others and this is an objective of the Centre.

More importantly, spending spare time in doing voluntary work will give old people a sense of satisfaction. People can further enhance their self-image through active participation in the tasks. It also helps them to find their own way and value in the society. Being a volunteer is not only about helping others, it is also about developing a more positive attitude in life. The contributions can in turn boost self-esteem accordingly.

Training Volunteers

There are briefing sessions and training for new volunteers, who may not be familiar with the nature of voluntary work. Experienced volunteers help them to understand the duty and scope of the related work.

Trainings are conducted by salaried staff and some professionals. Some volunteers need to have a longer period before they can put what they have learned into practice. Taking volunteers for the caring of dementia case as an example, they have to attend six lessons on the symptoms and precautions of dementia before rendering the service. Demented elderlies are relatively emotional by nature. Thus, volunteers need to learn how to handle the irrational reactions and have to be familiar with the games that help to slow down the development of dementia. Furthermore, before working at a dementia centre, volunteers are required to visit other dementia centres to learn from other carers in order to gain a better understanding of the expected caring skills.

Gatherings for volunteers are held once every two months. The aim is not only to build a sense of belonging and closer partnership among the volunteers, but also to review their performance in a relaxing way. Feedback and peer sharing help to optimise the performance of volunteers, and the quality of the voluntary service will thus be upgraded.

Apart from regular volunteers, some volunteers come from voluntary teams of other enterprises to provide project-based services together with Yan Oi Tong. "CHEER"is the program launched by Yan Oi Tong and the CLP Power Hong Kong Limited (CLP), one of the two electricity suppliers in Hong Kong. CLP's volunteers conduct home visits to identify electrical hazards and help to replace worn-out wires. In addition, educational sessions about how to use electronic devices in a safe and environmental-friendly way are held regularly.

Travel and Meal Allowance

Similar to some other voluntary agencies, volunteers receive an allowance which varies from project to project. For instance, in the Opportunities for the Elderly Project, an allowance based on service hours is given. For instance, a volunteer who has served for less than three continuous hours will receive HK$50 as a token honorarium. If the serving hours are more than three continuous hours, a volunteer will receive HK$65. On the other hand, the form of allowance varies in Yan Oi Tong. It can be a transport or a meal allowance. Nonetheless, even when allowances of any form are sometimes not provided, it is observed volunteers still actively participating in those voluntary works.

Reward and Recognition Systems

Two reward and recognition schemes have been introduced to commend volunteers with distinctive efforts and services. They are Yan Oi Tong's volunteer award system and the SWD Long Service Medal.

In the Yan Oi Tong scheme, service hours are calculated on a yearly basis. The hours that volunteers have served in the previous year determine the award they receive. Volunteers who have participated most actively are divided into different classes by their age and roles. They receive the Most Active Participant Award in each class. Volunteers having rendered service up to 300 hours get the "Diamond Award". "Gold Award" is given to those with services of 200 to 299 hours, while "Silver Award" is for those rendering services cumulative to the range of 100 to 199 hours. For services from 20 to 49 hours, a volunteer will receive a token recognition in the form of a Certificate of Appreciation.

In fact, SWD also runs a Long Service Medal Scheme for recognising the contributions of volunteers of all welfare agencies and NGOs in Hong Kong. Volunteers are nominated by their service units and, again, their service hours will be calculated annually. Three levels of certificates will be awarded. They are the Gold, Silver and Bronze Certificates, to those who have attained service hours cumulating to more than 200, 150 and 50 hours respectively.

Other than the Long Service Medal of the SWD, there is an award for individual voluntary groups. This award aims to encourage volunteers to contribute to the community with their friends and promote voluntarism. Volunteer groups are commended for their proposed voluntary activities and creativity too.

Challenges for Yan Oi Tong

In most voluntary agencies, it is a common trend that young people choose to join project-based voluntary works. They prefer to help in organizing monthly birthday parties or singing in some festival events as a group. The reason is due to their busy working schedule, whereas most elderly services involve mainly indoor activities and home visits which are less attractive to them. The Centre is now working very hard to find ways to recruit younger volunteers.

The age distribution of volunteer in elderly services inclines towards the younger elderlies. People retire at the age of 60 years and are still full of energy. They are in reasonably good physical health. This group of people is very devoted and dedicated to the voluntary work at Yan Oi Tong. Above all, developing different strategies on the empowerment of volunteers are the main concern of the Centre.

VOLUNTARY SERVICES IN OTHER ORGANISATIONS

The Evangelical Lutheran Church Social Service: Hong Kong

The Evangelical Lutheran Church Social Service - Hong Kong (ELCSS-HK) is one of the voluntary organisations providing elderly services in the Tuen Mun, Shatin and Kwai Chung Districts.

In the elderly centres, they provide supporting services with volunteers to underprivileged elderly people, carers, prospective retirees and their partners, as well as promote the message of health aging among the senior citizens; for example, delivering periodical on social policy to inform the residents and to facilitate them in utilising the social resources. The elderly people are encouraged to participate in diversified activities such as learning classes and voluntary work with the objectives to build a sense of worthiness and healthy social relationship. Playing an active role in the community promotes the positive self-image of the elderly people. It facilitates the establishment of a caring community.

The Day Care Centre and Care and Attention Home for the Elderly will provide day care services to the elderly people with illness, who have no one to take care of them during daytime. The elderly people can receive professional care services and join some leisure activities there. As a result, they can broaden their social network and improve their health. Meanwhile, it can relieve the pressure of family members when the elderly people are staying in the centre. The centre will also orangise courses to strengthen the carers' ability in elderly care. Training related to caring skills in a home setting are provided. Thus, Day Care Centre and Care and Attention Home benefit both the elderly people and the care providers.

Home and Community Care Services are home-based care services especially targeted for frail elderlies with moderate to severe impairment. Depending on the illness, different caring plans are designed to cover the needs of the elderly people. They can receive personal care as well as nutritional therapy at home. Through such tailor-made services, the quality of life in families with frail elderlies is maintained.

ELCSS-HK is one of the partner of ''Tuen Mun and Pok Oi Hospital integrated discharge support programme'' to provide six to eight weeks of community support when elderly patients are discharged for home convalescence. The elderly people are well looked after at home with a series of rehabilitation and transitional support services. If necessary, referral will be arranged to ensure that the elderly people will have a timely and appropriate care even when they are undergoing those prescribed convalescent stages at home (Evangelical Lutheran Church Social Service-Hong Kong, 2017a).

With the support from other organisations, ELCSS-HK acts as an intermediary between some private companies and the elderly people in need. For example, ELCSS-HK cooperates with CLP in ''Green Volunteers for Seniors Programme'' which is aiming at saving energy in the underprivileged households to promote the green message. With the assistance from ELCSS-HK, LED light bulbs are given out by CLP volunteer team to 180 needy over 60 year-olds in Tuen Mun District. The partnership between ELCSS-HK and CLP facilitates a better and meaningful allocation of voluntary manpower and social resources (Evangelical Lutheran Church Social Service-Hong Kong, 2017b).

ELCSS-HK recruit volunteers and provide training to them to serve the elderly people. Many retirees join as volunteers. They constitute the stable workforce in the elderly services, including rendering visits to the elderly people or providing general supports in a service centre. Young volunteers with tight working schedule, tend to provide services on a project basis.

The Pamela Youde Nethersole Eastern Hospital

In order to maximize of the service quality and quantity, voluntary services have been introduced to The Pamela Youde Nethersole Easter Hospital (PYNEH). The voluntary services of PYNEH are operated on hospital-based and divided into three parts: patients' concern and support services, ward/department support services and community services. Patients' concern and support services involve more interpersonal contact with patients than the other two services. For instance, volunteers at specialist outpatient clinics may provide escort services to elderly patients. For ward/department support services, volunteers are responsible for assisting rehabilitation shop operations, running the library or organizing festival events. PYNEH not only provides the voluntary services with its registered volunteers, but also co-operates with other NGOs, schools, religious groups and enterprises to provide services such as ward ambassadors and making caring calls to patients especially those elderly people living alone.

There are 1,200 retired elderlies involved in the PYNEH regular voluntary works. PYNEH's younger volunteers are more likely to participate in project-based voluntary work such as holding Christmas parties with patients. With the mental and social supporting services provided by volunteers, the quality and quantity of services can avoid the influence of manpower shortage.

The Senior Citizen Home Safety Association

The Senior Citizen Home Safety Association (SCHSA) is a NGO providing mainly community-based services. Parts of its services are provided by volunteers. Unlike other organisations, there is a service pledge that a volunteer should serve for no less than 30 hours in a year. Making caring calls to elderly people around the clock and all year round is what volunteers in SCHSA have to do. Through the calls, a better understanding of the conditions of elderly people can be obtained so that any need of referring them to other services can be identified. Besides, home visits are also part of the duty of volunteers. In addition to chatting with elderly people, volunteers also deliver clothes to them during winter. Volunteers of SCHSA may be required to handle clerical and administrative work such as making short films, performing information and photo search as well as supporting the operations of SCHSA. The voluntary service hours in total are more than 4,000 hours and more than 42,000 senior citizens have been benefited from their calls and care services in January, 2017. Through the community-based services provided, more elderly people's quality of life is thus improved (Senior Citizen Home Safety Association, 2015).

Volunteers Movement in Hong Kong Exchange and Clearing Limited

Apart from the NGOs, there are many private companies set up their volunteer teams. Hong Kong Exchange and Clearing Limited (HKEX) operates the securities and derivatives markets and their related clearing houses. It is the frontline regulator of listed companies in Hong Kong. Concerning community is one of its corporate social responsibilities. HKEX supports long-term community investment by establishing community partnerships and encouraging its employees to participate in volunteer work. Partnering with the SCHSA, the Tung Wah Group of Hospitals and the Haven of Hop Christian Service, HKEX volunteers participate in activities to support elderly services, including home visits, and gatherings as well as the provision of simple home maintenance. Every year, HKEX organizes an Annual Volunteer Recognition Ceremony to recognise its employees for their active participation in the volunteer work. In 2014, HKEX earned the SWD's Gold Award in appreciation of its contribution of more than 2,800 hours of volunteer services. The voluntary works provided from private companies are remarkable.

The Hong Kong Fire Services Department Volunteer Team

Governmental departments with the encourage by the Central Government also set up their volunteer team. The Hong Kong Fire Services Department Volunteer Team (HKFSDVT) was established in 2002 and has over 1,100 registered members comprising serving and retired uniformed fire and ambulance personnel as well as civilian staff members of different units. The mission of HKFSDVT includes supporting and helping the elderly in the community.

In the past few years, the HKFSDVT has had vigorous participation in charitable activities organised by community and voluntary agencies. More than 130,000 service hours in total have been contributed by the Team so far. Their team members provide household removal services to the elderly people who are living alone. They also pay visits to them with care and attention to their needs. The Team participates in general community services such as joining the festival events in elderly home.

The Hong Kong Jockey Club Volunteer Team

The Hong Kong Jockey Club (HKJC) has a volunteer team composed of their full-time, part-time and retired Club staff. The Team puts great emphasis on district-based programmes and is committed to serving each and every district of Hong Kong. The Team actively co-operates with local organisations in organising different kinds of volunteer activities. To reflect the characteristics of different districts of the city, the Team works hand in hand with local community to organise and design programmes that meet the special needs of local target groups. Examples are Chinese New Year lunch gatherings for elderly, elderly singles home visits and festive carnivals, etc.

OBSERVATIONS

Having studied and examined the services performed by various organizations and institutions of volunteers, it is observed that elderly services place emphasis on the following areas:

- **Organising Leisure and Cultural Activities:** Birthday parties, outings such as visits to Ocean Park, tours of New Territories, Chinese operas, folk dancing and Chinese kungfu (e.g. tai chi);
- **Provision of Supporting Work at the Voluntary Organisations:** Manning help desks at elderly centres, running mobile libraries at hospital, escorting patients in at outpatient clinics;
- **Paying Regular Home Visits:** Volunteers are sometimes divided into groups. For instance, a group can consist of two volunteers, led by a staff member of a voluntary organisation or a social worker to pay regular visits to elderly people who are weak and cannot go to an elderly centre. The volunteers attend to their well-being. In case of need, they will ask the family members of the elderly people to take the elderly people to a clinic or a hospital to consult a doctor and make necessary referrals;
- **Organising Special Projects Such as Home Cleaning and Repairs:** Such projects are common before Lunar New Year. For instance, having social responsibility and caring for the community are the core values of the CLP Hong Kong Limited. The repair of home electrical appliances is a well-known project organised by CLP volunteers, a voluntary Team initiated by the electric company in 1994; and
- **Conducting Health Talks and Other Health Promotional Activities:** Doctors and nurses will be regularly invited to give talks on common or chronic diseases at elderly centres. Talks on maintaining health and anti-degeneration conducted by Chinese medical practitioners are always welcomed by elderly people.

It is also observed that the services provided to elderly people do not place sufficient emphasis on their personal health problems. Can the demand for elderly care be met in the future if this situation continues?

"NEW" SERVICE AREAS REQUIRING FURTHER ATTENTION

Traditionally, medical services are provided by health professionals in hospitals. Since the inception of community nursing services (CNS) in 1967, patients have been able to receive nursing care services at home environment.

Community Nursing Service

The HA is responsible for community nursing service, and community centres are gradually being set up in each hospital cluster to provide a more comprehensive package of care services to outpatients. Community nurses conduct comprehensive health assessments, and they formulate, implement and evaluate nursing therapeutics for clients during regular visits according to their needs. The HA aims at providing skilled nursing care and enabling clients to remain in the community for the improvement of their health condition, through improving their self-care ability and knowledge and enhancing carers' skills. Patients in different age groups can benefit from CNS, especially those with difficulty to move or being unable to take care of themselves, e.g. patients with chronic illnesses who need case management in the community for better treatment outcomes (Hong Kong Community Nurses Association, 2012).

Pioneered by PYNEH, CNS is divided into five areas: patient care procedures, specialty care, education and counseling, information on community resources, chronic disease management and promotion of community health services. Patient care procedures refer to holistic home care services such as drug administration and monitoring of patients living in Eastern District. District community nurses also provide specialty care such as chronic disease care and hospice care. For the education and counseling work, educating patients and their families about self-care is one of the routine jobs of community nurses. They also provide information on community resources. For example, community nurses help with arrangement and referral of social resources such as medical equipment on loan service to enhance the self-care ability of elderly people. The enhanced care and support services enable patients to live at home in their community (Pamela Youde Nethersole Eastern Hospital, 2013).

Kowloon Hospital has more chronic patients than other hospitals because it provides rehabilitation services to patients in United Christian Hospital and Queen Elizabeth Hospital. Kowloon Hospital has set up a community service centre at Oi Man Estate in Ho Man Tin to provide chronic disease management, special care, drug counseling, nutrition and tube feeding care and community health education through home visits to reduce the reliance on hospital-based care. Community nurses normally visit patients once a week. Clients may ask for more visits according to their condition (Kowloon Hospital, 2015).

To draw an interim conclusion, it is observed that community nurses do provide valuable care services and give health advice to patients at their homes in order to maintain their health condition and mitigate the increasing demand for services offered by the public healthcare system. Can volunteers perform some of the duties of community nurses to look after elderly people with chronic diseases at their homes? This food for thought question can be inspiring to those involved in promoting healthcare volunteerism as a discipline of paramedic of modern days.

The answer could be that volunteers can definitely help, if the mindset and approach in broadening the service scope of volunteers is directed to addressing individual health issues. With more people and organisations realizing the importance and contributions of volunteers in taking care of elderly people at home, the International Federation of Red Cross and Red Cross Crescent Societies have compiled a report on Community-based Home Care for Older People after the South Eastern Europe Home Care Conference in 2011. The report points out that involvement of volunteers in community-based home care services for older people can be particularly significant, as it should contribute to more cohesive and inclusive communities and enhance the capacity of the Red Cross Red Crescent to address the main underlying causes of older people's vulnerability. The report further highlights the health and social services that volunteers can contribute. A volunteer can provide psychosocial support, assistance with social activities, preventing accident at home and providing respite opportunities for the carers (International Federation of Red Cross and Red Crescent Societies, 2011).

In this regard, it is considered that the following health related works can be carried out by trained / qualified volunteers during home visits.

Prevention of Falls and Home Accidents

In Hong Kong, one in five elders has at least one fall in a year. 75.2% and 7.2% of those elders suffered from sustaining injuries and serious injuries respectively (Luk, Chan, & Chan, 2015). Apart from the slow reaction, another reason is the hidden home hazards which are always overlooked by the elderly people and their family members. During home visits, volunteers can educate and remind the elderlies and caregivers the right concept and importance of home safety. Volunteers can help to check the physical environment such as the bathroom and the kitchen, and to identify potential hazards to reduce the risk of falls. By reducing the potential hazards more frequently, the risk of elderly fall and home accidents will decrease (Hospital Authority, 2016).

Prevention of Abuse

The relationship of an elderly with family members may become worse as a result of the effects and long-term impacts of chronic illness. Elderly people tend to be very demanding at home because of poor health, disability and functional and cognitive impairment. The pressure in providing long-term care may induce unstable emotion to a carer. It may lead to the occurrence of violence or abuse incidents. Abusive behaviour may happen when a carer does not cope well with the physical and mental incapacity of the old persons.

Physical abuse is the major type of elderly abuse cases that six in ten elderly victims are physically abused. Some abusive behaviour may not be easily observed. Volunteers should observe actions and behaviour of the old persons, talk with them and others involved to obtain more information such as bruises, pressure marks, unexplained withdrawal and fear of people. With the help of volunteers, more disclosure of the abusers can be revealed by the frequent home visits (Social Welfare Department, 2016).

Miscellaneous Preventive Measures

Apart from the above general health-related paramedic coverage, special tasks associated with some common chronic diseases can also be developed.

Hypertension

With the advancement of technology, the electronic blood pressure monitor can be easily used it to take blood pressure. Patients are advised to take their blood pressure at home every day. However, it is difficult to expect some old people to undertake this task competently and on an ongoing basis.

Community nurses pay regular visit to patients who are living alone. Depending on a patient's condition, the visit may be once in a week or more frequently. It is expected that volunteers can play an important role in serving these elderlies when they are trained to take blood pressure and to check drug administration practice of patients at their homes. In addition, volunteers can give general advice on food consumption and weight control to patients and their family members.

Diabetic Mellitus

It is common for diabetics to gauge their urine or blood sugar levels daily or before each meal at home. Some may need to have insulin injection according to their blood sugar levels. A volunteer with relevant training can monitor and guide patients to make sure they are properly following the instructions on testing of blood sugar levels and injection of insulin.

Diet control is also important in maintaining the health condition of patients with diabetes. Trained volunteers can give patients relevant health advice so that they can have proper diet control and avoid high-calorie food.

During a field visit to Yan Oi Tong, it was found that there were some healthy retired people in their early sixties who had demonstrated that they were capable of doing general voluntary works. They had the potential to be trained to carry out the above tasks for the patients who suffered from the two above-mentioned chronic diseases. Utilizing the talents and health knowledge of retired people will greatly help in health-related voluntary works, so as to ease the lack of human resources.

IMPORTANTCE OF TRAINING VOLUNTEERS

In all the above-mentioned organizations and agencies, volunteers normally go through some formal or informal training before they start providing services. They are under professional guidance and monitoring in order to maintain a reasonable level of service standard.

In line of the needs of services, systematic and organized training is considered crucial for the success of any voluntary service programme. A tailor-made training course should be conducted to suit, not only the service recipients but also the service providers, i.e. volunteers. This means that the background and interest of volunteers have to be considered when designing the course materials and training methods. Effective training can enrich volunteers' skills and knowledge, as well as their confidence.

The Auxiliary Medical Service (AMS) is a uniformed volunteer force within the ambit of Security Bureau of the Hong Kong Government, and is recognized as one of the more organized, trained and disciplined volunteer service in the community. It consists of 4,700 volunteers of professional medical and nursing background, and lay persons, plus around 100 full-time civil servants. Their main role is to augment the regular medical and health services in times of emergency.

All volunteer members are trained in first aid, management of infectious diseases, discipline and marching. Normally, volunteer members are deployed to provide first aid services at sports grounds, festive events and cycling tracks. They will also conduct health talks to the public. In times of emergency and natural disasters, AMS volunteer members provide first aid treatment to the injured and convey them to hospitals. AMS members also take care of patients at acute and convalescent hospitals. During the outbreaks of Severe Acute Respiratory Syndrome (SARS) in 2003, and other endemics, members had been deployed to isolation and quarantine camps to take care of contacts.

Volunteer members in AMS come from all walks of life. They have different educational qualifications and career backgrounds. The Headquarters arrange the basic training, followed by refresher training that consolidates the knowledge and skills. From the experience of AMS, the competency of volunteer members can be well maintained as long as they receive continuing training on a regular basis. Other important factors (which include well-designed training packages, working protocols and instructions on important tasks) are well integrated into their annual training curriculum.

Before joining the AMS, volunteer members do not necessarily have had a healthcare background. Upon taking training courses at different levels, members acquire the ability to take care of the sick. They also become proficient in taking body temperature and blood pressure, checking urine and blood sugar levels, performing oxygen and medication administration, and carrying out some simple nursing procedures such as tube feeding and wound dressings. During in influx of the Vietnamese Boat People in the 1990's, AMS volunteer members were deployed to the sick bay of detention centres to provide round-the -clock services to the refugees. Thus, members can render good assistance to regular health staff in taking care of the patients. They are capable to take up the task independently and to work efficiently under guidance.

During the outbreak of SARS in 2003 and avian influenza in recent years, AMS members have been deployed to quarantine centres to assist the Department of Health in taking care of the contacts. They have performed the duties effectively based on what they have learned in the handling of infectious diseases included in the centralised training courses. In view of the special role of AMS, volunteer members were also mobilised to the Hospital Authority Accident and Emergency Departments to cope with the Winter Surge in the past two years. Members provided assistance in the triage station, taking vital signs and provide general nursing care to patients. Members worked smoothly under the supervision of regular staff. Some experienced members could properly carry out simple nursing assignments in accordance to the written guidelines and protocols.

ENGAGEMENT OF TRAINED VOLUNTEERS

A voluntary organisation should be established with the appropriate organisational structure supported by sufficient funding to maintain its ongoing operations. Employment of suitable staff with sound administrative ability is indeed the basic and essential requirement. However, apart from the managerial skills, every staff member should be equipped with skills in volunteer management and engagement. They should be friendly with a sociable and outgoing personality and should seek to cultivate a close working relationship with volunteers who normally come from all walks of life.

Apart from the skeletal structure of salaried employees, many voluntary organisations are often supported by various sub-groups. In the Hong Kong Council of Social Service (HKCSS), salaried staff are responsible for the daily operations and report to the Executive Committee, which governs four Standing Committees, its volunteer sub-groups, and steers the development of their business. The Standing committees form different Specialised Committees to carry out related plans and programmes in their specific fields. Having a professional staff team and a governing committee structure, the HKCSS operates on a 2-tier structure, which enables HKCSS to run more smoothly (The Hong Kong Council of Social Service, n.d.).

Volunteer heads are the executive arms of an organisation. They are delegated the responsibility to oversee a service program. A salaried employee is responsible for monitoring and supporting the volunteer heads, who have important roles in managing the day-to-day operations and in interacting with frontline volunteers directly and frequently. Sometimes, volunteers quit an organisation because of the management style of their volunteer head, rather than that of the salaried employees. Special attention should be given to training those salaried employees and volunteer heads and to equipping them with the necessary skills in interacting with volunteers. Volunteers will leave an organisation if they feel that they are not respected.

Volunteers normally have their own jobs. They use their own holidays and spare times to serve the community. Their participation rate will be affected by their busy working schedules. In some projects, funding will be obtained to provide travel and meal allowances for volunteers. For example, an amount of HK$80 is given to a volunteer who has provided service for a full day. The amount of allowance can vary from project to project. For instance, patrons of Yan Oi Tong are willing to donate more money so that it can be used for allowances, which are a kind of gesture to thank volunteers for their contributions. On the other hand, allowance can also encourage volunteers to participate in more voluntary work.

However, motivation of volunteers is a more important factor in the success of a voluntary organization. It is always a challenge for every voluntary organisation to fully engage and sustain its volunteer services. Volunteer workforce engagement is a common issue for every voluntary agency. In the context of the theme of volunteerism of healthcare services to the aging population, it is particularly important to retain trained volunteers in providing services to the elderly people.

Workforce engagement is a common issue for every enterprise. As Jim Whitehurst, CEO of Red Hat, said that "It is the art of getting people to believe what you want them to believe." What kind of actions or activities do you think can help an organisation in convincing volunteers to believe what you want them to believe?

Sometimes, even when an organisation has its vision and mission statements, it is still not easy to change the mindset of a volunteer and influence him or her to work entirely towards the programme objectives. In this connection, engagement of volunteers is one of the top priority tasks of each voluntary organisation. Engagement of volunteers is a difficult and complicated issue.

Knowing the Volunteers

Housewives or the retired, students or those even on regular employment are willing to contribute themselves to voluntary work. Other than the hard data such as personal particulars, education and working experience of volunteers, a supervisor should find more chances to work with them in order to understand the personality and character of individual volunteer. This can facilitate the management to assign appropriate job to them as well as giving hints to a supervisor to maintain a close working relationship with them.

Nurturing the Volunteers

Tasks of any nature may affect a volunteer in carrying out the service with good standard, even in simple tasks. Every volunteer should start their work after proper training since they may have no previous knowledge about the work or they need to follow the laid down procedures in discharging their duty. If possible, it is better to team up volunteers in pairs so that an experienced volunteer can guide and supervise a junior one directly. Such arrangement is similar as the mentor system. The mentor system is extensively practiced in the health care sectors. It gives confidence to those new comers hence facilitating their self-learning process.

Continuing training and development helps the volunteers to grow. Regular training and experience sharing sessions should be conducted periodically so as to enhance their knowledge. Guest speakers of other voluntary organisations can help them broaden their insight in providing volunteers services. It is also a good opportunity for them to voice out what they want and ventilate their subtle feelings. When training needs or frustrations are identified, remedial actions should be taken immediately.

Involving the Volunteers

When an organisation is going to formulate policies and prepare action plans, it is better to get the concerned volunteers involved. Volunteers should be invited to participate in the decision making process wherever possible. Individual or group consultations can be applied to collects views and suggestions on important issues. Standing committees can also be set up and invite the volunteers to be involved in looking into complicated matters that are directly related to their immediate interests and welfare.

Volunteers are important assets of an organisation. At times, some volunteers even have a better service attitude than the salaried staff. They see work as a service rather than a job or an interest only. Every welfare organisation and NGO should pay efforts to nurture and sustain its volunteer workforce. The above-mentioned issues should be carefully and seriously considered, with reference to the norm and culture of each organisation. Maintaing a long-term sustainable programme is one of the vital tasks in each organisation.

CONCLUSION

In order to put these constructive ideas of volunteerism into practice on an ongoing basis, some complicated but very important issues need to be addressed first. Who has the authority to approve the training for volunteers? Is a training institution in a better position to conduct the courses? Who can be appointed as instructors? Are volunteers willing to take care of the elderly people? Do retirees have the ability to learn contents of tailor-made programmes? After training, can the volunteers be retained so that the services can be sustained? Will there be adequate doctors and nurses to man the hotline? Are there any legal implications that volunteers, doctors or nurses should be aware of and be dealt with appropriately?

Practically hypertension and diabetes are of the two most common chronic diseases among elderly people. The demand for home care services to elderlies and their family members will definitely be increasing significantly in the future. A survey of Organisation for Economic Cooperation and Development countries estimates that 8% to 16% of the population serves as family caregivers (Francesca, Ana, Jérôme, & Frits, 2011). Family caregivers are critical in optimising health and quality of life for older patient. With the assistance from trained volunteers, the workload of community nurses can potentially be reduced. Resources can be redirected to the more serious patients. Volunteers are capable of looking after some minor and stable cases after having received formal and systematic training.

In addition, written instructions and specific protocols of operations should be prepared to guide volunteers in handling different situations. Doctors or nurses can be invited to man an enquiry hotline. Volunteers can contact them through the hotline for advice when encountering problems during home visits. The setting up of a hotline should not be a major obstacle to this volunteerism concept. Doctors and nurses can be invited to man the hotline in their private volunteer capacity on a rotation basis, say, once in a week. With the aid of modern information and communication technology, onsite duty volunteers can even send photos via the internet to the hotline healthcare professionals by showing them the actual conditions of patients.

A pilot scheme can be developed with focuses on hypertension and diabetes to formally define the kinds of tasks that can be carried out by volunteers. Based on the scope of duties delineated, tailor-make training packages at different levels can then be designed for volunteers. A committee should be established to formulate standard working procedures and protocols, and to monitor the performance of the volunteers.

Volunteers are an asset to our community. It is strongly believed that the scope of services of volunteers in long-term care can be expanded by applying a new concept of volunteerism. Volunteers can play an important role in taking care of patients with chronic diseases, particularly those who have difficulty leaving their homes. The Food and Health Bureau can play a leading role in working with NGOs to launch some pilot schemes. Many NGOs are prepared to take up the challenges when a matching central policy of implementation is to be staged strategically.

FUTURE RESEARCH DIRECTIONS

The duties of CNS have been carried out by professional nurses for many years. As it has been mentioned, if volunteers are recruited, what kinds of duties should be assigned to them? Since the intention of the change is to alleviate the heavy workload of the CNS nurses, it is necessary to conduct a further in-depth research to define the areas and levels of work that are suitable for them. Training needs identification should also been done in order to design a suitable training programme for volunteers. The synergistic effect of professional nurses and volunteers working together is also meaningful as well as significant research topic that well deserves our further effort of investigation and collaboration by all stakeholders concerned in the future. The resulting and anticipated effectiveness of the proposed research theme can be measured by the health condition of the elderly population, the admission rate and other objective health data in the society as a whole. We, healthcare professionals, are yet to work harder towards this direction in the best interest of the future generations.

REFERENCES

Agency for Volunteer Service. (2009). *Survey of NGOs and NGO Volunteers*. Retrieved May 20, 2016 from http://www.avs.org.hk/symposium/pdf/AVS_BOOKlet_21.pdf

Agency for Volunteer Service. (n.d.). *About AVS.* Retrieved July 24, 2016 from http://www.avs.org.hk/en/intro

Census and Statistics Department. (2015). *Women and Men in Hong Kong Key Statistics.* Retrieved March 18, 2016 from http://www.statistics.gov.hk/pub/B11303032015AN15B0100.pdf

Centre of Health Protection. (2016). *Vital statistics.* Retrieved March 17, 2016 from http://www.chp.gov.hk/en/data/4/10/27/111.html

Evangelical Lutheran Church Social Service-Hong Kong. (2017a). *Elderly Services.* Retrieved February 20, 2017 from http://service.elchk.org.hk/eng/unit_service3.php

Evangelical Lutheran Church Social Service-Hong Kong. (2017b). *Support Us.* Retrieved February 20, 2017 from http://service.elchk.org.hk/eng/partner.php

Food and Health Bureau. (2016). *Life Expectancy.* Retrieved May 18, 2016 from http://www.fhb.gov.hk/statistics/en/statistics/life_expectancy.htm

Francesca, C., Ana, L. N., Jérôme, M., & Frits, T. (2011). *OECD health policy studies help wanted? Providing and paying for long-term care: providing and paying for long-term care* (Vol. 2011). OECD Publishing.

Hong Kong Community Nurses Association. (2012). *Newsletter 2012.* Retrieved July 14, 2016 from http://www.hkcnaltd.org.hk/2012.pdf

Hong Kong Fire Service Department Volunteer Team. (n.d.). *About Us.* Retrieved September 14, 2016 from http://www.hkfsdvt.org.hk/eng/establish.php

Hospital Authority. (2016). *Home care.* Retrieved August 23, 2016 from http://www21.ha.org.hk/smartelder/en/home_care.html

International Federation of Red Cross and Red Crescent Societies. (2011). *South Eastern Europe Home Care Conference.* Retrieved February 20, 2017 from https://www.cri.it/flex/cm/pages/ServeAttachment.php/L/IT/D/9%252F8%252Fe%252FD.ccbdf568ba9a2da44638/P/BLOB%3AID%3D10831/E/pdf

Joyce, B. T., & Bermanand, R. (2014). Formal and informal support of family caregivers managing medications for patients who receive end-of-life care t home: A cross –sectional survey of caregivers. *Palliative Medicine, 28*(9), 0269216314535963. doi:10.1177/0269216314535963 PMID:24854033

Kowloon Hospital. (2015). *Community Nursing Services.* Retrieved July 16, 2016 from http://www3.ha.org.hk/kh/ch/aboutus/introd.html

Luk, J. K., Chan, T. Y., & Chan, D. K. (2015). Falls prevention in the elderly: Translating evidence into practice. *Hong Kong Medical Journal, 21*(2), 165–171. PMID:25722468

Morris, S., Wilmot, A., Hill, M., Ockenden, N., & Payne, S. (2013). A narrative literature review of the contribution of volunteers in end-of-life care services. *Palliative Medicine, 27*(5), 428–436. doi:10.1177/0269216312453608 PMID:22833474

Movement, V. (n.d.). *About Volunteer Service.* Retrieved May 14, 2016 from http://www.volunteering-hk.org/aboutvs

Pamela Youde Nethersole Eastern Hospital. (2013). *Scope of Hospital Services*. Retrieved July 16, 2016 from http://www.ha.org.hk/pyneh/internet/Eng/scope/CNS/DOC/CNS.pdf

Perrels, A. J., Fleming, J., Zhao, J., Barclay, S., Farquhar, M., Buiting, H. M., & Brayne, C. (2014). Place of death and end-of-life transitions experienced by very old people with differing cognitive status: Retrospective analysis of a prospective population-based cohort aged 85 and over. *Palliative Medicine*, *28*(3), 220–233. doi:10.1177/0269216313510341 PMID:24317193

Po Leung Kok. (2011). *Our Services*. Retrieved May 20, 2016 from http://www.poleungkuk.org.hk/en/201408153461/social-services-department/Service.html

Senior Citizen Home Safety Association. (2015). *Volunteer Service*. Retrieved July 16, 2016 from https://www.schsa.org.hk/en/support_schsa/community_volunteer/volunteer/index.html

Social Welfare Department. (2005). *Central Office for Volunteer Service*. Retrieved May 14, 2016 from http://www.swd.gov.hk/en/index/site_pubsvc/page_supportser/sub_centraloff/

Social Welfare Department. (2016). *Services for Prevention and Handling of Elder Abuse*. Retrieved February 20, 2017 from http://www.swd.gov.hk/en/index/site_pubsvc/page_family/sub_listofserv/id_serabuseelder/

The Exchange and Clearing Limited. (2015). *Corporate Social Responsibility Report*. Retrieved September 14, 2016 from http://www.hkexgroup.com/-/media/HKEX-Group-Site/ssd/Investor-Relations/Regulatory-Reports/documents/2016/e160321csr.pdf

The Hong Kong Council of Social Service. (n.d.). *Organization structure*. Retrieved July 14, 2016 from http://www.hkcss.org.hk/e/fc_detail1.asp?fc_id=25

The Hong Kong Jockey Club. (n.d.). *Staff Volunteer Activities*. Retrieved September 14, 2016 from http://charities.hkjc.com/charities/english/connect-and-join/staff-volunteer-activities.aspx

The Samaritan Befrienders Hong Kong. (2016). *About us*. Retrieved May 20, 2016 from http://www.sbhk.org.hk/aboutus.php?lang=en

United Christian Nethersole Community Health Service. (2016). *Comprehensive Diabetes Mellitus Management Service*. Retrieved May 20, 2016 from http://www.ucn.org.hk/?l=e&c=comprehensive#

Volunteer Movement. (2008). *Volunteer Movement Volunteer GuideBook*. Retrieved May 20, 2016 from http://www.volunteering-hk.org/swdwebdata/tc_chi/resource/userguide/guidelines.pdf

Volunteer Movement. (2016). *Volunteer Movement Participating Organizations & Registered Volunteers*. Retrieved May 14, 2016 from http://www.volunteering-hk.org/aboutvs/vs_intro/vs_stat

Williams, E. L. (n.d.). *Effective Hospital Visitation*. Retrieved May 20, 2016 from http://enrichment-journal.ag.org/200403/200403_112_hospitalvisitation.cfm

Yan Oi Tong Limited. (2016). *Yan Oi Tong Annual Report 2015 – 2016*. Retrieved July 24, 2016 from http://www.yot.org.hk/download/annual-report/2015-16/2015_2016_Final.zip

Yi-Jung, L. (2010). Long-term Care Residents 'View About the Contributions of Christian-based Volunteer in Taiwan: A Pilot Study. *Journal of Religion and Health*, *51*(3), 709–722.

APPENDIX

Figure 1. The Yan Oi Tong elderly volunteer team

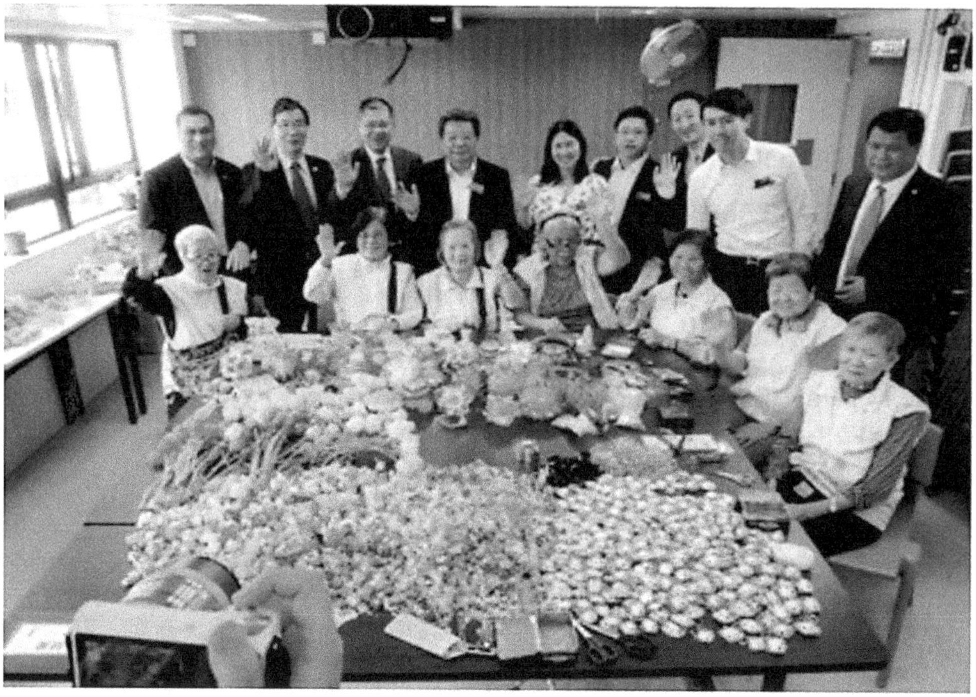

Section 3

Innovation in Practice

Chapter 13
SSLD and Senior Service:
A Comprehensive Model for Practice

Ka Tat Tsang
University of Toronto, Canada

Chui Fan Linus Ip
Centre for Learning and Change – Baycrest, Canada

ABSTRACT

This chapter introduces the SSLD (Strategies and Skills Learning and Development) System as a comprehensive model for practice in psychosocial service for seniors. The challenges and issues associated with aging are complex, and involve physical, biological, psychological, social, existential and spiritual dimensions. In order to address them in a comprehensive and balanced manner, we need to draw on an extensive set of knowledge, experience and skills taken from various healthcare and human service professions. The SSLD system is built on a meta-theoretical structure that interfaces well with both analytic and holistic conceptualizations of the human person within his or her life-world, or being-in-the-world. Principles and methods of SSLD practice are described through phases of intervention: engagement and problem translation, N3C assessment, 6D (domains of being-in-the-world) formulation, implementation, review and evaluation. These are illustrated with practice examples. Issues related to practice research and knowledge production are also explored.

INTRODUCTION

This chapter introduces the SSLD (Strategies and Skills Learning and Development) system (Tsang, 2013) as a conceptual and practice model for providing comprehensive service for seniors. The key idea of SSLD practice is to help people address their unmet human needs and achieve their desired goals in life through systematic learning and development of strategies and skills that are effective, appropriate, and relevant to their specific circumstances.

There are many theories and models for understanding the aging process as well as for informing practice. For example, in textbooks for specific disciplines such as social work, it is not uncommon to devote at least a chapter to major theories in that field (e.g., Youdin, 2014). In medicine, there are publications

DOI: 10.4018/978-1-5225-2633-9.ch013

on specialized theories regarding specific bio-medical processes such as cellular aging (e.g., Robert & Fulop, 2014). Whereas specialized accounts can offer more detailed knowledge and relatively in-depth exploration, human service practitioners are interested in more comprehensive or holistic frameworks because they are increasingly aware of the multi-faceted nature of the challenges they face, as well as the complex interactions between physical, psychological, and social factors. Authors trying to offer a more comprehensive perspective, therefore, often try to cover the physical, psychological, and social aspects (e.g., Morgan & Kunkel, 2016). Some practitioners believe that there are aspects of the human aging experience that go beyond the physical, psychological, and social, and they assert that existential, spiritual, artistic, and/or aesthetic dimensions are also significant (Bennett & Taylor, 2012; Moberg, 2008; Reker & Chamberlain, 2000).

A comprehensive review of these theories and models is beyond the scope of this chapter. In the following section, we will briefly introduce the key theoretical systems, and try to demonstrate how the SSLD system can be used as an integrative framework for understanding the aging process and for guiding professional intervention.

BIOMEDICAL MODELS

Biomedical models (e.g., Bowling & Dieppe, 2005; Rowe & Kahn, 1998) usually focus on the body and bodily functions. Bowling and Dieppe (2005), for instance, characterize usual aging as normal decline in physical, social, and cognitive functioning. They recognize the impact of external, environmental factors specific to the person, and the value of active engagement with life in order to achieve successful aging. These models, however, do not pay equal attention to the motivational and emotional experience of aging. The idea of successful aging is articulated as a set of objective criteria, and relatively little weight is assigned to subjective experience and individual agency. Some researchers have observed that a person's subjective assessment is often at odds with the medical definition (Strawbridge, Wallhagen & Cohen, 2002).

PSYCHOSOCIAL THEORIES

Erikson's (1950) stage theory is among the earliest attempts to articulate a theory of aging that is primarily psychological. His theory, in contrast to the biomedical models, focuses on the subjective experience of the individual and deals with the intellectual, emotional, and motivational domains. Ideally, individuals will explore life and find meaning, eventually attaining wisdom and developing integrity. The less successful ones may find themselves unproductive, feeling guilty or depressed, and their lives may be characterized by hopelessness or despair. In subsequent development of the theory, Joan Erikson (1982/1997) elaborated on the "ninth stage" in which biological decline and function loss take the individual back through the earlier eight stages, struggling with negative responses to their environments, such as mistrust, shame and guilt, isolation, and despair. The use of a stage approach, assuming there is homogeneity among people of the same age bracket, does not pay attention to cultural diversity and individual difference. In this approach, while biological decline is recognized, little attention is given to how the biology interacts with psychosocial processes. The role of environmental factors, including social systems, services and resources, as well as cultural and lifestyle differences, is not adequately explored.

Continuity Theory, also known as Personality Theory (Atchley, 1971, 1989, 2000), emphasizes the stable qualities of the individual and maintains that older adults will usually keep the same activities, behaviors, and relationships as they did in their earlier years of life. These are connected to the internal continuity of psychological characteristics, including self and identity. The theory focuses on external realities including the social environment and recognizes the interaction between the external and the internal processes (Nimrod & Kleiber, 2007). The theory has been criticized for its assumption of a universal normal aging process and its lack of attention to diversities related to gender, health status, and social circumstances (Quadagno, 2014).

First developed during the 1960s, Activity Theory (Havighurst, 1961; Neugarten, 1964) has remained influential within the social sciences (John, 1984). It focuses on human activity and relationships, and encourages seniors to stay active and engaged with interpersonal relationships and social life. The theory has been criticized for its lack of attention to how activity is understood and performed differently between men and women, and across different cultural and social contexts (Nimrod & Klieber, 2007).

Exchange Theory was originally derived from Social Exchange Theory (Dowd, 1975). It contends that individual behaviors are maintained by the rewards associated with them. According to this theory, people will only behave in a particular way when the rewards outweigh the cost. Applied to relationships, it follows that people will remain in a relationship when they derive certain rewards or satisfaction while the cost is not excessive. It is assumed that when people age, they will have less power and resources, including wealth, social capital, knowledge and skills. The decrease in such power and resources is supposed to put the aging person in a relatively imbalanced and disadvantaged position when they are negotiating relationships with others. This imbalance and disadvantage will render the aging person more vulnerable to becoming dependent and having less control in a relationship. Questions, however, can be raised against the assumption that aging persons necessarily have less power, as many of them do possess considerable wealth, knowledge, and social resources. As well, the assessment of reward and cost tends to be quite subjective, making empirical validation of the theory difficult (Davey & Eggebeen, 1998; John, 1984).

Disengagement Theory (Cumming & Henry, 1961), by focusing on the concept of roles, brings together important psychological and social processes associated with aging. It is an influential theory within the social sciences (Achenbaum & Bengtson, 1994). Disengagement theory almost unquestioningly accepts biological and functional decline as natural, and connects that with decreasing social participation. Such disengagement, however, is not framed as necessarily negative, as the process can serve useful personal and social functions. For the individual, reduced social role performance can mean less demand and pressure, and more personal freedom. Socially, disengagement by older people can open up roles and positions for younger and possibly more efficient or skilled people. While disengagement should ideally occur naturally as a process of mutual benefit to both the individual and society, disengagement is not necessarily chosen or voluntary, such as in the case of mandatory retirement, which is still practiced in many parts of the world.

CRITICAL ENGAGEMENT WITH SOCIAL, STRUCTURAL, AND POLITICAL REALITIES

Social realities include structural, institutional, and organizational aspects, and issues like power, public discourses, economics, and political processes are integral to any comprehensive conceptualization of the social. There is increasing awareness of structural and political issues among gerontologists (e.g., Dillaway & Byrnes, 2009). Riley's (1973, 1974, 1994) Age Stratification theory, for instance, addresses the relationship between age cohorts and social structures, taking into account the processes of social change and transition through the life course (Dannefer, Uhlenberg, Foner, & Abeles, 2005). The theory also recognizes structural realities and issues of inequality among groups based on race, class, and sex (Dowd, 1988). Feminist theories (e.g., Calasanti, 2004; Walker, 2012) usually pay attention to these structural issues as well, with a special focus on gender and sexuality. Feminist theorists also engage critically with socially constructed images of women, and the associated expectations and demands (Garner, 1999). Apart from gender and sexuality, ethnicity and race are critical issues taken up by an increasing number of authors (e.g., Karasik & Kishimoto, 2016; Torres, 2015; Zubair & Norris, 2015). These authors, while asserting the significance of ethnicity and race, usually adopt a dynamic and non-essentialist approach (Zubair & Norris, 2015) and recognize the value of conceiving different forms of diversity as intersecting (Torres, 2015).

Bengtson, Burgess and Parrott (1997) reviewed theory development in social gerontology in the early 1990s, which included theories covering micro and macro levels of analysis. They looked at social constructionism, social exchange, life course, feminism, age stratification, political economy of aging, and critical theory perspectives, and advocated for more methodical attention to theory development. Following their suggestion, the SSLD system offers a framework for bringing a diverse range of theoretical perspectives together, going beyond the confines of social gerontology. Up to this point, we have considered biomedical and psychological perspectives. We have also looked at theories that deal with the psychosocial domain, including the interaction between the individual and the social environment, as well as interpersonal and social relationships.

GEROTRANSCENDENCE: BEYOND THE PSYCHO-SOCIAL

Covering the biological, psychological, and social is considered a comprehensive approach to understanding human aging, but many human service practitioners, service providers, researchers, and scholars in the field of senior service find the bio-psycho-social construction inadequate, and maintain that a holistic understanding of the total being of the individual, while paying attention to existential, spiritual, and aesthetic dimensions is essential (e.g., Bennett & Taylor, 2012; Jewell & Nell, 2014; Moberg, 2008; Reker & Chamberlain, 2000).

Tornstam's (1989, 1996, 2005) idea of gerotranscendence has received much attention and generated a body of literature of both empirical studies and conceptual exploration (Jewell, 2014; Rajani, 2015, Topaz, Troutman-Jordan, & MacKenzie, 2014). Building on Disengagement Theory (Cumming & Henry, 1961), the Gerotranscendence Theory proposes that later in life, there will be changes in how people understand themselves, time, space, and social and individual relations (Tornstam, 1996). People will naturally shift toward values that are less materialistic and competitive, and their perspective will become more cosmic and transcendent (Tornstam, 1997). The theory asserts a more positive understanding of the aging process, and shifts people's focus away from death anxiety, and promotes meaningful activities and self-acceptance. It supports people's reflections on their relationships with people and the world, and facilitates their engagement with solitude, contributing to the development or realization of wisdom (Topaz, Troutman-Jordan, & MacKenzie, 2014). Jewell (2014) offered a critical review of the

Gerotranscendence Theory and questioned its universalist and essentialist assumptions, proposing that more attention should be paid to differences and diversity across cultures and religious systems.

Gerotranscendence involves the holistic concept of integrating all the biological, psychological, and social dimensions, and does not compartmentalize them. Transcendence implies going beyond the common-sense understanding of a metaphysical construction of the human person as an entity composed of physical, psychological, and social aspects (Moran, 2014). Transcendence is often understood in its existential, spiritual, and aesthetic dimensions, and these are usually explored in relation to the whole being or whole person, instead of confining them to specific biological, psychological, environmental or social domains.

SSLD: AN INTEGRATIVE CONCEPTUAL FRAMEWORK

The Person and the Lifeworld

The SSLD system offers a framework to conceptualize the physical, psychological, and social dimensions of human experience and activity, and allows for articulations that cover existential, spiritual, and aesthetic dimensions as well (Figure 1).

The term "lifeworld" refers to the totality of a person's lived experience. It is composed of six domains (6D): environment, body, motivation, cognition, emotion, and action. The environment refers to what is

Figure 1. Person and the lifeworld

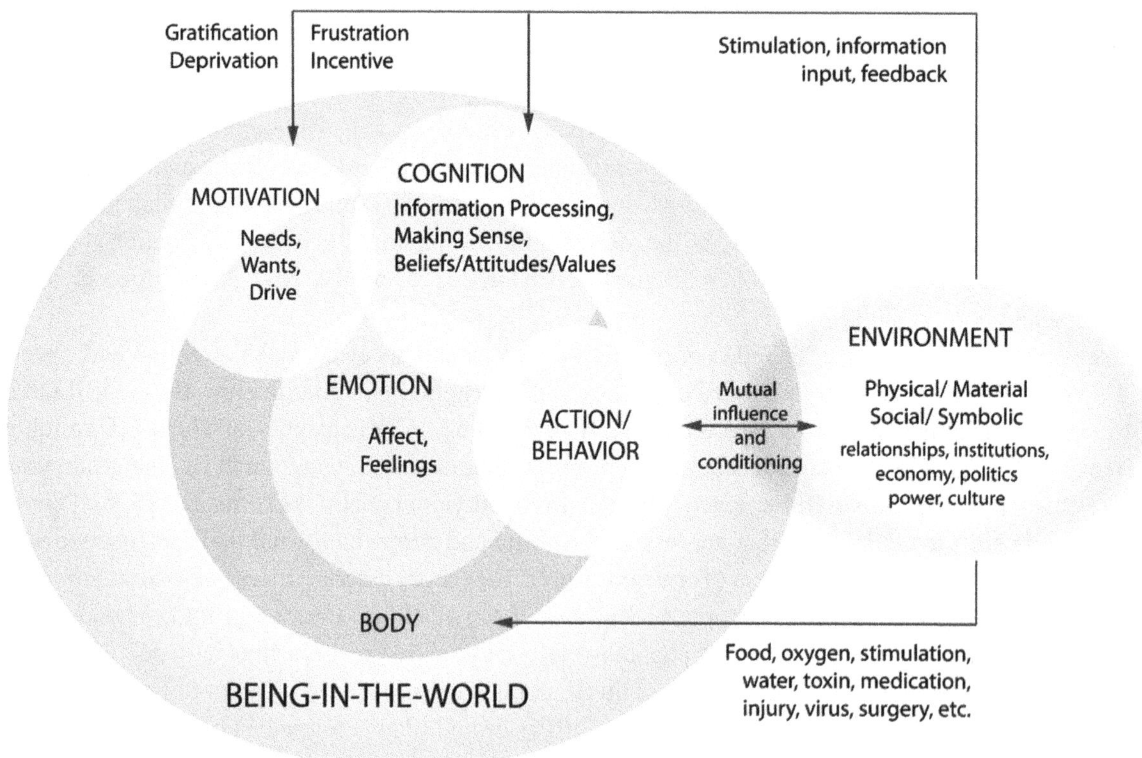

external to us, and includes the physical (e.g., geography, objects, air quality, material resources, etc.) and the social (e.g., economy, social systems, culture, politics, relationships, etc.). The body includes the biological aspects such as the anatomical, the physiological, and the genetic. It also includes our experience of the body, and the body as a socially constructed reality. Many philosophers argue that human existence is always embodied, and it is important to recognize the importance of embodiment when we talk about almost any aspect of human experience. Our psychological processes, including our thinking, feelings, desires and strivings, are all embodied, made possible and mediated through the body.

Our cognition, emotion, and motivation are usually considered psychological domains. Cognition includes our thoughts, intellectual activities, memory, knowledge, values, and beliefs. Emotion includes our feelings, mood, and affect. Motivation refers to our experience of what we need: our wants, desires, and strivings, including what some people refer to as drive. Behavior can also be understood as a psychological domain, and it includes all the things we do, what we say, and the actions we take. Human actions can be understood psychologically in relation to our motivation, cognition, and emotion; however, they are also performed with the involvement of the body, and usually have social implications. As well, human actions are often conditioned by physical and social realities.

The SSLD system emphasizes the interconnection and interaction among these six domains. It is not possible to imagine a human experience that is totally confined to one domain, or one that is purely cognitive, emotional, or otherwise. Other domains are always implicated. As will be illustrated later in this chapter, our experience of aging involves all these domains, and restricting ourselves to one or only a few of them will only provide an incomplete understanding.

Conceptual Interface: Metaphysical Trichotomy and Holistic Formulations

Most practitioners, service providers, researchers and scholars in the field of gerontology and senior service build their conceptual understanding on a metaphysical trichotomy that defines human reality in terms of the physical, psychological, and social. The popularly accepted definition of health by the World Health Organization (1946/ 2016) as a complete state of physical, psychological, and social well-being, is a good example. This metaphysical position is also popularly understood and used. Whereas most practice and research work in this area is framed in terms of this three-fold view, some people, including practitioners, service providers, researchers and scholars find this metaphysical register inadequate, and they find it helpful to use more holistic formulations to make sense of reality and to guide their actions.

Holistic or generic concepts, including notions of being, personhood, spirituality, aesthetics, citizenship, etc., are often used in human services and everyday discourse. The use of such holistic formulations counteracts the potential objectification of human beings, and the possible compartmentalization and fragmentation of human experience. Holistic formulations are supposedly more respectful of the integrity of the individual's being, personhood, or identity. Holistic language is also more suited for articulating the agentive, existential, spiritual, aesthetic, and similar dimensions of human reality or experience, which is often valued by practitioners and service users.

Some people experience a tension between the trichotomous metaphysical frame and holistic formulations, while some professionals are using both in their work or daily life. Taking a pragmatic position, the SSLD system offers an interface between these two language systems. We recognize the integrity and totality of human reality privileged by holistic formulations, and summarize them with the concept of *being-in-the-world*, which can be traced back to the German concept of *Dasein* (Heidegger 1927/1996; Moran, 2014), and sometimes expressed as person-in-environment in the human service literature.

These concepts usually refer to the human person as a whole, while recognizing his or her constitutive components such as embodiment, thoughts, feelings, desires and drives, human decision and action, as well as his or her relationship with the world and with other people.

The SSLD framework interfaces well with such concepts and articulations, bringing our attention to the component domains (Table 1). Experiences that are described in holistic terms such as existential, spiritual, or aesthetic, can usually be understood with reference to the six domains in SSLD analysis. The experience, first of all, will take place within a given environmental context, in terms of its physical location (e.g., in the woods, or in a temple, museum, or hospital) associated with specific economic, social, and cultural realities (e.g., Christian, Muslim, Chinese, or American; under autocratic rule or within a democracy). The holistic experience is usually understood as being embodied, and mediated through bodily sensations and experiences. There is usually a cognitive process to make sense of the holistic experience in question (e.g., poetic meanings, symbolization, musical structure). The experience is often associated with an emotional state (e.g., elation, ecstasy, awe). Motivational processes are also involved, such as personal needs, desires, cravings, or quest. Finally, the experience is almost always linked to specific human behavior (e.g., dance, painting, writing, worship). Translating holistic or transcendental experiences into the six domains usually leads to more clarity and a more comprehensive appreciation.

THE SSLD (STRATEGIES AND SKILLS LEARNING AND DEVELOPMENT) SYSTEM

The SSLD system (Tsang, 2013) was developed based on decades of direct practice experience. The System follows an educational and learning orientation rather than a medico-pathological approach. SSLD

Table 1. Conceptual interface with metaphysical trichotomy and holistic formulations

<table>
<tr><th rowspan="2">Conventional Metaphysical Frame</th><th colspan="2">SSLD</th></tr>
<tr><th>Analytic Domains</th><th>Holistic Formulations</th></tr>
<tr><td>Social</td><td>Environment</td><td rowspan="6">Being-in-the-World
Lifeworld
Selfhood/Identity
Existential
Spiritual
Aesthetic
Political/Citizenship</td></tr>
<tr><td>Biological</td><td>Body</td></tr>
<tr><td rowspan="4">Psychological</td><td>Motivation</td></tr>
<tr><td>Cognition</td></tr>
<tr><td>Emotion</td></tr>
<tr><td>Behavior</td></tr>
</table>

intervention, therefore, is not conceived with the practitioner as an individual actively implementing a treatment that the client passively receives. SSLD practice is always imagined as a collaborative process between the client and the practitioner, recognizing the subjectivity, the active input and contribution made by the client. An outline of key SSLD practice procedures is given in Table 2.

Engagement and Relationship Building

The primary importance of engagement and relationship cannot be overstated. Research in psychotherapy and counseling has consistently confirmed the significance of the client-practitioner relationship – sometimes called the therapeutic alliance or working alliance – which can be a more potent factor contributing to positive client change than the intervention method or the system of psychotherapy used (Barrett-Lennard, 1962; Gomes-Schwartz, 1978; Grencavage & Norcross, 1990; Hartley & Strupp, 1983; Lambert & Barley, 2002; Martin, Garske, & Davis, 2000; Norcross, 2010). Informed by this body of work, SSLD practice emphasizes the building of a relationship with the client, and collaborating with the client throughout the intervention process.

Initial engagement takes place within the context of a dialogue between the client and the practitioner, targeting the three key components of the working alliance (Bordin, 1979): (1) agreement on the goals

Table 2. SSLD intervention procedure

Engagement and Relationship Building	Engagement: Client-centered orientation to gain understanding
Problem Translation and Assessment	N3C (Needs, Circumstances, Characteristics, Capacity) Assessment
Implementation	Goal Setting Operationalize goals into specific tasks for learning and development Step-by-step experiential learning Instruction, demonstration, modeling Simulation and feedback, use of video recording, coaching Real-life practice, report back, review, and refinement (the 4Rs)
Evaluation and Review	Evaluation of outcome Review of learning process

of therapy; (2) agreement on the tasks needed to achieve the agreed-upon goals; and (3) the development of an interpersonal bond. The SSLD practitioner first tries to establish a shared understanding of the client's needs through collaborative review of the client's thoughts and actions, which will help to inform goal setting later. The second task in the engagement process is to facilitate the client's understanding of how SSLD procedures can address the agreed-upon goals. The third aspect of the engagement and alliance-building process is a positive emotional bond between the client and the practitioner. This can usually be achieved through an accepting and non-judgmental attitude, communication of empathic understanding of the client's experience, emotional attunement with the client, accurate understanding of the client's subjective meanings, emotional support, collaboration, and cultivation of positive expectancy with regard to the outcome of the intervention.

SSLD practice procedures lend themselves readily to the accomplishment of these engagement tasks. For instance, the problem translation procedure, which almost parallels the engagement process in terms of time, is a deliberate attempt to gain an empathic understanding of the client's experiences and underlying needs. The SSLD problem translation process is inherently non-judgmental as it reframes problems into needs, goals, and learning tasks. Recognizing the client's needs and efforts is, in itself, emotionally supportive and empowering. Finally, the action-orientated approach, and the extensive clinical experience and positive results associated with SSLD practice, can provide support to positive expectancy with regard to intervention outcomes (Tsang, 2013).

Problem Translation and Assessment

The SSLD system focuses on addressing and meeting client needs, as most forms of human problems reflect unmet needs. Challenges or difficulties experienced by clients are not seen as problems or pathology, but are construed as manifestations of unmet needs. For instance, when a resident in a long-term care facility is demonstrating aggressive behavior, we try to understand the function of such behavior, and what needs are being expressed. The aggressive behavior may be a functional attempt to gain mastery over one's physical environment or an interpersonal relationship, and this can be connected to a need for security and/or autonomy. The same act can also signify a need for affiliation, stimulation, or emotional regulation.

Appreciating the client's needs that motivate problem behaviors in the first place will allow us to formulate our understanding of the client's situation and set our intervention goals better. Instead of focusing on stopping or eliminating the problem behavior, we are focusing on how the underlying needs could be met. This process of reframing client problems in terms of unmet needs and setting corresponding goals is called *problem translation*. This approach can help us discover alternate behavioral strategies for addressing such needs. When the client learns and develops new strategies and skills that are effective in addressing the same needs, the dependence on the original problem behavior, such as aggression, will diminish.

N3C Assessment

Following this orientation, the key assessment framework of the SSLD system is summarised into the N3C-6D formulation. N3C stands for needs, circumstances, characteristics, and capacity; and 6D refers to the six domains of environment, body, motivation, cognition, emotion, and action. The N3C assessment is a parsimonious scheme that allows the practitioner to arrive at a relatively comprehensive

Figure 2. Replacing problem behavior with strategies and skills

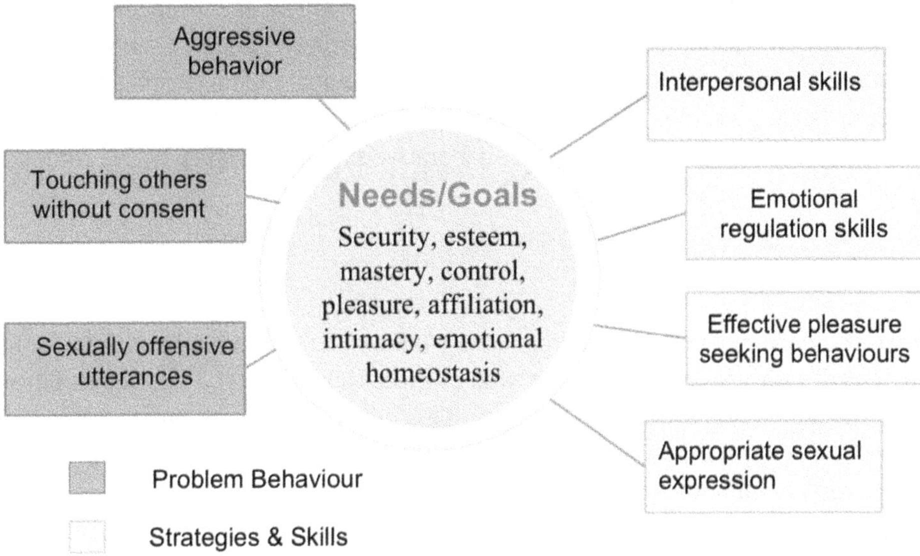

understanding of the client's experience and reality, which is individualized and easily summarised into a concise formulation. This assessment is person-centered and individualized, and takes us beyond the confines of diagnostic categories and the group-based view of human problems and challenges. People who have received the same diagnosis, be it Alzheimer's or depression, do not all experience the same reality and behave in the same way. They have different needs, circumstances, characteristics (having Alzheimer's or depression being just one of them), and capacity. People who manifest the same supposedly problematic behavior, such as substance use, aggression, or inappropriate sexual advances, are not driven by the exact same set of needs, and the relevant reality is again conditioned by circumstances, characteristics, and capacity of the person involved.

An elderly person manifesting aggressive behavior in a long-term care facility, for instance, can be reacting against sexual deprivation, expressing frustration at her lack of control over the environment, drawing attention to himself, or simply being bored and desiring some excitement by creating a conflict. Identifying the unmet needs of the client is a critical first step. The needs that lead to aggressive behaviors can vary from person to person, ranging from sex or emotional homeostasis to mastery and control, attention, stimulation, activity, and pleasure. Circumstances will include his or her financial situation, current health status, recent events such as loss of a loved one, prospective events such as institutionalization, or other ad hoc events such as a power outage, or being snowed in. Characteristics include gender, age, ethnicity, personality, specific behavioral patterns, and so on.

Capacity refers to skills, knowledge, resources, etc. Examples include being able to feed oneself, ability to move about using a walker or wheelchair, verbal communication, social skills, sense of humour, resilience, support network or social connections, and specific talents or skills such as singing or cooking. Technically speaking, capacity is a subset of characteristics. We set capacity aside to eliminate the risk of human service practitioners focusing on the client's problems, deficiencies, or pathology and neglecting the client's strengths, resources, and potentials.

An N3C assessment, as a collaborative process, not only provides information needed for formulation of the intervention plan, but simultaneously contributes to the engagement process as practitioner and client develop a shared understanding of the situation. The positive effects of empathic understanding of the client's needs, without implied judgment or pathologizing, cannot be overstated. Appreciating the client's circumstances, which is usually challenging, and recognizing the client's characteristics, and especially the client's capacity, all contribute to collaborative exploration and positive emotional bonding characterized by trust and understanding.

Case Example

Let us consider a case example of a client diagnosed with dementia who has been manifesting inappropriate sexual behavior towards other clients as well as professional caregivers, such as intrusive sexual utterances and touching the private parts of others. This client can also be quite irritable and become verbally aggressive and abusive at times. In our N3C assessment we find out that the client is not receiving adequate sensory stimulation, and there is not enough activity to keep him entertained. There is a strong need for interpersonal affiliation and attachment, plus the need for a sense of mastery and control, which the client is losing. Aggressive and abusive behaviors are often associated with frustration and helplessness, and ineffective emotional regulation. Our planned intervention will focus on his needs, which are often expressed and addressed through behaviors that are both ineffective and inappropriate. In our attempt to build alternative strategies to address these needs, we will take into consideration his circumstances, which includes his residence in a long-term care facility, his diabetic condition that impedes his sexual functioning, and his increasing isolation from his family and friends as he is receiving less frequent visits from them.

In terms of characteristics, this client is of East European background, and is only nominally religious. He used to be a successful accountant, and had his own firm. He has been preoccupied with order and control through much of his adult life, both professional and personal. Before retirement, he was used to getting what he wanted; additionally, his personal characteristics made it difficult for his wife and children to maintain a satisfying relationship with him. He is also prejudiced against people whom he considers to be unintelligent, and he had tremendous difficulty coming to terms with his dementia in the initial phase after formal diagnosis. He was in denial and did not look for service until functional deterioration had become more pronounced. Whereas it is understandable that staff and family caregivers have negative emotional response towards him, it is helpful for us to recognize his capacity, which we may want to mobilize in our intervention. His physical capabilities such as mobility and feeding himself are more visible assets. His verbal communication ability is another valuable resource. His needs for affiliation and attention can also be turn into positive motivational forces when we leverage them appropriately.

IMPLEMENTATION: THE 6 DOMAINS

After establishing a shared understanding of the client's N3C, we can move on to set realistic goals and design the intervention plan. In SSLD practice, the goals usually correspond with the client's needs. Recognizing the client's needs for order, control and mastery, attention, affiliation and attachment, pleasure, and emotional homeostasis, effective intervention would target them. There are multiple strategies available for each of these needs, and the client might not have chosen the most effective or appropriate responses. The following analysis is organized according to the 6D (domains of our being-in-the-world). It should be noted that these domains are not conceptualized as discrete and independent categories. Instead, they are overlapping and interconnected with one another, engaged constantly in ongoing interaction in a dynamic manner.

Environment

For instance, the need for order, mastery and control can be enhanced by reviewing the client's overall circumstances, identifying the areas that he could have increased control over. One of the things that institutionalization usually entails is dramatic decrease in the range of decisions a person can make about his life. Losing the opportunity to make decisions regarding everyday life such as the time to wake up, have meals, or go to bed, or simply the choice of food, or the choice of activities is, naturally, frustrating. Giving the client more opportunity to make choices can be a helpful environmental intervention.

Body

There are multiple strategies involving the body that can address the client's needs. The need for stimulation and pleasure can be addressed by physical activities such as the PID (Play Intervention for Dementia), which is an SSLD application (Tsang, 2013). The client may also benefit from tactile stimulation and interpersonal contact through services such as body massage. Physical workouts may also improve the general health and mental health status (Das, Do, Friedman, & McKenzie, 2008).

Motivation

People with the same needs do not necessarily have the same motivations. Some people are more likely to act on their needs than others. People may develop a lower level of motivation as a result of negative previous experiences, environmental constraints, or a generally pessimistic assessment of the prospect of fulfillment. Some people may lack energy because of a low activity lifestyle, and tiredness can also be a side effect of medications for dementia (e.g., Rivastigmine). Learned helplessness or depression, which is not uncommon among people with dementia (Flannery, 2002; Enache, Winblad, & Aarsland, 2011), can certainly impact the client's motivation as well. Strategies for improving motivation and energy levels include sufficient stimulation, activity, and interpersonal interaction. From an SSLD perspective, another key idea is to build successful experiences with the client, so that she can experience agency and mastery. By pursuing relevant tasks in an incremental manner, allowing clients to master tasks that are within their capacity and can lead to visible results (e.g., picking up small items with chopsticks, stretching, games and activities targeting bilateral coordination and integration), we can help the client to become more energized and motivated in general, likely associated with more positive expectancies.

Leveraging existing needs, such as those for affiliation and attachment, can help the client to channel energy into learning and performing more appropriate interpersonal and social behaviors. Clients often manifest anger and aggressive behavior because they are frustrated by their inability to attain what they need. When they can imagine how their action might lead to their desired goals in life, they would become less prone to use those less effective and inappropriate means.

Cognition

Many service programs for people with dementia focus on cognitive functions such as memory, counting and computation, sorting, speech, writing, sorting, concepts and reasoning. These are important functions to pay attention to. In SSLD practice, we also recognize the more generic and personal cognitive processes such as sense-making, searching for meaning, having a sense of self, and asserting personal significance and purpose. By conceptualizing the client holistically as a person and being respectful of his personhood, we support the client's development of agency and autonomy. Specifically, we try to give the client maximum space for self-expression and decision making, as well as the opportunity to develop and exercise cognitive functions that are significant for the client in his life. Cognitive functions such as self-awareness, self-reflection, and self-expression will be supported and enhanced. This may involve expanding the media and channels for the client's story-telling, narrativization, self-account, creative and symbolic processes such as art, poetry, music, fantasy and so on.

It is expected that enhanced cognitive engagement with oneself, other people, and the environment in general, will contribute positively to the overall functioning of the client. Improved self-awareness, making better sense of the environment, and better appreciation of interpersonal and social realities can all contribute to the client's sense of mastery, and development of interpersonal and social skills, leading to better adjustment and less reliance on inappropriate behaviors to address his needs.

Emotions

Emotions are arguably at the centre of human experience. In addition to understanding what people think and do, appreciating their emotional experience is critical to successful psychosocial intervention. Starting with the positive emotional bond between client and practitioner in the engagement phase and the building of a working alliance, empathic understanding of the client's feelings can go a long way in facilitating positive change. Clients showing behaviors that are considered problematic usually arouse negative emotions such as disappointment, resentment, or disgust among the people around them, including professional and family caregivers. At the same time, the client may be experiencing emotional difficulties such as pain, loss, fear, frustration, confusion, anger, and sadness. These emotions have to be dealt with by all parties concerned to facilitate meaningful client-practitioner collaboration.

Recognizing the emotional meaning and significance behind problematic acts such as aggressive and inappropriate sexual behavior allows us to engage with the client's subjective experience. In a context that is non-judgmental, where the client's emotional difficulties are understood and cared for, problematic behaviors usually would not exacerbate. If alternate channels are made available for the client to express his emotions without fear of reprimand, space for positive transformation can be created. Instead of telling the client what he did was wrong or unacceptable, we may want to communicate to him that we understand his pain, frustration, and fear, and we are committed to help him make changes so that he can eventually feel better about his life.

Action/Behavior

Psychologists tend to talk about human action in terms of behavior. The word action amplifies the agentive aspect, and its connection to the human subject. Much of SSLD practice is about building new sets of actions, often called strategies and skills, that can address the client's needs effectively. A person who is angry and resorts to verbal or even physical aggression may have to learn to get in touch with her feelings, and to express her feelings and needs in a way that is more likely to bring about understanding, engagement, and help instead of turning people off. Effective strategies and skills in this case can also include effective communication, relationship building, and pleasure seeking activities, which can include activities that directly address sexual needs. An SSLD program on sexuality and intimacy among seniors (Tsang, Chu, Liu, Ip, and Mak, 2014), for instance, has listed many specific activities ranging from self-regulation and cognitive control to the direct use of sex service (pp. 47-48).

COMING BACK TO THE PERSON: BEING-IN-THE-WORLD

The case above illustrates how the SSLD system can be applied analytically to inform assessment, goal setting, and an intervention plan. As mentioned above, the N3C-6D analytic frame can also interface with a more holistic conceptualization of the person. We do not lose sight of the wholeness and integrity of the personhood of the client, and we value the client's subjectivity, agency, and autonomy throughout. As a result of our intervention, not only will the client's needs be more effectively addressed, we also expect to see the personhood of the client being enhanced, associated with an improved sense of self, increased self-efficacy and an expanded repertoire of strategies and skills. In our experience, positive changes are usually observed in the client's interpersonal and social functioning as well.

It should also be noted that such a person-centered approach allows practitioners to address issues related to diversities and differences related to gender, ethnicity, class, sexual orientation, ability, and so on. The N3C-6D framework is sensitive both to shared conditions and characteristics as well as individual differences, enabling practitioners to manage them in a flexible and dynamic manner. The SSLD system has been applied in many different cultural and professional contexts internationally, and valuable experience is accumulated on an ongoing basis.

EVALUATION AND REVIEW

Given the focus on individual needs, a key outcome measure for SSLD intervention is how well the needs are met. In senior service, like in most other human service contexts, there is usually a preference for objective measures with established psychometric properties. In SSLD practice, we recognize the value of such measures, especially in terms of allowing quantification, easy comparison, and statistical analysis. In direct practice, it is usually helpful to complement such measures with assessment or accounts capturing experiences that are significant to the client, and these can include changes that are directly observable as well as those that are more private or subjective. For instance, a decrease or complete elimination of behaviors considered to be problematic, such as aggression, is usually amenable to direct observation, scaling and measurement. Certain subjective experiences, such as depressive feelings, can be assessed and quantified through self-report instruments.

There are, however, experiences that can be quite idiosyncratic but are of high significance to the client, and there may not be appropriate measures available. For example, a client becomes more accepting of her own sexual needs and feels comfortable expressing them. We can also be looking at a client with dementia whose speech was stereotypic and non-communicative for years becoming verbally communicative, showing initiative in interpersonal engagement, use of humor, and increased future orientation in his utterances. It can also be a client who used to show extreme resistance and aggression when asked to take a shower becoming cooperative with the caregiver, and even showing appreciation and gratitude. We can also share a client's excitement over an aesthetic experience associated with the rediscovery of romantic love, or with poetry, painting, music, or other art forms.

Congruent with our conceptualization of the people as subjects and our engagement with their being-in-the-world, we value significant events and happenings in their lives, how they experience and make sense of them, and their subjective sense of satisfaction. These experiences can be accessed through our participation, our observation, conversations with them, their narratives, their artwork, and/or various forms of direct and symbolic expression. We may also access these indirectly through caregivers, family members, practitioners, or other informants. Combining such information with objective and self-report measures can offer us a more complete picture of the client's overall reality, within which we assess the role played by our intervention.

SSLD AND THE PRACTICE REALITY

In the section above, we have used a case example to illustrate the SSLD intervention procedure. In actual practice, the SSLD system has been used with individuals, couples, families, groups, organizations, and communities. The limited space in this chapter does not permit detailed description of these applications, however, readers can refer to other SSLD publications (Tsang, 2013; Tsang et al., 2014; Tsang & Li, in press) and the website (http://ssld.kttsang.com/) for more information. In the area of senior service, a good example is an organizational change initiative to develop positive policy and practice with regards to intimacy and sexual needs of seniors (Chu, Liu, Leung, Ip, & Tsang, 2015).

The seniors' sexuality and intimacy initiative (Chu et al., 2015) is an example of a multi-level intervention using the SSLD system. The initiative is carried out in one of the largest publicly funded senior service systems in Canada since 2009. This initiative includes the following components:

1. Articulating an organizational policy for managing sexuality and intimacy issues of clients, including specific practice guidelines.
2. Professional development programs to enable staff to acquire the requisite knowledge and skills to manage such issues competently and ethically, including training workshops and case conferences, specific skills training for staff, and production of instruction and learning material (educational videos and a practice manual) (Tsang et al., 2014).
3. Extensive engagement with clients and family caregivers, including meetings with family caregivers and clients to share the issues and challenges they face, and to explore effective strategies for addressing them (experiential interactive groups). There were also individual and family system interventions to resolve issues.
4. Bringing about change in the community will involve disseminating knowledge and skills through distribution of instructional material, offering training workshops for professionals, and ongoing case conferences for practicing professionals.

This initiative involves the application of SSLD principles and methods at the organizational level, both in terms of policy formulation and building in-house knowledge and skills through staff development and team building. Services were delivered through community education and consultation, as well as direct intervention with individual clients and their families and, additionally, group programs. Core SSLD principles and methods are applied, including engagement and relationship building, N3C-6D formulations, developing alternative strategies and skills to address unmet needs, and close collaboration with clients and client systems in learning and development.

EBP3.0: PRACTICE-BASED RESEARCH AND DEVELOPMENT (PBRD)

The PID (Play Intervention for Dementia) program is another example of SSLD application in senior service. The program was first conceived in 2013. A typical PID session consists of a number of play or activity segments targeting different areas of functioning affected by dementia, including: gross-motor activities, neuro-corporal integration, fine sensory-motor coordination, cognitive operations, emotional regulation, interpersonal synchronization, engagement and communication, social participation, etc. The program was initially developed through experimenting with new ways of playing with seniors with dementia who participated in adult day programs, drawing upon practice experience as well as research and knowledge developed in the areas of neuroscience, psychology of learning, gerontology, and group dynamics.

The program conceptualization and design combine knowledge and skills from SSLD, neuroscience, learning psychology, and group dynamics. N3C assessment of the clients are taken into account while the program design is informed both by the 6D analysis and holistic conceptualization of being and sense of self, agency, autonomy, existential and spiritual issues (purpose, meaning, transcendence), aesthetics, etc. The games and activities are designed to optimize the selfhood, subjectivity, agency, and autonomy of the participants as they learn and develop new responses, skills, and strategies through the activities and games, and through interactions with other participants and staff.

The PID program has been piloted at 5 service sites in Canada and Asia, with encouraging results. Observed benefits include: decreased deterioration, reduced disruptive behavior, functional recovery, learning and development, positive affect, increased energy and motivation, interpersonal engagement, enhanced agency and autonomy, and pro-social behavior, etc. The specific intervention procedures, including the literal game plans for each session, are continuously reviewed and refined, based on careful observation of in-session responses of the clients, with due regard to their respective and collective N3Cs. Knowledge development activities include direct practice experience and reflection, video-recording and review, systematic observation and documentation, case studies, case conferences and consultation sessions, focus groups with staff and family caregivers, and so on. Funding for program development has been awarded by the Trillium Foundation of Ontario, Canada (2014-2016), and the Hong Kong Polytechnic University has funded an initial outcome study (2016-2017). Encouraging outcome data are now emerging.

As a practice-based research and development (PBRD) initiative, PID follows a third-generation evidence-based practice (EBP3.0) framework (Tsang, 2013). This framework recognizes the contribution of clients and practitioners both in bringing about positive outcomes and in the process of knowledge production. It does not assume that it is only the assumed active ingredients of intervention method that cause positive client change. It engages with both the subjective realities constructed and shared by clients and practitioners as well as objective measures and assessment procedures. The research and knowledge production process is grounded in the site of practice, linked to the knowledge needs of the clients and the practitioners. It follows contingency-based thinking and pursues an ongoing revision and refinement process, responding to the ever-changing realities and challenges of direct practice. This approach to practice research and development is used in many other SSLD applications.

CONCLUSION

The SSLD system recognizes and values the personhood of the seniors and seeks to empower them by enhancing their agency, autonomy, and self-efficacy. We attempt to simultaneously offer analytic tools such as the N3C-6D formulations as well as engaging with holistic experiences in their various dimensions, including the existential, spiritual, aesthetic, political, and so on. The system has been applied to a wide range of human service contexts. In the area of senior service, it aims at providing a more optimistic and proactive approach to offset the pessimism often found among clients, families, caregivers, practitioners, and service providers. The system has extensive applicability and can support practitioners working with individuals, families, groups, organizations, and communities. It has already been used in managing challenging issues in senior service such as sexuality and intimacy issues, dementia, and associated psychosocial challenges. SSLD programs in senior service include direct practice programs with clients, support and education services for family and caregivers, volunteers training and development, professional education and development for staff, organizational development, and community education. The system is expected to go through ongoing review, revision, and refinement through practice-based research and development, drawing on the collaborative input of clients, caregivers, volunteers and community members, practitioners, service providers, researchers and scholars.

REFERENCES

Achenbaum, W. A., & Bengtson, V. L. (1994). Re-engaging the disengagement theory of aging: On the history and assessment of theory development in gerontology. *The Gerontologist*, *34*(6), 756–763. doi:10.1093/geront/34.6.756 PMID:7843604

Atchley, R. C. (1971). Retirement and leisure participation: Continuity or crisis? *The Gerontologist*, *11*(1), 13–17. doi:10.1093/geront/11.1_Part_1.13 PMID:5579223

Atchley, R. C. (1989). A continuity theory of normal aging. *The Gerontologist*, *29*(2), 183–190. doi:10.1093/geront/29.2.183 PMID:2519525

Atchley, R. C. (2000). *Continuity and adaptation in aging: Creating positive experiences*. Baltimore, MD: Johns Hopkins University Press.

Barrett-Lennard, G. T. (1962). Dimensions of therapist response as causal factors in therapeutic change. *Psychological Monographs*, *76*(43), 1–36. doi:10.1037/h0093918

Bengtson, V. L., Burgess, E. O., & Parrott, T. M. (1997). Theory, explanation, and a third generation of theoretical development in social gerontology. *The Journals of Gerontology. Series B, Psychological Sciences and Social Sciences*, *52B*(2), S72–S88. doi:10.1093/geronb/52B.2.S72 PMID:9060987

Bennett, A., & Taylor, J. (2012). Popular music and the aesthetics of ageing. *Popular Music, 31*(2), 231–243. doi:10.1017/S0261143012000013

Bordin, E. S. (1979). The generalizability of the psychoanalytic concept of the working alliance. *Psychotherapy (Chicago, Ill.), 16*(3), 252–260. doi:10.1037/h0085885

Bowling, A., & Dieppe, P. (2005). What is successful ageing and who should define it? *British Medical Journal, 331*(7531), 1548–1551. doi:10.1136/bmj.331.7531.1548 PMID:16373748

Calasanti, T. (2004). New directions in feminist gerontology: An introduction. *Journal of Aging Studies, 18*(1), 1–8. doi:10.1016/j.jaging.2003.09.002

Chu, M. L. S. C., Liu, K. Y., Ip, C. F., Leung, E., & Tsang, A. K. T. (2015). Transforming organizational culture using the SSLD system to address the taboo of sexuality and intimacy needs of seniors. *Journal of Contemporary Management, 4*(4), 15–23.

Cumming, E., & Henry, W. E. (1961). *Growing old.* New York: Basic.

Dannefer, D., Uhlenberg, P., Foner, A., & Abeles, R. P. (2005). On the shoulders of a giant: The legacy of Matilda White Riley for gerontology. *The Journals of Gerontology. Series B, Psychological Sciences and Social Sciences, 60*(6), S296–S304. doi:10.1093/geronb/60.6.S296 PMID:16260711

Das, J., Do, Q.-T., Friedman, J., & McKenzie, D. (2008). *Mental Health Patterns and Consequences: Results from Survey Data in Five Developing Countries.* Policy Research Working Paper; No. WPS 4495. World Bank, Washington. Retrieved from https://openknowledge.worldbank.org/handle/10986/6376

Davey, A., & Eggebeen, D. J. (1998). Patterns of intergenerational exchange and mental health. *The Journals of Gerontology. Series B, Psychological Sciences and Social Sciences, 53*(2), 86–95. doi:10.1093/geronb/53B.2.P86 PMID:9520925

Dillaway, H., & Byrnes, M. (2009). Reconsidering successful aging. *Journal of Applied Gerontology, 28*(6), 702–722. doi:10.1177/0733464809333882

Dowd, J. J. (1975). Aging as exchange: A preface to theory. *Journal of Gerontology, 30*(5), 584–594. doi:10.1093/geronj/30.5.584 PMID:1181364

Dowd, J. J. (1988). The reification of age: Age stratification theory and the passing of the autonomous subject. *Journal of Aging Studies, 1*(4), 317–335. doi:10.1016/0890-4065(87)90008-9 PMID:25195842

Enache, D., Winblad, B., & Aarsland, D. (2011). Depression in dementia. *Current Opinion in Psychiatry,* 462–472. doi:10.1097/yco.0b013e32834bb9d4 PMID:21926624

Erikson, E. H. (1950). *Childhood and society.* New York: Norton.

Erikson, E. H., & Erikson, J. M. (1982/1997). *The life cycle completed: Extended version.* New York: Norton.

Flannery, R. B. (2002). Treating learned helplessness in the elderly dementia patient: Preliminary inquiry. *American Journal of Alzheimers Disease and Other Dementias, 17*(6), 345–349. doi:10.1177/153331750201700605 PMID:12501481

Garner, J. D. (1999). Feminism and feminist gerontology. *Journal of Women & Aging*, *11*(2-3), 3–12. doi:10.1300/J074v11n02_02 PMID:10568093

Gomes-Schwartz, B. (1978, October). Effective ingredients in psychotherapy: Prediction of outcome from process variables. *Journal of Consulting and Clinical Psychology*, *46*(5), 1023–1035. doi:10.1037/0022-006X.46.5.1023 PMID:701541

Grencavage, L. M., & Norcross, J. C. (1990). Where are the commonalities among the therapeutic common factors? *Professional Psychology, Research and Practice*, *21*(5), 372–378. doi:10.1037/0735-7028.21.5.372

Hartley, D., & Strupp, H. H. (1983). The therapeutic alliance: Its relationship to outcome in brief psychotherapy. In J. Masling (Ed.), *Empirical studies of psychoanalytic theories* (Vol. 1, pp. 1–38). Hillsdale, NJ: Lawrence Erlbaum.

Havighurst, R. J. (1961). Successful Aging. *The Gerontologist*, *1*(1), 8–13. doi:10.1093/geront/1.1.8

Heidegger, M., & Stambaugh, J. (1996). *Being and time: a translation of Sein und Zeit*. Albany, NY: State University of New York Press.

Jewell, A., & Nell, E. (2014). Gerotranscendence. *Rural Theology*, *12*(2), 96–105. doi:10.1179/14704 99414Z.00000000029

Jewell, A. J. (2014). Tornstams notion of gerotranscendence: Re-examining and questioning the theory. *Journal of Aging Studies*, *30*, 112–120. doi:10.1016/j.jaging.2014.04.003 PMID:24984914

John, R. (1984). Prerequisites of an adequate theory of aging: A critique and reconceptualization. *Mid-American Review of Sociology*, *9*(2), 79–108.

Karasik, R. J., & Kishimoto, K. (2016). Is gerontology ready for anti-racist pedagogy? A survey of educators practices and perspectives. *Gerontology & Geriatrics Education*, *37*(1), 1–18. doi:10.1080/0 2701960.2015.1115984 PMID:26886051

Lambert, M. J., & Barley, D. E. (2002). Research summary on the therapeutic relationship and psychotherapy outcome. In J. C. Norcross (Ed.), *Psychotherapy relationships that work* (pp. 17–32). New York: Oxford University Press; doi:10.1037//0033-3204.38.4.357

Martin, D. J., Garske, J. P., & Davis, M. K. (2000). Relation of the therapeutic alliance with outcome and other variables: A meta-analytic review. *Journal of Consulting and Clinical Psychology*, *68*(3), 438–450. doi:10.1037/0022-006X.68.3.438 PMID:10883561

Moberg, D. O. (2008). Spirituality and aging: Research and Implications. *Journal of Religion, Spirituality and Aging*, *20*(1-2), 95–134. doi:10.1080/15528030801922038

Moran, D. (2014). What does Heidegger mean by the transcendence of Dasein? *International Journal of Philosophical Studies*, *22*(4), 491–514. doi:10.1080/09672559.2014.948717

Morgan, L. A., & Kunkel, S. R. (2016). *Aging, society, and the life course* (5th ed.). New York, NY: Springer.

Newgarten, B. L. (1964). *Personality in the middle and late life*. New York: Atherton Press.

Nimrod, G., & Kleiber, D. A. (2007). Reconsidering change and continuity in later life: Toward an innovation theory of successful aging. *International Journal of Aging & Human Development*, *65*(1), 1–22. doi:10.2190/Q4G5-7176-51Q2-3754 PMID:17703747

Norcross, J. C. (2010). The therapeutic relationship. In B. L. Duncan, S. D. Miller, B. E. Wampold, & M. A. Hubble (Eds.), *The heart & soul of change: Delivering what works in therapy* (2nd ed.; pp. 113–141). Washington, DC: American Psychological Association; doi:10.1037/12075-004

Quadagno, J. (2014). *Aging and The Life Course: An Introduction to Social Gerontology* (6th ed.). New York: McGraw-Hill.

Rajani, F. (2015). Theory of Gerotranscendence: An Analysis. *European Psychiatry*, *30*, 1467. doi:10.1016/S0924-9338(15)31138-X

Reker, G. T., & Chamberlain, K. (Eds.). (2000). *Exploring existential meaning: Optimizing human development across the life span*. Thousand Oaks, CA: Sage.

Riley, M. W. (1973). Aging and cohort succession: Interpretations and misinterpretations. *Public Opinion Quarterly*, *37*(1), 35–49. doi:10.1086/268058

Riley, M. W. (1974). The perspective of age stratification. *The School Review*, *83*(1), 85–91. doi:10.1086/443174

Riley, M. W. (1994). Aging and society: Past, present, and future. *The Gerontologist*, *34*(4), 436–446. doi:10.1093/geront/34.4.436 PMID:7959099

Robert, L., & Fulop, T. (Eds.). (2014). *Aging: Facts and theories*. Basel, Switzerland: Karger. doi:10.1159/isbn.978-3-318-02653-5

Rowe, J. W., & Kahn, R. L. (1998). *Successful aging*. New York: Pantheon Book.

Strawbridge, W. J., Wallhagen, M. I., & Cohen, R. D. (2002). Successful aging and well-being: Self-rated compared with Rowe and Kahn. *The Gerontologist*, *42*(6), 727–733. doi:10.1093/geront/42.6.727 PMID:12451153

Topaz, M., Troutman-Jordan, M., & MacKenzie, M. (2014). Construction, deconstruction, and re-construction: The roots of successful aging theories. *Nursing Science Quarterly*, *27*(3), 226–233. doi:10.1177/0894318414534484 PMID:24951524

Tornstam, L. (1989). Gero-transcendence; A Meta-theoretical Reformulation of the Disengagement Theory. *Aging: Clinical and Experimental Research (Milano)*, *I*(1), 55–63.

Tornstam, L. (1996). Gerotranscendence – a theory about maturing into old age. *Journal of Aging and Identity*, *1*, 37–50.

Tornstam, L. (1997). Gerotranscendence: The contemplative dimension of aging. *Journal of Aging Studies*, *11*(2), 143–154. doi:10.1016/S0890-4065(97)90018-9

Tornstam, L. (2005). *Gerotranscendence: A developmental theory of positive aging*. New York: Springer Pub. Co.

Torres, S. (2015). Expanding the gerontological imagination on ethnicity: Conceptual and theoretical perspectives. *Ageing and Society*, *35*(5), 935–960. doi:10.1017/S0144686X14001330

Tsang, A. K. T. (2013). *Learning to change lives: The strategies and skills learning and development system*. Toronto, ON, Canada: University of Toronto Press.

Tsang, A. K. T. (2014). Managing sexuality and intimacy issues among seniors: The SSLD approach. Toronto: Yee Hong Centre for Geriatric Care.

Tsang, A. K. T., & Li, B. (in press). Building a practice system for working with immigrants and refugees: The SSLD approach. In M. C. Yan & U. Anucha (Eds.), *Working with immigrants and refugees: A handbook for social work and human services*. Toronto: Oxford University Press.

Walker, L. (2012). The future of femme: Notes on femininity, aging and gender theory. *Sexualities*, *15*(7), 795–814. doi:10.1177/1363460711417482

World Health Organization. (1946/ 2016). *Constitution of WHO: Principles*. Retrieved from http://www.who.int/about/mission/en/

Youdin, R. (2014). *Clinical gerontological social work practice*. New York, NY: Springer.

Zubair, M., & Norris, M. (2015). Perspectives on ageing, later life and ethnicity: Ageing research in ethnic minority contexts. *Ageing and Society*, *35*(5), 897–916. doi:10.1017/S0144686X14001536 PMID:25937682

KEY TERMS AND DEFINITIONS

6D: The six domains of human experience: environment, body, motivation, cognition, emotion, action/behavior.

Being-in-the-World: The totality of a person's being, including all the experience the person has within his or her lifeworld.

EPB3.0: Third generation evidence-based practice, a practice-based research and development approach that emphasized inter-subjectivity between client and practitioner, dynamic involvement of multiple contingencies in bringing about positive outcome, epistemological eclecticism and methodological pluralism.

Lifeworld: The totality of a person's lived reality, including both internal and external realities, and their objective and subjective aspects.

N3C: Needs, circumstances, characteristics and capacity.

Neuroplasticity: The brain's ability to reorganize itself by generating new neurons and forming new neural connections. Neuroplasticity allows the brain to compensate for lost or compromised functions due to injury or disease.

PBRD: Practice-based research and development.

Problem Translation: Reformulating the client's presenting problem through assessing the client's N3C (needs, circumstances, characteristics, and capacity) and setting realistic goals to be attained.

Chapter 14
Aging in Place

Ben Yuk Fai Fong
The Hong Kong Polytechnic University, Hong Kong

Vincent T. Law
The Hong Kong Polytechnic University, Hong Kong

ABSTRACT

Aging is a function of time and is a natural and integral part of the life cycle. Aging process differs among individuals and brings all kinds of changes, affecting not just the physical body and its functions, but also to the social, psychological and financial situations to individuals. Aging in place (AIP) is a common preference among older people for remaining in their local community and maintaining their social networks throughout the aging process. Issues about appropriateness of aging in place, long-term care, and residential homes are discussed. Some models and recommendations are discussed, completed with thoughts on future studies.

INTRODUCTION

Life, aging, sickness and death are the four phases in life. People enjoy life. Everyone strikes to avoid sickness, but nobody can escape aging and death. Aging is a function of time and is a natural and integral part of the life cycle. However, the aging process differs among individuals, depending on genetic inheritance, early life development, nutritional status, degenerative bodily workload, healthy lifestyle, psychological wellness, etc. Death is the ultimate end-point to all living creatures, and human beings are no exception.

Aging is associated with the gradual accumulation of a wide variety of molecular and cellular damage at the biological level (Steves et al., 2012). Aging brings all kinds of changes, affecting not just the physical body and its functions, but the social, psychological, and financial situations to individuals. Dynamics in the family, personal life and work alter with age. Understanding the changes and knowing how to deal with the inevitable changes in life are learnable essential skills. The elderly encounter decrease in strength and endurance of the body frame, impairment in vision and hearing, compromise in immunity, deterioration of brain functions and reactions, etc., leading to risks of falls, restricted mobility and more frequent illnesses, including degenerative chronic conditions like high blood pressure, heart

DOI: 10.4018/978-1-5225-2633-9.ch014

disease, diabetes, arthritis, and dementia. Undoubtedly healthy aging will have far reaching affections on the elderly by balancing the interaction between the body, mind, social and economic status, as well as between life and environment (Fenton & Draper, 2014).

Definitions of Aging in Place

"Aging in place" (or "age in place") is a contested concept (Rowles, 1993) and the term is widely used in aging policy and research but underexplored with the elderly themselves (Wiles et al., 2012). Golant (2015) even suggested that aging in place (AIP) has been romanticized while its associated challenges minimized.

Rowles (1993) refers aging in place to the ability to remain in one's residence of choice as one ages, avoiding unwanted relocation associated with age-related personal or environmental limitations. Aging in place is the ability to live in one's own home and community safely, independently, and comfortably, regardless of age, income, or ability level (Centers for Disease Control and Prevention, 2013). It emphasizes that older people to remain living in the locality with which they are familiar for as long as they wish (Chui, 2008). Some view aging in place as the situation whereby older adults remain at home or a similar preferred setting for as long as possible with as much ability and dignity as possible (Benefield & Holtzclaw, 2014).

This chapter presents the perspectives of aging in place and illustrate two models as the appropriate solutions for AIP. Living in own homes and long-term care are discussed. Finally, problems arising from relocation to residential care homes and to another country will be described.

BACKGROUND

Many industrialized countries are facing with population aging. The World Health Organization (2007) estimated the number of people aged 60 and over will be doubled from 11% of the global population in 2006 to 22% by 2050. Many retirees will be expected to live for another 25 years for men and 30 years for women after their economically productive time is over. The elderly will be a burden to the society in terms of health services and daily care.

Traditionally, in an extended family, three and more generations live under the same roof. With the large population living in limited developed lands in Hong Kong, nuclear families become the norm in the younger generation, who are much influenced by the Western culture. Even the unmarried grow-ups do not live with their parent. Therefore, many of the elderly are likely to live with their spouse or alone. These old people will remain at home while aging. There are elderly who chose to relocate to residential care homes or to another country.

Aging in Place vs. Relocation

Aging in place and relocation is a complex topic of age-related subjective considerations in the everyday lives of older people (Lofqvist et al., 2013). Older people desire choices about their living arrangements and access to services and amenities (Wiles et al., 2012). Decision-making process about aging in place and relocation includes mixed feelings and negotiations about personal health and housing aspects (Sim et al., 2012). The process takes place over a long period of time throughout the aging process (Nygren

& Iwarsson, 2009). Perceived availability of community services is related to decision of AIP or relocation (Tang & Pickard, 2008). For very old people (aged more than 80), decline in health is a predictor in making the decision to relocate (Stoeckel & Porell, 2010). Relocation is a stressful major life event (Sergeant et al., 2008). Old people tend to struggle with justifying the decision whether to move to a residential home (Soderberg et al., 2012). Thoughts of relocation for very old people involve diverse, complex, and ambivalent matters (Lofqvist et al., 2013).

Aging in place is a common preference among older people for remaining in their local community and maintaining their social networks throughout the aging process (World Health Organization, 2015). Older people want to age and remain in place (Deloitte and Touche, 1996; Wahl, 2010; Lofqvist et al., 2013). The specific elements necessary for individuals to age in place depend largely on their situation and level of functionality (Wiles et al., 2012). However, numerous factors threaten possibilities for safe and sound health in the residence of the elderly (Benefield & Holtzclaw, 2014). Successful aging in place depends on individual capacity in handle demands from their environments (Lawton et al., 1997).

In 2002, The World Health Organization (WHO) recommended a framework for active aging, which is the lifelong process of optimizing opportunities for health, participation and security, to enhance quality of life as people age. There are many ways for older people to age in place. It may mean continuing to live in the same home, or moving to a unit that is safer or more adapted to their needs while maintaining vital connections with their community, friends and family. In all cases the older persons should age in a place which is right for them, while maintaining the quality of life as they age. They continue to stay in the community even though there is increasing fragility and associated problems. It also entails independency in an appropriate housing. The elderly can have the services and supports, per their needs that may change over time, but they avoid the trauma of moving to a costly but inappropriate, unfamiliar, and dependent facility (Wong, 2012).

Where a person lives often occurs as "a matter of life" or naturally, or with planning. Aging in place can be a continuation of living in the same place and house, or can be part of a retirement plan, including relocation to a more suitable home and migration, or demigration, for various reasons and causes. In addition to having a place to live and access to services, there are other concerns in aging in place. Well-being, both in the body and mind, is essential to keep the life machine functioning. Keeping the individual elderly's identity, dignity, independence, and autonomy are all important to all old people. This is more so in achieving optimization and fulfilment of life, which is certainly limited for this group of formerly active members of the community and country. Academics and professionals have advocated active aging, despite the often "ignored" existence of unfavorable elderly policy for aging in place in many societies, where there is a service gap, resulting in failure to fulfill the needs of the retirees.

Some elderly regard quality of life as the top priority after retirement. They do not want to become a burden to their children, family, and the society. The more educated middle class people plan their retirement. Often they continue to live in their own homes. They are still mentally active and begin to take up creative hobbies, interest classes, traveling, volunteer services, paid or non-paid consulting works, teaching, etc. Most of these endeavors help the elderly to maintain their identity, dignity, and respect. After all, people should be able to enjoy the last phase of life.

The Hong Kong Housing Authority has schemes to encourage young residents to live with or live nearby their elderly generation. This will help to promote mutual family support and care for the elderly in public rental residential estates. On the other hand, the Hong Kong Housing Society has implemented the "Aging-in-Place" Scheme in its rental units to improve the living environment and facilities for the elderly residents, enabling them to age in place (Hong Kong SAR Government, 2016 LCQ 13).

When people get old and retire, they look for a place to spend the rest of their life. This is a very important, but complex and demanding, phase in life. Aging in place has been a common issue of concern to the community, families, service providers, health professions, politicians, and most of all, the government. In Hong Kong, "Aging in place as the core, institutional care as back-up" is the policy on elderly care (Hong Kong SAR Government, 2017).

AGING IN PLACE

Aging population drives serious advanced planning (Benefield & Holtzclaw, 2014). A significant portion of the population may experience functional limitations due to advanced age (Brown et al., 2012). Place is a broad and complex conceptual matrix that embraces both the physical and social environment (Chippendale & Bear-Lehman, 2010).

Aging in place aims at maintaining independence to the fullest extent possible without compromising safety (Wiles et al., 2012). It is generally viewed as better for the elderly and may gain significant financial advantages in terms of healthcare expenditure (Marek et al., 2012). AIP can facilitate people's engagement in their local neighborhoods and communities, reduce the costs of aged care, as well as fulfill the goals and aims of many older people to remain in their own homes (Baldassar, 2017).

Social capital is an important factor associated with successful aging in place (Lin, 1999). People who successfully age in place tend to have larger social networks (Chippendale & Bear-Lehman, 2010). Social networks and social resources in the community allow the elderly to make informed decisions about their "place" (Chippendale & Bear-Lehman, 2010). Long-term emotional attachments to environmental surroundings promote well-being in old age (Taylor, 2001).

Culture

People's culture and identity influence the understanding of aging, which is not necessarily ethnically neutral. The elderly's norms, perceptions, and self-awareness of the reality of aging vary among different cultures. A Taiwanese study has shown elder Chinese would adopt a healthy lifestyle, think positively, promote family and inter-personal relationships, and build up financial resources. There exist intergenerational ties, which entail the relationship and the levels of supports offered by children to their parents (Fenton & Draper, 2014). The Hong Kong government promotes aging in place with the objective of "intergenerational harmony" (Hong Kong SAR Government, 2016 LCQ 13).

Psychological and Social Aspects

The most common psychological condition in old age is depression (Jones, 1984). Psychological distress in older people may be due to life stressors such as bereavement, drop in socioeconomic status with retirement, or disability and chronic condition. The World Health Organization (2016) also suggests that 1 in 10 old people experience elder abuse, including physical, sexual, psychological, emotional, financial and material abuse, leading to long-lasting psychological consequences. Appropriate AIP should bring emotional wellness and happiness. Social network, connection, and interaction should be facilitated even when elderly lives at home.

Location and Environment

Attention to selection of the right physical location will make a difference to the elderly in AIP. Ideally, and naturally, old people prefer to live in the home and familiar environment they have spent years and are familiar with it. However, if there is a lack of services and support in the locality, then relocation is inevitable. The elderly should feel comfortable and safe with environment, which is conducive for active and healthy aging, even to those living alone.

Community

Everyone would choose a safe community to live in. This is an important AIP consideration for old people, who also look for clanship so that they feel belonging and being attached to the surrounding community. Health and active aging are affected by family caregiver support, adequate financial resources, access to social and community resources, as well as safe neighborhoods (Benefield & Holtzclaw, 2014). The traditional reliance on children as primacy caretakers fade with time (Cheng et al., 2013). Caregivers of the elderly face many challenges, including insufficient caregiver support, absence of eldercare leave, inflexible work arrangements, and significant stress (Chin & Phua, 2016). Informal sources of support such as neighbors have also been long-standing (Vasunilashorn et al., 2012). Mutual support among neighbors is driven by the values of interdependence and reciprocity (Gardner, 2011). Neighborhood effects show linkage between the quality of one's neighborhood environment and the mental health status of older adults (Ivey et al., 2015), their physical health (Yen et al., 2009), and perceived safety (Oh & Kim, 2009).

The government should provide supporting services for caregivers to sustain the current level of informal care. To successfully implement aging in place, the capability of community support and home help services for dependent elderly needs should be expanded (Deloitte and Touche, 1996). Community centers should be well designed and planned to meet the needs of the local elderly population, who wish to live in harmony. The Hong Kong government is carrying out the "Hong Kong 2030+: Towards a Planning Vision and Strategy Transcending 2030" initiative to update the long-term development strategy, and to study how urban planning, building design, and so on can meet the challenges arising from the aging population (Hong Kong SAR Government, 2016 LCQ 13). The New South Wales (NSW) state government in Australia has established grants to local councils to build age-friendly local communities as local solutions to accessibility of town centers, meeting facilities and social connections for old adults (DFCS, 2016). An American team suggests that a community may engage healthy elders as key volunteers to keep them active and connected, and to help improving the life of the community. Volunteer capacity needs efforts in recruitment, training, and support (Knickman & Snell, 2002).

Livability of Elderly

The NSW government has collaborated with the building industry to adopt the Livable Housing Design Guidelines, aiming to build a variety of age-friendly housing that requires minimal or no adaptation as people age (DFCS, 2016). The Hong Kong Housing Society (2017a) has pledged to promote and improve the "Aging in Place" concept through three aspects: (i) *proper living environment*: with focus on the mental and physical needs of the elderly, and the latest information of living environment and related services; (ii) *healthy and active aging*: better understanding of the aging process, facing retirement life positively and optimistically, and having a happy and enjoyable golden age; and (iii) *safety living habit*: recognizing the hidden dangers at home and risky habits which may lead to accidents. While there is no single perfect housing solution for all old people, improving the structure of housing for the elderly is an important social policy measure (Howden-Chapman et al., 1999).

Services

Achieving age in place needs many supporting services. These include health and medical services, particularly in long-term care (LTC) and mental wellness; commercial services in hair dressing, clothing, cleaning; food services such as groceries, supermarkets, restaurants; sporting and recreational amenities; as well as domestic services for daily living needs, whether provided by formal, informal agencies, or volunteers. All services are geared to support successful AIP. They need to be well planned and properly implemented to ensure appropriateness, accessibility, and affordability to the elderly. Joint venture partnership among the local government, business sector, community organizations, local seniors and their families is paramount in undertaking concerted efforts in the provision of in-home services and the promotion of the community care for the older people (Chui, 2008).

APPROPRIATE AIP: SOLUTIONS

Life is beautiful. Aging is a natural biological process. The main objective of getting old is to continue to live happily in optimal health, and to increase the quality and years of healthy life (Fenton & Draper, 2014). Chinese says that "good birds select the wood to live".

Longevity does not necessarily equate to better health or life quality. Aging involves some life-course transitions within individuals, including acquiring some new and different social roles, diminishing community and social people's network, relocating residence, and retiring from regular jobs. These changes may lead to isolation, loneliness, and social withdrawal in the elderly. A key way to cope with these negative consequences and to lead to a fulfilling life is staying connected to the community through social activities. A Singaporean study found that living arrangements, such as size of households, living alone, were important determinants in self-care management, social support and use of social services, and in the older adults' coping skills (Chokkanathan et al., 2015).

The Institute of Active Aging at The Hong Kong Polytechnic University encourages people aged 50 years or above to continue engaging actively with the society in their Project for the Third Age. These elderly have free time after retirement and have influence on the social and economic development of the society with their wisdom and life-long experiences. Not only will they boost self-actualization, self-belief, self-image and self-worth, they will also help others, who will benefit from acquiring new knowledge and skills, and will be equipped to take up paid work and voluntary services. These "teachers" and "learners", through meaningful activities, can demonstrate to the society their worthiness as valuable members with much to offer even as old adults, in such a social network of mutual trust, respect and reciprocal relationships (Institute of Active Aging, 2017).

United Nations Principles for Older Persons designate six imperatives for any social policy for older people: independence, participation, care, dignity, self-fulfillment, and dignity (United Nations, 1991). Policymakers need to understand that societies have the duty to protect dignity of older people and cater for their needs (Cheng et al., 2013). Policy advocacy can encourage city adoption of innovations that affect the mobility and quality of life of the elderly (Lehning, 2012). Aging in place should be realized in both policy and actual practice (Chi et al., 2011). Solutions should be practical. The elderly should have a choice to live safely in their home and neighborhood. Policies on aging and related services differ across countries in Asia, but there should a goal to encourage elderly to age within the family in a comfortable and familiar environment (Chokkanathan et al., 2015).

The NSW Government has the vision for their residents to experience the benefits of living longer and enjoy opportunities to participate in, contribute to, and be included in their communities. Five priority areas are regarded as important in AIP: (i) health and wellbeing, (ii) working and retiring, (iii) housing choices, (iv) getting around, and (v) inclusive communities (DFCS, 2016).

In the United States, the Office of Policy Development and Research (PD&R, 2016) has studied two community-centered models as solutions for aging at home, namely (i) Naturally Occurring Retirement Community (NORC) Supportive Services Programs, and (ii) Villages. The elderly become more active and are aware of available supportive services that fill the service gaps to prevent or delay moves to institutional settings.

Naturally Occurring Retirement Community Supportive Services Programs

The first NORC program was founded in 1986 in a large, moderate income cooperative housing complex in New York City (Vladeck, 2004). NORCs are not planned or designed but the number of old adults has the advantage of the economies of scale in delivering elderly-specific services in the NORC SSP model. The model is defined as a "community-based intervention designed to reduce service fragmentation and create healthy, integrated communities in which seniors living in NORCs are able to age in place with greater comfort and security in their own homes." NORC programs are typically led by private, nonprofit organizations, with professional staff responsible for overseeing the day-to-day operations (Greenfield et al., 2013). NORC Supportive Services Programs have made communities more livable for aging residents. These programs focus on older adults as active contributors to their own and others' well-being (Bookman, 2008).

A national evaluation in 2007 demonstrated increased socialization, effectiveness in linking older adults to services, and improved volunteerism among the elderly. Local initiatives include a walking club, a transportation coupon program, health and wellness program, neighbor-to-neighbor program, home repairs, workshops on health and safety topics, etc. Social and educational activities, transportation, and information and referral services are used most frequently by the elderly. NORC Supportive Services Programs reflect the efforts of a broad spectrum of the community in working towards AIP objectives. It relies heavily on volunteers, community partnerships, and in-kind contributions. Such communities incorporate all aspects of the natural, built, and social urban environment, with accessible public transportation, and security at home and at outdoor spaces (Gonzales & Morrow-Howell, 2009; Plouffe & Kalache, 2010). The older people are not only consumers of services but are rather a social capital that contributes to the well-being of the whole community.

The Village Model

The Village model is a grassroots initiative and has emerged as an alternative to traditional approaches that depend on private social services or government agencies. Villages are typically founded and governed by older adults in a neighborhood or town. They try to avoid forced moves or institutionalization in the future (Greenfield et al., 2012). Villages provide opportunities for social engagement and many support services (Graham et al., 2016). The elderly design their own lifestyles and create their own futures as they plan the support systems for successful AIP. Programs take the whole-person approach, to meet the emotional, intellectual, bodily, social, and spiritual needs of individuals, by building community around shared interests, addressing member service and information needs, and promoting healthy aging.

These communities must ensure the continuation of necessary resources, energies, and investments of members, staff, volunteers, and community partnerships. Board of directors with diverse backgrounds are instrumental in the development of aging-friendly communities, through active committees that work on planning, programming, health and wellness, fundraising, marketing, communications, and technology support. Volunteers-first philosophy steers services as in maintenance projects, health and fitness activities, routine telephone check-ins, transportation, convenience services, technology assistance, and gardening advice and help.

Moreover, collaboration with services agencies and community organizations will avoid duplicating services and works while adding value to the partnerships. Another challenge lies with securing financial resources to sustain the programs through fundraising for specific initiatives, funds from philanthropies, with a degree of uncertainty, and sometimes from the government. In these models, housing choices of aging individuals are respected while integrated communities are created by closing service gaps, building partnerships among participating institutions, and adding cross-generational engagement by involving more young volunteers.

Many age-friendly community initiatives emphasize both the physical environment, and social environment and structures to support and enable people to age actively through the wide range of capacities and resources among older people. The needs and preferences of the elderly and their decisions and lifestyle choices are taken into consideration by adopting a bottom-up participatory approach. More importantly, their contribution to all areas of community life are conveyed and expressed to the government in formulation of pertinent policies (Hanson, 2006; World Health Organization, 2007).

Satisfactory and sustainable AIP requires the attention to a number of interlocking issues, including locality, housing design, barrier-free access, fall prevention, home supports, public security, community amenities, formal and information services, teamwork, inter-disciplinary approaches, government policy, legislation, land use, town planning, re-vitalization of old districts, transportation, accessibility and affordability of services, social engagement, health promoting program, quality of life, quality of care, integration of services and supports, comprehensiveness, co-ordination, partnership and collaboration, case management, etc.

LIVING IN OWN HOME

It is a clear preference amongst the elderly to remain living in their own home, whether owned or rental, instead of in an institution, or at least in their own communities (Knickman & Snell, 2002; Chui et al., 2009). Older people generally have a subtle and realistic perspective on their residential decisions (WHO, 2016). Housing options allow continuation of links to family and friends (Wiles et al., 2012). Planning on housing can help communities become better places to age in place (Warner et al., 2017). Older people should be provided with adequate and appropriate housing and accommodation which they are familiar with (Chui, 2008). Promoting aging in place within supportive housing may contain features such as communal settings, shared living space, on-site support, independent apartment living, and off-site mobile support (Henwood et al., 2015). Designing homes for aging in place need to consider neighborhood, community, as well as housing aspects (Cagney & Cornwell, 2010). Aging in place can be facilitated by assisted living technologies (ALTs) which include home and environmental modifications - technologies or modifications that can be installed or used within a home to promote independent living (Graybill et al., 2014). Information generated by assistive technology help early identification of changing conditions and ongoing customized monitoring (Demiris et al., 2008).

Homes require some modifications to suit the activities of daily living (ADL) of old adults for them to get around in the residence safely. The facilities may be purposely designed and built and are barrier free. Sunken shower, non-slippery floor, power sockets at one meter above floor level, bright décor, etc. are essential for appropriate AIP. Attention to fire prevention, fall prevention, cleaning and maintenance should be at the top priority in home design. In Hong Kong, tailor-made housing flats for the elderly are only provided in the public sector. Private developers do not respond actively to the housing needs of the elderly. However, the Building Ordinance stipulates design requirements to ensure that suitable barrier-free access and facilities are provided in buildings, as stated in the Design Manual, which was first published in 1984 and updated regularly to include the advancements in building designs, technologies and construction methods, and the latest overseas regulatory controls and standards (Hong Kong SAR Government, 2016 LCQ 13).

RELOCATION

Residential Care Homes

When staying in one's own home is no longer adequate to meet the changing needs arising from declining health, mobility, self-care abilities, lack of caregivers, the next choice is the highly institutionalized formal care in residential care homes (RCH), often not by preference. RCHs are operated by charity, non-government organizations (NGO) or private companies. They are generally purpose-built and equipped for the care of the elderly by trained supportive and professional staff. They offer places that may be subvented or on contract with the government, and may be entirely private and self-financing. RCHs are usually situated in convenient spots in the cities to allow for easy access by the family and visitors. They tend to be crowded, particularly in densely populated cities like Hong Kong. Those located in the suburban and rural parts promote their tranquility and natural surroundings that are most suitable for the aged.

In Hong Kong, there is an undesirably high institutionalization rate of 6.8% of population aged 60 and above, and this is more than doubled that of Japan, and more than three times that of Singapore and Taiwan, even though the health status and "activities of daily living" abilities of Hong Kong's elderly are similar to the elderly in these countries (Chui et al., 2009). This is due to an imbalance between residential LTC and community based LTC in terms of volume and government financing (Sau Po Center on Aging, 2011), despite the long-standing government policy of "aging in place" (Lou, 2014; Chan & Pang, 2007; Kwong & Kwan, 2002). Waiting time for a place in subsidized care and attention homes is up to 36 months, and 26 months for nursing homes (Social and Welfare Department, 2017). In 2014, 5568 of elderly applicants who were on the waiting list passed away before being offered a place (Legislative Council Secretariat, 2015).

Being institutions, RCHs are known to provide impersonal and substandard care. While there are good homes, there are also badly managed ones that received many complaints. Some fail to achieve accreditation standards, and even licensing requirements by failing in meeting the basic provisions in nutrition and safety. Quality control does not exist. Violation of standards is common, especially during after-hours. Inadequate staffing and unsatisfactory staff skills are becoming the major concerns and challenge in developed countries like Australia and United States. It is difficult for home care agencies and other providers to find and retain qualified caregivers in these formal settings. So many workers are not trained at all and they earn close to the minimum wage. Staff morale is low and turnover is high. New incentives and organizational structures are suggested. Many residential care homes in Australia are relying on migrant labor to deal with the shortfall. Furthermore, operators can also be part of the problem (Knickman & Snell, 2002; Choice, 2016). Some homes lack adequate and safety equipment or sufficient facilities for caring the elderly.

Another Country

Migration to another country as a preparation for retirement is also considered as a form of "lifestyle migration" (Benson & O'Reilly, 2009). Such move aims to search for "self-fulfillment" or the "good life" (Oliver, 2007). Individuals have their own motives to move to another country, either of similar or different cultures. Some are looking for environmental and housing comfort. Some wish to enjoy a better quality of life away from where they have lived and worked for years. However, people still retain a strong dependence on family living in the homeland, and friends and community organization in the new place, originally from the same homeland, particularly for care, as found by a study on British retiring to Spain. This group of migrating retirees is described as "transmigrants". Furthermore, migrants tend to return to their home country when things go wrong, when they cannot live independently, or lacking of support in the host country. Care is the utmost reason for returning home, and many would do so because of crisis situation or deteriorated health (Hall & Hardill, 2016).

In Hong Kong, many elderly have relocated from different parts of the Chinese Mainland, during the phased migration starting over half of a century ago. Most have raised their families and their children, but many of these non-Hong Kong born elderly have their root in their homeland in the Chinese Mainland. Some have chosen cross-the-border place, mostly in the Guangdong Province, for retirement. About 70,000 Hong Kong retirees have moved to live in the Chinese Mainland because of the much cheaper, affordable, and spacious housing units and the comparatively lower living expenses (Census and Statistics Department, 2017). They face a major problem of affordable health care services. The full charges in the Chinese Mainland are much higher than those in Hong Kong. There are two nursing homes in Guangdong operated by Hong Kong charity groups, but they are remote and far from Western medicine services. Sick elderly return to Hong Kong for medical treatment, including long-term medications. Furthermore, elderly living in the Chinese Mainland are not qualified for the Old Age Living Allowance scheme, which will require a change of policy by the Hong Kong government.

LONG-TERM CARE

Most old adults enjoy a healthy life. However, there is a high prevalence of chronic diseases, degenerative illness, mental health problems and cognitive impairments, progressing with age, and associated with psychosocial problems arising from family disharmony, social exclusion, alienation, insecurity, demanding behavior, suspicion, etc. These chronic conditions become a significant burden on the individual elderly, the family, as well as the medical, community, caregiving and support services. Primary care and family medicine are the most effective service models to take care of the medical and health aspects, while community services cater for the functional, social and domestic care and support. Day care centers, also known as day hospitals in some societies, and community centers provide a continuing care to all those who can reach these facilities, either by themselves or being assisted. At times referrals to the specialists are necessary. Likewise, hospitalization is unavoidable when conditions become acute or deteriorated.

In some places, like Hong Kong, the existing service model for long-term elderly care is highly "acute care-centric" being led by hospital-based geriatricians. Public funding for health care services is under the Food and Health Bureau while that for LTC and social services is under the Labor and Welfare Bureau. Resources from the heavily funded acute health care will not cater much for the LTC. The absence of a single government body to oversee both acute and long-term care contributes to compartmentalization and gross inefficiencies in service provision. Planning and adoption of innovative models of care are hindered by the lack of an integrated approach within the government. Moreover, the lack of medical staff in LTC facilities has also resulted in frequent visits to the high-cost Accident and Emergency Departments of public hospitals (Yuen, 2014).

There is a lack of well-developed primary care systems, despite evidence that stronger primary health care results in better health of the population at a much lower cost and greater user satisfaction (Atun, 2004; Woo, 2007). To promote aging in place, there should be a more holistic and comprehensive approach in the provision of elderly care, home care services, and health services. Such community-based programs are designed to promote better physical, emotional and social health conditions in the familiar environment the elderly have lived for decades. Again, the government should co-ordinate and oversee a well-orchestrated inter-disciplinary approach, drawing on the expertise, wisdom and collaboration of all stakeholders, including the community organizations, NGOs, business sector, health professionals, and the elderly themselves.

On the other hand, there is a decline in the traditional form of family support, common in nearly all developed cites. This has resulted in government interventions in the development of community-based services, residential care services and long-term care services for the aged population. However, even when such services are made available, affordability, accessibility, or quality are not guaranteed. Some advocates have recommended the need for bottom-up integrated services, instead of the current popular model, which is piecemeal and top-down (Chokkanathan et al., 2015). Knickman and Snell (2002) suggest a socioeconomic approach, in which the challenges are (i) developing better payment and insurance systems for long-term care, (ii) adopting the medical advancement and improvements in behavioral health to keep the elderly healthy and active, (iii) organizing community services to provide more accessible care, and (iv) altering the cultural view of aging to integrate all ages into the routines of community life. Social and public policy changes are required to meet the long-term care needs, and the associated financial and social service burdens.

FUTURE RESEARCH DIRECTIONS

Most writers agree that care of elderly people should put emphasis on aging in place. Many studies on the social and community aspects of living arrangements have been conducted, but there should be some focus on physical home environment and facilities and designs, which are equally important to the elderly in a fulfilling AIP.

Financing elderly and long-term care and delivery models are important to appropriate AIP. Yuen in his chapter, *The Economics of Long Term Care: Key Concepts and Major Financing and Delivery Models*, has urged a clear understanding of the economic concepts to underpin major transformation of existing systems and policies. Studies on the costs and savings of AIP will help the elderly to make an "informed" choice.

At the policy level, interdisciplinary and intersectoral research on social and health policies for healthy aging and long-term care are needed, particularly in the Asia Pacific. Policy makers, academics, and providers should join hand in steering AIP in preparation of an expected fast growth of the aging populations in the coming two decades (Chokkanathanet et al., 2015).

CONCLUSION

Aging in place appears to be a matter of fact and a matter of life to many old adults. It is not because they do not have a choice but to stay in the same house or unit they have lived for the entire life, but because most people do not plan for aging until it happens. Practically AIP should be planned and organized, in view of the inevitable changes in the body, mind, spirit, and mental status arising from aging in the natural life cycle.

Government policy on elderly determines how AIP may lead to active and healthy aging in age or elderly-friendly communities, where care and residential environment should co-exist. These places are also safe and appropriately planned to engage the elderly, together with contribution by all stakeholders, including the old adults themselves, families, caregivers, local government, businesses, community organizations, health professionals, funders, academics and volunteers, in an interdisciplinary approach with the objective of achieving residential and community normalcy.

Integration and continuum of care, supported by the latest technologies in medicine, monitoring and communication, is the ultimate goal for a fulfilling experience of AIP. The elderly should be taken care of well for happiness and good health. They should enjoy every moment of the last stage of life, without any concern of uncertainty, anxiety, and worries. There are some commonly adopted models of AIP. Each community should work out the most suitable and applicable local solution in a smart manner. In addition, sustainable solutions which aim at creating a livable residential, social, and caring environment for the elderly members to live to the end of life should also be in place. After all, every human should be able to age successfully and happily in the best possible place on earth.

REFERENCES

Atun, R. (2004). *What are the advantages and disadvantages of restructuring a health care system to be more focused on primary care services?* Copenhagen: WHO Regional Office for Europe, Health Evidence Network report. Retrieved February 1, 2017, from http://www.euro.who.int/document/e82997.pdf

Baldassar, L., Wilding, R., Boccagni, P., & Merla, L. (2017). Aging in place in a mobile world: New media and older peoples support networks. *Transnational Social Review*, *7*(1), 2–9. doi:10.1080/21931674.2016.1277864

Benefield, L. E., & Holtzclaw, B. J. (2014). Aging in Place: Merging Desire with Reality. *The Nursing Clinics of North America*, *19*(2), 123–131. doi:10.1016/j.cnur.2014.02.001 PMID:24846462

Benson, M., & O'Reilly, K. (Eds.). (2009). Lifestyle Migration: Expectations, Aspirations and Experiences. Ashgate, UK: Aldershot.

Bookman, A. (2008). Innovative models of aging in place: Transforming our communities for an aging population. *Community Work & Family*, *11*(4), 419–438. doi:10.1080/13668800802362334

Brown, R. T., Kiely, D. K., Bharel, M., & Mitchell, S. L. (2012). Geriatric syndromes in older homeless adults. *Journal of General Internal Medicine*, *27*(1), 16–22. doi:10.1007/s11606-011-1848-9 PMID:21879368

Cagney, K. A., & Cornwell, E. Y. (2010). Neighborhoods and health in later life: The intersection of biology and community. *Annual Review of Gerontology & Geriatrics*, *30*(1), 323–348. doi:10.1891/0198-8794.30.323

Census and Statistics Department. (2017). *Statistics on Hong Kong residents usually staying in Guangdong*. Hong Kong: Hong Kong Special Administrative Region Government. Retrieved February 1, 2017, from http://www.censtatd.gov.hk/hkstat/sub/sp150.jsp?productCode=D5320188

Centers for Disease Control and Prevention. (2013). *Healthy places terminology.* Retrieved March 18, 2017, from https://www.cdc.gov/healthyplaces/terminology.htm

Chan, H. M., & Pang, S. (2007). Long-Term Care: Dignity, Autonomy, Family Integrity, and Social Sustainability: The Hong Kong Experience. *The Journal of Medicine and Philosophy*, *32*(5), 401–424. doi:10.1080/03605310701631661 PMID:17924269

Cheng, S. T., Lum, T., Lam, L. C. W., & Fung, H. H. (2013). Hong Kong: Embracing a Fast Aging Society With Limited Welfare. *The Gerontologist*, *53*(4), 527–533. doi:10.1093/geront/gnt017 PMID:23528290

Chi, I., Lam, Z., & Chan, P. (2011). *Consultancy Report on Community Support Services for the Elderly People in Hong Kong*. Hong Kong: The University of Hong Kong.

Chin, C. W. W., & Phua, K. H. (2016). Long-Term Care Policy: Singapores Experience. *Journal of Aging & Social Policy*, *28*(2), 113–129. doi:10.1080/08959420.2016.1145534 PMID:26808468

Chippendale, T. L., & Bear-Lehman, J. (2010). Enabling aging in place for urban dwelling seniors: An adaptive or remedial approach? *Physical & Occupational Therapy in Geriatrics*, *28*(1), 57–62. doi:10.3109/02703180903381078

Choice. (2016). *Failing standards in nursing homes and aged care.* Retrieved February 1, 2017, from https://www.choice.com.au/health-and-body/healthy-aging/aging-and-retirement/articles/nursing-home-problems

Chokkanathan, S., Morrow-Howell, N., & Chen, H. (2015). Older adults in the community: Capacities and engagement for aging in place. *Asia Pacific Journal of Social Work and Development*, *25*(4), 183–185. doi:10.1080/02185385.2015.1119534

Chui, E. W. T. (2008). Ageing in Place in Hong Kong – Challenges and Opportunities in a Capitalist Chinese City. *International Ageing*, *32*(3), 167–182. doi:10.1007/s12126-008-9015-2

Chui, W. T. E., Chan, K. S., Chong, M. L., Ko, S. F., Law, S. C. K., Law, C. K., . . . Ng, Y. T. (2009). *Elderly Commission's Study on Residential Care Services for the Elderly - Final Report*. Retrieved February 1, 2017, from http://www.elderlycommission.gov.hk/en/download/library/Residential%20Care%20Services%20-%20Final%20Report(eng).pdf

Deloitte and Touche Consulting Group. (1996). *Consultancy Study on Needs of Elderly in Hong Kong for Community Support and Residential Care Services*. Retrieved March 19, 2017, from http://www.legco.gov.hk/yr98-99/english/panels/ws/papers/ws14093d.pdf

Demiris, G., Oliver, D. P., Dickey, G., Skubic, M., & Rantz, M. (2008). Findings from a participatory evaluation of a smart home application for older adults. *Technology and Health Care*, *16*(2), 111–118. PMID:18487857

Department of Family and Community Services (DFCS), NSW Government. (2012). *The NSW Aging Strategy 2016-2020*. Retrieved February 1, 2017, from https://www.adhc.nsw.gov.au/__data/assets/file/0011/257276/1282_ADHC_NSW-AgeingStrategy_WEB.pdf

Department of Family and Community Services (DFCS), NSW Government. (2016). *The NSW Aging Strategy 2016-2020*. Retrieved February 1, 2017, from https://www.facs.nsw.gov.au/participation-and-inclusion/the-nsw-ageing-strategy-2016-2020

Fenton, S., & Draper, H. (2014). *Cultural differences in aging in the UK - A significant knowledge gap*. Birmingham Policy Commission. Retrieved March 13, 2017, from http://www.birmingham.ac.uk/Documents/research/policycommission/healthy-aging/2-Cultural-differences-in-aging-in-the-UK-a-significant-knowledge-gap.pdf

Gardner, J. (2011). Natural neighborhood networks: Important social networks in the lives of older adults aging in place. *Journal of Aging Studies*, *25*(3), 263–271. doi:10.1016/j.jaging.2011.03.007

Golant, S. M. (2015). *Aging in the right place*. Baltimore, MD: Health Professions Press.

Gonzales, E., & Morrow-Howell, N. (2009). Productive engagement in aging-friendly communities. *Generations (San Francisco, Calif.)*, *33*(2), 51–58.

Graham, C., Scharlach, A. E., & Kurtovich, E. (2016). Do Villages Promote Aging in Place? Results of a Longitudinal Study. *Journal of Applied Gerontology*, 1–22. doi:10.1177/0733464816672046 PMID:27708072

Graybill, E. M., McMeekin, P., & Wildman, J. (2014). Can Aging in Place Be Cost Effective? A Systematic Review. *PLoS ONE*, *9*(7), e102705. doi:10.1371/journal.pone.0102705 PMID:25058505

Greenfield, E. A., Scharlach, A. E., Graham, C., Davitt, J., & Lehning, A. (2012). *A national overview of Villages: Results from a 2012 organizational survey*. New Brunswick, NJ: Rutgers University. Retrieved March 21, 2017, from http://www.neighborsnetworkfl.org/media/2012-Village-Org-Survey.pdf

Greenfield, E. A., Scharlach, A. E., Lehning, A. J., Davitt, J. K., & Graham, C. L. (2013). A tale of two community initiatives for promoting aging in place: Similarities and differences in the national implementation of NORC programs and villages. *The Gerontologist*, *53*(6), 928–938. doi:10.1093/geront/gnt035 PMID:23626371

Hall, K., & Hardill, I. (2016). Retirement migration, the other story: Caring for frail elderly British citizens in Spain. *Ageing and Society*, *36*(3), 562–585. doi:10.1017/S0144686X14001342 PMID:26962269

Hanson, D., & Emlet, C. A. (2006). Assessing a communitys elder friendliness. *Family & Community Health*, *29*(4), 266–278. doi:10.1097/00003727-200610000-00005 PMID:16980802

Henwood, B. F., Katz, M. L., & Gilmer, T. P. (2015). Aging in place within permanent supportive housing. *International Journal of Geriatric Psychiatry*, *30*(1), 80–87. doi:10.1002/gps.4120 PMID:24737594

Hong Kong S. A. R. Government. (2016a). *The 2016 Policy Address*. Retrieved March 13, 2017, from http://www.policyaddress.gov.hk/2016/eng/pdf/leaflet_community.pdf

Hong Kong S. A. R. Government. (2016b). *LCQ13: Housing for elderly*. Retrieved March 13, 2017, from http://www.info.gov.hk/gia/general/201604/13/P201604130432.htm

Hong Kong S. A. R. Government (2017). *The 2017 Policy Address*. Retrieved March 18, 2017, from http://www.policyaddress.gov.hk/2017/eng/p173.html

Hong Kong Housing Society. (2017a). *"Aging in Place" Concept*. Retrieved March 13, 2017, from http://www.hkhselderly.com/en/aboutus

Hong Kong Housing Society. (2017b). *Universal Design Guidebook for Residential Development in Hong Kong*. Retrieved March 13, 2017, from http://www.hkhs.com/eng/wnew/udg.asp

Howden-Chapman, P., Signal, L., & Crane, J. (1999). Housing and Health in Older People. *Social Policy Journal of New Zealand, 13*. Retrieved March 13, 2017, from http://www.msd.govt.nz/about-msd-and-our-work/publications-resources/journals-and-magazines/social-policy-journal/spj13/housing-and-health-in-older-people.html

Institute of Active Aging. (2017). *Project for the Third Age*. Retrieved March 13, 2017, from http://iaa.fhss.polyu.edu.hk/Project_Third_Age.html

Ivey, S. L., Kealey, M., Kurtovich, E., Hunter, R., Prohaska, T. R., Bayles, C. M., & Satariano, W. A. (2015). Neighborhood characteristics and depressive symptoms in an older population. *Aging & Mental Health, 19*(8), 713–722. Retrieved from http://www.tandfonline.com/loi/camh20#.V0cWX1c01FI doi ;10.1080/13607863.2014.962006

Jones, K. (1984). Psychological Problems in the Elderly. *Canadian Family Physician Medecin de Famille Canadien*, *30*, 591–593. PMID:21279076

Knickman, J. R., & Snell, E. K. (2002). The 2030 Problem: Caring for Aging Baby Boomers. *Health Services Research*, *37*(4), 849–884. doi:10.1034/j.1600-0560.2002.56.x PMID:12236388

Kwong, E. W. Y., & Kwan, A. Y. H. (2002). A Review of Private Residential Care in Hong Kong. *Journal of Aging & Social Policy*, *13*(4), 73–89. doi:10.1300/J031v13n04_05 PMID:12418383

Lawton, M. P., Weisman, G. D., Sloane, P., & Calkins, M. (1997). Assessing environments for older people with chronic illness. *Journal of Mental Health and Aging*, *3*, 83–100.

Legislative Council Secretariat. (2015). *Challenges of population aging*. Retrieved March 13, 2017, from http://www.legco.gov.hk/research-publications/english/1516rb01-challenges-of-population-aging-20151215-e.pdf

Lehning, A. J. (2012). City Governments and Aging in Place: Community Design, Transportation and Housing Innovation Adoption. *The Gerontologist*, *52*(3), 345–356. doi:10.1093/geront/gnr089 PMID:21900505

Lin, N. (1999). Building a network theory of social capital. *Connections*, *22*(1), 28–51.

Lofqvist, C., Granbom, M., Himmelsbach, I., Iwarsson, S., Oswald, F., & Haak, M. (2013). Voices on Relocation and Aging in Place in Very Old Age - A Complex and Ambivalent Matter. *The Gerontologist*, *53*(6), 919–927. doi:10.1093/geront/gnt034 PMID:23626372

Lou, V. W. Q. (2014). Case Management in Community-based Long-term Care: Good Practices and Challenges in Hong Kong. In K. W. Tong & K. N. K. Fong (Eds.), *Community Care in Hong Kong: Current Practices, Practice-research Studies and Future Directions* (pp. 17–36). Hong Kong: City University of Hong Kong Press.

Marek, K. D., Stetzer, F., Adams, S. J., Popejoy, L. L., & Rantz, M. (2012). Aging in place versus nursing home care: Comparison of costs to Medicare and Medicaid. *Research in Gerontological Nursing*, *5*(2), 123–129. doi:10.3928/19404921-20110802-01 PMID:21846081

Nygren, C., & Iwarsson, S. (2009). Negotiating and effectuating relocation to sheltered housing in old age: A Swedish study over 11 years. *European Journal of Ageing*, *6*(3), 177–189. doi:10.1007/s10433-009-0121-0

Office of Policy Development and Research (PD&R). (2016). *Community-Centered Solutions for Aging at Home*. Retrieved February 1, 2017, from https://www.huduser.gov/portal/periodicals/em/fall13/highlight3.html#title

Oh, J. H., & Kim, S. (2009). Aging, neighborhood attachment, and fear of crime: Testing reciprocal effects. *Journal of Community Psychology*, *37*(1), 21–40. doi:10.1002/jcop.20269

Oliver, C. (2007). Imagined communitas: older migrants and aspirational mobility. In V. Amit (Ed.), *Going First Class? New Approaches to Privileged Travel and Movement* (pp. 126–143). Oxford: Berghahn.

Plouffe, L., & Kalache, A. (2010). Towards global age-friendly cities: Determining urban features that promote active aging. *Journal of Urban Health*, *87*(5), 733–739. doi:10.1007/s11524-010-9466-0 PMID:20549569

Rowles, G. D. (1993). Evolving images of place in aging and 'Aging in Place'. *Generations (San Francisco, Calif.)*, *17*(2), 65–70.

Sau Po Center on Aging and Department of Social Work & Social Administration, The University of Hong Kong. (2011). *Consultancy Study on Community Care Services for the Elderly: Final Report* (Elderly Commission report). Retrieved February 1, 2017, from http://www.elderlycommission.gov.hk/en/download/library/Community%20Care%20Services%20Report%202011_eng.pdf

Sergeant, J. F., Ekerdt, D. J., & Chapin, R. (2008). Measurement of late-life residential relocation: Why are rates for such a manifest event so varied? *The Journals of Gerontology. Series B, Psychological Sciences and Social Sciences*, *63*(2), S92–S98. doi:10.1093/geronb/63.2.S92 PMID:18441274

Sim, J., Liddle, J., Bernard, M., Scharf, T., & Bartlam, B. (2012). Home from home? A mixed-methods study of relocation within a purpose built retirement community. *Journal of Housing for the Elderly*, *26*(4), 372–394. doi:10.1080/02763893.2012.724375

Social and Welfare Department. (2013). *Legislative Council Paper CB(2)673/12-13(01) Long-term Care Policy for the Elderly and Persons with Disabilities*. Paper presented to the Joint Subcommittee on Long Term Care Policy.

Social and Welfare Department. (2017). *Overview of Residential Care Services for Elders*. Retrieved February 1, 2017, from http://www.swd.gov.hk/en/index/site_pubsvc/page_elderly/sub_residentia/id_overviewon/

Soderberg, M., Stahl, A., & Emilsson, U. M. (2012). Independence as a stigmatizing value for older people considering relocation to a residential home. *European Journal of Social Work*, *16*(3), 1–16.

Steves, C. J., Spector, T. D., & Jackson, S. H. (2012). Ageing, genes, environment and epigenetics: What twin studies tell us now, and in the future. *Age and Ageing*, *41*(5), 581–586. doi:10.1093/ageing/afs097 PMID:22826292

Stoeckel, K. J., & Porell, F. (2010). Do older adults anticipate relocation? *Journal of Applied Gerontology*, *29*(2), 231–250. doi:10.1177/0733464809335595

Tang, F., & Pickard, J. G. (2008). Aging in place or relocation: Perceived awareness of community-based long-term care and services. *Journal of Housing for the Elderly*, *22*(4), 404–422. doi:10.1080/02763890802458429

Taylor, S. A. P. (2001). Place identification and positive realities of aging. *Journal of Cross-Cultural Gerontology*, *16*(1), 5–20. doi:10.1023/A:1010673000367 PMID:14617990

United Nations. (1991). *Principles for Older Persons*. Retrieved March 19, 2017, from http://www.ohchr.org/Documents/ProfessionalInterest/olderpersons.pdf

Vasunilashorn, S., Steinman, B. A., Liebig, P. S., & Pynoos, J. (2012). Aging in place: Evolution of a research topic whose time has come. *Journal of Aging Research*, *2012*, 1–6. doi:10.1155/2012/120952 PMID:22175020

Vladeck, F. (2004). *A good place to grow old: New York's model for NORC supportive service programs*. New York: United Hospital Fund.

Wahl, H. W., Schmitt, M., Danner, D., & Coppin, A. (2010). Is the emergence of functional ability decline in early old age related to change in speed of cognitive processing and also to change in personality? *Journal of Aging and Health*, *22*(2), 691–712. doi:10.1177/0898264310372410 PMID:20495152

Warner, M. E., Homsy, G. C., & Morken, L. J. (2017). Planning for Aging in Place: Stimulating a Market and Government Response. *Journal of Planning Education and Research*, *37*(1), 29–42. doi:10.1177/0739456X16642824

Wiles, J. L., Leibing, A., Guberman, N., Reeve, J., & Allen, R. E. S. (2012). The Meaning of Aging in Place to Older People. *The Gerontologist*, *52*(3), 357–366. doi:10.1093/geront/gnr098 PMID:21983126

Wong, K. K. (2012). *Aging in place for the Hong Kong Housing Society public rental housing elderly* (Unpublished Master of Housing Management dissertation). University of Hong Kong, Hong Kong.

Woo, J. (2007). Development of elderly care services in Hong Kong: Challenges and creative solutions. *Clinical Medicine (London, England)*, *6*(6), 548–550. doi:10.7861/clinmedicine.7-6-548 PMID:18193700

World Health Organization. (2007). *Global Age-friendly Cities: A Guide*. Retrieved March 13, 2017, from http://www.who.int/aging/publications/Global_age_friendly_cities_Guide_English.pdf

World Health Organization. (2015). *World Report on Ageing and Health 2015*. Retrieved March 19, 2017, from http://apps.who.int/iris/bitstream/10665/186463/1/9789240694811_eng.pdf

World Health Organization. (2016). *Mental health and older adults*. Retrieved February 1, 2017, from http://www.who.int/mediacentre/factsheets/fs381/en/

Yen, I. H., Michael, Y. L., & Perdue, L. (2009). Neighborhood environment in studies of health of older adults: A systematic review. *American Journal of Preventive Medicine*, *37*(5), 455–463. doi:10.1016/j.amepre.2009.06.022 PMID:19840702

Yuen, P. P. (2014). Financing Health and Long Term Care in a Rapidly Aging Context: Assessing Hong Kong's Readiness. *Public Policy and Administration*, *17*(1), 56–64.

ADDITIONAL READING

Carr, A. J., Higginson, I. J., & Robinson, P. G. (Eds.). (2003). *Quality of life*. London, UK: BMJ Books.

Lum, T. Y. S., Lou, V. W. Q., Chen, Y., Wong, G. H. Y., Luo, H., & Tong, T. L. W. (2016). Neighborhood Support and Aging-in-Place Preference Among Low-Income Elderly Chinese City-Dwellers. *The Journal of Gerontology: Psychological Sciences and Social Sciences*, *71*(1), 98–105. doi:10.1093/geronb/gbu154 PMID:25384636

O'Neill, P. A. (Ed.). (2002). *Caring for the older adult: a health promotion perspective*. Philadelphia, Pennsylvania: Sauders.

Victor, C. R. (Ed.). (2010). *Ageing, health and care*. Bristol, UK: The Policy Press.

Chapter 15
Preferred Place of Care and Death Among the Terminally Ill:
Asian Perspectives and Implications for Hong Kong

Raymond Kam-wing Woo
Caritas Medical Centre, Hong Kong

Annie Oi Ling Kwok
Caritas Medical Centre, Hong Kong

Doris Man Wah Tse
Caritas Medical Centre, Hong Kong

ABSTRACT

The research on patients' preferred place of care and death has received increasing attention in recent decades. In palliative care, one of the main goals is to facilitate patients to stay in their preferred place of care, and to die in the place of their choice. Although 'home' is often quoted as the most preferred place of care and death among the terminally-ill in other places, local studies suggested otherwise. In Hong Kong, death is highly institutionalized with the vast majority of deaths occurring in public hospitals. Local culture, health care system and its provision and accessibility, presence of public health care policy on palliative care and care for the terminally-ill are among the factors affecting patients' preferred and actual place of care and death. This chapter is going to provide an overview of the recent studies and to discuss the topic from the Asian perspectives, and to highlight on the debates on the related policies.

BACKGROUND

To receive care and die in one's own preferred place is regarded as one of the indicators of "good death" for individual patient (Khan, Gomes, &Higginson, 2014). From a systematic review involving more than 100,000 people in 33 countries, most people prefer dying at home, a place where patients may feel more comfortable physically and psychologically (Gomes, Calanzani, Gysels, Hall, & Higginson, 2013).

DOI: 10.4018/978-1-5225-2633-9.ch015

A century ago, most deaths occurred at home in Chinese societies. Home death is regarded as the natural way of death in the traditional Chinese belief. "To die in one's own bed" is regarded as the most glorious and fortunate way of death (Tang, 2000). "Falling leaf returns to the root soil described that home death is as natural as fallen leaves (Yao et al., 2007).

While Hong Kong is now highly modernized, Hong Kong is still a place where traditional Chinese culture prevails. Despite the remarkable economic growth in Hong Kong throughout all these years, the total health expenditure is only 5.5% of the GDP, lagging behind other developed economics. Nonetheless, the public services under the Hospital Authority (HA) provide a safety net in health care, which is heavily utilized by the general public. More than 90% of deaths in Hong Kong occurred in public hospitals. In 2014, there were about 46,000 registered deaths, and with the rapidly aging population, the annual deaths would rise to 69,000 by 2035 and to 92,000 by 2046 (Leung, 2016). Cancer remains the top killer in Hong Kong, accounting for almost one-third of all deaths. However, the prevalence of chronic organ failure is increasing and deaths from chronic diseases and cancer account for more than half of total deaths (Department of Health, 2015).

Western Medicine has evolved on the basis of body organs and systems. However, the needs of the dying are hardly organ-based and therefore the role of organ-specific interventions diminishes as death is near. Modern palliative care has risen against this background and has evolved with time to meet the needs of patients and their families. According to the World Health Organisation's (WHO) definition, palliative care is no longer limited to the last days of life but is applicable in the earlier stages of the disease trajectory. Moreover, the application is no longer limited to terminal cancer patients, but also to patients with life limiting chronic diseases (Connor & Sepulveda Bermedo, 2014). Hospice care was formally established in the Hospital Authority (HA) in the 1980's. United Kingdom is the first place to recognize Palliative Medicine as a specialty in the world, followed by Hong Kong in 1987, under the Hong Kong College of Physicians. "Palliative care" is now a commonly used term, but in the local context the term "hospice care" is sometimes used interchangeably. In Hong Kong, palliative care service in HA supports the terminal cancer patients by a comprehensive range of services including inpatient, outpatient, home care, day care and bereavement care. The recommended palliative care coverage for cancer deaths by WHO is 80%, while for Hong Kong, the percentage of cancer deaths in HA who ever received palliative care was less than 70% in the 2012-13 review (Leung, 2016). Among the cancer deaths in HA, only a proportion of them died in palliative care beds, more died in the acute settings, and very few died at home or in institutions. Palliative care for non-cancer patients, however, only began to develop in HA in 2010.

In developed countries, policies on palliative care are being established to recognize that care for the dying is about meeting the basic needs and not a luxury for the patients. Accessibility, equity and being cared for and die in patient's preferred place are important issues to address. Such policies are often perceived as a "litmus paper" in modernized health care. In Hong Kong, although the degree of matching patients' expressed choices and the actual place of care and death is not known, it is important for a modern society like Hong Kong to provide choices so that patients who wish to die in place are being facilitated or supported to do so (Lam, 2013; Luk, Liu, Ng, Beh, & Chan, 2011).

BENEFITS OF ACTUALIZATION OF PREFERRED PLACE OF CARE AND DEATH

Where patients stay in their last days of life is important to their well-being and also to their caregivers. A survey conducted in Japan has reported that home death is associated with higher quality of death and dying when compared with death in other settings. Home death is associated with lower overall caregiver burden as well as financial burden as compared with hospital death (Kinoshita et al., 2015). Another study in UK has shown that cancer patients dying at home are more peaceful in their last week of life as compared with those dying in hospitals. The grief of bereaved caregivers from the home death group are also less intense than the hospital death group (Gomes, Calanzani, Koffman, & Higginson, 2015).

In a multi-site, prospective, longitudinal study conducted in the United States, patient's quality of life is negatively affected by dying in the intensive care unit (ICU), or hospital setting and more aggressive medical care (Wright et al., 2008, 2010). Bereaved caregivers of patients who die in the hospitals are at higher risk of developing prolonged grief disorder (Wright et al., 2010).

DYING AT HOME = GOOD DEATH?

Hoare et al. (2015) have challenged the belief that home death is the most preferred option. Their systematic review concluded that "the proportion of patients who preferred home death or elsewhere" should be unknown in view of considerable missing data in the studies under review. They have also concluded that the preferences expressed by the respondents are very much affected by the place of interview. For example, home death would be more preferred if the respondents were from a community-based sample, but less preferred among the respondents from hospices and hospitals.

Early studies have shown that home death is associated with higher psychological distress experienced by the bereaved caregivers as compared to death in other sites (Addington-Hall & Karlsen, 2000). However, the latest studies have suggested the contrary (Gomes et al., 2015). In Taiwan, Yao et al. (2007) have reported that the good-death score is higher among the home death group when compared with those dying in hospitals. However, the "place of death" is not an independent predictor of good death on multiple regression analysis.

In Hong Kong, a survey was conducted in 2004 by the Society for the Promotion of Hospice Care on the general public. A total of 738 Chinese adults were asked to rate their agreement against 14 statements regarding good death from 0 (totally disagree) to 10 (totally agree). 'Dying at home' was rated as least important for good death with a score of 2.72, which was even lower than having an extravagant funeral. The three "physical factors" including "no physical torture", "a painless death" and "not dependent on others" were rated as the most agreed indicators and their mean scores were 8.78, 8.59 and 7.93 respectively. (Chan et al., 2004) It was postulated that the general public was less concerned about the "post-mortem" items as compared with the "physical factors" (Chan, Tse, & Chan, 2006). As the medical experience of the cohort was not taken into consideration, views of the general might not represent that of the sick patients.

Pollock has warned the risk of distraction from attending the dying experience of patients and family members by focusing on place of death as the key indicator of quality of care for the dying (Pollock, 2015). She argues that dying at preferred place might not be the priority for the public or even for the dying patients. She describes the idealization of home death as "preoccupation" and it could be guilt-promoting if death occurs in other settings. She calls for actions to improve the experience of dying in hospital given that this is the most frequent place where deaths occur.

MODERNIZATION AND CHANGES IN CARE SETTINGS

Development in Asian Countries

Modernization has changed the context and settings in caring for the terminally ill, including their dying phase. Death becomes highly institutionalized and the actual dying process is largely unknown to the general public. Death is often perceived as failure in the light of technological advances in modern medicine, with many aiming at prolonging life. This is also the case in Asian countries that have undergone rapid socio-economic development after World War II.

Gu and colleagues have postulated a "three-stage hypothesis on place of death" (Table 1) to explain the pattern of transition of death settings with the socioeconomic development (Gu, Liu, Vlosky, & Yi, 2007).

Nonetheless, among the Asian countries, the pace and magnitude of economic growth, and the development of their health care systems, including that of their palliative care movements, differ. Results from studies or surveys in various Asian countries also show considerable variations in patients' preferences and their actual place of death, even among places being influenced by Chinese culture such as China, Taiwan and Hong Kong.

Singapore

In Singapore, a densely populated country without "urban-rural differentiation", emergency hospitals can be reached within half an hour for all residents (Hong et al., 2011). A pilot survey in Singapore has shown that about half of interviewed cancer patients have preferred home death while one-third have preferred hospital death (Lee & Pang, 1998). In a cross-sectional study of Singapore Cancer Registry, more than 52,000 deaths from 2000 to 2009 were analyzed. More than half of the deaths occurred in

Table 1. Transition pattern of death settings with socioeconomic development

First stage	Most people died at home	• Limited care resources • Under-developed medical technologies
Second stage	Most people died in hospital	• Improved medical techniques • Greater access to health care resources
Third stage	More and more people are choosing to die at home	• Quality of care at end-of-life highly emphasized • Presence of modern hospice movement • Increased home death due to increased home-based care • Home-based care are more accessible and affordable

hospital, and 3 out of 10 deaths occurred at home while one-tenth occurred in hospice beds (Hong et al., 2011). Factors associated with home deaths instead of hospital deaths include older age, female, Malay in ethnics (as compared to Chinese), cancer as the primary cause of death as well as duration of illness from 1 to 5 years. Factors favouring hospice death over home death include being old age, presence of distance metastasis and dying from non-cancer illness, while suffering from haematological malignancy and being young age are consistently associated with hospital death.

Taiwan

In Taiwan, with a population mainly of Chinese in ethnicity, home death is a tradition. From a retrospective population-based study involving nearly 700,000 elderly deaths between 1995 and 2004, two-thirds of deaths occurred at home and one-third occurred in hospital (Lin, Lin, Liu, Chen, & Lin, 2007). Patients living in administrative area with more hospital beds per population, as well as most urbanized communities, were associated with higher odds of hospital death. In a more recent survey of 2,188 terminally ill cancer patients from 24 hospitals, 54.7% of the participants have expressed the preference to die at home. The adjusted odds of preferring to die at home are greater for participants described by one or more of the following factors, including participant's preference for place of death made known to family, participants with awareness of prognosis, greater functional dependency, cancer of liver/pancreas/head/neck, and education level below junior high school (Chen, Lin, Liu, & Tang, 2014).

South Korea

A survey has also been conducted in South Korea through internet. A total of 277 elderly women participated in the study and more than 60% of respondents have preferred hospital death and only one-third have preferred home death. "Reducing the children's burden" is the most common reason behind the choice of hospital death (Choi, Lee, &SH, 2001). Another Korean study on cancer patients and family members has found that living in rural area increases the odds of preferring home death (Choi et al., 2005). Regarding the actual place of death, the proportion of hospital deaths had increased from one-sixth in 1992 to almost 40% in 2001 as reported by a retrospective review of a 10-year death registration database from the Korean National Statistical Office on over 2.4 million deaths. Factors of being in the younger age groups, having higher education, living in metropolitan area, living in area with more hospital beds being available, dying from cancer, ischaemic heart disease, and chronic lower respiratory diseases, have increased the odds of dying in hospital rather than at home (Yun, Lim, Choi, & Rhee, 2006).

Japan

In Japan, where the life expectancy is comparable to that of Hong Kong, one in eight deaths occurs at home. A population-based national survey involving 1,042 citizens in Japan has identified the preferred place of death among the general public as 40%, 20% and 15% for home, palliative care unit and hospitals respectively. Factors favouring hospital care rather than home based care include being a female, older age, regular hospital visits, experience of relative's death due to cancer, being unfamiliar with home care nursing and the 24-hour home care support system (Fukui, Yoshiuchi, Fujita, Sawai, & Watanabe, 2011).

Going across the border, the scene is very different in China as compared with Hong Kong. The Chinese Longitudinal Healthy Longevity Survey studied 6,444 deceased patients who died at the age of

80 to 105 years, majority (92%) of them died at home. However, the authors showed that an increase of 1 additional hospital bed per thousand population would increase the chance of hospital death by 25%, while a one percent point increase in non-agriculture population was associated with a 2% increase in hospital death (Gu et al., 2007).

Hong Kong Scenario

Several local studies have explored the preferred place of care and death among Hong Kong patients and the general population. (Table 2)

These studies were conducted among different populations and findings could be heterogeneous. Findings have suggested that the preferred place of care need not be the preferred place of death. Among the two studies conducted in advanced cancer patients receiving palliative care, PCU is the most preferred place of death (Hong et al., 2010; Woo et al., 2013). It is postulated that medical experience, especially that of hospitalization, could affect patient's choice. Moreover, palliative care is an unfamiliar concept among the public. A local survey on Hong Kong people's attitudes on death and dying has found that only 10.5% of respondents would like to receive information about hospice care (Mjelde-Mossey &Chan, 2007). On the other hand, enrollment in palliative care service might enable patients and family to have more understanding of palliative care service and gain more acceptance.

Table 2. Local Hong Kong studies on the preferred place of care and death

Years and First Author	Cohort	Study Period	Findings
Woo et al., 2013	102 advanced cancer patients followed-up in Palliative Care Unit (PCU) of Caritas Medical Centre	Feb to June 2012	PCU was the most preferred place of care and death (42.2% and 53.9% respectively); Home as a choice in 22.5% and 12.7% respectively
Hong et al., 2010	121 advanced cancer patients under the care of Palliative Care Unit (PCU) of United Christian Hospital	Jan to Jun 2009	Home was the most favourable place of care in pre-terminal stage (37%) followed by hospital (28%) and PCU (17%). However, for preferred place of death, PCU was the most favourite setting (40%) followed by hospital (26%) and home (19%)
Society for the Promotion of Hospice Care, 2011	1,015 general public	Sept 2011	Preferred place of care · 14.6% hospital · 40.9% home · 24.0% in-patient hospice · 6.6% rehabilitation setting
Chu et al., 2011	1600 cognitively normal residents in 140 old age homes	1st July 2007 to 16th July 2008	· 34.75% respondents agreed or totally agreed with the statement "I wish to die at the present nursing home". · 42.18% disagreed or totally disagreed with this statement
Chung et al., 2017	1067 adults contacted through residential telephone line using random sampling	---	· 31.2% of participants would choose to die at home · Among them, 19.5% would still prefer to die at home even if they do not have sufficient support

In Hong's and Woo's studies, the choice of home as the preferred place of care is reported by 37% and 22% of patients respectively, but the home as the place of death is only preferred by 19% and 12% respectively. Patients, who prefer to die in old age home, are less than 5%. These findings contradict with those reported by Chu et al. (2011), which has shown that one-third of elderly home residents prefer to pass away in their residential homes. By logistic-regression, it is found that independent predictors of preferring receiving community end-of-life care and dying in the institution are older age, not having siblings in Hong Kong, Catholics religion, non-believers of traditional Chinese religion, not receiving any old age allowance, lower depressive symptoms, and being residents of subvented nursing homes. However, when interpreting these results, it should be noted that around 80% of respondents in Chu's study are independent walkers with good performance in activities of daily living as measured by Barthel Index with mean score of 18.45 (maximum score 20), and 70.6% perceive their health as good or fairly-good. They represent a group of relatively healthy elders. Furthermore, the face to face interviews take place in the residential homes where the respondents are staying. This factor of place of interview may have impact on the findings.

A recent population survey performed by Chung et al. (2017) found that 31.2% of respondents preferred to die at home. Among these 329 respondents, only 64 respondents opt for home death in case there is not sufficient family, social or medical professional support. Among 726 respondents who did not choose home as preferred place of death, the most agreed concerns include "do not want to trouble the family" (80.4%), "lack of professional nursing and medical support" (45.9%), and "lack of technological support" (22.5%).

Beyond Asia

Beyond Asia, the association of hospital bed provision and hospital deaths instead of home deaths is also evident. In the systematic review performed by Gomes and Higginson (2006), which included 58 studies with over 1.5 million patients from 13 countries, living in the rural area is associated with home death, while living in the areas with greater hospital support is associated with hospital death. Living in the city with more than 100,000 residents is associated with hospital death, according to the Mexican Health and Aging Study (Cárdenas-Turanzas, Torres-Vigil, Tovalín-Ahumada, & Nates, 2011). In Botswana where two-thirds of the population die at home, living in city and town are associated with less proportion of home death when compared with the rural area (Lazenby & Olshvevski, 2012).

A study in the Marie Curie Hospice of Edinburgh has found that while 80% of patients with no hospice admissions have expressed their wish to die at home, 79% of patients, who have previous hospice admissions, have expressed their wish to die in the hospice (Arnold, Finucane, & Oxenham, 2015). Another study in New Zealand has found that patients initially transferred to hospice for respite care are associated with dying in the hospice unit (Taylor, Ensor, & Stanley, 2012).

In summary, patients may have different preferences for place of care and place of death. Factors affecting patients' preferences are multiple and may include, but not exhaustive of the following: age, gender, social culture, availability and accessibility of health care services, past medical experience and palliative care service utilization. Most studies conducted are cross-sectional and the stability of patients' choices have not been explored. Also, the preferences of the caregivers could be different from that of the patients.

ACTUALIZATION OF PATIENTS' PREFERRED PLACE OF CARE AND DEATH AND WHAT PROMOTES HOME DEATH

In the systematic review performed by Gomes and Higginson, they have identified 17 factors significantly influencing the place of death (Gomes & Higginson, 2006). These factors are classified into different categories (Table 3).

A study among Japanese patients with advanced malignancy and their caregivers have identified 10 factors that would increase the chance of home death, relative to hospital death. Their model has an excellent accuracy in predicting the actual place of death up to 94.4%. The factors can be classified into (1) *patient factors*, including lack of crisis-related re-hospitalization, and being total bedridden; (2) *caregiver factors*, including caregiver expressing wish for home care, caregivers with low psychological distress, caregivers being able to assist medicine infusion and patient's bowel opening; (3) *medical factors*, including caregivers being able to confirm patients' preferred place of death during the stable phase, frequent home visits by home care nurses (at least 3 times per week in the introductory phase and at least 5 times per week in the dying phase), and caregivers having been informed by home care nurses about the dying process. Presence of medical crisis leading to re-hospitalization is the strongest predictor of failure to achieve home death in this study (Fukui, Fukui, & Kawagoe, 2004).

The medical factors conducive to home death, including the increasing professional support when death is near and lack of crisis events, can be interpreted in the light of what we know about the disease trajectories. Cancer patients run a relatively predictable rapid downhill course in the last 3 months of life, and the diagnosis of "dying phase" is not difficult (Lynn, 2003). The symptom profile also changes as disease progresses. While some symptoms, including pain, are generally well controlled even in the dying phases, there are symptoms that may become more refractory or more intense in the final days, e.g. dyspnoea, delirium and fatigue. Managing these difficult symptoms often requires timely interventions with medical assessment and input, as death will not wait. Lack of necessary support in the dying phase could be very distressing for the family, and caregivers and they would call for hospital admission despite the initial choice of home death. For patients suffering from non-cancer illness such as organ failure, the trajectory could be more unpredictable. Among the progressive decline, there may be acute episodes

Table 3. Factors influencing the place of death

Category	Favoring Home Death	Favoring Hospital Death
Illness-related factors	Non-solid tumors	• Long duration of illness • Lower functional status
Individual factors	• Good social condition • Patient's preference	Ethnic minorities
Environment factors • Healthcare input • Social support • Macrosocial factors	• Use of home care • Intensity of home care • Rural environment • Living with relatives • Extended family support • Being married • Caregiver's preference • Historical trend	• Availability of inpatient bed • Previous admission to hospital • Areas with greater hospital provision

of exacerbations, which may or may not be salvageable with medical interventions. Such acute events, such as acute coronary event in a patient with end-stage renal failure, often trigger hospital admissions as prognostic telling is far more difficult.

In Hong Kong, many factors could have contributed to hospital deaths, including progressive decline of household size in past years with more elders living alone, increase in woman labour work force, lack of day time caregivers and easy access to public hospitals. In an earlier study among the 1,300 patients under palliative home care from 1999 to 2003, only 6 patients had achieved to die at home, a place of their choice (Liu, 2006; Liu & Lam, 2005). The common characteristics of these 6 patients were having female family members, who were young and educated and being available 24 hours a day, living in spacious homes, and well supported by other family members and financially. At the same time, the caregivers of these 6 patients had access to professional experts with knowledge, skill and experience in care for the dying and were prepared to pay visits as needed. In fact, according to Chung's recent population survey (2017), around 80% of respondents who initially chose to die at home will change their mind in case there is not enough family, social and professional support.

Studies in other places have also generated similar findings. A study in Germany has shown that living together with a relative and having a non-working relative increased the odds to die in the preferred place (Escobar Pinzon et al., 2011). In Denmark, lower household income is associated with lower preference of home death (Schou-Andersen, Ullersted, Jensen, & Neergaard, 2015). A study in the United States has found that lower household income is associated with less likelihood to die at home (Barclay, Kuchibhatla, Tulsky, & Johnson, 2013). In fact, financial affairs has been regarded as one of the five important end-of-life care domains for family members (Virdun, Luckett, Davidson, & Phillips, 2015).

SOME SOLUTIONS AND RECOMMENDATIONS

The choice of home death or staying at home as far as possible till the final hours, however, should not be limited to the privileged. It should be a realistic option for patients who choose to die at home. To make it a real option, we have to remove the obstacles, to provide necessary support and care, and to empower our patients and their family members (Lau, 2010). Public health care policies, either in favour of home or institutional death, need to address the issue of availability of community based support, including professional support, education, and social culture.

Professional Support in the Community

A multidisciplinary approach is adopted in palliative care. However, in paying the home visits, it is commonly the task of the palliative care nurses, and far less by other team members. One of the objectives of the palliative home care nurses is to empower the patients and their caregivers at home with acknowledgment of the difficulties that they are facing. Local studies have shown that caregivers, apart from coping with the physical demand in care giving, are also experiencing difficulties in handling emotional reactions and relationship with patients. The caring process also mean restrictions of the caregivers' social life (Loke, Liu, & Szeto, 2003). Younger caregivers experience more difficulties in caregiving, particularly in the maintenance of social and family ties, while caregivers of younger patients experience more difficulty in most aspects of caregiving tasks (Chan, & Chang, 2000).

In a qualitative study on empowerment of patients and caregivers at home, home care nurses empower them by establishing an engaged relationship through commitment, accessibility and involvement, as well as providing information, knowledge and skills on physical care and identifying dying, affirming self-worth, and reassurance that patient is receiving good care in order to reduce guilt and uncertainties (Mok, Chan, Chan, & Yeung, 2002).

Although the palliative home care service is often valued by our patients and their caregivers, the coverage limited to office hours and the general lacking of doctors' visits are the existing pitfalls in Hong Kong if home death is contemplated. Availability of home care team support has been shown to be the key of success implementation of home care and death (Costa, 2014; Gomes & Higginson, 2006). Familiarity with the 24-hour home care support system (Fukui et al., 2011) and intensifying home visits in the dying phases (Fukui et al., 2004), home visits by family physicans (Brazil, Howell, Bedard, Krueger, & Heidebrecht, 2005) favour actualization of home death.

Timely intervention is also important when crisis occurs (Fukui et al., 2004). A recent study in Kent has revealed that the implementation of Hospice Rapid Response Service doubled the odds to achieve dying in the preferred place (Gage, Holdsworth, Flannery, Williams, & Butler, 2015). The service provides 24/7 crisis intervention in patient's homes, as well as nursing homes, with basic medical and practical supports on site. The team consists of experienced health care assistants, who are experienced and trained in hospice, and they are supported by a full hospice multidisciplinary team.

Education and Training: Dissemination of General Skills and Knowledge in Caring for the Dying

As death is highly institutionalized, the dying scene is one of the unknowns that the public is facing. Such unknowns generate anxiety, myths and avoidance. Before we consider on-job, undergraduate or post graduate training, inculcating life and death education in secondary, or even primary school curriculum, is considered an important strategy in some places. In a local qualitative study, university students have revealed that death is seldom talked about, despite having experiences of loss and death. Most participants express a need to have death education at a younger age (Mak, 2010).

In an aging population with high prevalence of multiple chronic diseases like Hong Kong, the role of informal caregivers cannot be over-emphasized. In traditional Chinese families, females are natural caregivers (Holroyd &Mackenzie, 1995). As the female labour participation rate increases for all adult age groups, it is a common phenomenon that caregiving tasks are dedicated to household maids or helpers in the old age homes (Census and Statistics Department, 2012). Few of them are equipped to care for the dying. The provision of training to residential care home for the elderly (RCHE) staff is a recent initiative of HA to target at this gap. Apart from training of RCHE staff, the program, delivered with collaboration of geriatrics and palliative care team, aims to facilitate advance care planning among the residents, to increase on-site nursing support, and to facilitate direct clinical admissions to hospitals.

At the professional level, post-graduate training is available to doctors and nurses. However, it is unrealistic for a finite group of specialists to look after all the deaths in HA. Moreover, stratification of needs with matching of expertise is important in planning health care services. As such, it is prudent for health care professionals, especially those who shall manage the terminally ill or the dying patients in their settings, to be equipped with the general skills and knowledge in adopting a palliative care approach. The considerations are "Who, When and How?" Exposure to care for the dying should be an integral part of the undergraduate curriculum in training doctors and nurses. However, the magnitude of exposure is subject to the time allocated to various competing learning objectives.

Rotation of junior doctors to palliative care units serves to provide basic training in this area. In the United Kingdom, general practitioners are among the key supporters of the terminally ill patients in the community. However, training in palliative medicine is not a compulsory module for family medicine training here in Hong Kong. Kung (2013), as a family physician, has challenged the adequacy of palliative medicine training in both basic and higher family physician training, and has called for more training opportunities. Interestingly, a survey among the primary physicians in Hong Kong has shown that having a primary qualification from Canada increases the odds of palliative care provision (Hong, Lam, & Chao, 2013). Rotation of junior physicians to palliative care units also helps to cultivate their interest in this area so that more doctors will join the higher training to become Palliative Medicine specialists (Subcommittee of Palliative Medicine, 2008).

Legal Constraints and Practicalities

The current legal procedure for patients dying in the community can be a barrier of promoting home and residential home death (Luk et al., 2011). According to the Coroners Ordinance (Cap. 504), certain types of deaths must be reported to the Coroner via the Police. Reportable death implies the circumstances may demand a fuller investigation, e.g. autopsy, and to hold death inquests. Although "no registered medical practitioner has attended the person during his last illness within 14 days prior to his death" is a reportable death, patients, who have the diagnosis of terminal illness, are exempted (Chang, 2013).

Death at home is not a reportable death provided the following conditions are fulfilled: (i) a doctor, who has attended the patient during his last illness, to personally view the body to be satisfied that death has occurred, and sign Form 18 (certificate of cause of death); (ii) informant to report to Death Registry office within 24 hours with the signed Form 18 and the necessary information regarding the date and place of death and the deceased (Chang, 2013). Finding a doctor who is willing to pay such home visits could be difficult in Hong Kong. A recent survey has indicated that only 14% of local primary physicians will provide home visits (Hong et al., 2013).

Removal of the dead body is another practical problem for the bereaved family to handle. The removal is only allowed after obtaining the Certificate of Registration of Death from the Death Registry, upon the presentation of Form 18 or obtaining a permit from the nearest police station. Failure to report death within 24 hours and premature removal of dead bodies are both criminal offences, as stipulated in the Births and Deaths Registration Ordinance (Cap. 174).

For deaths in institutions, those in registered nursing homes are exempted from reporting to the Coroner, but deaths in residential care homes are reportable cases as these are premises in which residents are being cared for with rewards, including financial considerations. Keeping the dead body in the residential care home could be more problematic practically.

Given the complexity of the process and the legislations, most people do not know what to do when deaths occur at home or RCHE. What is legally required for the bereaved family members to follow could be a mundane or distress for those who are moaning. Amendment of legislations is hoped for to overcome some of the hurdles for dying in place.

Quality Care for the Dying as a Public Health Care Policy

Care for the dying is not a luxury, nor something that we can put on the back burner. With a rapidly aging population and an overloaded public health care system, it is imperative to define the future strategy. Hospice care in the old days was missionary or charitable in nature, but contemporary palliative care is part of main stream medicine, being evidence based and supported by government in most developed countries, where good care at the end-of-life is recognized as basic needs of the patients. Indeed care for the dying should not rely on the merciful acts but the responsibility of the government in developed places. However, providing quality care for the dying is not confined to the effort of health care providers, other needs, including dying in their preferred place, require involvement and coordination of various bodies and stakeholders to provide system and legislative supports for building up a holding society for deaths to occur at home.

CONCLUSION

Death is highly "hospitalized" in Hong Kong. More studies are needed to define the preferences of the terminally ill patients and their families, including the preferred places of care and death. Preliminary small scale studies have shown that patients, who received palliative care, prefer to be cared for and die in palliative care beds. Home death in Hong Kong is low in terms of actualization and expressed preference though more would like to be cared for at home. Preferences to die in old age homes vary in the local studies. There is no "standard" place with respect to good death. However, it is important that patient's choice can be respected and facilitated by removing the barriers and fitting in the enablers, so that patient's comfort could be promoted to the fullest, irrespective of the place of death.

Although dying in place is something to look forward to, dying well is not automatic with dying in place. For those who wish to stay or die at home or in old age homes, timely professional and practical supports for the patients and families are critical in maintaining patients to stay in the community and in enhancing the quality of dying. With an aging population and increasing number of deaths per year, quality care for the dying should be on the priority agenda of the public health care policy.

REFERENCES

Addington-Hall, J., & Karlsen, S. (2000). Do home deaths increase distress in bereavement? *Palliative Medicine*, *14*(2), 161–162. doi:10.1191/026921600674991350 PMID:10829152

Arnold, E., Finucane, A. M., & Oxenham, D. (2015). Preferred place of death for patients referred to a specialist palliative care service. *BMJ Supportive & Palliative Care*, *5*(3), 294–296. doi:10.1136/bmjspcare-2012-000338 PMID:24644165

Barclay, J. S., Kuchibhatla, M., Tulsky, J. A., & Johnson, K. S. (2013). Association of hospice patients income and care level with place of death. *JAMA Internal Medicine*, *173*(6), 450. doi:10.1001/jamainternmed.2013.2773 PMID:23420383

Brazil, K., Howell, D., Bedard, M., Krueger, P., & Heidebrecht, C. (2005). Preferences for place of care and place of death among informal caregivers of the terminally ill. *Palliative Medicine*, *19*(6), 492–499. doi:10.1191/0269216305pm1050oa PMID:16218162

Cárdenas-Turanzas, M., Torres-Vigil, I., Tovalín-Ahumada, H., & Nates, J. L. (2011). Hospital versus home death: Results from the Mexican Health and Aging Study. *Journal of Pain and Symptom Management*, *41*(5), 880–892. doi:10.1016/j.jpainsymman.2010.07.007 PMID:21146354

Census and Statistics Department. (2012). *2011 Population Census - Summary Results. Census and Statistics Department*. Retrieved July 1, 2016 from http://www.census2011.gov.hk/pdf/summary-results.pdf

Chan, C. W., & Chang, A. M. (2000). Experience of palliative home care according to caregivers' and patients' ages in Hong Kong Chinese people. *Oncology Nursing Forum*, *27*(10), 1601–1605. PMID:11103379

Chan, W. C. H., Chan, H. Y., Chan, F. M. Y., Tin, A., & Chan, C. L. W. (2004). *Perceptions of good death: how does it affect end-of-life care decisions?* Paper presented at the 11th Hong Kong International Cancer Congress, Hong Kong.

Chan, W. C. H., Tse, H. S., & Chan, T. H. Y. (2006). What is Good Death: Bridging the Gap between Research and Intervention. In C. L. W. Chan & A. Y. M. Chow (Eds.), *Death, dying and bereavement -- A Hong Kong Chinese experience* (pp. 127–135). Hong Kong: Hong Kong University Press.

Chang, W. (2013). *Legal Issues relating to End-of-life and Palliative Care*. Paper presented at the Asia Pacific Regional Conference on End-of-life and Palliative Care in Long Term Care Settings, Hong Kong.

Chen, C. H., Lin, Y. C., Liu, L. N., & Tang, S. T. (2014). Determinants of Preference for Home Death among Terminally Ill Patients with Cancer in Taiwan. *The Journal of Nursing Research*, *22*(1), 37–44. doi:10.1097/jnr.0000000000000016 PMID:24517898

Choi, J. H., Byeon, J., & Lee, S., & Sh, H. (2001). Preferred place of death of elderly women in Seoul. *Journal of Korean Academy of Family Medicine*, *22*(6), 939–945.

Choi, K. S., Chae, Y. M., Lee, C. G., Kim, S., Lee, S., Heo, D. S., & Yun, Y. H. et al. (2005). Factors influencing preferences for place of terminal care and of death among cancer patients and their families in Korea. *Supportive Care in Cancer*, *13*(8), 565–572. doi:10.1007/s00520-005-0809-4 PMID:15812653

Chu, L. W., Luk, J. K. H., Hui, E., Chiu, P. K. C., Chan, C. S. Y., Kwan, F., & Woo, J. et al. (2011). Advance Directive and End-of-Life Care Preferences Among Chinese Nursing Home Residents in Hong Kong. *Journal of the American Medical Directors Association*, *12*(2), 143–152. doi:10.1016/j.jamda.2010.08.015 PMID:21266291

Chu, L. W., McGhee, S. M., Luk, J. K., Kwok, T., Hui, E., Chui, P. K., ... Woo, J. (2011). Advance directive and preference of old age home residents for community model of end-of-life care in Hong Kong. *Hong Kong Medical Journal*, *17*(852), 13–5.

Chung, R. Y., Wong, E. L., Kiang, N., Chau, P. Y., Lau, J. Y., Wong, S. Y., & Woo, J. et al. (2017). Knowledge, Attitudes, and Preferences of Advance Decisions, End-of-Life Care, and Place of Care and Death in Hong Kong. A Population-Based Telephone Survey of 1067 Adults. *Journal of the American Medical Directors Association*, *18*(4), 367. doi:10.1016/j.jamda.2016.12.066 PMID:28214237

Connor, S. R., & Sepulveda Bermedo, M. C. (2014). *Global atlas of palliative care at the end of life*. World Health Organization.

Costa, V. (2014). The Determinants of Place of Death: An Evidence-Based Analysis. *Ontario Health Technology Assessment Series*, *14*(16), 1–78. PMID:26351550

Department of Health. (2015). *Health Facts of Hong Kong*. Retrieved July 1, 2016 from http://www.dh.gov.hk/english/statistics/statistics_hs/files/Health_Statistics_pamphlet_E.pdf

Escobar Pinzon, L. C., Claus, M., Zepf, K. I., Letzel, S., Fischbeck, S., & Weber, M. (2011). Preference for place of death in Germany. *Journal of Palliative Medicine*, *14*(10), 1097–1103. doi:10.1089/jpm.2011.0136 PMID:22004148

Fukui, S., Fukui, N., & Kawagoe, H. (2004). Predictors of place of death for Japanese patients with advanced-stage malignant disease in home care settings: A nationwide survey. *Cancer*, *101*(2), 421–429. doi:10.1002/cncr.20383 PMID:15241842

Fukui, S., Yoshiuchi, K., Fujita, J., Sawai, M., & Watanabe, M. (2011). Japanese peoples preference for place of end-of-life care and death: A population-based nationwide survey. *Journal of Pain and Symptom Management*, *42*(6), 882–892. doi:10.1016/j.jpainsymman.2011.02.024 PMID:21689901

Gage, H., Holdsworth, L. M., Flannery, C., Williams, P., & Butler, C. (2015). Impact of a hospice rapid response service on preferred place of death, and costs. *BMC Palliative Care*, *14*(1), 75. doi:10.1186/s12904-015-0065-4 PMID:26701763

Gomes, B., Calanzani, N., Gysels, M., Hall, S., & Higginson, I. J. (2013). Heterogeneity and changes in preferences for dying at home: A systematic review. *BMC Palliative Care*, *12*(1), 7. doi:10.1186/1472-684X-12-7 PMID:23414145

Gomes, B., Calanzani, N., Koffman, J., & Higginson, I. J. (2015). Is dying in hospital better than home in incurable cancer and what factors influence this? A population-based study. *BMC Medicine*, *13*(1), 235. doi:10.1186/s12916-015-0466-5 PMID:26449231

Gomes, B., & Higginson, I. J. (2006). Factors influencing death at home in terminally ill patients with cancer: Systematic review. *BMJ (Clinical Research Ed.)*, *332*(7540), 515–521. doi:10.1136/bmj.38740.614954.55 PMID:16467346

Gu, D., Liu, G., Vlosky, D. A., & Yi, Z. (2007). Factors Associated With Place of Death Among the Chinese Oldest Old. *Journal of Applied Gerontology*, *26*(1), 34–57. doi:10.1177/0733464806296057

Hoare, S., Morris, Z. S., Kelly, M. P., Kuhn, I., & Barclay, S. (2015). Do Patients Want to Die at Home? A Systematic Review of the UK Literature, Focused on Missing Preferences for Place of Death. *PLoS ONE*, *10*(11), e0142723. doi:10.1371/journal.pone.0142723 PMID:26555077

Holroyd, E. A., & Mackenzie, A. E. (1995). A review of the historical and social processes contributing to care and caregiving in Chinese families. *Journal of Advanced Nursing*, *22*(3), 473–479. doi:10.1046/j.1365-2648.1995.22030473.x PMID:7499614

Hong, C. Y., Chow, K. Y., Poulose, J., Jin, A. Z., Devi, A., Chee, E. M. F., & Goh, C. (2011). Place of death and its determinants for patients with cancer in Singapore: An analysis of data from the Singapore Cancer Registry, 20002009. *Journal of Palliative Medicine, 14*(10), 1128–1134. doi:10.1089/jpm.2011.0092 PMID:21966990

Hong, T. C., Lam, T. P., & Chao, D. V. (2013). Barriers facing family physicians providing palliative care service in Hong Kong - A questionnaire survey. *The Hong Kong Practitioner, 35*(2), 36–51.

Hong, T. C., Yau, L. M., Ng, C. C., Au Yeung, H. Y., Ma, S. Y., Ng, H. Y., . . . Chao, D. V. K. (2010). *Attitudes and expectations of patients with advanced cancer towards community palliative care service in Hong Kong*. Paper presented at The 2010 Hospital Authority Convention, Hong Kong.

Khan, S. A., Gomes, B., & Higginson, I. J. (2014). End-of-life care--what do cancer patients want? *Nature Reviews. Clinical Oncology, 11*(2), 100–108. PMID:24281062

Kinoshita, H., Maeda, I., Morita, T., Miyashita, M., Yamagishi, A., Shirahige, Y., & Eguchi, K. et al. (2015). Place of death and the differences in patient quality of death and dying and caregiver burden. *Journal of Clinical Oncology, 33*(4), 357–363. doi:10.1200/JCO.2014.55.7355 PMID:25534381

Kung, K. (2013). Family medicine and palliative care: Is there a missing link? *The Hong Kong Practitioner, 35*(2), 33–34.

Lam, P. T. (2013). Practical challenges in ambulatory palliative care service in a regional hospital in Hong Kong. *The Hong Kong Practitioner, 35*(2), 52–58.

Lau, K. S. (2010). Facilitating home death. *HKSPM Newsletter,* (2), 24–25.

Lazenby, J. M., & Olshvevski, J. (2012). Place of death among Botswana's oldest old. *Omega, 65*(3), 173–187. PMID:23057243

Lee, A., & Pang, W. S. (1998). Preferred place of death--a local study of cancer patients and their relatives. *Singapore Medical Journal, 39*(10), 447–450. PMID:9885706

Leung, P. Y. (2016). *Chief Executive Speech -- Travelling life's journeys together*. Paper presented at the Hospital Authority Convention 2016, Hong Kong.

Lin, H. C., Lin, Y. J., Liu, T. C., Chen, C. S., & Lin, C. C. (2007). Urbanization and place of death for the elderly: A 10-year population-based study. *Palliative Medicine, 21*(8), 705–711. doi:10.1177/0269216307083033 PMID:18073257

Liu, F. C. F. (2006). Community palliative care in Hong Kong. In C. L. W. Chan & A. Y. M. Chow (Eds.), Death, dying and bereavement -- A Hong Kong Chinese experience (pp. 183–193). Hong Kong: Hong Kong University Press.

Liu, F. C. F., & Lam, C. (2005). Preparing cancer patients to die at home. *Hong Kong Nursing Journal, 4*(1), 7–14.

Loke, A. Y., Liu, C. F. F., & Szeto, Y. (2003). The difficulties faced by informal caregivers of patients with terminal cancer in Hong Kong and the available social support. *Cancer Nursing, 26*(4), 276–283. doi:10.1097/00002820-200308000-00004 PMID:12886118

Luk, J., Liu, A., Ng, W., Beh, P., & Chan, F. (2011). End-of-life care in Hong Kong. *Asian Journal of Gerontology & Geriatrics*, *6*(2), 103–106.

Lynn, J., & Adamson, D. M. (2003). *Living well at the end of life. Adapting health care to serious chronic illness in old age*. Santa Monica, CA: RAND.

Mak, M. H. J. (2010). Quality insights of university students on dying, death, and death education--a preliminary study in Hong Kong. *Omega*, *62*(4), 387–405. PMID:21661541

Mjelde-Mossey, L., & Chan, C. (2007). Survey on death and dying in Hong Kong: Attitudes, beliefs, and preferred end-of-life care. *Social Work in Health Care*, *45*(1), 49–65. doi:10.1300/J010v45n01_04 PMID:17804347

Mok, E., Chan, F., Chan, V., & Yeung, E. (2002). Perception of empowerment by family caregivers of patients with a terminal illness in Hong Kong. *International Journal of Palliative Nursing*, *8*(3), 137–145. doi:10.12968/ijpn.2002.8.3.10250 PMID:11923742

Pollock, K. (2015). Is home always the best and preferred place of death? *BMJ (Clinical Research Ed.)*, *351*(October), h4855. PMID:26446163

Schou-Andersen, M., Ullersted, M. P., Jensen, A. B., & Neergaard, M. A. (2015). Factors associated with preference for dying at home among terminally ill patients with cancer. *Scandinavian Journal of Caring Sciences*, *2015*(Sept), 22. PMID:26395354

Society for the Promotion of Hospice Care. (2011). *Opinion on End-of-life Care and Advance Care (Chinese version)*. Retrieved March 1, 2017 from http://www2.hospicecare.org.hk/wp-content/uploads/2011/10/20111003acpsurvey-whd11.pdf

Subcommittee of Palliative Medicine, Hong Kong College of Physicians. (2008). *Palliative Care: Setting the scene for the future. A position paper of Hong Kong College of Physicians*. Retrieved July 1, 2016 from http://www.hkcp.org/docs/News/Position%20paper%20in%20Palliative%20Medicine.pdf

Tang, S. T. (2000). Meanings of dying at home for Chinese patients in Taiwan with terminal cancer: A literature review. *Cancer Nursing*, *23*(5), 367–370. doi:10.1097/00002820-200010000-00007 PMID:11037957

Taylor, E. J., Ensor, B., & Stanley, J. (2012). Place of death related to demographic factors for hospice patients in Wellington, Aotearoa New Zealand. *Palliative Medicine*, *26*(4), 342–349. doi:10.1177/0269216311412229 PMID:21697264

Virdun, C., Luckett, T., Davidson, P. M., & Phillips, J. (2015). Dying in the hospital setting: A systematic review of quantitative studies identifying the elements of end-of-life care that patients and their families rank as being most important. *Palliative Medicine*, *29*(9), 774–796. doi:10.1177/0269216315583032 PMID:25921707

Woo, K. W., Kwok, O. L. A., Ng, K. H. D., Khemlani, M. H., Yau, W. S. C., Poon, Y. C., & Tse, M. W. D. (2013). *The preferred place of care and death in advanced cancer patients under palliative care services*. Paper presented at the 10th Hong Kong Palliative Care Symposium, Hong Kong.

Wright, A. A., Keating, N. L., Balboni, T. A., Matulonis, U. A., Block, S. D., & Prigerson, H. G. (2010). Place of death: Correlations with quality of life of patients with cancer and predictors of bereaved caregivers mental health. *Journal of Clinical Oncology*, *28*(29), 4457–4464. doi:10.1200/JCO.2009.26.3863 PMID:20837950

Wright, A. A., Zhang, B., Ray, A., Mack, J. W., Trice, E., Balboni, T., & Prigerson, H. G. et al. (2008). Associations between end-of-life discussions, patient mental health, medical care near death, and caregiver bereavement adjustment. *Journal of the American Medical Association*, *300*(14), 1665–1673. doi:10.1001/jama.300.14.1665 PMID:18840840

Yao, C. A., Hu, W. Y., Lai, Y. F., Cheng, S. Y., Chen, C. Y., & Chiu, T. Y. (2007). Does Dying at Home Influence the Good Death of Terminal Cancer Patients? *Journal of Pain and Symptom Management*, *34*(5), 497–504. doi:10.1016/j.jpainsymman.2007.01.004 PMID:17629664

Yun, Y. H., Lim, M. K., Choi, K. S., & Rhee, Y. S. (2006). Predictors associated with the place of death in a country with increasing hospital deaths. *Palliative Medicine*, *20*(4), 455–461. doi:10.1191/0269216306pm1129oa PMID:16875117

Chapter 16
Community-Based Rehabilitation in Hong Kong:
Opportunities and Challenges

Kar-wai Tong
City University of Hong Kong, Hong Kong

Kenneth N. K. Fong
The Hong Kong Polytechnic University, Hong Kong

ABSTRACT

Community care is one of the worldwide strategies for governments to manage contemporary healthcare challenges and long-term care. In response to an ageing population, the Hong Kong government has been promoting the concepts of community care and made initiatives, inter alia, in community-based rehabilitation (CBR). Despite these new drives, there is insufficient supply of CBR services. Provisions of CBR are currently fragmented, project-based, or on a self-financed basis. The authors argue that there is a lack of longer-term plan on CBR and that the government still relies on the heavily subsidized public hospital system. In this chapter, the authors share their views on the opportunities and challenges of CBR in Hong Kong.

INTRODUCTION

Contemporary societies have been exploring appropriate approaches to promote and sustain health (World Health Organization ("WHO"), 2005) and identifying healthcare strategies to help those in suffering (Arnott & Koubel, 2012). Community care is one of the healthcare choices to take care of the needs of those requiring long-term care (Campbell et al., 2016), to manage inherent rising costs (Chappell, Dlitt, Hollander, Miller, & McWilliam, 2004) and to address issues arising from an ageing population (Sau Po Center on Ageing & Department of Social Work & Social Administration, 2011). Other tactics may include patients' self-management, telemedicine, cross-disciplinary disease management programmes, care paths, and financial incentives to minimize preventable admissions to casualties, etc. (Bardsley, Steventon, Smith, & Dixon, 2013).

DOI: 10.4018/978-1-5225-2633-9.ch016

Developing countries welcome the concept of community care. In Thailand, for instance, community care provisions such as "the Bangkok 7 Model" have been in place to integrate health care and social services (Kespichayawattana & Jitapunkul, 2008). In China, in view of the increasing social care demand for older people, scholars have advocated that more emphasis should be placed on community care and partnering with families, whereas institutional care should be the last recourse (Zhou & Walker, 2016); and the Chinese government has been developing community care since 2004 to provide care at levels of provinces, municipalities, and counties (Li & Chui, 2016). A number of other developing countries have also realized the need for community care and established national strategies to manage mental patients (Jacob, 2001) and support patients with tuberculosis (WHO, 2003), for example.

Developed jurisdictions have also advocated community care for decades. In the UK, for instance, the policy debate on community care could be dated back to mid-1950s (Smith et al., 1993) and a recent successful story in practice involved a National Health Service foundation trust which satisfactorily piloted a community-based therapy scheme, allowing patients to receive treatment at home or at a health centre to help save bed days ("Antibiotic clinics provide 'incredible' community care", 2015). In the United States, section 10202 of the Patient Protection and Affordable Care Act 2010 has provided for a "State Balancing Incentive Payments Program" to increase financial incentives for states offering home and community-based services as a long-term care alternative to nursing homes. In Canada, the government expanded community care as one of the tactics to ease the financial pressure in the 1990s (Naylor, 1999) and it has become "a vital part of health systems in Canada" (The Conference Board of Canada, 2012, p. i). In Western Australia, community care has been regarded as a non-inpatient means to improve the overall efficient flow of patients and alleviate hospital pressure on space and equipment, on top of increased staff satisfaction gained through new models of community care (Health Reform Implementation Taskforce of Western Australia, 2007). In Japan, the government has put in place an integrated model of community care as a national long-term care policy to facilitate ageing in place (Nakanishi, Shimizu, Murai, & Yamaoka, 2015). In Hong Kong, "[a]geing in place as the core, institutional care as back-up" is the guiding principle of the elderly care policy (Labour and Welfare Bureau ("LWB") & Social Welfare Department of Hong Kong ("SWD"), 2014, paragraph 2). In this chapter, the authors discuss community care, with a special focus on the opportunities and challenges of community-based rehabilitation ("CBR") in Hong Kong.

COMMUNITY CARE

Health is a resource for everyday life (the Ottawa Charter for Health Promotion, cited in WHO, 1986). Various modes of care delivery have impacts to different degrees on the quality of life and the cost effectiveness . Elders in institutionalized care, for instance, may feel alienated from their usual living environments and practices, thus resulting in a drop of their perceived quality of life (Kong, Fang, & Lou, 2016). In terms of healthcare financing, home-based care may be more cost-effective than hospital-based care in a shorter term of health maintenance (Knapp et al., 1998). In fact, care shifting from hospitals to the community has been a global trend (Royal College of Nursing of the UK, 2014).

Community care is defined by the WHO (2004, p. 16) as "[s]ervices and support to help people with care needs to live as independently as possible in their communities". The WHO Centre for Health Development has further elaborated the meaning of community care from the perspective of elderly care (WHO, 2004, p. 3):

Community health care aims to add new scope and value to the existing primary health care approach in providing integrated health and social services by public and private partnership to meet the increasing health and welfare needs of older persons and their families at community level.

Community care complements the concepts of active ageing, i.e. "the process of optimizing opportunities for health, participation and security in order to enhance quality of life as people age", as advocated by the WHO (2002, p. 12) and active ageing allows older people to make full use of their potential and thus less dependent on family members and societies (United Nations Economic Commission for Europe / European Commission, 2015). In Hong Kong, there is no principle for active ageing and supports to services for the ageing population are provisioned on an incremental approach across various government bureaus and departments (Legislative Council Secretariat, 2015a).

In practice, service scopes of community care programmes vary on a case-by-case basis and are subject to changes over time (Means, Richards, & Smith, 2008). For example, Murphy (1987) reported that the British community care policies served four overlapping groups of people, namely the aged with physical or mental problems, patients with mental handicap, those with chronically mentally illness, and physically disabled younger people. Sharkey (2007) suggested two decades later a broader perspective of community care to serve not only mental and physical health issues, but include at least three elements, namely people previously living in long-stay institutions, vulnerable persons such as the aged and the disabled with a preference of being cared in a community rather than in institutions, and volunteer support from carers like relatives, friends, and neighbours. In 2014, the UK government outlined a new multispecialty community care model in the "Five-Year Forward View for the NHS" (National Health Service of the UK, 2014), allowing general medical practitioners to work with other healthcare practitioners and social care providers to set up a cross-disciplinary community network to provide integrated out-of-hospital care.

COMMUNITY-BASED REHABILITATION

Developments of CBR

CBR is one of the models of community care (Chatterjee, Patel, Chatterjee, & Weiss, 2003). It has been attracting academic attention for decades, as reflected in the increased number of academic publications on CBR (Finkeflügel, Wolffers, & Huijsma, 2005; Cleaver & Nixon, 2014). At the international level, following the concept of managing health issues in the community as stipulated in the Declaration of Alma-Ata (1978; Article VII(2)) and the principle of making care accessible to all people in the community through their full participation and at affordable costs (Article VI), the WHO commenced the development of CBR strategies, with an aim to integrate rehabilitation, health care, and other development activities at the community level (WHO, 1994). Subsequently in 1979, the WHO published a CBR manual in collaboration with other United Nations agencies, and this manual was translated into thirty languages (Helander, Mendis, Nelson, & Goerdt, 1989). In the 1994, the WHO issued *Joint Position Paper on CBR* with the International Labour Organization ("ILO") and the United Nations Educational, Scientific and Cultural Organization ("UNESCO") to address the concept of CBR (ILO, UNESCO, &WHO, 2004). In 2003, these three UN specialized agencies worked with the International Disability and Development and developed a set of CBR guidelines (WHO, n.d.(b)). One year later, the same three

UN agencies made further revisions to the aforesaid joint paper and issued *Joint Position Paper 2004*, describing CBR in the title of the paper as "a strategy for rehabilitation, equalization of opportunities, poverty reduction and social inclusion of people with disabilities" (ILO, UNESCO, & WHO 2004). In 2006, the United Nations General Assembly adopted the Convention on the Rights of Persons with Disabilities, where its Article 19 requires member states to recognize the equal right of all persons with disabilities to live in the community. Throughout these decades, CBR has been developed from a focus solely on rehabilitation to advocating people's access to education, employment, health care, as well as social services, and more than ninety countries in the world have optimized their CBR programmes (WHO & the Gulbenkian Global Mental Health Platform, 2015).

Concepts and Service Scopes of CBR

CBR is a concept subject to different interpretations (WHO & Swedish Organizations of Disabled Persons International Aid Association, 2002). It involves basically three components. "Community" in healthcare sense may refer to groups of people who are connected "through culture, occupation, conditions based on a common workplace, prognosis, stage in the care process, intensity of care needed, and more", and people having a particular disease is one of the examples of a healthcare community (Institute of Medicine, 2013, p. 206). The second component is "community-based care", which is in general described by the WHO (2004, p. 16) in the way below:

The blend of health and social services provided to an individual or family in his/her place of residence for the purpose of promoting, maintaining or restoring health or minimizing the effects of illness and disability. These services are usually designed to help older people remain independent and in their own homes. They can include senior centres, transportation, delivered meals or congregate meals sites, visiting nurses or home health aides, adult day care and homemaker services.

For the last component, i.e. "rehabilitation", CBR is more than the conventional understanding of functional or health-related rehabilitation, and it has been re-defined to incorporate a broader sense in accordance with the Convention on the Rights of Persons with Disabilities (2006) (Geiser & Boersma, 2013), where its Article 26 requires member states to "organize, strengthen and extend comprehensive habilitation and rehabilitation services and programmes, particularly in the areas of health, employment, education and social services". The WHO (n.d.(a)) considers CBR a multiparty strategy to satisfy the basic needs and promote the quality of life of the disabled and their families through the concerted efforts of various stakeholders in the areas of health care, education, vocational training, and social services, thus enhancing the public's access to rehabilitation services in the community and creating social integration and equitable opportunities for needy people for inclusion in the society.

CBR differs from the traditional institutional-based rehabilitation in that CBR is based in community settings, and programmes of which are planned and evaluated subject to the perceptions of the community (Sharma, 2007). CBR is not confined to people with disability but serves also the elderly as well, as the prevalence of disability increases, among other factors, with the rising number of ageing population (Paudel, Bhandari, & Bhandari, 2017). The scope of CBR covers, for example, social, educational and vocational rehabilitation, early interventions to geriatric care, disease and disability prevention, intensive individualized rehabilitation, and sports rehabilitation, etc. (Hoeman, 1992). Programmes under CBR include, for instance, training for the welfare of patients and families, educational assistance, improving physical access, referral services, financial assistance, social and recreational support, as well as facilitating employments (Shrivastava, Shrivastava, & Ramasamy, 2005).

In Hong Kong, "Enhanced Home and Community Care Services" and "Integrated Home Care Services" are local examples of CBR (Lai et al., 2009). Both programmes materialize the concepts of "ageing in place" from a perspective of continuous care. The former caters for frail or ordinary elders' needs to allow them to age at home as well as to provide support to carers and to strengthen family cohesion (SWD, 2016(a)). The latter takes care of elders (assessed to be of moderate or severe level of impairment), people with disabilities, and families in need in a community by experienced and trained professional staff through a network of collaborative and supportive services in the community (SWD, 2016(b)), services of which include basic and special nursing care, personal care, home rehabilitation exercise, day care services, carer support services, day respite service, counselling services, 24-hour emergency support, environment risk assessment and home modifications, home–making and meals-on-wheels services, as well as transportation and escort services, etc.

A BRIEF ABOUT HONG KONG

Hong Kong runs a dual-track health care system consisting both public and private sectors (Hong Kong government, 2013). There is a significant imbalance between the two sectors, with the public sector shouldering 87% of total hospital beds and approximately 90% of in-patient services (Food and Health Bureau of Hong Kong ("FHB", 2013). Also, the public healthcare services in Hong Kong are heavily subsidized by tax and the government charges, for instance, only HK$100 per day of hospitalization for an acute general beds with a cost estimated at HK$4,910 in 2015/16 (FHB, 2015b).

Population ageing is a primary concern leading to reforms of health care and welfare provisions (Duff, 2001). Hong Kong is no exception as it is a society with very long life expectancy, if not the longest, in the world (Census and Statistics Department of Hong Kong ("CSD", 2016b). The proportion of people aged 65 or above in Hong Kong jumped from 8% in 1986 through 12% in 2006 to 16% in 2016 (CSD, 2016a), and it is further projected to rocket to 36% in 2064 (CSD, 2015a). To further exacerbate the situation, the reduction in fertility rate continues. The total number of live births per 1,000 women in Hong Kong is estimated to drop from 1,355 in 1994 through 1,234 in 2014 to 1,182 in 2064 (CSD, 2015a). The combined effect of an ageing population and continuously decreasing fertility rate leads to a rise of median age of the population from 39.6 in 2006 through 41.7 in 2011 to 43.4 in 2016 (CSD, 2016b).

The demographic changes make healthcare financing an imminent challenge in longer term in Hong Kong. It is projected that there will be fewer and fewer people paying tax in the future as a result of the ageing population with low fertility rate. Together with the heavy subsidy from the government (FHB, 2014 & 2015b) and the narrow tax base in Hong Kong (Financial Secretary of Hong Kong, 2015), these phenomena will affect the sustainability of its healthcare financing system (Tong & Fong, 2014), especially when the underlying principle of healthcare policy in Hong Kong is that "no person should be prevented, through lack of means, from obtaining adequate medical treatment" (section 4(d) of the Hospital Authority Ordinance). There is a genuine worry as elders in Hong Kong consume six times the inpatient bed-day resources (FHB, 2010) and nine times in general specialty bed utilization than non-elderly patients below the age of 65 years (Hospital Authority of Hong Kong, 2012). To give a further example, as far as residential services are concerned, as at 31 July 2016, there were a total of 34,749 elders waiting for various subsidized residential care services and the waiting time may last for as long as 38 months (SWD, 2016(d)).

Hong Kong is keen on managing how to sustain its healthcare system arising from the ageing population due to increased longevity and low fertility, as well as other contemporary challenges such as escalating healthcare costs and rising public expectations (Tong & Fong, 2014). Demographic changes, together with the underlying principle of healthcare policy in Hong Kong, require the government to take care of the healthcare needs of people, especially those of the expanding elderly community, in a practical, feasible, and sustainable manner (Yip, Lee, & Law, 2006). In particular, long-term strategies for healthcare financing have been one of the burning challenges in Hong Kong and the government explicitly announced the impracticability to increase public healthcare expenditure indefinitely (Chief Executive of Hong Kong, 2007). The present strategies to tackle healthcare issues are diverse, including, for example, the establishment of a central health education unit with a vision to build a healthy society (Central Health Education Unit of Hong Kong, 2015), the development of reference frameworks for preventive care for children and the aged in primary care settings (Task Force on Conceptual Model and Preventive Protocols, Working Group on Primary Care, & FHB, 2012(a) & 2012(b)), promotion of preventive health screening services for well people like breast cancer (Cancer Expert Working Group on Cancer Prevention and Screening & Department of Health of Hong Kong ("DH"), 2016), the then controversial policy to encourage Mainland mothers to give births in Hong Kong to address the issues of low fertility rate and ageing population (Chief Secretary for Administration's Office of Hong Kong, 2012), as well as the enhancement of public-private partnership initiatives and a HK$200-billion ten-year blueprint for hospital development (Chief Executive of Hong Kong, 2016), etc. Furthermore, the government has also developed initiatives in the context of community care, though the supply of such services is limited.

Snapshots of the Current Status

The ageing population has called for the need of CBR. In an ageing society, there is a rising demand for care in connection with the elderly's losses of physical, functional, and mental abilities and such impairments will in turn enhance their reliance on others' assistances (Cox, 2005). In Hong Kong, the old aged persons have had common health problems in areas of dementia, stroke, bones and joints, cancer, digestive, urinary and sexual problems, hypertension, heart diseases, infections, and mental illness (DH, 2016a). A few observations arising from these common diseases are shared below.

Chronic Diseases and Disability

The increase in number of chronic patients and persons with disabilities is alarming. In 2013, there were about 1.38M persons with chronic diseases (19.2% of the total population), equivalent to a rise of 20% from 2007; and among them, 0.7M with hypertension (9.9% of the total population), 0.32M with diabetes mellitus (4.4%), and 0.14M with heart diseases (2%) (CSD, 2015b). Also, the number of persons with disabilities (excluding those with intellectual disability) in 2013 was estimated at approximately 0.6M (8.1% of the total population), representing an increase of 60% in comparison with the corresponding data in 2007; among them, 0.32M with restrictions in body movement (4.5% of the total population),

0.18M with seeing difficulty (2.4%), and 0.16M with hearing difficulty (2.2%) (CSD, 2015b). Woo and colleagues (1997) studied 1,902 recipients of the age and disability allowance schemes in Hong Kong and revealed that disease burden was the highest for arthritis, hypertension, cardiac disease, and peptic ulcer for people falling into the age group of 70-79.

Healthcare and Social Burden from Stroke Patients

In Hong Kong, it was estimated that stroke patients alone would require HK$1,900M in 2001 for treatments in hospitals owing to the insufficiently developed primary healthcare system (Woo et al. 1997). The direct medical expenditures (e.g. hospitalization, outpatient services, rehabilitation, and community allied health services) for stroke patients was projected to increase to HK$3,979M per annum by 2036 (Yu, Chau, McGhee, & Chau et al., 2012). The Hong Kong government also acknowledged that with longer life expectancy, the number of chronic patients with non-communicable diseases like diabetes mellitus, heart diseases, cancer, etc. has increasingly become a burden to patients themselves, their families, and the society as a whole (DH, 2008). CBR may help reduce the financial burdens and enhance patients' wellbeing, as reported by the study of Legg and colleagues (2004) that therapy-based rehabilitation services for selected stroke patients residing in the community could improve their daily-activity abilities and decrease the risk of further deterioration in ability.

Healthcare and Social Burden from Dementia Patients

An ageing population inevitably leads to a prevalent population of dementia patients (National Institute on Aging, National Institutes of Health, & WHO, 2011). In Hong Kong, the life expectancies at birth for male and female in 2016 were respectively 81.2 and 87.3 years old (DH, 2016b), and the number of mild dementia patients increased with age from 0.8% in people aged 60-64 to 19.1% in people aged 85 and above (Centre for Health Protection of the DH, 2012),. The number of dementia patients at 60 years old or above was projected from 103,433 in 2009 to 332,688 in 2039, representing a rise of 222% (Yu, Chau, McGhee, & Cheung et al., 2012).

In fact, dementia has been considered a healthcare and social burden in developed countries (Wimo, Jonsson, & Winblad, 2006). In a systematic review of 27 previous studies from fourteen healthcare systems, Schaller and colleagues (2015) estimated that the total costs for each dementia patient per annum may go as high as US$70,911, with an average annual total cost estimate per capita at US$30,554, and a significant portion of such costs come from informal costs arising from home-based long term care and nursing home care, instead of direct medical expenditures. Despite this review did not include Hong Kong, the financial burden of dementia patients arouses a real concern in Hong Kong as its public health services and social welfare are heavily subsidized by the government (FHB, 2014; Financial Secretary of Hong Kong, 2016(a)).). In another study, the number of people aged 60 or above with dementia in Hong Kong was estimated in 2010 to be 105,069 and the expenditure for their institutional care was at HK$ 1,624M, which was projected to rise to approximately HK$4,212M per annum for 273,449 elders with dementia in 2036; and the corresponding costs for informal care were estimated at HK$10,368M in 2010, with a projected increase to HK$27,000M by 2036 (Yu et al., 2010). Unfortunately, there is a general ignorance of this disease (Chan, 2012).

OPPORTUNITIES

The Hong Kong government has made some improvements to pave the way for the future to tackle foreseeable healthcare and social challenges. A few examples are cited below.

Empowerment of Patients-Led Support Groups

The concepts of community care and CBR are not new to Hong Kong. Dating back to 1990, the Hong Kong government suggested in a key policy paper entitled *Health for All – The Way Ahead* to provide quality care in the community for the elderly (Working Party on Primary Health Care of Hong Kong, 1990). In 2000, the Hong Kong government articulated in another consultation document bearing a title of *Lifelong Investment in Health* to improve the outcomes and cost efficiency of health care through, among others, a community-focused, patient-centred and knowledge-based health care system (Health and Welfare Bureau of Hong Kong, 2000). The Hong Kong Society for Rehabilitation, a non-government organization ("NGO"), provided a good example of such a care system when it set up the Community Rehabilitation Network ("CRN") in 1994 (Poon, So, & Loong, 2014). There are six CRN centres in different regions of Hong Kong subsidized by the Social Welfare Department since 1997 (Hong Kong Society for Rehabilitation, n.d.). The CRN provides a very good linkage and resource support to most of the patients-led support groups in the society.

Centre-Based CBR in the Community

The Hong Kong government has made some initiatives for community-based care and CBR since the publication of a further consultation document in 2005, *Building a Healthy Tomorrow* (Health and Medical Development Advisory Committee of Hong Kong, 2005), which was considered the first attempt to outline a future healthcare model by better differentiating the roles of primary, secondary and tertiary care as well as home care and community support (Lam, 2005). For example, in his *2005-06 Policy Address*, the Chief Executive of Hong Kong (2005) announced the plans to strengthen community support services to the disabled and their family members, including, for example, transitional residence, day training, as well as nursing and support services for people with severe disabilities, continuous day rehabilitation and infirmary care for discharged patients with mental, physical or neurological impairments, and a new scheme for visiting doctors for the disabled residing in rehabilitation facilities, etc. Since 2007, the Social Welfare Department (n.d.) has also funded the development of four community rehabilitation day centres ("CRDCs"), aiming at providing goal-oriented and time-defined rehabilitation services for discharged patients from the Hospital Authority, with a view to enhancing their independent living in the community and social integration. The original idea of setting up CRDCs is good. With payments to services comparable to the charges of outpatient rehabilitation in public hospitals, the establishment of CRDCs aims at building up patients' physical functioning and self-maintenance abilities, reinforcing their domestic living and community living skills, and facilitating them to redesign a healthy lifestyle and productive life roles to assist their integration into the community; more than that, CRDCs provides respite care service and education for patients' families and caregivers to improve their quality of living (SWD, n.d.). In addition to CRDCs, following the direction stated in the *2008-09 Policy Address* to explore the use of community health centres to enhance primary care (Chief Executive of Hong Kong,

2008), the Hong Kong government set up the Tin Shui Wai (Tin Yip Road) Community Health Centre, which was built and designed based on the primary care development strategy and service model of the government, opened in 2012, and is a one-stop centre to provide comprehensive primary care services by multi-disciplinary primary care professionals in the community (Hong Kong government, 2012a).

Ambulatory Care and Support

Since 2009, an elderly healthcare voucher scheme has been launched (FHB, 2015a) under the concept of "money follows patients" (Elderly Commission of Hong Kong, 2009) to enable elders aged 70 or above to choose primary care services in the community (Chief Executive of Hong Kong, 2007), and this scheme has become a recurrent support programme and the vouchers can be used for rehabilitation services (Chief Executive of Hong Kong, 2014). The Chief Executive of Hong Kong (2015) further promoted the concepts of community care in his *2015 Policy Address* by, for instance, providing more choices for the elderly via other voucher schemes in the contexts of community care services and residential care services, building mutual help community networks among residents of new public rental housing estates, along with encouraging active ageing through senior volunteerism, a HK$2 public transport fare concession scheme, and residences and reverse mortgage programmes for the aged. The importance of developing an age-friendly city and promoting active ageing in Hong Kong and the use of community resources to improve home care services, elderly services, ambulatory care, primary care and community care were iterated again in his *2016 Policy Address* (Chief Executive of Hong Kong, 2016). In the *2017 Policy Address*, the Chief Executive (2017, paragraph 173) also reported that the public and different stakeholders in general supported the principle of "ageing in place as the core, institutional care as back-up" and recognized the need to strengthen community care services. To follow the Chief Executive's policy directions, the Financial Secretary of Hong Kong (2016(b)) announced a series of initiatives, e.g. the establishment of three new community health centres at the district level to provide additional 410,000 general outpatient attendances annually, and appropriation of additional recurrent budgets of HK$170 million and HK$17 million respectively in 2015-16 and 2016-17 for the provision of 1,600 and 160 extra places for the Enhanced Home and Community Care Services to strengthen the support for the overarching principle of "ageing in place". The Community Care Fund (2016) also provides pilot schemes on subsidy for people with severe disabilities, and living allowance for low-income caregivers of people with disabilities (SWD, 2016(c)).

CHALLENGES

The opportunities mentioned above have laid a foundation stone, but there are still barriers on the road to a nourished supply of community care. A few limitations are elaborated below.

Lack of a Longer-Term Policy

Social policy and healthcare policy serve as a mechanism to redistribute resources and make use of intersectional health actions to reduce inequities in health status (Baum, 2008). The resource allocation targets to meet a society's dominant values, which means in practice the underpinning values of the government of the day (Jamrozik, 2001). Without a longer-term policy, the current strategies used in community-based care and CBR may be changed subject to the values of the government of the day. This anticipated change is not theoretical but real, as exemplified by the development of private hospitals in Hong Kong. Mr. Donald Tsang, the second Chief Executive of Hong Kong, announced in his *Policy Address* for two years that the government had reserved four pieces of land to develop private hospitals (Chief Executive of Hong Kong, 2008; 2009). However, the direction of developing private hospitals has been changed after Mr. Tsang's stepping down from the government. Out of the four pieces of land, only the land in Wong Chuk Hang is used for building a new 500-bed private hospital, whilst the site in Tseung Kwan O is reserved for the construction of a self-financing public Chinese medicine hospital (Chief Executive of Hong Kong, 2014), and the land in Tai Po has been returned to the Development Bureau for other development purposes (Legislative Council Secretariat, 2015b). The use of the fourth piece of land in North Lantau is not clear. Hong Kong needs a longer-term community-based care policy.

Heavy Reliance on Public Hospital Services

As mentioned above, the most important principle of healthcare policy in Hong Kong is that no one is to be deprived of access to adequate medical treatment because of lack of means (section 4(d) of the Hospital Authority Ordinance). It is also projected that the number of taxpayers will be decreasing because of the ageing population and low fertility rate. In Taiwan, Lee (2002) projected that the supply of long-term care could not meet the ever-increasing demand and suggested expanding community care instead of continuing to rely on institutionalized care as well as Taiwanese government reviewing financing options and integrating various fragmented services. In fact, the Taiwanese government has recently launched a "10-year long-term care 2.0 plan" to facilitate ageing in place through a comprehensive community care service system (Executive Yuan of Taiwan, 2017). Hong Kong faces similar issues as those in Taiwan. However, rather than going to the direction of community-based services as per the basic principle of the elderly care policy that ageing in place should be the core with a back-up by institutional care (LWB & SWD, 2014), it seems that the government continues to rely on public hospital services which are heavily subsidized by tax payers' money (FHB, 2014), as shown by the allocation of HK$200 billion for hospital development in the ten years up to 2026, on top of other hospital development projects already in the pipeline such as the expansion of the United Christian Hospital and the re-development of Kwong Wah Hospital (FHB, 2016). The study of Tin and colleagues (2016) further supports the authors' viewpoints about the Hong Kong government's reliance on hospital services, where they found that the expenditures for rehabilitative and extended care as a percentage of the total health expenditure in Hong Kong in the period of 1989/90-2012/2013 increased from 2.3% in 1989/90 to a peak at 4.2% in 2003/04 and then gradually reduced to 3.5% in 2012/13, and similar pattern of ups-and-downs was also observed in the expenditures for long-term care in the same period of time, with the lowest share at 2.3% in 1998/90 and the highest at 5.5% in 2002/03 before it dropped to 4.5% in 2012/13, whilst the corresponding expenditures in hospitals were 28.2% of the total health expenditure in 1989/90 to 46.8% in 2002/03, with subsequent reduction to 42%-44% in the period 2005/06-2012/13. A significant proportion of the total health expenditures in the past few decades were spent in hospitals and less than 10% were allocated for rehabilitative and extended care and long-term care. It seems that this trend will continue as discussed above.

Attitude of the Hong Kong Government

Attitude of the Hong Kong government may be an issue. In 2007, the Rehabilitation Advisory Committee published a document entitled *Hong Kong Rehabilitation Programme Plan*, setting out two major strategic directions for rehabilitation services to establish (a) individual capacity of persons with disabilities and their family members through social investment, and (b) an appropriate environment socially, economically and physically to facilitate full integration of these persons into community; and among proposed specific measures, one was to provide a barrier-free environment for access and transport services for full integration of persons with disabilities into the society (Health, Welfare and Food Bureau of Hong Kong, 2007). However, as a result of ineffective implementation of this special transport measure, a number of people in need took unauthorized rehabilitation transport services, and pursuant to the Ombudsman Ordinance, the Ombudsman of Hong Kong (2014) subsequently conducted a direct investigation into it. In early 2017, the Ombudsman (2017) pointed out explicitly the passive attitude of the Hong Kong government in carrying out this measure, as reflected in the following observations: (a) the LWB setting no timeframe to implement the policy of "Transport for All"; (b) treating the policy of "Transport for All" as a concept by the LWB and the Transport Department; (c) the failure of the Transport Department in proactively and professionally supporting the subvented rehabilitative vehicle services, i.e. the Rehabus services; and (d) the failure of the Transport Department in adjusting its mentality about the demand for special transport services. In the investigation report, the Ombudsman (2017) made a few findings: (a) serious under-supply of the Rehabus; (b) government's failure in seriously assessing the demand and setting targets for the special transport services; (c) government's failure in making full coordination for effective use of the special transport services; and (d) government's failure in adequately managing the issues of unlicensed rehabilitation vehicles. The Ombudsman recommended that government continue to introduce wheelchair accessible taxis and minibuses and make more efforts in publicity and public education.

In response, the government expressed that it has been promoting "Building a City for All" by providing barrier-free access in public transportation and pedestrian pathways to every destination. The Hong Kong government (2017b) issued a press release with a headline of "Ombudsman recommendations noted" and stated that the LWB and the Transport Department would enhance the rehabilitative services for the physically repaired accordingly. In another press release issued on the same day, the LWB iterated its commitments to develop barrier-free transport for persons in need, particularly the Rehabus under government subvention, and would examine the investigation report of the Ombudsman seriously and make a new rehabilitation programme plan including the long-term strategy for special transport services when the Elderly Commission has formulated the elderly services programme plan in the second quarter of 2017 (Hong Kong government, 2017a). As mentioned before, success of community-based care and CBR depends on multi-sectoral collaborations, not just confined to healthcare providers but also the assistance of stakeholders in other fields such as education, vocational training, social services, communities, concerned government departments, and NGOs, etc. (WHO, n.d. (a); Iemmi et al., 2013). The findings of the Ombudsman shown above illustrate the importance of the multiparty strategy in community-based care as advocated by the WHO (n.d.(a)) and the significant roles played by the Hong Kong government.

Coordination of Inter-Sectors in the Government

The Hong Kong government may wish to review its policies in health care and elderly care, which are now managed respectively by two bureaus, and strike an optimal balance between hospital developments and community-based care. To facilitate the aged to live and function less dependently in the community as far as possible requires multi-sectoral cooperations among, for instance, people with disabilities, family members, communities, concerned government departments, and NGOs in the fields of health care, education, career development, and social services, etc. (Iemmi et al., 2013), and one of the underlying principles of community care is its flexibility in implementation, so as to cope with local contexts and take into account any local chances and limitations (Davies & Challis, 1986). In the UK, for instance, Bernard and Phillips (2000) advocated an integrated social policy to take care the broad needs of an ageing society in contrast to those narrowly defined services for specific age groups or cohorts with particular problems or stigmas. In fact, Hong Kong attempted to formulate a central policy about ageing services in the 1980s and 1990s but the difficulty in making inter-departmental coordination made issues of ageing focus on health and personal social services and become the responsibility of the then Health and Welfare Bureau (Chan & Phillips, 2002). After the changeover of sovereignty from the UK to China, the government machinery responsible for health and social welfare issues in Hong Kong has changed a number of times. The "Health and Welfare Branch" before 1997 was restructured to establish the "Health and Welfare Bureau", which was subsequently re-named the "Health, Welfare and Food Bureau" in 2002 under the Principal Officials Accountability System (Ma, 2007). In 2007, it was further re-named the "Food and Health Bureau" and the welfare function was transferred to the "Labour and Welfare Bureau" (FHB, 2008). In accordance with the CBR strategy developed by ILO, UNESCO and WHO (2004) to consider collectively rehabilitation, equality of chances, poverty reduction and social inclusion, these hierarchical changes in the government structure could not help improve the inter-departmental coordination for community-based care, not to mention CBR.

In recent years, it appears that the government has realized the importance of inter-departmental coordination and participation by different parties, as illustrated by a government setup with a name of "Energizing Kowloon East Office", which was set up in 2012 to coordinate the work of relevant departments in the government machinery and more importantly, to play the role of place-maker, and to serve as a platform for all walks of life to work together to generate innovate ideas for the optimal use of public space and environmental improvement in the Kowloon East region of Hong Kong (Hong Kong government, 2012b). As reported in a panel of the Legislative Council, "Energizing Kowloon East Office" serves as an advisor and facilitator for development projects of both public and private sectors in Kowloon East, and it has so far provided one-stop advisory and coordinating services among all concerned government department for over sixty private development projects and has had extensive engagements and cooperations with the public and different stakeholders at various stages of initiatives and projects (Development Bureau of Hong Kong, 2016). Another example is the establishment of a tripartite platform to mend the broken relationship between the government, doctors, and patient advocates after the failure of the Medical Registration (Amendment) Bill 2016 to pass through the Legislative Council in July 2016 (Hong Kong government, 2016). In rehabilitation services, the government has proposed to upgrade the rank of and strengthen the role of the Commissioner for Rehabilitation (Chief Executive of Hong Kong, 2014), who is responsible for making rehabilitation policy for the disabled persons and enhancing coordination with other government bureau and departments, public organizations and NGOs in the provision and formulation of rehabilitation services (LWB, 2014). The realization of better coordination of inter-sectors, particularly the role delineation of the FHB and the LWB in rehabilitation, may help break down the current compartmentalization and fragmentation of health care and community care.

Domiciliary Services

In 2014, only 1.05% of persons aged 60 and over in Hong Kong lived in institutions including homes for the aged, care and attention homes, and nursing homes (The Hong Kong Council of Social Service, 2017). Given that most of the elderly live with their families and not in institutions, the ageing-in-place concept has been advocated by the Hong Kong government in recent years to enable older people to remain living in a familiar and preferred environment. Ageing-in-place is a world-wide trend that even vulnerable older people can live in their own domestic housing with community-based in-home support services and innovative housing designs to meet their needs when they become aged and frailer (Chui, 2008). At present, clients of both "Enhanced Home and Community Care Services" and "Integrated Home Care Services" have to be assessed and arranged by the Standardized Care Need Assessment Mechanism (SCNAM) for Elderly Services through multidisciplinary teams consisting of accredited assessors from various professional disciplines such as nurses, social workers, occupational therapists, and physiotherapists, etc. who have gone through training and accreditation on the use of assessment tools (SWD, 2017). The SCNAM teams also serve as a gatekeeper to cover applications for residential services such as admissions to homes for the aged, care and attention homes, nursing homes, day care centres for the elderly, enhanced home and community care services, and integrated home care services (for disabled and frail cases). There are only 5 SCNAM teams in Hong Kong and the current level of manpower and resources may not be enough to serve the increasing number of elders in the population, which may increase the waiting time under the Central Waiting List, particularly for those who are in urgent health and care needs.

Centre-Based CBR in the Community

With regard to the CRDC project, it still operates on a trial basis since its inauguration a decade ago. At present, there are only four CRDCs in four districts (Kwun Tong, Wanchai, Shatin, and Tuen Mun) funded by the Social Welfare Department (n.d.) since 2007, the services provided are far less than the demand of people with disabilities. There are no district centres in the Kowloon West and the Central districts, for instance, and each existing centre may not be able to cope with the demand of rehabilitation needs from people with chronic diseases and physical disabilities. To cite an example, most of the clients visiting the CRDCs are stroke survivors, and this is not surprising as the incidence of stroke cases increases in an ageing population as the risk of stroke increase with age (Sheppard & Ko, 2009). In Hong Kong, there was an average of 25,247 people yearly suffered from stroke in the period of 2008-12 and among them, there was an average of 21,813 survivors per year with a survival rate about 86% (Hospital Authority of Hong Kong, 2014). Most of them might end up with various degrees of sensorimotor impairments, physical and cognitive disabilities, and require varying degrees of rehabilitation. It is not difficult or unreasonable to infer that services offered by only four CRDCs are insufficient. As regards other subsidy schemes from the Community Care Fund for people with severe disabilities, they are also on a pilot basis.

Self-Management of Chronic Diseases by Patients

The Chronic Disease Self-Management Programme ("CDSMP") facilitates patients with chronic diseases to gain self-management skills and behavior based on the theory of self-efficacy, social learning, mastery of skills, and problem-solving (Bodenheimer, Lorig, Holman, & Grumbach., 2002), and is a 6-week standardized programme to help participants to join in self-management skills training and set up health action plans (Chan, Siu, Poon, & Chan, 2005). However, to the best knowledge of the authors, there has been no plan to implement the CDSMP in the long run. The Hospital Authority has also partnered with NGOs since 2010 to offer a patient empowerment programme as a pilot public-private-partnership project, mainly for patients with diabetes mellitus and high blood pressure with an aim to enhancing their disease specific knowledge and self-care capabilities, and an enhanced model with more emphasis on personalization has commenced since April 2016 (Hospital Authority of Hong Kong, 2016). There is no indication either as to whether such a pilot project would become recurrent in the near future.

NGOs' Running CBR Programmes on a Project Basis

In addition to the call for enhanced coordination within the government, there is also a need to strengthen the coordination of NGOs which are playing an important role in the provisions of community-based care and CBR. The Hong Kong government allocates resources to NGOs in accordance with the Lump Sum Grant Subvention System, which was introduced in 2001 and is considered as a "a major revamp of the public funding and management" of NGOs in the social welfare sector (Lump Sum Grant Independent Review Committee, 2008). In terms of community care, sustainability is a concern. There may not be empirical studies on the number of self-financed community-based services in Hong Kong, and according to the authors' personal observations, a number of community-based programmes run by NGOs in Hong Kong are operated on a project or self-financed basis, e.g. self-financing day care centres for elders with dementia (SWD, 2012), and when budget is exhausted, the programmes concerned have to put a stop to provisions of services. The authors argue that because of the sustainability concern, NGOs may see other counterparts as competitors rather than partners, and this has created a further stumbling block to the development of community care in Hong Kong.

CONCLUSION

Ageing population has been challenging governments to give new initiatives and policies in the provision of care (WHO, 2013). This requires linking comprehensive and consistent policies, services, and other supports together (Cox, 2005) in a sustainable manner. Hong Kong is no exception.

To enable healthy ageing and reduce the number of chronic patients, the Hong Kong government must reduce the reliance on hospital and institutional care and considers increasing community care in the long run for frail aged persons (Chu & Chi, 2006). Although there have been some social programmes by NGOs and public healthcare programmes in place in Hong Kong, CBR and other community-based services are still limited and fragmented, as exemplified by the facts that there is a lack of a longer-term policy of community-based services, that the Hong Kong government continues to rely on public hospital services, that there is still room to improve coordination of inter-sectors, and that NGOs are running community-based programmes on a project or self-financing basis, the services of which are susceptible to termination when funding is exhausted, not to mention the need to strengthen inter-departmental coordination within the Hong Kong government (Chan & Phillips, 2002), interagency coordination between the government, the Hospital Authority, the Social Welfare Department, and NGOs, and, last but not least, inter-NGOs coordination.

Hong Kong goes in a similar direction of community care as other contemporary societies, but without a longer-term policy in Hong Kong, the so-called guiding principle of "ageing in place as the core, institutional care as back-up" (LWB & SWD, 2014, paragraph 2) is far words more than action. The authors suggest that the Hong Kong government make community-based care a longer-term policy which is free of interruptions because of changes of government leaders, and for the sake of long-term sustainability of Hong Kong, review the present heavy reliance on public hospital services and revamp the existing financing model to optimize the imbalance between hospital care and community care. In practice, to strengthen the Hong Kong government's coordinating role, in addition to the upgrade of the rank of the Commissioner for Rehabilitation, the authors further recommend that the government make reference to the success of the "Energizing Kowloon East Office" (Hong Kong government, 2012b) and establish an appropriate coordination mechanism among different policy bureaus to allow different stakeholders like practitioners in the health care and community care fields, NGOs, and patient advocates, to join hands to discuss and improve the longer-term planning in community care to rectify the current fragmented approach. Once an appropriate context of community-based care is in place in Hong Kong, the authors are confident that there should be no doubt as to the quality of care provisions, as evidenced by the very long life expectancy of citizens (CSD, 2016b).

REFERENCES

Antibiotic clinics provide 'incredible' community care. (2015). *Nursing Standard, 29*(40), 10. doi: 10.7748/ns.29.40.10.s11

Arnott, J., & Koubel, G. (2012). Interprofessional working and the community care conundrum. In G. Koubel & H. Bungay (Eds.), *Rights, risks and responsibilities: Interprofessional working in health and social care* (pp. 159–178). Basingstoke, UK: Palgrave Macmillan. doi:10.1007/978-0-230-36907-8_10

Bardsley, M., Steventon, A., Smith, J., & Dixon, J. (2013). *Evaluating integrated and community-based care: How do we know what works?* London, UK: Nuffield Trust. Retrieved March 20, 2017 from https://www.nuffieldtrust.org.uk/files/2017-01/evaluating-integrated-community-care-web-final.pdf

Baum, F. (2008). The social determinants of health inequity. In F. Baum (Ed.), *The new public health* (3rd ed.). Melbourne, Australia: Oxford University Press.

Bernard, M., & Phillips, J. (2000). The challenge of ageing in tomorrows Britain. *Ageing and Society, 20*(1), 33–54. doi:10.1017/S0144686X99007576

Bodenheimer, T., Lorig, K., Holman, H., & Grumbach, K. (2002). Patient self-management of chronic disease in primary care. *Journal of the American Medical Association, 288*(19), 2469–2475. doi:10.1001/jama.288.19.2469 PMID:12435261

Campbell, J., Ikegami, N., Gori, C., Barbabella, F., Chomik, R., d'Amico, F., & Theobald, H. (2016). *Long-term care reforms in OECD countries: Successes and failures* (C. Gori, J.-L. Fernandez, & R. Wittenberg, Eds.). Bristol, UK: Policy Press.

Cancer Expert Working Group on Cancer Prevention and Screening, & Department of Health of Hong Kong. (2016). *Prevention and screening for breast cancer: Information for women and their families.* Hong Kong: Department of Health. Retrieved March 20, 2017 from http://www.chp.gov.hk/files/pdf/breast_ca_en.pdf

Census and Statistics Department of Hong Kong. (2015a). *Hong Kong populations projections 2015-2064.* Retrieved March 20, 2017 from http://www.statistics.gov.hk/pub/B1120015062015XXXXB0100.pdf

Census and Statistics Department of Hong Kong. (2015b). *Hong Kong monthly digest of statistics: January 2015.* Hong Kong: Author. Retrieved March 20, 2017 from http://www.statistics.gov.hk/pub/B71501FB2015XXXXB0100.pdf

Census and Statistics Department of Hong Kong. (2016a). *2016 population by-census: Summary results.* Hong Kong: Author. Retrieved March 20, 2017 from http://www.bycensus2016.gov.hk/data/16bc-summary-results.pdf

Census and Statistics Department of Hong Kong. (2016b). Statistics and you. Retrieved March 20, 2017 from http://www.censtatd.gov.hk/statistical_literacy/educational_materials/statistics_and_you/

Central Health Education Unit of Hong Kong. (2015). *The Central Health Education Unit.* Retrieved March 20, 2017 from https://www.cheu.gov.hk/eng/aboutus/index.htm

Centre for Health Protection of the Department of Health of Hong Kong. (2012). Brain health. *Non-communicable Diseases Watch, 5*(12), 1-6. Retrieved March 20, 2017 from http://www.chp.gov.hk/files/pdf/ncd_watch_dec2012.pdf

Chan, A. C. M., & Phillips, D. R. (2002). Policies on ageing and long-term care in Hong Kong. In D. R. Phillips & A. C. M. Chan (Eds.), Ageing and long-term care: National policies in the Asia-Pacific (pp. 23-67). Singapore: Institute of Southeast Asian Studies.

Chan, S. C. C., Siu, A. M. H., Poon, P. K. K., & Chan, C. C. H. (2005). Chronic disease self-management program for Chinese patients: A preliminary multi-baseline study. *International Journal of Rehabilitation Research. Internationale Zeitschrift fur Rehabilitationsforschung. Revue Internationale de Recherches de Readaptation, 28*(4), 351–354. doi:10.1097/00004356-200512000-00008 PMID:16319561

Chan, W. M. (2012). Policy implication and the way forward. *Asian Journal of Gerontology and Geriatrics, 7*(1), 59–63.

Chappell, N. L., Dlitt, B. H., Hollander, M. J., Miller, J. A., & McWilliam, C. (2004). Comparative costs of home care and residential care. *The Gerontologist, 44*(3), 389–400. doi:10.1093/geront/44.3.389 PMID:15197293

Chatterjee, S., Patel, V., Chatterjee, A., & Weiss, H. A. (2003). Evaluation of a community-based rehabilitation model for chronic schizophrenia in rural India. *The British Journal of Psychiatry, 182*(1), 57–62. doi:10.1192/bjp.182.1.57 PMID:12509319

Chief Executive of Hong Kong. (2005). *The 2005-06 policy address: Strong governance for the people.* Retrieved March 20, 2017 from http://www.policyaddress.gov.hk/05-06/eng/pdf/speech.pdf

Chief Executive of Hong Kong. (2007). *The 2007-08 policy address: A new direction for Hong Kong.* Retrieved March 20, 2017 from http://www.policyaddress.gov.hk/07-08/eng/docs/policy.pdf

Chief Executive of Hong Kong. (2008). *The 2008-09 policy address: Embracing new challenges.* Retrieved March 20, 2017 from http://www.policyaddress.gov.hk/08-09/eng/docs/policy.pdf

Chief Executive of Hong Kong. (2009). *The 2009-10 policy address: Breaking new ground together.* Retrieved March 20, 2017 from http://www.policyaddress.gov.hk/09-10/eng/docs/policy.pdf

Chief Executive of Hong Kong. (2014). *The 2014 policy address: Support the needy, let youth flourish, unleash Hong Kong's potential.* Retrieved March 20, 2017 from http://www.policyaddress.gov.hk/2014/eng/pdf/PA2014.pdf

Chief Executive of Hong Kong. (2015). *The 2015 policy address: Uphold the rule of law, seize the opportunities, make the right choices.* Retrieved March 20, 2017 from http://www.policyaddress.gov.hk/2015/eng/pdf/PA2015.pdf

Chief Executive of Hong Kong. (2016). *The 2016 policy address: Innovate for the economy, improve livelihood, foster harmony, share prosperity.* Retrieved March 20, 2017 from http://www.policyaddress.gov.hk/2016/eng/pdf/PA2016.pdf

Chief Executive of Hong Kong. (2017). *The 2017 Policy Address: Make best use of opportunities, develop the economy, improve people's livelihood, build an inclusive society.* Retrieved March 20, 2017 from http://www.policyaddress.gov.hk/2017/eng/pdf/PA2017.pdf

Chief Secretary for Administration's Office of Hong Kong. (2012). *Steering Committee on Population Policy – Progress report 2012* (File Ref.: CSO/ADM CR 1/3581/12). Retrieved March 20, 2017 from http://www.legco.gov.hk/yr08-09/english/hc/sub_com/hs52/papers/hs520605-csoadmcr1358112-e.pdf

Chu, L.-W., & Chi, I. (2006). Long-term care and hospital care for the elderly. In G. M. Leung & J. Bacon-Shone (Eds.), *Hong Kong's health system: Reflections, perspectives and visions* (pp. 223–252). Hong Kong: Hong Kong University Press.

Chui, E. (2008). Ageing in place in Hong Kong – challenges and opportunities in a capitalist Chinese city. *Ageing International*, *32*(3), 167–182. doi:10.1007/s12126-008-9015-2

Cleaver, S., & Nixon, S. (2014). A scoping review of 10 years of published literature on community-based rehabilitation. *Disability and Rehabilitation*, *36*(17), 1385–1394. doi:10.3109/09638288.2013.845257 PMID:24151820

Cox, C. B. (2005). *Community care for an aging society.* New York, NY: Springer.

Davies, B., & Challis, D. (1986). *Matching resources to needs in community care: An evaluated demonstrations of a long-term care model.* Hants, UK: Gower Publishing.

Department of Health of Hong Kong. (2008). *Promoting health in Hong Kong: A strategic framework for prevention and control of non-communicable diseases*. Retrieved March 20, 2017 from http://www.change4health.gov.hk/filemanager/common/image/strategic_framework/promoting_health/promoting_health_e.pdf

Department of Health of Hong Kong. (2016a). *Common health problems*. Retrieved March 20, 2017 from http://www.elderly.gov.hk/english/common_health_problems/index.html

Department of Health of Hong Kong. (2016b). *Health facts of Hong Kong* (2016 edition). Retrieved March 20, 2017 from http://www.dh.gov.hk/english/statistics/statistics_hs/files/Health_Statistics_pamphlet_E.pdf

Development Bureau of Hong Kong. (2016). *Legislative Council Panel on Development: Extending the operation of Energizing Kowloon East Office* (Paper No. LC Paper No. CB(1)133/16-17(04)). Retrieved March 20, 2017 from http://www.ekeo.gov.hk/filemanager/content/public/en/dev20161122cb1-133-4-e.pdf

Duff, J. (2001). Financing to foster community health care: A comparative analysis of Singapore, Europe, North America and Australia. *Current Sociology, 49*(3), 135–154. doi:10.1177/0011392101049003009

Elderly Commission of Hong Kong. (2009). *Minutes of the 56th meeting*. Retrieved March 20, 2017 from http://www.elderlycommission.gov.hk/en/download/meeting/Min-56(22.1.09)_e.pdf

Executive Yuan of Taiwan. (2017). *Executive Yuan passes 10-year long-term care 2.0 plan*. Retrieved March 20, 2017 from http://english.ey.gov.tw/News_Hot_Topic.aspx?n=FE8C5966F81D8273&sms=BBB420E471DAF6C0

Financial Secretary of Hong Kong. (2015). *The 2015-16 budget*. Retrieved March 20, 2017 from http://www.budget.gov.hk/2015/eng/pdf/e_budgetspeech2015-16.pdf

Financial Secretary of Hong Kong. (2016a). *2016-17 budget (media sheet)*. Retrieved March 20, 2017 from http://www.budget.gov.hk/2016/eng/pdf/2016-17_Media_Sheet.pdf

Financial Secretary of Hong Kong. (2016b). *The 2016-17 budget*. Retrieved March 20, 2017 from http://www.budget.gov.hk/2016/eng/pdf/e_budgetspeech2016-17.pdf

Finkeflügel, H., Wolffers, I., & Huijsma, R. (2005). The evidence base for community-based rehabilitation: A literature review. *International Journal of Rehabilitation Research. Internationale Zeitschrift fur Rehabilitationsforschung. Revue Internationale de Recherches de Readaptation, 28*(3), 187–201. doi:10.1097/00004356-200509000-00001 PMID:16046912

Food and Health Bureau of Hong Kong. (2008). *Environmental Report, 2007*. Retrieved from http://www.epd.gov.hk/epd/english/how_help/tools_epr/files/fhb_ER2007e.pdf

Food and Health Bureau of Hong Kong. (2010). *Legislative Council Panel on Health Services: Healthcare service reform – primary care development strategy* (Paper No. CB(2)1995/09-10(01)). Retrieved March 20, 2017 from http://www.legco.gov.hk/yr09-10/english/panels/hs/papers/hs0712cb2-1995-1-e.pdf

Food and Health Bureau of Hong Kong. (2013). *Legislative Council Panel on Health Services Subcommittee on Health Protection Scheme: Role and development of public and private healthcare services* (Paper No. CB(2)448/12-13(02)). Retrieved March 20, 2017 from http://www.legco.gov.hk/yr12-13/english/panels/hs/hs_hps/papers/hs_hps0114cb2-448-2-e.pdf

Food and Health Bureau of Hong Kong. (2014). *Consultation document on voluntary health insurance scheme*. Retrieved March 20, 2017 from http://www.vhis.gov.hk/doc/en/full_consultation_document/consultation_full_eng.pdf

Food and Health Bureau of Hong Kong. (2015a). *Legislative Council Panel on Health Services: 2015 Policy Address – Policy initiatives of the Food and Health Bureau* (LC Paper No. CB(2)612/14-15(03)). Retrieved March 20, 2017 from http://www.legco.gov.hk/yr14-15/english/panels/hs/papers/hs20150119cb2-612-3-e.pdf

Food and Health Bureau of Hong Kong. (2015b). *Report of the Steering Committee on Review of Hospital Authority*. Retrieved March 20, 2017 from http://www.legco.gov.hk/yr14-15/english/panels/hs/papers/hs20150720cb2-1907-1-e.pdf

Food and Health Bureau of Hong Kong. (2016). *Legislative Council Panel on Health Services: An update on public hospital developments* (LC Paper No. CB(2)652/15-16(04)). Retrieved March 20, 2017 from http://www.legco.gov.hk/yr15-16/english/panels/hs/papers/hs20160118cb2-652-4-e.pdf

Geiser, P., & Boersma, M. (2013). The role of the community in CBR. In G. Musoke & P. Geiser (Eds.), *Linking CBR, disability and rehabilitation* (pp. 24–35). Bangalore, India: CBR Africa Network.

Health and Medical Development Advisory Committee of Hong Kong. (2005). *Building a healthy tomorrow: Discussion paper on the future service delivery model for our health care system*. Retrieved March 20, 2017 from http://www.info.gov.hk/archive/consult/2005/hmdac_paper_e.pdf

Health and Welfare Bureau of Hong Kong. (2000). *Lifelong investment in health: Consultation document on health care reform*. Hong Kong: Author. Retrieved March 20, 2017 from http://www.hpdo.gov.hk/en/doc/lifelong_investment_in_health_eng.pdf

Health Reform Implementation Taskforce of Western Australia. (2007). *Ambulatory and community-based care: A framework for non-inpatient care*. Retrieved March 20, 2017 from http://zanran_storage.s3.amazonaws.com/www.health.wa.gov.au/ContentPages/19041594.pdf

Health, Welfare and Food Bureau of Hong Kong. (2007). *LegCo Panel on Welfare Services – 2007 rehabilitation programme plan* (LC Paper No. CB(2)2348/06-07(01)). Retrieved March 20, 2017 from http://www.legco.gov.hk/yr06-07/english/panels/ws/papers/ws0709cb2-2348-1-e.pdf

Helander, E., Mendis, P., Nelson, G., & Goerdt, A. (1989). *Training in the community for people with disabilities*. Geneva, Switzerland: World Health Organization. Retrieved March 20, 2017 from http://www.who.int/disabilities/publications/cbr/training/en/

Hoeman, S. P. (1992). Community-based rehabilitation. *Holistic Nursing Practice*, *6*(2), 32–41. doi:10.1097/00004650-199206020-00007 PMID:1735743

Hong Kong government. (2012a, June 5). *Opening ceremony held for Tin Shui Wai (Tin Yip Road) Community Health Centre (with photos)* [Press release]. Retrieved March 20, 2017 from http://www.info.gov.hk/gia/general/201206/05/P201206050459.htm

Hong Kong government. (2012b, June 7). *Transformation of Kowloon East in full swing with inception of Energizing Kowloon East Office* [Press release]. Retrieved March 20, 2017 from http://www.info.gov.hk/gia/general/201206/07/P201206070322.htm

Hong Kong government. (2013, April 9). *HK healthcare is a dual-track system.* Retrieved March 20, 2017 from http://www.news.gov.hk/en/record/html/2013/04/20130409_190409.shtml

Hong Kong government. (2016, July 16). *Medical platform to be formed.* Retrieved March 20, 2017 from http://www.news.gov.hk/en/categories/health/html/2016/07/20160716_111123.lin.shtml

Hong Kong government. (2017a, March 9). *LWB's response to Ombudsman's direct investigation report* [Press release]. Retrieved March 20, 2017 from http://www.info.gov.hk/gia/general/201703/09/P2017030900515.htm

Hong Kong government. (2017b, March 9). *Ombudsman recommendations noted* [Press release]. Retrieved March 20, 2017 from http://www.news.gov.hk/en/categories/health/html/2017/03/20170309_141809.shtml

Hong Kong Society for Rehabilitation. (n.d.). *Community rehabilitation network* . Retrieved March 20, 2017 from http://www.rehabsociety.org.hk/dccs/crn/wp-content/uploads/sites/4/2016/01/crn_社區復康網絡服務介紹單張.pdf (in Chinese)

Hospital Authority of Hong Kong. (2012). *Hospital Authority strategic plan 2012–2017.* Retrieved March 20, 2017 from http://www.ha.org.hk/upload/publication_29/359.pdf

Hospital Authority of Hong Kong. (2014). *Hospital Authority statistical report 2012-2013.* Retrieved March 20, 2017 from https://www.ha.org.hk/upload/publication_15/491.pdf

Hospital Authority of Hong Kong. (2016). *Update on Hospital Authority's public-private partnership programmes* (paper no. AOM-P1180). Retrieved March 20, 2017 from https://www.ha.org.hk/haho/ho/cad_bnc/AOM-P1180.pdf

Iemmi, V., Suresh Kumar, K., Blanchet, K., Gibson, L., Hartley, S., Murthy, G. V. S., & Kuper, H. et al. (2013). Community-based rehabilitation for people with physical and mental disabilities in low- and middle-income countries. *Cochrane Database of Systematic Reviews*, *7*, 1–15. doi:10.1002/14651858.CD010617

Institute of Medicine. (2013). *Best care at lower cost: The path to continuously learning health care in America.* Washington, DC: The National Academies Press.

Jacob, K. S. (2001). Community care for people with mental disorders in developing countries: Problems and possible solutions. *The British Journal of Psychiatry*, *178*(4), 296–298. doi:10.1192/bjp.178.4.296 PMID:11282806

Jamrozik, A. (2001). *Social policy in the post-welfare state: Australians on the threshold of the 21st century.* Frenchs Forest: Longman.

Kespichayawattana, J., & Jitapunkul, S. (2008). Health and health care system for older persons. *Ageing International*, *33*(1), 28–49. doi:10.1007/s12126-009-9028-5

Knapp, M., Marks, I., Wolstenholme, J., Beecham, J., Astin, J., Audini, B., & Watts, V. et al. (1998). Home-based versus hospital-based care for serious mental illness. Controlled cost-effectiveness study over four years. *The British Journal of Psychiatry*, *172*(6), 506–512. doi:10.1192/bjp.172.6.506 PMID:9828991

Kong, S.-T., Fang, C. M.-S., & Lou, V. W. Q. (2016, August 7). published online). Solving the personhood jigsaw puzzle in residential care homes for the elderly in the Hong Kong Chinese context. *Qualitative Health Research*, *27*(3), 421–433. doi:10.1177/1049732316658266

Labour and Welfare Bureau, & Social Welfare Department of Hong Kong. (2014). *Legislative Council Panel on Welfare Services: Home care and community support services for the elderly and persons with disabilities* (LC Paper No. CB(2)2077/13-14(05)). Retrieved March 20, 2017 from http://www.legco.gov.hk/yr13-14/english/panels/ws/papers/ws0725cb2-2077-5-e.pdf

Labour and Welfare Bureau of Hong Kong. (2014). *Item for Establishment Subcommittee of Finance Committee Head 141– Government Secretariat: Labour and Welfare Bureau Subhead 000 Operational expenses* (Paper No. EC(2014-15)2). Retrieved March 20, 2017 from http://www.legco.gov.hk/yr13-14/english/fc/esc/papers/e14-02e.pdf

Lai, W. W. L., Chan, J. P. Y., Choi, P. K. K., Ngai, L. C. T., Mar, C. S. F., Chan, E. Y. L., & Lam, F. N. Y. et al. (2009). Occupational therapy in the integrated elderly and community support services for the elderly in Hong Kong. *Hong Kong Journal of Occupational Therapy*, *19*(1), 27–30. doi:10.1016/S1569-1861(09)70041-5

Lam, C. L. K. (2005). The role of the family doctor in building a healthy tomorrow. *The Hong Kong Practitioner*, *27*, 363–367.

Lee, S.-D. (2002). Exploring policy and financing options for long-term care in Taiwan. *Journal of Aging & Social Policy*, *13*(2-3), 203–216. doi:10.1300/J031v13n02_14 PMID:12216356

Legg, L., & Langhorne, P. (2004). Rehabilitation therapy services for stroke patients living at home: Systematic review of randomised trials. *Lancet*, *363*(9406), 352–356. doi:10.1016/S0140-6736(04)15434-2 PMID:15070563

Legislative Council Secretariat. (2015a). Challenges of population ageing. *Research Brief*, *2015-2016*(1). Retrieved March 20, 2017 from http://www.legco.gov.hk/research-publications/english/1516rb01-challenges-of-population-ageing-20151215-e.pdf

Legislative Council Secretariat. (2015b). *Panel on Health Services – Updated background brief prepared by the Legislative Council Secretariat for the meeting on 16 March 2015: Private hospital development* (LC Paper No. CB(2)993/14-15(04)). Retrieved March 20, 2017 from http://www.legco.gov.hk/yr14-15/english/panels/hs/papers/hs20150316cb2-993-4-e.pdf

Li, Y., & Chui, W.-E. (2016). Community care for adults with severe mental disorders in rural China: A case study. *International Journal of Social Welfare*, *25*(3), 273–282. doi:10.1111/ijsw.12201

Lump Sum Grant Independent Review Committee. (2008). *Review Report on the Lump Sum Grant Subvention System*. Retrieved March 20, 2017 from http://www.lwb.gov.hk/eng/consult_paper/Review%20Report%20on%20Lump%20Sum%20Grant%20Subvention%20System.pdf

Ma, N. (2007). *Political development in Hong Kong: State, political society, and civil society*. Hong Kong: Hong Kong University Press.

Means, R., Richards, R., & Smith, R. (2008). *Community care: policy and practice* (4th ed.). Basingstoke, UK: Palgrave Macmillan. doi:10.1007/978-1-137-07383-9

Murphy, E. (1987). Community care I: Problems. *British Medical Journal, 295*(6612), 1505–1508. doi:10.1136/bmj.295.6612.1505-a PMID:3122879

Nakanishi, M., Shimizu, S., Murai, T., & Yamaoka, A. (2015). Ageing in place policy in Japan: Association between the development of an integrated community care system and the number of nursing home placements under the public long-term care insurance program among municipal governments. *Ageing International, 40*(3), 248–261. doi:10.1007/s12126-014-9215-x

National Health Service of the UK. (2014). *Five-year forward view for the NHS*. Retrieved March 20, 2017 from https://www.england.nhs.uk/wp-content/uploads/2014/10/5yfv-web.pdf

National Institute on Aging, National Institutes of Health, & World Health Organization. (2011). *Global health and aging*. Retrieved March 20, 2017 from http://www.who.int/ageing/publications/global_health.pdf

Naylor, C. D. (1999). Health care in Canada: Incrementalism under fiscal duress. *Health Affairs, 18*(3), 9–26. doi:10.1377/hlthaff.18.3.9 PMID:10388197

Paudel, S., Bhandari, L., & Bhandari, D. B. (2017). Disability: A case screening program approach. *Journal of Biosciences and Medicines, 5*(2), 10–21. doi:10.4236/jbm.2017.52002

Poon, P. K.-k., So, A., & Loong, E. L.-c. (2014). Self-management in community-based rehabilitation programmes for persons with chronic disease. In K.-w. Tong & K. N.-k. Fong (Eds.), *Community care in Hong Kong: Current practice, practice research studies, and future directions* (pp. 53–73). Hong Kong: City University of Hong Kong Press.

Royal College of Nursing of the UK. (2014). *Moving care to the community: An international perspective* (Policy briefing 12/13 March 2013 (updated December 2014)). RCN Policy and International Department, Royal College of Nursing. Retrieved March 20, 2017 from https://www2.rcn.org.uk/__data/assets/pdf_file/0006/523068/12.13_Moving_care_to_the_community_an_international_perspective.pdf

Sau Po Center on Ageing, & Department of Social Work & Social Administration, the University of Hong Kong. (2011). *Consultancy study on community care services for the elderly: Final report*. Hong Kong: Authors. Retrieved March 20, 2017 from http://www.elderlycommission.gov.hk/en/download/library/Community%20Care%20Services%20Report%202011_eng.pdf

Schaller, S., Mauskopf, J., Kriza, C., Wahlster, P., & Kolominsky-Rabas, P. L. (2015). The main cost drivers in dementia: A systematic review. *International Journal of Geriatric Psychiatry, 30*(2), 111–129. doi:10.1002/gps.4198 PMID:25320002

Sharkey, P. (2007). *The essentials of community care* (2nd ed.). New York, NY: Palgrave.

Sharma, M. (2007). Evaluation in community based rehabilitation programmes: A strengths, weaknesses, opportunities and threats analysis. *Asia Pacific Disability Rehabilitation Journal, 18*(1), 46–62.

Sheppard, L., & Ko, K. F. (2009). A new stroke unit: Implementation issues. *The Hong Kong Physiotherapy Journal, 27*(1), 7–10. doi:10.1016/S1013-7025(10)70003-8

Shrivastava, S., Shrivastava, P., & Ramasamy, J. (2015). Exploring the scope of community-based rehabilitation in ensuring the holistic development of differently-abled people. *African Health Sciences, 15*(1), 278–280. doi:10.4314/ahs.v15i1.36 PMID:25834559

Smith, R., Gaser, L., Harrison, L., Martin, L., Means, R., & Thistlethwaite, P. (1993). *Working together for better community care*. Bristol, UK: School for Advanced Urban Studies.

Social Welfare Department of Hong Kong. (2012). *List of self-financing day care centres for the dementia elderly* (June 2012). Retrieved March 20, 2017 from http://www.swd.gov.hk/doc/elderly/List%20of%20Self-financing%20Day%20Care%20Centre%20for%20the%20Dementia%20Elderly_Jun%202012(1).pdf

Social Welfare Department of Hong Kong. (2016a). *Enhanced home and community care services*. Retrieved March 20, 2017 from http://www.swd.gov.hk/en/index/site_pubsvc/page_elderly/sub_csselderly/id_enhancedho/

Social Welfare Department of Hong Kong. (2016b). *Integrated home care services*. Retrieved March 20, 2017 from http://www.swd.gov.hk/en/index/site_pubsvc/page_elderly/sub_csselderly/id_618/

Social Welfare Department of Hong Kong. (2016c). *Pilot scheme on living allowance for low-income carers of persons with disabilities*. Retrieved March 20, 2017 from http://www.swd.gov.hk/en/index/site_pubsvc/page_supportser/sub_PWD/

Social Welfare Department of Hong Kong. (2016d). *Waiting list for subsidised residential care services for the elderly*. Retrieved March 20, 2017 from http://www.swd.gov.hk/doc/elderly/ercs2/LTC%20statistics%20HP-Eng(201607).pdf

Social Welfare Department of Hong Kong. (2017). *Standardised care need assessment mechanism for elderly services*. Retrieved March 20, 2017 from http://www.swd.gov.hk/en/index/site_pubsvc/page_elderly/sub_standardis/

Social Welfare Department of Hong Kong. (n.d.). *Community rehabilitation day centre*. Retrieved March 20, 2017 from http://www.swd.gov.hk/doc/rehab/Service%20brief_CRDC_Eng.pdf

Task Force on Conceptual Model and Preventive Protocols, Working Group on Primary Care, & Food and Health Bureau of Hong Kong. (2012a). *Hong Kong reference framework for preventive care for children in primary care settings 2012*. Retrieved March 20, 2017 from http://www.pco.gov.hk/english/resource/files/ref_framework_children.pdf

Task Force on Conceptual Model and Preventive Protocols, Working Group on Primary Care, & Food and Health Bureau of Hong Kong. (2012b). *Hong Kong reference framework for preventive care for older adults in primary care settings 2012*. Retrieved March 20, 2017 from http://www.pco.gov.hk/english/resource/files/ref_framework_adults.pdf

The Community Care Fund. (2016). *Assistance programmes under the fund*. Retrieved March 20, 2017 from https://www.communitycarefund.hk/en/assistance.asp

The Conference Board of Canada. (2012). *Home and community care in Canada: An economic footprint*. Ottawa, Canada: Author. Retrieved March 20, 2017 from http://carewatchtoronto.org/wp-content/uploads/2012/05/12-306_HomeandCommunityCare_PRT.pdf

The Convention on the Rights of Persons with Disabilities (2006).

The Declaration of Alma-Ata (1978).

The Hong Kong Council of Social Service. (2017). *Social indicators of Hong Kong*. Retrieved March 20, 2017 from http://www.socialindicators.org.hk/en/indicators/elderly/31.12

The Hospital Authority Ordinance (Cap 113) of Hong Kong.

The International Labour Organization, the United Nations Educational, Scientific and Cultural Organization, & the World Health Organization. (2004). *CBR: A strategy for rehabilitation, equalization of opportunities, poverty reduction and social inclusion of people with disabilities*. Joint position paper 2004. Geneva, Switzerland: World Health Organization. Retrieved March 20, 2017 from http://apps.who.int/iris/bitstream/10665/43060/1/9241592389_eng.pdf

The Ombudsman of Hong Kong. (2014, November 20). *Ombudsman probes government regulation of rehabilitation transport services to persons with mobility difficulties* [Press release]. Retrieved March 20, 2017 from http://ofomb.ombudsman.hk/abc/en-us/press_releases/detail/45

The Ombudsman of Hong Kong. (2017). *Executive summary: Direct investigation into government regulation of special transport services to persons with mobility difficulties*. Retrieved March 20, 2017 from http://ofomb.ombudsman.hk/abc/files/IR360_ES_E-9_3_2017.pdf

The Patient Protection and Affordable Care Act 2010 of the United States.

Tin, K. Y. K., Song, W., Tsoi, P. K. O., Lee, Y. H., Chong, D. S. Y., Lam, D. W. S., & Maw, C. K. C. et al. (2016). Hong Kong domestic health spending: Financial years 1989/90 to 2012/13. *Hong Kong Medical Journal*, *22*(Supplement 3), S2–S23. PMID:27389870

Tong, K.-w., & Fong, K. N.-k. (2014). Introduction: Challenges in healthcare and community care in Hong Kong. In K.-w. Tong & K. N.-k. Fong (Eds.), *Community care in Hong Kong: Current practice, practice research studies, and future directions* (pp. 3–16). Hong Kong: City University of Hong Kong Press. doi:10.1142/9789814566582_0016

United Nations Economic Commission for Europe / European Commission. (2015). *Active ageing index 2014: Analytical report*. Report prepared by Asghar Zaidi of Centre for Research on Ageing, University of Southampton and David Stanton, under contract with United Nations Economic Commission for Europe (Geneva), co-funded by European Commission's Directorate General for Employment, Social Affairs and Inclusion (Brussels). Retrieved March 20, 2017 from http://www.age-platform.eu/images/stories/Publications/AAI_2014_Report.pdf

Wimo, A., Jonsson, L., & Winblad, B. (2006). An estimate of the worldwide prevalence and direct costs of dementia in 2003. *Dementia and Geriatric Cognitive Disorders, 21*(3), 175–181. doi:10.1159/000090733 PMID:16401889

Woo, J., Ho, S. C., Chan, S. G., Yu, A. L., Yuen, Y. K., & Lau, J. (1997). An estimate of chronic disease burden and some economic consequences among the elderly Hong Kong population. *Journal of Epidemiology and Community Health, 51*(5), 486–489. doi:10.1136/jech.51.5.486 PMID:9425456

Working Party on Primary Health Care of Hong Kong. (1990). *Health for all – The way ahead.* Hong Kong: Government Printer.

World Health Organization. (1986). *Ottawa Charter for Health Promotion.* Retrieved March 20, 2017 from http://www.who.int/healthpromotion/conferences/previous/ottawa/en/

World Health Organization. (1994). *Community-based rehabilitation and the health care referral services* (WHO/RHB/94.1). Retrieved March 20, 2017 from http://www.who.int/management/community/services/CommunityBasedRehabilitation.pdf

World Health Organization. (2002). *Active ageing: A policy framework.* Geneva, Switzerland: World Health Organization Noncommunicable Disease Prevention and Health Promotion Ageing and Life Course. Retrieved March 20, 2017 from http://apps.who.int/iris/bitstream/10665/67215/1/WHO_NMH_NPH_02.8.pdf

World Health Organization. (2003). *Community contribution to TB care: Practice and policy* (WHO/CDS/TB/2003.312). Geneva: Author. Retrieved March 20, 2017 from http://apps.who.int/iris/bitstream/10665/67865/1/WHO_CDS_TB_2003.312.pdf

World Health Organization. (2004). *A glossary of terms for community health care and services for older persons* (WHO Centre for Health Development: Ageing and Health Technical Report, Volume 5, WHO/WKC/Tech.Ser./04.2). Retrieved March 20, 2017 from http://www.who.int/kobe_centre/ageing/ahp_vol5_glossary.pdf

World Health Organization. (2005). *Sustainable health financing, universal coverage and social health insurance: World Health Assembly Resolution 58.33.* Retrieved March 20, 2017 from http://apps.who.int/iris/bitstream/10665/20383/1/WHA58_33-en.pdf?ua=1

World Health Organization. (2013). *Global action plan for the prevention and control of NCDs 2013-2020.* Retrieved March 20, 2017 from http://apps.who.int/iris/bitstream/10665/94384/1/9789241506236_eng.pdf?ua=1

World Health Organization. (n.d.a). *Disabilities and rehabilitation: Community-based rehabilitation (CBR).* Retrieved March 20, 2017 from http://www.who.int/disabilities/cbr/en/

World Health Organization. (n.d.b). *Disabilities and rehabilitation: Community-based rehabilitation guidelines.* Retrieved March 20, 2017 from http://www.who.int/disabilities/cbr/guidelines/en/

World Health Organization, & the Gulbenkian Global Mental Health Platform. (2015). *Promoting rights and community living for children with psychosocial disabilities*. Geneva, Switzerland: World Health Organization. Retrieved March 20, 2017 from http://apps.who.int/iris/bitstream/10665/184033/1/9789241565004_eng.pdf

World Health Organization, & Swedish Organizations of Disabled Persons International Aid Association. (2002). *Community-based rehabilitation as we have experienced it ... voices of persons with disabilities*. Geneva, Switzerland: World Health Organization. Retrieved March 20, 2017 from http://apps.who.int/iris/bitstream/10665/42629/1/9241590432.pdf

Yip, P., Lee, J., & Law, C. K. (2006). Implications of the demographic transition. In G. M. Leung & J. Bacon-Shone (Eds.), *Hong Kong's health system: Reflections, perspectives and visions* (pp. 61–80). Hong Kong: Hong Kong University Press.

Yu, R., Chau, P. H., McGhee, S. M., Chau, J., Lee, C. H., Chan, M. Y., . . . Woo, J. (2012). *Trends of disease burden consequent to stroke in older persons in Hong Kong: Implications of population ageing*. Hong Kong: The Hong Kong Jockey Club. Retrieved March 20, 2017 from https://hub.hku.hk/bitstream/10722/161124/1/Content.pdf?accept=1

Yu, R., Chau, P. H., McGhee, S. M., Cheung, W. L., Chan, K. C., Cheung, S. H., . . . Woo, J. (2010). *Dementia trends: Impact of the ageing population and societal implications for Hong Kong*. Hong Kong: The Hong Kong Jockey Club. Retrieved March 20, 2017 from https://hub.hku.hk/bitstream/10722/138520/1/Content.pdf

Yu, R., Chau, P. H., McGhee, S. M., Cheung, W. L., Chan, K. C., Cheung, S. H., ... Woo, J. (2012). Trends in prevalence and mortality of dementia in elderly Hong Kong population: Projections, disease burden, and implications for long-term care. *International Journal of Alzheimer's Disease, 2012*. doi: 10.1155/2012/406852

Zhou, J., & Walker, A. (2016). The need for community care among older people in China. *Ageing and Society*, *36*(6), 1312–1332. doi:10.1017/S0144686X15000343

Chapter 17
Chinese Herbal Medicine in the Management of Atherosclerosis-Related Chronic Conditions in an Aging Population

Enoch Chan
University of New South Wales, Australia

Tsoi Ming Au Yeung
Hong Kong Community College, Hong Kong

Sai Wang Seto
Western Sydney University, Australia

Gabriel Hoi Huen Chan
Hong Kong Community College, Hong Kong

ABSTRACT

Chronic conditions are important problems for an aging society. They impede on healthy aging and increases the cost of living due to increased medical cost. The most prevalent chronic conditions faced by the elderly population are hypertension, high cholesterol and diabetes mellitus. They increase the risk of developing atherosclerosis, a chronic condition which causes heart attack and stroke. This chapter provides a review on existing therapeutics for the treatment of cardiovascular disease, and briefly discusses their side effects. This chapter also provides a brief introduction to Traditional Chinese Medicine (TCM), and its development in ancient China. This will be followed by a discussion on the recent research on the use of Chinese herbal medicine (CHM) in the treatment of cardiovascular diseases, and the potentials and challenges of incorporating CHM in mainstream healthcare system.

INTRODUCTION

Chronic conditions are the major obstacles to healthy aging. They impact on the quality of life and increase the cost of living. The top three most prevalent chronic conditions in the elderly population are hypertension, high cholesterol and diabetes mellitus (Census and Statistics Department Hong Kong SAR, 2014). These chronic conditions are the main contributing factors to atherosclerosis, which can

DOI: 10.4018/978-1-5225-2633-9.ch017

manifest as ischemic heart disease and stroke, the two most common causes of death in the world (World Health Organization, 2014). Chinese Herbal Medicine (CHM) has been used for thousands of years in China. In recent years, there is greater recognition of CHM due to advances in pre-clinical and clinical research leading to mounting evidence of its efficacy.

This chapter will first highlight the important public health problems faced by an aging and westernizing Chinese community – ischemic heart disease and stroke; and an outline of conventional therapeutics being used to manage ischemic heart disease and stroke. Then the pitfalls of existing therapeutics will be discussed, followed by a brief introduction to CHM and generic examples of the use of CHM in health maintenance; and a review on pre-clinical and clinical studies on using CHM or integrative Western and Chinese Medicine specifically in managing ischemic heart disease and stroke. The readers will gain an appreciation of how CHM being combined with modern Western medicine or on its own can be used to manage ischemic heart disease and stroke, and ultimately promoting healthy aging. It also hopes to encourage medical professionals and policymakers to consider how to better engage Chinese medicine practitioners when devising treatment regime for their patients where appropriate to bring about the best outcome for patients.

BACKGROUND

There has been an increasing life expectancy in the populations of most developed countries in the last decade. From 2004 to 2014, life expectancy for both male and female increased by 2 years in most countries including Hong Kong (Food and Health Bureau, 2016). Moreover, in Hong Kong approximately 15% of the population are aged 65 years or older at the end of 2015 (Census and Statistics Department Hong Kong SAR, 2016). It is expected to double and reach approximately 30% in the next 20 years (Census and Statistics Department Hong Kong SAR, 2015), and by then the median age will shift to 50. The increase in life expectancy and the aging of population over the past decades have led to a substantial increase in age-related cardiac, arterial and microvascular diseases in developed countries. It is well documented that aging is closely associated with the progressive decline in normal physiological functions and has significant impact on the heart and vascular system. The incidence of ischemic heart disease and stroke increases exponentially with aging.

According to the World Health Organization (WHO) (2014), ischemic heart disease and stroke were the top two leading causes of death in 2012, accounting for 7.4 million and 6.7 million of deaths, respectively. In Hong Kong, diseases of heart and cerebrovascular diseases were both listed among the top four causes of death in Hong Kong for elderly people aged 65 and over (Census and Statistics Department Hong Kong SAR, 2014).

In a recent study in Hong Kong, total direct medical cost for a patient newly diagnosed with stable ischemic heart disease is approximately HK$ 89,700 (US$ 11,500) in the first-year, where the cost can be significantly higher if the patients required surgical procedures for their conditions (Lee et al., 2013). These costs are currently not being covered under the Public healthcare in Hong Kong, and the patients are often required to pay out of pocket. The ongoing cost in managing chronic conditions is also likely to increase, due to an extended lifespan of individuals and inflation. In the coming years, the society will be facing an increase in the proportion of elderly people and the decrease in the number of working population. Moreover, the public healthcare sectors face shortage of doctors and the lack of hospital beds in public hospitals. Therefore, there is a pressing need to develop more effective medications to combat aging-related cardiovascular diseases, as well as effective ways to prevent cardiovascular complications once chronic conditions, such as diabetes and high cholesterol level, are detected.

Traditional Chinese Medicine (TCM) has had a very long and rich history in the Chinese community, and is third oldest form of medicine the world has ever known. It originated and developed over thousands of years in ancient China. In the pre-historical time, *Shennong*, who was the deity of agriculture in Chinese mythology, was said to have used himself as test subject and tried various herbs and tested the medicinal effects. A major milestone in the developmental history of CHM occurred in the Ming dynasty, when Li Sizhen authored the *Ben Cao Gang Mu* (Compendium of Materia Medica). It provided detailed diagrams for each herb and until today it remains the most comprehensive herbal encyclopedia in the history of Chinese medicine. Throughout history, Chinese herbal medicine provided a solid foundation for the development of other forms of traditional medicines in Asia, including *Kampo* in Traditional Japanese Medicine and Traditional Korean Medicine. However, being isolated in east Asia throughout its developmental history, the development of TCM in other parts of the world was limited. To date, TCM is considered an alternative medicine in modern world due to the lack of scientific evidence to prove its effectiveness, and the fact that in TCM, physiology and pathophysiology are explained in ways that are radically different from modern medical science. In fact, physiology and pathophysiology are founded on the Chinese theories of Yin and Yang, *Wu-Xing* (Five Elements), *Zang-Fu* (Organs) and *Qi* (Energy).

There has been a marked increase in the popularity of CHM in both Western and Asian countries over the past few decades (Hao et al., 2015; Karalliedde & Kappagoda, 2009). It is reported that over 65% of the Australian population have used complementary and alternative medicine, including CHM, to alleviate chronic or recurrent conditions (Team et al., 2011). In addition, herbal medicines have been approved as treatment for cardiovascular diseases in both Germany and Japan (Karalliedde & Kappagoda, 2009). There has also been a growing acceptance of CHM.

MANAGEMENT OF CHRONIC DISEASES IN AGING

Chronic Diseases in Aging Population

Advanced age is one of the major risk factors of cardiovascular and cerebrovascular diseases as demonstrated by numerous epidemiological studies (Fleg et al., 1995; Lakatta, 2003). As reported by WHO (2014), the number of deaths due to ischemic heart disease in the world for individuals aged 60 or above is approximately 4 times higher than that in individuals of other ages, while the number of deaths due to stroke for individuals aged 60 or above is approximately 5.5 times higher.

Hypertension is a major risk factor for cardiovascular diseases (Špinar, 2012). The risk of stroke in elderly patients increases by more than double when systolic blood pressure is 160 mm Hg or higher, compared to those of less than 140 mm Hg (Cressman & Gifford, 1983). In fact, among hypertensive patients, stroke is a more common complication than heart attack (Kjeldsen, Julius, Hedner, & Hansson, 2001).

High cholesterol and triglycerides levels are also major problems faced by elderly people (Census and Statistics Department Hong Kong SAR, 2014). In recent years, Western fast food with high fat content has become much more accessible by most individuals in urban Chinese cities because of accelerated globalization, busier lifestyle and longer working hours. A clinical study indicates that "Westernized" Chinese adults have higher LDL-cholesterol compared to their rural counterparts (Woo et al., 1999).

In addition, the lack of exercise also correlates with higher LDL-cholesterol level (Gordon et al., 2008; Prabhakaran, Dowling, Branch, Swain, & Leutholtz, 1999). Increased cholesterol and triglycerides levels are important risk factors for cardiovascular disease (Yarnell et al., 2001).

Diabetes mellitus is another major problems faced by elderly people (Census and Statistics Department Hong Kong SAR, 2014). It is a chronic condition in which the body cannot regulate glucose in the blood, resulting in high glucose levels. In 2015, approximately 9.3% of adults in Asia Pacific region, aged between 20-79, had diabetes. In the same year, 1.9 million people in this region died due to diabetes, and 65% of this group were aged above 60. It was estimated that 12% of global health expenditure was due to diabetes (International Diabetes Federation, 2015). It is expected that in 2040, the prevalence of diabetes in Asia Pacific region will increase to 11.9%. Diabetes increases the risk of ischemic heart disease and stroke by 2 to 4-folds (Beckman, Creager, & Libby, 2002).

Underlying ischemic heart disease and stroke is a pathological condition called "atherosclerosis" – the buildup of fatty material in blood vessels (Kumar, Abbas, & Aster, 2013). Atherosclerosis can start in early adolescence without presenting any signs and symptoms (McGill et al., 2000). However, with advancing age, the symptoms may appear. The progression of atherosclerosis in blood vessels narrows the passage for blood flow. Atherosclerosis usually gives rise to no significant symptoms unless it becomes vulnerable and ruptures. The rupture of an atherosclerotic lesion leads to clotting of blood, and may result in the complete obstruction of blood flow. In the worse scenario, the obstruction may occur in the important blood vessels that supply blood to the heart or the brain, and this would cause a heart attack or a stroke (Kumar, et al., 2013).

Moreover, the heart and blood vessel structure and function alter progressively as part of the normal aging process even without the presence of atherosclerosis or hypertension, the major contributing factors of cardiovascular dysfunction (Susic, & Frohlich, 2008). In the heart, a series of notable changes, such as decrease in the elasticity of the heart wall, thickening of the heart valves, impaired intracellular calcium handling and cardiac muscle cell apoptosis, are commonly observed, hence affecting the ability of the heart to pump blood efficiently (Shah et al., 2012; Stern, Behar, & Gottlieb, 2003). Similarly, blood vessels also undergo significant changes, including stiffening, wall thickening and endothelial dysfunction. Although these cardiovascular changes are deemed to be part of the normal aging process, when combined with other risk factors, such as type 2 diabetes, hypertension, dyslipidemia, obesity and smoking, which are commonly present in the aged population, can lead to cardiovascular diseases. Even though aging is an inevitable and intractable process, it is thought that aging can be slowed down by various interventions including dietary, nutraceutical and pharmacological agents that may delay or prevent a range of age-associated diseases.

Conventional Management of Cardiovascular Diseases in Elderly

While pharmacological therapy remains the most commonly used interventions for elderly patients with cardiovascular conditions, the use of cardiovascular medication is more challenging among older patients. Age-related changes in renal functions, hepatic blood flow, muscle mass and end-organ responsiveness can affect the efficacy of cardiovascular drugs. For example, older patients are more likely to develop orthostatic hypotension with the use of nitrates and α-adrenergic blockers due to reduced cardiovascular responses to catecholamine and the carotid sinus baroreceptor sensitivity (Fleg, 2008). Indeed, it is not uncommon that older patients present with multiple disease states concurrently. Moreover, polypharmacy, the use of four or more medications, is another major concern when prescribing cardiovascular medicine to older patients. Studies have shown more than 50% of older patients receive five or more prescription medicines for the treatment of hypertension, heart failure and diabetes (Fleg, Aronow, & Frishman, 2011; Jyrkkä, Vartiainen, Hartikainen, Sulkava, & Enlund, 2006). The higher number of medications used in older patients has considerably increased the possibility of both drug-drug interaction as well as drug-disease interaction, highlighting the importance of knowledge in age-related physiological changes and the need of a holistic approach in the use of cardiovascular drugs in elderly. The following section is an overview of drugs commonly used in elderly for cardiovascular diseases.

Blood Pressure-Lowering Drugs

The angiotensin converting enzyme inhibitor (ACEI) blocks the generation of the powerful vasoconstrictor angiotensin II (Ang II) both systemically and locally, reducing blood pressure without reflex stimulation of heart rate. It is one of the most frequently administered drugs in elderly, given the fact that it can influences three diseases (coronary artery disease, hypertension and diabetes) simultaneously. A meta-analysis of 109 studies has shown that ACEI are more effective than other antihypertensive agents in reducing left ventricle (LV) mass (Dahlöf, Pennert, & Hansson, 1992). Numerous clinical studies have demonstrated that ACEI reduces risk of cardiovascular events to a similar extent as other antihypertensive agents (Lennart Hansson et al., 1999). Another study showed that ACEI is more effective than diuretics in reducing cardiovascular events in elderly (Wing et al., 2003). Although ACEI has been recommended as the standard therapy for most elderly patient with significant LV systolic dysfunction with or without chronic heart failure (CHF), it is important to be aware of the possible deterioration of renal function, palpitations and cardiac rhythm disorder and hypotension when initiation ACEI treatment in elderly patients (Pfeffer et al., 1992; Yusuf et al., 1992). Hyperkalemia can also occur in elderly patients with renal insufficiency. Therefore, treatment with ACEI should be started at low dose after correction and titrated gradually to avoid overdiuresis and hypotension.

Angiotensin receptor I blocker (ARB) inhibits the effects of Ang II by blocking of the angiotensin receptor, thus exhibit very similar and comparable effects to ACEI in hypertension, diabetes, and CHF (Grossman, Messerli, & Neutel, 2000; Okereke & Messerli, 2001). It is noteworthy that ARB has fewer side-effects, more tolerable with minimal first-dose hypotension when comparing to ACEI (Elliott, 2000; Tadevosyan, MacLaughlin, & Karamyan, 2011). Hence, they have been considered as safer and a more superior option for elderly patient with type 2 diabetes mellitus, hypertension and CHF (Brenner et al., 2001; Lindholm et al., 2002).

β-blockers have been used to treat hypertension for decades and have been shown to be an effective anti-anginal agents in both young and elderly patients (Frishman, Chiu, Landzberg, & Weiss, 1998; Sica, 1999). In controlled clinical trials, β-blockers have been shown to reduce cardiovascular morbidity and mortality, particularly older hypertensive patients with myocardial infraction, angina pectoris, arrhythmias or hypertrophic cardiomyopathy (Chobanian et al., 2003; Sica, 1999; Teo, Yusuf, & Furberg, 1993). It is also worth to point out that despite some studies showing no or limited beneficial effects of β-blockers monotherapy in reducing the incidence of stroke, coronary events and total cardiovascular events, β-blockers could have a role in combination therapy (Dahlöf et al., 1991; L Hansson, 1990). When co-administrated with diuretics and ACEI, β-blockers significantly reduced mortality in older patients with CHF (Aronow, Ahn, & Kronzon, 1997, 2001; Flather et al., 2005). In some elderly patient, even a very small dose of β-blockers can induce disordered of atrioventricular conduction and severe bradycardia (Kubesova, Weber, Meluzinova, Bielakova, & Matejovsky, 2013). Moreover, the β-blockers should be used carefully in elderly CHF patient with chronic obstructive pulmonary disease (COPD) to avoid further deterioration of myocardium contractility and manifest heart failure. Finally, drug interaction should be considered when prescribing β-blockers to elderly patient (Frishman, et al., 1998).

Diuretics have been the mainstay for blood pressure management in elderly. They are commonly used due to their low cost and are generally well-tolerated. Serum electrolytes must be closely monitored when treating elderly with diuretics to prevent hypokalemia and hypomagnesemia which can lead to ventricular arrhythmias and/or digitalis toxicity (Franse et al., 2000). Also, hyponatremia is occurring more frequently in older patients under diuretics therapy and has been associated with fatigue, cognitive impairment, gait, falls and even increased mortality in elderly patients (Hoorn & Zietse, 2011; Kengne, Andres, Sattar, Melot, & Decaux, 2008; Liamis, Filippatos, Liontos, & Elisaf, 2016). Age-related impairment in renal function may reduce the efficacy of conventional doses of diuretics in elder patients. In several randomized controlled trials (RCTs), diuretics have been shown to reduce cardiovascular events when combined with ACEI or β-blockers in elderly patients (Beckett et al., 2008; Chobanian, et al., 2003). In addition, recent meta-analysis has demonstrated that diuretic antihypertensive drugs are associated with reduction in dementia risk in elderly (Tully, Hanon, Cosh, & Tzourio, 2016).

Lipid-Lowering Drugs

Dyslipidemia is a major risk factor for cardiovascular diseases in aging population. Total cholesterol and LDL levels are strongly correlated with fatal coronary heart disease across all age groups, including individuals aged over 65. The statins are the most popularly used lipid lowering drugs due to its effectiveness and good tolerance. Its effectiveness in lowering serum LDL as well as reduction in major coronary events and death has been demonstrated (Scandinavian Simvastatin Survival Study Group, 1994). Later study has shown that the effects in reducing both all-cause mortality in individual aged between 65-70 is two times greater than individuals younger than 65 (Miettinen et al., 1997). Similarly, a RCT study of 8,804 patients has demonstrated the reduction of LDL level by 34% in individual aged between 72-80 years, and the reduction of coronary heart disease death and nonfatal myocardial infraction (Shepherd, 2002). Many other studies have also reported similar results, highlighting the benefits of statins in reducing cardiovascular event in the elderly (Heart Protection Study Collaborative Group, 2002; Lewis et al., 1998). Although statins are generally considered well-tolerated and safe, side effects, including headache, insomnia, myalgia, rhabdomyolysis and dyspepsia, are more frequently observed in elderly patients. These side effects (Kevelaitiene & Slapikas, 2007)

Anticoagulants

Anticoagulants are commonly used to manage various cardiovascular conditions such as nonvalvular atrial fibrillation, venous thromboembolism, ischemic heart disease, stroke and mechanical heart valve. Given the fact that these conditions increase with advancing age, anticoagulants are one of the most frequently prescribed drugs used in the older population. For example, the prevalence of arterial fibrillation (AF) increased from less than 1% in individuals aged 50 and under to 10% in octogenarians. Stroke, caused by embolization of clots from atrium to the brain, is one of the major complications of AF in the older population. AF contributes to 23.5% of stroke in the patients over 80 years of age (Wolf, Abbott, & Kannel, 1991). Numerous clinical trials have demonstrated that anticoagulants prevent stroke in AF

(Bajorek, Magin, Hilmer, & Krass, 2014; Ford et al., 2007; Olsson & Halperin, 2005). When administrating anticoagulant to elderly patients, it is important to be aware of drug-drug interactions that can increase the risk of bleeding, because older patients tends to receive multiple medications. In addition, the anticoagulant response to certain anticoagulation agents such as warfarin increases with age.

THE POTENTIAL OF USING CHINESE HERBAL MEDICINE FOR HEALTH MAINTENANCE IN THE ELDERLY

In Hong Kong, from 2008 to 2012, there has been a 6-fold increase in the total number of chronic disease patients who reported using Chinese medicine regularly, both exclusively and together with Western medicine. To the public, CHM is considered to have milder pharmacological effects than Western medicine with fewer the side effects. For example, when facing communicable diseases such as flu or common cold, Western medicine is usually seen as the preferred first-line treatment. Also, CHM is sometimes considered as an "alternative" therapy when Western medicine fails (Lam, 2001). Interestingly, CHM has the advantages over some abstract complaints of mild symptoms that are not regarded as problematic by Western medicine practitioners. For example, elderly people may complain about "fungus-like substances" growing on the tongue or bitterness in the mouth. Apart from being poisoned or stimulated by certain kind of chemicals, such symptoms are hardly diagnosed by Western medicine practitioners. However, in TCM, these are very common "symptoms" indicating sub-optimal health, indicating "humidity" in the body and gastrointestinal tract upset. They can be treated by CHM formulae known as "dehumidifying tea" and "tea for relieving stagnancy". These formulae can be prescribed based on the overall health status of the patients, highlighting the fact that TCM practitioners treat their patients in a holistic and personalized approach, in contrast to Western medicine which manages sickness and diseases symptomatically.

Western medicine has been the standard for the treatment of infectious diseases. The discovery by Alexander Fleming has marked a milestone in the development of Western medicine, because antibiotics are selectively working on the disease-causing bacteria (Drago et al., 2016; Gruson et al., 2000). However, the use of antibiotics poses an evolutionary pressure to pathogens, and this can give rise to "super-pathogen" that are resistant to antibiotics (Davies & Davies, 2010). Elderly patients are the group of the main risk with methicillin-resistant *Staphylococcus aureus* (MRSA) infection (Y. Ge, 2014). On the other hand, mounting experimental evidence shows that Chinese herbal medicine can be effective in treating even infectious diseases. TCM is usually composed of very complicated components and antibiotic resistances is not easily developed towards numerous amounts of active ingredients. For anti-viral activities, CHM may be a better candidate for therapy because traditional anti-viral drugs have notorious side effects. Compared to Western medicine, TCM has the advantages of rich resources, low price and less adverse effects (Huang, Su, Feng, Liu, & Song, 2014). Elderly people, especially the Chinese ethnic groups, prefer taking TCM (Kong & Hsieh, 2012).

In addition, according to the WHO traditional medicine strategy, the cost to treat neck pain with physiotherapy or care provided by a general practitioner is more expensive and it is believed that many governments recognize the need to develop a cohesive and integrative approach, so that the TCM therapy can be provided in a safe, respectful, cost-efficient and effective manner (World Health Organization, 2014).

Research on the Use of Chinese Herbal Medicines in Cardiovascular Diseases

As mentioned previously, most of the drugs used in western medicine have well defined composition, chemical structure, pharmacological properties and mechanisms of actions. Although Western medicines have been shown to reduce cardiovascular mortality effectively, a substantial proportion of elderly still remains at high risk of cardiovascular events. The situation may be due to the fact that the majority of western cardiovascular medicines focus only on the management of the 'hard' clinical outcomes rather than the improvement of the quality of life, that might be of a greater concern for the elderly patients. Furthermore, it has been a major issue among the elderly for not adhering to prescription drugs, i.e. poor drug compliance, due to the increased adverse effects arising from polypharmacy, or use of multiple drugs (MacLaughlin et al., 2005).

In contrast, CHMs has been used for thousands of years in the management of diseases, maintenance of health and prolongation of life. Chinese medicine practitioners often adopt a holistic approach in treating patients, managing cardiovascular conditions through integrated care; nourishing and strengthening the body functions rather than focusing solely on relieving clinical symptoms. For example, hypertensive patients may receive CHM that "strengthens" heart, liver, spleen, lung or kidney according to TCM theory. Nonetheless, there are a large body of evidence suggesting that many CHMs and their active ingredients possess cardiovascular protective properties with minimal and few adverse reactions (Hong et al., 2009; Liu et al., 2014; Ravera et al., 2016). It comes no surprise that there has been a marked increase in the popularity of CHM in both the Western and Asian countries over the past few decades (Hao, et al., 2015; Karalliedde & Kappagoda, 2009). In Australia, over 65% of the population have used complementary and alternative medicine, including CHM, to alleviate chronic or recurrent conditions (Team, Canaway, & Manderson, 2011). In addition, herbal medicines have been approved to treat cardiovascular diseases in both Germany and Japan (Karalliedde & Kappagoda, 2009). There has also been an increasing trend of acceptance of CHM.

Numerous basic and clinical studies have demonstrated the beneficial effects of CHMs on cardiovascular diseases. A recent population-based retrospective study in Taiwan showed there was a 33% decreased risk of stokes among 1,049 type 2 diabetic patients that used CHMs (Lee et al., 2016). In a multi-centre, randomized, double-blind, placebo-controlled trial involving 4,870 Chinese patients with a history of myocardial infractions, *xuezhikang*, a partially purified extract of red yeast rice significantly decreased cardiovascular and all-cause mortality by 30% and 33% respectively. Moreover, the same study also showed that long term treatment of *xuezhikang* significantly lowered serum levels of total and LDL cholesterol and prevented the occurrence of coronary events in patients with a history of myocardial infraction (Lu et al., 2008). Many CHMs and their active components, such as *Coptis chinensis*, *Scutellaria baicalensis*, *Panax ginseng* and *Ganoderma lucidum*, have been shown to have anti-arrhythmic property (Hao, et al., 2015). In particular, *Scutellaria baicalensis* has also been shown to protect against myocardial infarction in a rat model (Chan et al., 2011).

In a randomized, double blind, placebo-controlled multi-centre trial, a 4-week treatment with *shensong-yangxin* significantly increased the heart rate in patients with atrioventricular block. More importantly, only minimal side effects were observed (0.8%) in the treated group (Liu, et al., 2014). These results highlighted the usefulness of CHMs in normalizing heart rhythm in patients with bradycardia, given the fact that almost all current clinical available western anti-arrhythmic drugs have notable adverse effects (Brignote, Auricchio, & Baron-Esquivias, 2013). It is interesting to note that in a prospective cohort study involving 13,655 diabetic patients, the rate of coronary artery disease admission of diabetic patients received CHMs is not significantly different from those receiving western medicine (Fang et al, 2015), suggesting that CHMs could have similar therapeutic effects as western medicine.

A pre-clinical study has demonstrated that *Panax notoginseng saponin* has more superior vascular protective effects than aspirin via the inhibition of platelet adhesion and apoptosis in both endothelial cells and platelets and downregulates the atherosclerosis-promoting genes (Wang et al., 2016; Chan et al., 2013). In addition, *Lingzhi* is also shown to decrease blood glucose level in animal model of type 2 diabetes (Seto et al., 2009). However, it is important to point out that, although there are mounting reports indicating the beneficial role of CHMs in cardiovascular managements, some reports have suggested otherwise. For example, Panahi et al. (2011) have failed to show any significant benefit of supplementation with *H. persicum* extract in patients with minimal coronary artery disease, despite several pharmacological studies have indicated that *H. persicum* could be important in the prevention of atherosclerosis and the promotion of cardiovascular health due to its anti-oxidative, anti-inflammatory and lipid-modifying properties (Firuzi et al., 2010; Hajhashemi, Sajjadi, & Heshmati, 2009; Panahi, Pishgoo, & Sahebkar, 2015). Moreover, many clinical trials on CHMs suffer from the shortcomings of small sample size, short follow-up period and diverse outcome results.

Incorporation of Chinese Herbal Medicine in the Modern Healthcare System

A national survey in China in 2004 reported 71.2% and 18.7% of patients preferred integrative medicine, i.e. TCM combined with Western medicine, and TCM respectively (Chen & Lu, 2006). Integrative medicine has been shown to have effects in alleviating clinical symptoms and in improving the quality of life in cardiovascular patients (Chu, Wang, Yao, & Li, 2010; Zhang et al, 2009). In a clinical study involving 108 unstable angina patients, 4 weeks of combined therapy of Yiqi Yangyin Decoction (YQYYD) and conventional medicine showed more significant improvement in clinical symptoms and quality of life when compared to patient received conventional treatment only (He et al., 2010). Similarly, another study showed that combined therapy of CHM Xinyue Capsule plus Composite Salvia Tablet with conventional medical treatment could markedly improve myocardial perfusion in acute myocardial infarction patients after revascularization (Li et al., 2009). These clinical studies highlight a great potential in incorporating Chinese Herbal Medicine in the Modern Healthcare System.

Historically, there is great abundance of written resources on TCM, and the training of Chinese medicine practitioners in Hong Kong was mostly carried out in a master-apprentice model. Since the early 20th centuries, TCM training become formalized and has been incorporated in the university education. Most TCM training in universities takes 6 years at the undergraduate entry, or 4 years at the graduate entry. Knowledges on TCM are usually delivered alongside with modern medical sciences, including anatomy, physiology, pharmacology and pathology, and internal medicine, complemented with clinical internship. Chinese medicine practitioners go through rigorous training both in theory and practice, and are required to have a working understanding of modern medical sciences and medicine.

In in Mainland China and Taiwan, there are universities offering integrated program of Bachelor of Chinese medicine, Bachelor of Medicine and Bachelor of Surgery, enabling graduates to be registered as both Chinese medicine practitioner and Western medical practitioner. In Hong Kong, Chinese medicine programs are offered by three public universities, namely the Chinese University of Hong Kong, the University of Hong Kong and the Hong Kong Baptist University. The curriculum at these institutions are designed as per the accreditation requirements of the Chinese Medicine Council of Hong Kong. The degree programs typically cover basic theories of Chinese medicine as well as specialist disciplines of

Chinese medicine including diagnostics, Chinese materia medica, Chinese medicinal formulary; internal medicine, external medicine, gynecology, pediatrics, orthopedics and traumatology, acupuncture and moxibustion. These contents are delivered alongside conventional biomedical sciences, providing the graduates the knowledge and skill set to bridge the gap between TCM and Western Medicine.

In Hong Kong, in order to become a registered Chinese Medicine Practitioner, one is required to sit for and pass the licensing examination conducted by the Chinese Medicine Practitioners Board of the Chinese Medicine Council of Hong Kong. According to section 61 of chapter 549 of *Chinese Medicine Ordinance 2000* (Hong Kong), an eligible candidate is a person who "satisfies the Practitioners Board that at the time of the application he has satisfactorily completed such undergraduate degree course of training in Chinese medicine practice or its equivalent as is approved by the Practitioners Board". This applies to candidates who completed undergraduate degree in Chinese Medicine in Hong Kong and other countries.

Potential Challenges of Chinese Herbal Medicine in Health Protection in Elderly

Difficulties in Defining the Mechanism of Action

The pharmacology of CHM is complicated and is difficult to be studied by conventional scientific methods. Moreover, the different complicated components in the Chinese herbal formula are difficult to be identified with. Some examples of herbs and their multi-functions are shown in Table 1.

TCM usually are not prescribed in a single herb form but in the form of a formulation. This makes it extremely difficult to analyse the combination of all ingredients and the net pharmacological effect. Like *Liu wei di huang wan* and *Shen qi wan*, the basic composition is the same. With the addition of new ingredients and alteration of the percentage of individual components, the medicinal effects may not be the same.

Liu wei di huang wan has multi-functions. In a clinical study, it was found that this formula may reduce the risk of diabetic ketoacidosis in patients with type 1 diabetes mellitus (Lien et al., 2016). On the other hand, *Shen qi wan* was reported to retard the progression of renal failure and alleviate flank pain or tenderness in urolithiasis patients (Lin et al, 2016).

Table 1. Five commonly used herbs in Chinese medicine and their multi-functions

English Name	Latin Name	Functions
Balloon flower root	*Platycodon grandiflorus*	Anti-bloating effects, relieve cough, reduce phlegm, relieve throat pain, anti-bleeding
Puffball Mushroom	*Lasiosphaera calvatia*	Anti-bleeding, smoothing burning throat
Sweet Wormwood herb	*Artemisiae Annuae herba*	Anti-malaria, breast cancer, antibacterial and antifungal activity
Capillary Wormwood Herb	*Artemisiae Scopariae*	Diuretic, excrete dampness and alleviate jaundice, clear heat and remove toxicity
Ginseng	*Panax ginseng*	Loss of appetite, weakness, vomiting, lack of "yang", lower cholesterol

Table 2. The ingredients of Liu wei di huang wan and Shen qi wan

Liu wei di huang wan (Six-Ingredient Rehmannia Pill)	Shen qi wan (Kidney Qi Pill)
shou di huang (*Rehmanniae Radix Praeparata*) 160g	shou di huang (*Rehmanniae Radix Praeparata*) 160g
shan zhu yu (*Corni Fructus*) 80g	shan zhu yu (*Corni Fructus*) 80g
mu dan pi (*Moutan Cortex*) 60g	mu dan pi (*Moutan Cortex*) 60g
shan yao (*Dioscoreae Rhizoma*) 80g	shan yao (*Dioscoreae Rhizoma*) 80g
ze xie (*Alismatis Rhizoma*) 60g	ze xie (*Alismatis Rhizoma*) 60g
fu ling (Poria) 60g	fu ling (Poria) 120g
	rou gui (Cinnamon) 20g
	fu zi (*Aconiti Radix Lateralis Praeparata*) 20g
	niu xi (*Achyranthis Bidentatae Radix*) 40g
	che qian zi (*Plantaginis Semen*) 40g

Quality and Safety of Chinese Medicinal Herbs

Though there are potential benefits of Chinese Herbal Medicine in health protection in elderly, people may not be aware of possible side effects of TCM (Hon et al., 2004). For example, an investigation has shown the samples of TCM being contaminated with microorganisms, pesticides and heavy metals (Melchart, Hager, Dai, & Weidenhammer, 2016), and may link to liver injury, and gastrointestinal upset. Moreover, although the Chinese government has implemented quality control systems such as the Good Agricultural Practice (GAP), Good Laboratory Practice (GLP), Good Manufacturing Practice (GMP) on the production of Chinese medicinal herbs, there are still rooms for improvement on the quality of TCM. (Xu & Yang, 2009).

In Hong Kong, the Chinese Medicine Council of Hong Kong was set up in accordance with the Chinese Medicine Ordinance (Cap. 549F) to rigorously regulate the sales and manufacturing of propriety Chinese medicines, as well as potent or toxic CHMs (Schedule 1). The safety, efficacy, quality as well as the dispensation and labeling of CHMs are assessed before the products can be registered and be available to the practitioners and consumers.

Herb-Drug Interactions

Stemming from the fact that it is not easy to define the pharmacology of Chinese herbal medicine, it is even more difficult to specifically identify the herb-drug interactions, as in Western medicinal preparations. With the raising popularity of CHM and the advances in CHM research, there are more cases and studies to link the adverse events to the unwanted herb-drug interactions. For example, there are quite a few herbs known to affect the efficacy of warfarin. The first example is ginseng (Lee et al., 2008). *Radix Puerariae lobatae* (Gegen) has also been shown to offset the anticoagulant effects of warfarin via accelerating the clearance of warfarin from human body (Ge, Zhang, & Zuo, 2016).

On the other hand, some herbs such as *Ephedrae herba* contains ephedrine, which itself is a stimulant and a chemical precursor for the production of methamphetamine (Liu et al, 1993). This herb is harmful to the cardiovascular disease patients in particular, as it can counteract the anti-hypertensives, increasing the blood pressure, and causing tachycardia and palpitation (Haller & Benowitz, 2000). Other known examples of herb-drug interaction include the effect of *Artemisia capillaris Thunb* on the metabolism of paracetamol, and excessive bleeding in co-administration of Ginkgo biloba and aspirin (Gardner et al, 2007). These adverse events highlight the practical and clinical importance of collaborative efforts between Western and Chinese medicine practitioners to design the medical treatment regime with the best outcomes for the patients.

It is worth to note that various counties have their own systems for reporting of adverse reaction, such as the China Food and Drug Administration (CFDA) in China and the Health Sciences Authority Adverse Event Monitoring Unit in Singapore. In Hong Kong, adverse drug reactions are governed by the Drug and Poison Information Bureau, established in 1987 and run by the Division of Clinical Pharmacology of the Chinese University of Hong Kong at Prince of Wales Hospital, its teaching hospital. It gives advice to health care professionals on the diagnosis and treatment of all forms of poisoning and adverse reactions to medicines, and on drug usage in general. It is staffed by nurses, pharmacists, junior physicians, and is backed up by an on-call consultant physician with a specialist interest in clinical pharmacology and toxicology. The bureau has access to various international databases with a listing of over 500,000 drugs, chemical entities and other items. The scope of its experience ranges from modern medicines, traditional Chinese and other remedies, to seafood and pesticide poisoning. All these monitoring systems play an important role to ensure patient and public safety and to serve as the basics for further researches on drug-herb and herb-herb reactions.

DISCUSSION

Over the last two decades, Chinese herbal medicine has been widely spread throughout the world. Its enormous therapeutic potentials have been accepted and well recognized, not only in the Asian population such as China, Taiwan, Hong Kong, Japan, Korea and Singapore, but in many non-Asian and Western counties, including Germany, Australia, Canada, United Kingdom and the United States. For example, a TCM hospital was opened in Germany in 1991 with TCM physicians from China to provide treatment according to traditional practice (Melchart et al., 1999). In Australia, the National Institute of Complementary Medicine at Western Sydney University was established by the Australian Federal and New South Wales State Governments in 2007, with a focus on Chinese medicine research and translation into practice.

In Hong Kong, despite the great influence from the British culture for over 100 years, the use of CHMs remains an important and integral part of the Hong Kong health care services and community culture in seeking medical therapies. Indeed, the government of Hong Kong has been keen to strengthen the status of Chinese medicine and integration of Chinese medicine and conventional medicine in Hong Kong and the setup of the Chinese Medicine Council of Hong Kong in September 1999. It is responsible for the implementation of regulatory measures for Chinese medicine and the registration of Chinese medicine practitioners in Hong Kong. Moreover, the vital role of Chinese medicine in Hong Kong was clearly highlighted in several recommendations in the Consultation Document on Healthcare Reform issued by the Hong Kong Food and Health Bureau in 2000. They include the incorporation of Chinese medicine into the public healthcare system, such as the provision of outpatient Chinese medicine service in the public sector in all the 18 districts, the introduction of Chinese medicine practice in selected public hospitals and to facilitate the development of the integration of western and Chinese medicines.

The emerging role of Chinese and integrative medicine in Hong Kong is clearly reflected by the establishment of the Chinese Medicine Research and Service Centre at the Queen Elizabeth Hospital in 2006 to provide out-patient consultations where patients can choose to receive Chinese or combined treatment of Chinese and Western medicine. Moreover, two integrated Chinese and Western medicine centers were established on the same year at Kwong Wah Hospital and Tung Wah Hospital to provide Chinese medicine service to in-patients in some selected clinical conditions. The Chinese Medicine Development Committee set up in 2013 to give recommendations to the government concerning the direction and long-term strategy of the future development of Chinese medicine in Hong Kong. The Hong Kong government proposed, in the 2014 Policy Address, to develop a Chinese medicine hospital to provide Chinese medicine inpatient services.

Despite the growing importance of Chinese medicine in Hong Kong, some of the major issues, such as the lack of robust Evidence-Based perspectives and safety issue, are hindering its acceptance and integration with conventional medicine. In 2000, a multidisciplinary team consisting of pharmacist, chemical pathologist, scientist and physician, was formed to provide advisory service on herbal safety to health professionals to address the safety issue CHMs. In addition, a recent report has suggested that Chinese medicine and inter-professional programs should be scaled up to all medical, nursing and allied health professional in Hong Kong in order to facilitate the interaction between Chinese Medicine Practitioners and conventional clinicians towards an inter-professional referral mechanisms (Brosnan, Chung, Zhang, & Adams, 2016). All in all, with the growing popularity, Evidence-Based researches and quality education of Chinese medicine in Hong Kong and around the world, CHMs will continue to extend their coverage for the treatment and management of chronic conditions (e.g. cardiovascular diseases) and impact the evolution of our healthcare system.

CONCLUSION

This chapter has provided a review of the important public health challenges in the aging society, and highlighted that the medical cost on chronic conditions like ischemic heart disease and stroke is likely to increase in the future. A brief review on conventional medications for the management of cardiovascular diseases was provided and their side-effects were discussed. Recent research on CHM has proven its effectiveness in managing chronic diseases, particularly cardiovascular diseases. The increasing public interest in CHM, in the midst of the potential adverse events due to inappropriate co-consumption of CHM with Western medicine, highlights the need for: (1) more research input, and (2) actual collaboration between Western and Chinese medicine practitioners to design the best medical treatment regime. The latter can be achieved right now, with more Chinese medicine practitioners being equipped with knowledge of Western medicine and modern medical sciences, and the administrative support from the Government.

REFERENCES

Aronow, W. S., Ahn, C., & Kronzon, I. (1997). Effect of propranolol versus no propranolol on total mortality plus nonfatal myocardial infarction in older patients with prior myocardial infarction, congestive heart failure, and left ventricular ejection fraction≥ 40% treated with diuretics plus angiotensin-converting enzyme inhibitors. *The American Journal of Cardiology*, *80*(2), 207–209. doi:10.1016/S0002-9149(97)00320-2 PMID:9230162

Aronow, W. S., Ahn, C., & Kronzon, I. (2001). Effect of beta blockers alone, of angiotensin-converting enzyme inhibitors alone, and of beta blockers plus angiotensin-converting enzyme inhibitors on new coronary events and on congestive heart failure in older persons with healed myocardial infarcts and asymptomatic left ventricular systolic dysfunction. *The American Journal of Cardiology*, *88*(11), 1298–1300. doi:10.1016/S0002-9149(01)02092-6 PMID:11728359

Bajorek, B., Magin, P., Hilmer, S., & Krass, I. (2014). A cluster-randomized controlled trial of a computerized antithrombotic risk assessment tool to optimize stroke prevention in general practice: A study protocol. *BMC Health Services Research*, *14*(1), 55. doi:10.1186/1472-6963-14-55 PMID:24507462

Beckett, N. S., Peters, R., Fletcher, A. E., Staessen, J. A., Liu, L., Dumitrascu, D., & Bulpitt, C. J. et al. (2008). Treatment of hypertension in patients 80 years of age or older. *The New England Journal of Medicine*, *358*(18), 1887–1898. doi:10.1056/NEJMoa0801369 PMID:18378519

Beckman, J. A., Creager, M. A., & Libby, P. (2002). Diabetes and atherosclerosis: Epidemiology, pathophysiology, and management. *Journal of the American Medical Association*, *287*(19), 2570–2581. doi:10.1001/jama.287.19.2570 PMID:12020339

Brenner, B. M., Cooper, M. E., de Zeeuw, D., Keane, W. F., Mitch, W. E., Parving, H.-H., & Shahinfar, S. et al. (2001). Effects of losartan on renal and cardiovascular outcomes in patients with type 2 diabetes and nephropathy. *The New England Journal of Medicine*, *345*(12), 861–869. doi:10.1056/NEJMoa011161 PMID:11565518

Brignote, M., Auricchio, A., & Baron-Esquivias, G. (2013). ESC guidelines on cardiac pacing and cardiac resynchronization therapy. *European Heart Journal*, *34*, 2281–2329. PMID:23801822

Brosnan, C., Chung, V. C., Zhang, A. L., & Adams, J. (2016). Regional Influences on Chinese Medicine Education: Comparing Australia and Hong Kong. *Evidence-Based Complementary and Alternative Medicine*. PMID:27379170

Census and Statistics Department Hong Kong SAR. (2014). *Thematic Household Survey Report No. 58*. Retrieved March 28, 2016, from http://www.statistics.gov.hk/pub/B11302582015XXXXB0100.pdf

Census and Statistics Department Hong Kong SAR. (2015). *Hong Kong Population Projections*. Retrieved March 28, 2016, from http://www.censtatd.gov.hk/hkstat/sub/sp190.jsp?productCode=B1120015

Census and Statistics Department Hong Kong SAR. (2016). *Table 002: Population by Age Group and Sex*. Retrieved March 28, 2016, from http://www.censtatd.gov.hk/hkstat/sub/sp150.jsp?tableID=002&ID=0&productType=8

Chan, E., Liu, X. X., Guo, D. J., Kwan, Y. W., Leung, G. P., Lee, S. M., & Chan, S. W. (2011). Extract of Scutellaria baicalensis Georgi root exerts protection against myocardial ischemia-reperfusion injury in rats. *The American Journal of Chinese Medicine*, *39*(04), 693–704. doi:10.1142/S0192415X11009135 PMID:21721150

Chan, G. H. H., Law, B. Y. K., Chu, J. M. T., Yue, K. K. M., Jiang, Z. H., Lau, C. W., & Wong, R. N. S. et al. (2013). Ginseng extracts restore high-glucose induced vascular dysfunctions by altering triglyceride metabolism and downregulation of atherosclerosis-related genes. *Evidence-Based Complementary and Alternative Medicine*, *2013*, 1–13. doi:10.1155/2013/812096 PMID:24194784

Chen, K. J., & Lu, A. P. (2006). Situation of integrative medicine in China: Results from a National Survey in 2004. *Chinese Journal of Integrative Medicine*, *12*(3), 161–165. doi:10.1007/BF02836514 PMID:17005073

Chinese Medicine Ordinance, Cap 549, Laws of Hong Kong (2000).

Chobanian, A. V., Bakris, G. L., Black, H. R., Cushman, W. C., Green, L. A., Izzo, J. L., et al. (2003). Seventh report of the joint national committee on prevention, detection, evaluation, and treatment of high blood pressure. *Hypertension, 42*(6), 1206-1252.

Chu, F. Y., Wang, J., Yao, K. W., & Li, Z. Z. (2010). Effect of Xuefu Zhuyu Capsule on the symptoms and signs and health-related quality of life in the unstable angina patients with blood-stasis syndrome after percutaneous coronary intervention: A randomized controlled trial. *Chinese Journal of Integrative Medicine*, *16*(5), 399–405. doi:10.1007/s11655-010-9999-9 PMID:20535581

Cressman, M. D., & Gifford, R. W. Jr. (1983). Hypertension and stroke. *Journal of the American College of Cardiology*, *1*(2), 521–527. doi:10.1016/S0735-1097(83)80083-7 PMID:6826961

Dahlöf, B., Hansson, L., Lindholm, L., Schersten, B., Ekbom, T., & Wester, P. (1991). Morbidity and mortality in the Swedish trial in old patients with hypertension (STOP-Hypertension). *Lancet*, *338*(8778), 1281–1285. doi:10.1016/0140-6736(91)92589-T PMID:1682683

Dahlöf, B., Pennert, K., & Hansson, L. (1992). Reversal of left ventricular hypertrophy in hypertensive patients a metaanalysis of 109 treatment studies. *American Journal of Hypertension*, *5*(2), 95–110. doi:10.1093/ajh/5.2.95 PMID:1532319

Davies, J., & Davies, D. (2010). Origins and evolution of antibiotic resistance. *Microbiology and Molecular Biology Reviews*, *74*(3), 417–433. doi:10.1128/MMBR.00016-10 PMID:20805405

Drago, F., Ciccarese, G., Broccolo, F., Sartoris, G., Stura, P., Esposito, S., & Parodi, A. et al. (2016). A new enhanced antibiotic treatment for early and late syphilis. *Journal of Global Antimicrobial Resistance*, *5*, 64–66. doi:10.1016/j.jgar.2015.12.006 PMID:27436469

Elliott, W. J. (2000). Therapeutic trials comparing angiotensin converting enzyme inhibitors and angiotensin II receptor blockers. *Current Hypertension Reports*, *2*(4), 402–411. doi:10.1007/s11906-000-0045-8 PMID:10981176

Fang, H. S., Liu, C. C., Jia, C. H., Chen, Y. H., & Li, C. Y. (2015). Risk of Developing Coronary Artery Disease in Patients with Type 2 Diabetes Receiving Traditional Chinese Medicine Therapy. *Journal of Alternative and Complementary Medicine (New York, N.Y.)*, *21*(10), 604–609. doi:10.1089/acm.2014.0079 PMID:26247098

Firuzi, O., Javidnia, K., Gholami, M., Soltani, M., & Miri, R. (2010). Antioxidant activity and total phenolic content of 24 Lamiaceae species growing in Iran. *Natural Product Communications, 5*(2), 261-264.

Flather, M. D., Shibata, M. C., Coats, A. J., Van Veldhuisen, D. J., Parkhomenko, A., & Borbola, J. (2005). Randomized trial to determine the effect of nebivolol on mortality and cardiovascular hospital admission in elderly patients with heart failure (SENIORS). *European Heart Journal*, *26*(3), 215–225. doi:10.1093/eurheartj/ehi115 PMID:15642700

Fleg, J. L. (2008). Improving Exercise Tolerance in Chronic Heart Failure. *Journal of the American College of Cardiology*, *51*(17), 1672–1674. doi:10.1016/j.jacc.2008.01.027 PMID:18436119

Fleg, J. L., Aronow, W. S., & Frishman, W. H. (2011). Cardiovascular drug therapy in the elderly: Benefits and challenges. *Nature Reviews. Cardiology*, *8*(1), 13–28. doi:10.1038/nrcardio.2010.162 PMID:20978470

Fleg, J. L., O'connor, F., Gerstenblith, G., Becker, L., Clulow, J., & Schulman, S. et al.. (1995). Impact of age on the cardiovascular response to dynamic upright exercise in healthy men and women. *Journal of Applied Physiology*, *78*(3), 890–900. PMID:7775334

Food and Health Bureau. (2016). *Life expectancy at birth.* Retrieved March 28, 2016, from http://www.fhb.gov.hk/statistics/en/statistics/life_expectancy.htm

Ford, G. A., Choy, A. M., Deedwania, P., Karalis, D. G., Lindholm, C.-J., Pluta, W., & Olsson, S. B. et al. (2007). Direct Thrombin Inhibition and Stroke Prevention in Elderly Patients With Atrial Fibrillation. *Stroke*, *38*(11), 2965–2971. doi:10.1161/STROKEAHA.107.488007 PMID:17885258

Franse, L. V., Pahor, M., Di Bari, M., Somes, G. W., Cushman, W. C., & Applegate, W. B. (2000). Hypokalemia associated with diuretic use and cardiovascular events in the Systolic Hypertension in the Elderly Program. *Hypertension*, *35*(5), 1025–1030. doi:10.1161/01.HYP.35.5.1025 PMID:10818057

Frishman, W. H., Chiu, R., Landzberg, B. R., & Weiss, M. (1998). Medical therapies for the prevention of restenosis after percutaneous coronary interventions. *Current Problems in Cardiology*, *23*(10), 533–635. doi:10.1016/S0146-2806(98)80002-9 PMID:9805205

Gardner, C. D., Zehnder, J. L., Rigby, A. J., Nicholus, J. R., & Farquhar, J. W. (2007). Effect of Ginkgo biloba (EGb 761) and aspirin on platelet aggregation and platelet function analysis among older adults at risk of cardiovascular disease: A randomized clinical trial. *Blood Coagulation & Fibrinolysis*, *18*(8), 787–793. doi:10.1097/MBC.0b013e3282f102b1 PMID:17982321

Ge, B., Zhang, Z., & Zuo, Z. (2016). Radix Puerariae lobatae (Gegen) suppresses the anticoagulation effect of warfarin: A pharmacokinetic and pharmacodynamics study. *Chinese Medicine*, *11*(1), 7. doi:10.1186/s13020-016-0078-9 PMID:26925159

Ge, Y. (2014). Interpretation of 'Expert consensus on methicillin-resistant Staphylococcus aureus infection prevention and control'. *Chinese Clinical Oncology*, *42*, 11–12.

Gordon, L. A., Morrison, E. Y., McGrowder, D. A., Young, R., Fraser, Y. T. P., Zamora, E. M., & Irving, R. R. et al. (2008). Effect of exercise therapy on lipid profile and oxidative stress indicators in patients with type 2 diabetes. *BMC Complementary and Alternative Medicine*, *8*(1), 21. doi:10.1186/1472-6882-8-21 PMID:18477407

Grossman, E., Messerli, F. H., & Neutel, J. M. (2000). Angiotensin II receptor blockers: Equal or preferred substitutes for ACE inhibitors? *Archives of Internal Medicine*, *160*(13), 1905–1911. doi:10.1001/archinte.160.13.1905 PMID:10888965

Gruson, D., Hilbert, G., Vargas, F., Valentino, R., Bebear, C., Allery, A., & Cardinaud, J. P. et al. (2000). Rotation and restricted use of antibiotics in a medical intensive care unit: Impact on the incidence of ventilator-associated pneumonia caused by antibiotic-resistant gram-negative bacteria. *American Journal of Respiratory and Critical Care Medicine*, *162*(3), 837–843. doi:10.1164/ajrccm.162.3.9905050 PMID:10988092

Hajhashemi, V., Sajjadi, S. E., & Heshmati, M. (2009). Anti-inflammatory and analgesic properties of Heracleum persicum essential oil and hydroalcoholic extract in animal models. *Journal of Ethnopharmacology*, *124*(3), 475–480. doi:10.1016/j.jep.2009.05.012 PMID:19467316

Haller, C. A., & Benowitz, N. L. (2000). Adverse cardiovascular and central nervous system events associated with dietary supplements containing ephedra alkaloids. *The New England Journal of Medicine*, *343*(25), 1833–1838. doi:10.1056/NEJM200012213432502 PMID:11117974

Hansson, L. (1990). How far should blood pressure be lowered? What is the importance of the J-curve phenomenon? *Giornale Italiano di Cardiologia*, *20*(1), 1. PMID:2184071

Hansson, L., Lindholm, L. H., Niskanen, L., Lanke, J., Hedner, T., Niklason, A., & Björck, J.-E. et al. (1999). Effect of angiotensin-converting-enzyme inhibition compared with conventional therapy on cardiovascular morbidity and mortality in hypertension: The Captopril Prevention Project (CAPPP) randomised trial. *Lancet*, *353*(9153), 611–616. doi:10.1016/S0140-6736(98)05012-0 PMID:10030325

Hao, P. P., Jiang, F., Chen, Y. G., Yang, J., Zhang, K., Zhang, M. X., & Zhang, Y. et al. (2015). Evidence for traditional Chinese medication to treat cardiovascular disease. *Nature Reviews. Cardiology*, *12*(6), 374–374. doi:10.1038/nrcardio.2014.177-c2 PMID:25917155

He, Q. Y., Wang, J., Zhang, Y. L., Tang, Y. L., Chu, F. Y., & Xiong, X. J. (2010). Effect of Yiqi Yangyin Decoction on the quality of life of patients with unstable angina pectoris. *Chinese Journal of Integrative Medicine*, *16*(1), 13–18. doi:10.1007/s11655-010-0013-3 PMID:20131030

Heart Protection Study Collaborative Group. (2002). MRC/BHF Heart Protection Study of cholesterol lowering with simvastatin in 20 536 high-risk individuals: A randomised placebocontrolled trial. *Lancet*, *360*(9326), 7–22. doi:10.1016/S0140-6736(02)09327-3 PMID:12114036

Hon, E. K., Lee, K., Tse, H. M., Lam, L. N., Tam, K. C., Chu, K. M., & Leung, T. F. et al. (2004). A survey of attitudes to Traditional Chinese Medicine in Hong Kong pharmacy students. *Complementary Therapies in Medicine*, *12*(1), 51–56. doi:10.1016/j.ctim.2003.12.002 PMID:15130573

Hong, S. J., Wan, J. B., Zhang, Y., Hu, G., Lin, H. C., Seto, S. W., & Lee, S. M.-Y. et al. (2009). Angiogenic effect of saponin extract from Panax notoginseng on HUVECs in vitro and zebrafish in vivo. *Phytotherapy Research*, *23*(5), 677–686. doi:10.1002/ptr.2705 PMID:19107746

Hoorn, E. J., & Zietse, R. (2011). Hyponatremia and mortality: How innocent is the bystander? *Clinical Journal of the American Society of Nephrology; CJASN*, *6*(5), 951–953. doi:10.2215/CJN.01210211 PMID:21493744

Huang, J., Su, D., Feng, Y., Liu, K., & Song, Y. (2014). Antiviral herbs-present and future. *Infectious Disorders-Drug Targets (Formerly Current Drug Targets-Infectious Disorders), 14*(1), 61-73.

International Diabetes Federation. (2015). *IDF Diabetes Atlas* (7th ed.). Retrieved March 28, 2016, from http://www.diabetesatlas.org/

Jyrkkä, J., Vartiainen, L., Hartikainen, S., Sulkava, R., & Enlund, H. (2006). Increasing use of medicines in elderly persons: A five-year follow-up of the Kuopio 75+ Study. *European Journal of Clinical Pharmacology*, *62*(2), 151–158. doi:10.1007/s00228-005-0079-6 PMID:16408226

Karalliedde, L. D., & Kappagoda, C. T. (2009). The challenge of traditional Chinese medicines for allopathic practitioners. *American Journal of Physiology. Heart and Circulatory Physiology*, *297*(6), H1967–H1969. doi:10.1152/ajpheart.00944.2009 PMID:19855052

Kengne, F. G., Andres, C., Sattar, L., Melot, C., & Decaux, G. (2008). Mild hyponatremia and risk of fracture in the ambulatory elderly. *QJM*, *101*(7), 583–588. doi:10.1093/qjmed/hcn061 PMID:18477645

Kevelaitiene, S., & Slapikas, R. (2007). A new approach to the treatment of dyslipidemia. *Medicina (Kaunas, Lithuania)*, *44*(5), 407–413. PMID:18541958

Kjeldsen, S. E., Julius, S., Hedner, T., & Hansson, L. (2001). Stroke is more common than myocardial infarction in hypertension: Analysis based on 11 major randomized intervention trials. *Blood Pressure*, *10*(4), 190–192. doi:10.1080/08037050152669684 PMID:11800055

Kong, H., & Hsieh, E. (2012). The social meanings of traditional Chinese medicine: Elderly Chinese immigrants health practice in the United States. *Journal of Immigrant and Minority Health*, *14*(5), 841–849. doi:10.1007/s10903-011-9558-2 PMID:22160808

Kubesova, H. M., Weber, P., Meluzinova, H., Bielakova, K., & Matejovsky, J. (2013). Benefits and pitfalls of cardiovascular medication in seniors. *Wiener Klinische Wochenschrift*, *125*(15-16), 425–436. doi:10.1007/s00508-013-0395-2 PMID:23846454

Kumar, V., Abbas, A. K., & Aster, J. C. (2013). *Robbins basic pathology*. Elsevier Health Sciences.

Lakatta, E. G. (2003). Arterial and cardiac aging: Major shareholders in cardiovascular disease enterprises. *Circulation*, *107*(3), 490–497. doi:10.1161/01.CIR.0000048894.99865.02 PMID:12551876

Lam, T. P. (2001). Strengths and weaknesses of traditional Chinese medicine and Western medicine in the eyes of some Hong Kong Chinese. *Journal of Epidemiology and Community Health*, *55*(10), 762–765. doi:10.1136/jech.55.10.762 PMID:11553662

Lee, A. L., Chen, B. C., Mou, C. H., Sun, M. F., & Yen, H. R. (2016). Association of traditional Chinese medicine therapy and the risk of vascular complications in patients with type II diabetes mellitus: A nationwide, retrospective, Taiwanese-registry, cohort study. *Medicine*, *95*(3), e2536. doi:10.1097/MD.0000000000002536 PMID:26817897

Lee, S. H., Ahn, Y. M., Ahn, S. Y., Doo, H. K., & Lee, B. C. (2008). Interaction between warfarin and Panax ginseng in ischemic stroke patients. *Journal of Alternative and Complementary Medicine (New York, N.Y.)*, *14*(6), 715–721. doi:10.1089/acm.2007.0799 PMID:18637764

Lee, V. W., Lam, Y. Y., Yuen, A. C., Cheung, S. Y., Yu, C.-M., & Yan, B. P. (2013). Direct medical cost of newly diagnosed stable coronary artery disease in Hong Kong. *Heart Asia*, *5*(1), 1–6. doi:10.1136/heartasia-2012-010168 PMID:27326062

Lewis, S. J., Moye, L. A., Sacks, F. M., Johnstone, D. E., Timmis, G., & Mitchell, J. et al.. (1998). Effect of pravastatin on cardiovascular events in older patients with myocardial infarction and cholesterol levels in the average range: Results of the Cholesterol and Recurrent Events (CARE) trial. *Annals of Internal Medicine*, *129*(9), 681–689. doi:10.7326/0003-4819-129-9-199811010-00002 PMID:9841599

Li, Y. Q., Jin, M., Qiu, S. L., Wang, P. L., Zhu, T. G., Wang, C. L., & Shi, D. Z. et al. (2009). Effect of Chinese drugs for supplementing Qi, nourishing yin and activating blood circulation on myocardial perfusion in patients with acute myocardial infarction after revascularization. *Chinese Journal of Integrative Medicine*, *15*(1), 19–25. doi:10.1007/s11655-009-0019-7 PMID:19271165

Liamis, G., Filippatos, T., Liontos, A., & Elisaf, M. (2016). Hyponatremia in patients with liver diseases: not just a cirrhosis-induced hemodynamic compromise. *Hepatology International, 10*(5), 762-772.

Lien, A. S. Y., Jiang, Y. D., Mou, C. H., Sun, M. F., Gau, B. S., & Yen, H. R. (2016). Integrative traditional Chinese medicine therapy reduces the risk of diabetic ketoacidosis in patients with type 1 diabetes mellitus. *Journal of Ethnopharmacology*, *191*, 324–330. doi:10.1016/j.jep.2016.06.051 PMID:27340102

Lin, P. H., Lin, S. K., Hsu, R. J., Cheng, K. C., & Liu, J. M. (2016). The Use and the Prescription Pattern of Traditional Chinese Medicine Among Urolithiasis Patients in Taiwan: A Population-Based Study. *Journal of Alternative and Complementary Medicine (New York, N.Y.)*, *22*(1), 88–95. doi:10.1089/acm.2015.0116 PMID:26359806

Lindholm, L. H., Ibsen, H., Dahlöf, B., Devereux, R. B., Beevers, G., de Faire, U., & Snapinn, S. et al. (2002). Cardiovascular morbidity and mortality in patients with diabetes in the Losartan Intervention For Endpoint reduction in hypertension study (LIFE): A randomised trial against atenolol. *Lancet*, *359*(9311), 1004–1010. doi:10.1016/S0140-6736(02)08090-X PMID:11937179

Liu, Y., Li, N., Jia, Z., Lu, F., & Pu, J. (2014). Chinese medicine shensongyangxin is effective for patients with bradycardia: Results of a randomized, double-blind, placebo-controlled multicenter trial. *Evidence-Based Complementary and Alternative Medicine*. PMID:24527049

Liu, Y. M., Sheu, S. J., Chiou, S. H., Chang, H. C., & Chen, Y. P. (1993). A comparative study of commercial samples of Ephedrae Herba. *Planta Medica*, *59*(04), 376–378. doi:10.1055/s-2006-959706 PMID:17235993

Lu, Z., Kou, W., Du, B., Wu, Y., Zhao, S., Brusco, O. A., & Capuzzi, D. M. et al. (2008). Effect of Xuezhikang, an extract from red yeast Chinese rice, on coronary events in a Chinese population with previous myocardial infarction. *The American Journal of Cardiology*, *101*(12), 1689–1693. doi:10.1016/j.amjcard.2008.02.056 PMID:18549841

MacLaughlin, E. J., Raehl, C. L., Treadway, A. K., Sterling, T. L., Zoller, D. P., & Bond, C. A. (2005). Assessing medication adherence in the elderly. *Drugs & Aging*, *22*(3), 231–255. doi:10.2165/00002512-200522030-00005 PMID:15813656

McGill, H. C., McMahan, C. A., Herderick, E. E., Malcom, G. T., Tracy, R. E., & Strong, J. P. et al.. (2000). Origin of atherosclerosis in childhood and adolescence. *The American Journal of Clinical Nutrition*, *72*(5), 1307s–1315s. PMID:11063473

Melchart, D., Hager, S., Dai, J., & Weidenhammer, W. (2016). Quality control and complication screening programme of Chinese medicinal drugs at the first German hospital of traditional Chinese medicine-a retrospective analysis. *Forschende Komplementärmedizin/Research in Complementary Medicine*, *23*(Suppl. 2), 21-28.

Melchart, D., Linde, K., Weidenhammer, W., Hager, S., Liao, J., Bauer, R., & Wagner, H. (1999). Use of traditional drugs in a hospital of Chinese medicine in Germany. *Pharmacoepidemiology and Drug Safety*, *8*(2), 115–120. doi:10.1002/(SICI)1099-1557(199903/04)8:2<115::AID-PDS412>3.0.CO;2-I PMID:15073936

Miettinen, T. A., Pyörälä, K., Olsson, A. G., Musliner, T. A., Cook, T. J., Faergeman, O., & Group, S. S. S. et al. (1997). Cholesterol-lowering therapy in women and elderly patients with myocardial infarction or angina pectoris. *Circulation*, *96*(12), 4211–4218. doi:10.1161/01.CIR.96.12.4211 PMID:9416884

Okereke, C. E., & Messerli, F. H. (2001). Efficacy and safety of angiotensin II receptor blockers in elderly patients with mild to moderate hypertension. *The American Journal of Geriatric Cardiology*, *10*(1), 42–49. doi:10.1111/j.1076-7460.2001.90855.x PMID:11413935

Olsson, S. B., & Halperin, J. L. (2005). Prevention of stroke in patients with atrial fibrillation. *Seminars in Vascular Medicine*, *5*(03), 285–292. doi:10.1055/s-2005-916168 PMID:16123916

Panahi, Y., Pishgoo, B., Beiraghdar, F., Araghi, Z. M., Sahebkar, A., & Abolhasani, E. (2011). Results of a randomized, open-label, clinical trial investigating the effects of supplementation with Heracleum persicum extract as an adjunctive therapy for dyslipidemia. *TheScientificWorldJournal*, *11*, 592–601. doi:10.1100/tsw.2011.43 PMID:21403978

Panahi, Y., Pishgoo, B., & Sahebkar, A. (2015). Angiographic findings after supplementation with Heracleum persicum extract: Results of a randomized controlled trial. *Heart Views: The Official Journal of the Gulf Heart Association*, *16*(3), 85. doi:10.4103/1995-705X.164462 PMID:27326348

Pfeffer, M. A., Braunwald, E., Moyé, L. A., Basta, L., Brown, E. J. Jr, Cuddy, T. E., & Hawkins, C. M. et al. (1992). Effect of captopril on mortality and morbidity in patients with left ventricular dysfunction after myocardial infarction: Results of the Survival and Ventricular Enlargement Trial. *The New England Journal of Medicine*, *327*(10), 669–677. doi:10.1056/NEJM199209033271001 PMID:1386652

Prabhakaran, B., Dowling, E. A., Branch, J. D., Swain, D. P., & Leutholtz, B. C. (1999). Effect of 14 weeks of resistance training on lipid profile and body fat percentage in premenopausal women. *British Journal of Sports Medicine*, *33*(3), 190–195. doi:10.1136/bjsm.33.3.190 PMID:10378072

Ravera, A., Carubelli, V., Sciatti, E., Bonadei, I., Gorga, E., Cani, D., & Lombardi, C. et al. (2016). Nutrition and cardiovascular disease: Finding the perfect recipe for cardiovascular health. *Nutrients*, *8*(6), 363. doi:10.3390/nu8060363 PMID:27314382

Scandinavian Simvastatin Survival Study Group. (1994). Randomised trial of cholesterol lowering in 4444 patients with coronary heart disease: The Scandinavian Simvastatin Survival Study (4S). *Lancet*, *344*(8934), 1383–1389. PMID:7968073

Seto, S., Lam, T., Tam, H., Au, A., Chan, S., Wu, J., & Kwan, Y. W. et al. (2009). Novel hypoglycemic effects of Ganoderma lucidum water-extract in obese/diabetic (+ db/+ db) mice. *Phytomedicine*, *16*(5), 426–436. doi:10.1016/j.phymed.2008.10.004 PMID:19109000

Shah, A. B., Morrissey, R. P., Baraghoush, A., Bharadwaj, P., Phan, A., & Hamilton, M. et al.. (2012). Failing the failing heart: A review of palliative care in heart failure. *Reviews in Cardiovascular Medicine*, *14*(1), 41–48. PMID:23651985

Shepherd, J. (2002). Resource management in prevention of coronary heart disease: Optimising prescription of lipid-lowering drugs. *Lancet*, *359*(9325), 2271–2273. doi:10.1016/S0140-6736(02)09299-1 PMID:12103306

Sica, D. A. (1999). Old antihypertensive agents-diuretics and β-Blockers: Do we know how and in whom they lower blood pressure? *Current Hypertension Reports*, *1*(4), 296–304. doi:10.1007/s11906-999-0037-2 PMID:10981081

Špinar, J. (2012). Hypertension and ischemic heart disease. *Cor et Vasa, 54*(6), e433-e438.

Stern, S., Behar, S., & Gottlieb, S. (2003). Aging and diseases of the heart. *Circulation*, *108*(14), e99–e101. doi:10.1161/01.CIR.0000086898.96021.B9 PMID:14530186

Susic, D., & Frohlich, E. D. (2008). The aging hypertensive heart: A brief update. *Nature Clinical Practice. Cardiovascular Medicine*, *5*(2), 104–110. doi:10.1038/ncpcardio1091 PMID:18223542

Tadevosyan, A., MacLaughlin, E. J., & Karamyan, V. T. (2011). Angiotensin II type 1 receptor antagonists in the treatment of hypertension in elderly patients: focus on patient outcomes. *Patient Related Outcome Measures, 2*, 27.

Team, V., Canaway, R., & Manderson, L. (2011). Integration of complementary and alternative medicine information and advice in chronic disease management guidelines. *Australian Journal of Primary Health*, *17*(2), 142–149. doi:10.1071/PY10013 PMID:21645469

Teo, K. K., Yusuf, S., & Furberg, C. D. (1993). Effects of prophylactic antiarrhythmic drug therapy in acute myocardial infarction: An overview of results from randomized controlled trials. *Journal of the American Medical Association*, *270*(13), 1589–1595. doi:10.1001/jama.1993.03510130095038 PMID:8371471

Tully, P. J., Hanon, O., Cosh, S., & Tzourio, C. (2016). Diuretic antihypertensive drugs and incident dementia risk: A systematic review, meta-analysis and meta-regression of prospective studies. *Journal of Hypertension*, *34*(6), 1027–1035. doi:10.1097/HJH.0000000000000868 PMID:26886565

Wang, M. M., Xue, M., Xu, Y. G., Miao, Y., Kou, N., Yang, L., & Shi, D. et al. (2016). Panax notoginseng saponin is superior to aspirin in inhibiting platelet adhesion to injured endothelial cells through COX pathway in vitro. *Thrombosis Research*, *141*, 146–152. doi:10.1016/j.thromres.2016.03.022 PMID:27043068

Wing, L. M., Reid, C. M., Ryan, P., Beilin, L. J., Brown, M. A., Jennings, G. L., & West, M. J. et al. (2003). A comparison of outcomes with angiotensin-converting–enzyme inhibitors and diuretics for hypertension in the elderly. *The New England Journal of Medicine*, *348*(7), 583–592. doi:10.1056/NEJMoa021716 PMID:12584366

Wolf, P. A., Abbott, R. D., & Kannel, W. B. (1991). Atrial fibrillation as an independent risk factor for stroke: The Framingham Study. *Stroke*, *22*(8), 983–988. doi:10.1161/01.STR.22.8.983 PMID:1866765

Woo, K. S., Chook, P., Raitakari, O. T., McQuillan, B., Feng, J. Z., & Celermajer, D. S. (1999). Westernization of Chinese adults and increased subclinical atherosclerosis. *Arteriosclerosis, Thrombosis, and Vascular Biology*, *19*(10), 2487–2493. doi:10.1161/01.ATV.19.10.2487 PMID:10521379

World Health Organization. (2014). *WHO traditional medicine strategy: 2014-2023*. Retrieved July 14, 2016, from http://www.who.int/medicines/publications/traditional/trm_strategy14_23/en/

Yarnell, J., Patterson, C., Sweetnam, P., Thomas, H., Bainton, D., Elwood, P. C., & Miller, N. E. et al. (2001). Do total and high density lipoprotein cholesterol and triglycerides act independently in the prediction of ischemic heart disease? *Arteriosclerosis, Thrombosis, and Vascular Biology*, *21*(8), 1340–1345. doi:10.1161/hq0801.093505 PMID:11498463

Yusuf, S., Pepine, C. J., Garces, C., Pouleur, H., Rousseau, M., Salem, D., & Pitt, B. et al. (1992). Effect of enalapril on myocardial infarction and unstable angina in patients with low ejection fractions. *Lancet*, *340*(8829), 1173–1178. doi:10.1016/0140-6736(92)92889-N PMID:1359258

Zhang, Y. C., Chen, R. M., Lu, B. J., Zhao, M. H., & Rong, Y. Z. (2009). Influence of Shengmai Capsule on recovery of living capacity in patients after myocardial infarction. *Chinese Journal of Integrative Medicine*, *15*(5), 333–336. doi:10.1007/s11655-009-0333-3 PMID:19802535

KEY TERMS AND DEFINITIONS

Angina Pectoris: Also known as “angina”, it is caused by insufficient blood flow to heart muscles, and often it presents as chest pain, feel of pressure or squeezing.

Anticoagulants: They are medicines that help prevent or remove blood clots.

Arrhythmia: It occurs when there are changes in the normal sequence of electrical impulses within the heart. This causes changes in the heart rhythm, either by beating too fast, too slowly or irregularly.

Atherosclerosis: The accumulation of fats, cholesterol and pro-inflammatory white blood cells within the artery wall, leading to a formation of plaques. It causes obstruction of blood flow and the hardening of blood vessels.

Cardiomyopathy: It refers to the malfunctioning of heart muscle which causes insufficient supply of blood to the rest of the body. It presents as breathlessness, tiredness and swelling in legs and/or abdomen.

Dyslipidemia: An abnormal level of blood lipids, and in developed countries, it often presents as elevated blood triglycerides and/or cholesterol.

Hypertension: High blood pressure, usually defined as blood pressure above 140/90.

Myocardial Infarction: A condition that underlies heart attack. It is caused by an obstruction of coronary artery which supplies blood to the heart muscle, which leads to death of a portion of the heart muscle.

Nutraceuticals: Products derived from food sources that are recognized to provide health benefits in addition to the nutritional value.

Chapter 18
Eating Habits of Young Persons for Healthy Aging:
An Exploratory Study Involving University Students in Hong Kong

Simon T. Cheung
The Hong Kong Polytechnic University, Hong Kong

Susan Dawkes
Edinburgh Napier University, UK

ABSTRACT

Fruits and vegetables are important parts of healthy eating and they provide excellent sources of vitamins, minerals, and dietary fiber in our diet. Those who consume fruits and vegetables regularly have a reduced risk of many chronic diseases. According to the WHO, inadequate consumption of fruits and vegetables may have contributed to as much as 14% of gastrointestinal cancer deaths and 11% of deaths resulted from ischemic heart disease worldwide. Since 2011, Hong Kong has been promoting a "2 Plus 3 a day" diet campaign aiming to raise the general public's awareness on consuming a minimum of 2 portions of fruits and 3 portions of vegetables a day. However, recent statistics showed that nearly 81% of people aged 18 – 64 failed to meet this requirement. This paper focuses on investigating the determinants of fruits and vegetables consumption behavior among university students in Hong Kong.

INTRODUCTION

Ageing has become an urgent socioeconomic issue around the world in the last decade. In less than 15 years from now, researchers estimate that the number of people aged 65 years and over in the global population will increase to more than one billion, meaning that there will be one elderly person for every eight people. In Hong Kong, the population of people aged 65 years and over is projected to rise markedly from 13% in 2011 to 30% in 2041. Correspondingly, the median age would rise from 41.7 in 2011 to 49.9 in 2041. The changing age structure of the projected population can also be reflected in

DOI: 10.4018/978-1-5225-2633-9.ch018

the overall dependency ratio which is defined as the number persons aged 15 and below, and those aged 65 and over per 1000 persons aged 15 – 64. The ratio is projected to rise from 333 in 2011 to 645 in 2041 (Census and Statistics Department, 2012). This rapid ageing tendency will not only change family and workforces structures, increase the burden on the productive part of the population to maintain the upbringing of economically dependent people, but also result in increased demand for social security matters such as pensions, housing, and healthcare. This increased demand will in turn lead to higher public healthcare expenditures. Nonetheless, a healthy lifestyle that consists of multiple healthy behaviours such as adopting a healthy diet with high intakes of fruits and vegetables, exercising regularly, avoid drinking alcohol and smoking, can play a significant role in healthy and active ageing, reducing the overall demand for healthcare services (Glanz, 2008).

As people age, their health deteriorates and the risk of contracting diseases increases correspondingly. Chronic conditions affect a significant proportion of society and, although they are commonly associated with older people, the prevalence of them is increasing in all age groups (Conn, 2011). A recent cross-sectional study found that over 42% of Scots living in the United Kingdom had one or more co-morbidity with almost a quarter of those studied being classed as 'multi-morbid' (>2 co-morbidities) (Barnett et al., 2012). Around 70% of healthcare expenditure in the United Kingdom and Australia is spent on providing care for people with chronic conditions and the elderly population account for a significant proportion of this (College of Medicine, 2013). As the global population ages, the prevalence of people with chronic conditions is set to increase. A healthy lifestyle can also enhance individuals' perceptions of being healthy, and have an impact on mortality and morbidity as a result (Mossey, & Shapiro, 1982). Hence, promoting healthy behaviours and forming healthy lifestyles would be a sound investment from the health policy makers' perspective.

In this chapter, the perceptions and dietary habits of university students and how this may impact on their social responsibility in promoting health, will be explored, and also the long-term consequences of poor fruit and vegetable intake will be discussed. Instead of providing guidelines and suggestions, it is hoped that this chapter will not only provide new perspectives to the role higher education plays with regard health promotion and education, but it also aims at generating reflection and discussion among readers on the topic of health promotion.

THE CASE OF HONG KONG

The Hong Kong health system has often been admired by others for its ability in providing some of the best vital statistics when compared to other developed countries. In 2015, the average life expectancy at birth in Hong Kong was 87.3 for women and 81.2 for men, being one of the highest in the world; while the infant mortality rate in Hong Kong was 2 per 1,000 live births, being one of the lowest in the world (Food and Health Bureau, 2016). Healthcare services are relatively affordable in Hong Kong in which all of its citizens are eligible to receive care from public hospitals and clinics at a heavily subsidized rate.

In spite of these strengths and a currently well-endowed service provision ($ 57 billion HKD in 2016-17), the Hong Kong health system is facing challenges with an increasing demand for services driven by an over-dependence on acute care, changing patient culture and most important of all, an ageing population. According to some of the recent projections by Chung et al. (2009), the population of Hong Kong is ageing much more rapidly than previously expected. Other statistics predicted that population ageing in Hong Kong is expected to be most rapid in the coming two decades with the proportion of population over 65 years old reaching 23% in 2024 and 30% in 2034 (Census and Statistics Department, 2015). The speed and magnitude of population ageing is bound to have significant repercussions on the financing, and delivery systems of health and long-term care (Yuen, 2014). Various efforts such as the proposal of the Health Protection Scheme (HSP), the Voluntary Health Insurance Scheme (VHIS) or various public hospital redevelopment projects were made by the Government in attempt to provide sustainable solutions to the ageing population. Besides these short-term efforts, it is worthwhile to do some long-term planning on how we can approach the issue more proactively. As the conventional wisdom goes "prevention is better than cure". If we were able to engage the young population now in adopting healthy lifestyles, then healthy ageing may become possible for them in the future.

Many longitudinal studies suggest that healthy behaviours formed at a younger age are much better carried forward to later life. Even though it is never too late to change behaviour, it would be preferable to have a healthy diet and be physically active from an early age in order to promote optimal growth and development adulthood, and this applies to cases of consuming sufficient fruits and vegetables (McAleese, & Rankin, 2007). In a recent study carried out by Gooding et. al (2015), it was shown that adults who reach middle age with ideal blood pressure, cholesterol, and blood glucose level (i.e. the ideal cardiovascular health [CVH] profile) and without cardiovascular disease (CVD) enjoy exceedingly long life spans in good health. Studies have shown that even the adoption of healthy lifestyles at mid-age from 45 to 59 years old would help to reduce the incidence of chronic diseases such as diabetes and, cancer, and vascular diseases in an old age of 75 to 89 years (Elwood et. al., 2013). Other studies have also confirmed that people who exhibit greater numbers of health behaviours including a healthy diet that is rich in fruits and vegetables, being physically active, and non-smoking in adolescence and young adulthood, are more likely to reach later adulthood with lower blood pressure, cholesterol, and blood glucose levels and lower favorable intermediate markers of CVD (Laitinen et. al., 2012; Liu et. al., 2012; Spring et. al., 2014). Healthy diets and physical activities are well known lifestyle factors important for healthy ageing. It is universal knowledge that healthy diets consist of sufficient intake of fruits and vegetables as they provide excellent sources of vitamins, minerals, and dietary fiber.

Those who consume fruits and vegetables regularly have a reduced risk of many chronic diseases. According to the World Health Organisation (WHO), inadequate consumption of fruits and vegetables may have contributed to as much as 14% of gastrointestinal cancer deaths and 11% of deaths resulted from ischemic heart disease worldwide. Higher risk of all-cause mortality is associated with insufficient intake of fruits and vegetables (Wang et. al 2014; WHO, 2015). Therefore, in order to better understand the current healthy behaviours of young adults in Hong Kong, it would be appropriate to first explore their current habits of fruits and vegetables consumption. Since 2011, the Hong Kong Department of Health has been promoting a "2 Plus 3 a day" diet campaign aiming to raise the general public's awareness on consuming a minimum of 2 portions of fruits and 3 portions of vegetables a day. However, recent statistics showed that nearly 81% of people aged 18 – 64 failed to meet this requirement. It is evident that adequate consumption of fruits and vegetables have many health benefits, however, the underlying determinants affecting people's consumption of fruits and vegetable are much less investigated (Department of Health, 2016).

Research Design

Cross sectional surveys were conducted in person from mid-October to mid-November, 2015 and a total of 600 random subjects were selected from different universities in Hong Kong. It was hoped that the findings of the research could provide some insights on the current fruits and vegetables consumption among young adults. A review of the literature showed that various factors including socio-demographic factors such as age, gender, income, personal factors such as taste preferences, and family factors such as parental intake and availability and accessibility to fruits and vegetables, all played different roles in affecting the consumption behaviours (Blanchette, & Brug, 2005; Rasmussen et al., 2006). In addition, parenting styles were also thought to play a role in a child's eating behaviour as indicated in some studies (Fisher et al., 2002). Due to a limitation in time and recourses, the study mainly focused on some of the determinants including gender, preferences, knowledge, parental intakes, home availability, time costs, and price as it was perceived that these important data would provide meaningful insight for educators to potentially develop health promotional programmes that are practical to changing the consumption behaviours amongst students.

Results

In terms of sample size, a total of 600 university students responded to the questionnaires with no exclusion of participants. Table 1 summarized the demographic data of participants in this study: 260 (43.3%) participants were males and 340 (56.7%) were females; for the three faculties, 226 (37.7%) participants were grouped into Sciences, 261 (43.5%) participants were Arts, and 113 (18.8%) were Commerce.

Table 1. Demographic data of university students; Consumption behavior of university students (n = 600) on daily consumption frequency and amount of fruits and vegetables were categorized by gender and faculty. 14 major disciplines were induced into 3 faculties: Sciences, Arts and Commerce

Demographic Perception / Measurements	Gender		Faculty		
	Male	Female	Sciences	Arts	Commerce
n (% of Total)	260 (43.3)	340 (56.7)	226 (37.7)	261 (43.5)	113 (18.8)
Frequency[a]					
< 1 time/day	9 (3.5)	6 (1.8)	6 (2.7)	9 (3.4)	0 (0)
1 time/day	124 (47.7)	165 (48.5)	103 (45.6)	129 (49.4)	57 (50.4)
2 times/day	79 (30.4)	129 (37.9)	80 (35.4)	87 (33.3)	41 (36.3)
3 times/day	23 (8.8)	30 (8.8)	16 (7.1)	24 (9.2)	13 (11.5)
4 times/day	10 (3.8)	3 (0.9)	5 (2.2)	8 (3.1)	0 (0)
≥ 5 times/day	15 (5.8)	7 (2.1)	16 (7.1)	4 (1.5)	2 (1.8)
Amount[b]					
< 1 Portion/day	16 (6.2)	19 (5.6)	13 (5.8)	19 (7.3)	3 (2.7)
1-4 Portions/day	202 (77.7)	273 (80.3)	181 (80.1)	196 (75.1)	98 (86.7)
5-7 Portions/day	40 (15.4)	46 (13.5)	32 (14.2)	42 (10.6)	12 (10.6)
> 7 Portions/day	2 (0.8)	2 (0.6)	0 (0)	4 (1.5)	0 (0)

[a] There are differences in between gender and frequency (χ^2 = 15.65, P < .01), as well as faculty and frequency (χ^2 = 21.25, P < .05)

[b] There are no differences in between gender and amount (χ^2 = 0.63, P > .05), as well as faculty and amount (χ^2 =11.13, P > .05)

Consumption Behavior

In terms of consumption behaviour, Table 1 also summarized the consumption behaviors of participants. Data analysis by 2 x 6χ2 related gender and frequency [χ2 (5, N = 600) = 15.65, P < .01, C = .16], 3 x 6χ2 related faculty and frequency [χ2 (10, N = 600) = 21.25, P < .05, C = .19]. Consumption frequency of fruits and vegetables for all variances in gender and faculty were mostly once per day (more than 45%), followed by twice per day (more than 30%). Consumption amount of fruits and vegetables for all groups in gender and faculty were mostly less than 5 portions per day (more than 80%). In fact, observed frequencies in consumption amount has no meaning difference among genders [χ2 (3, N = 600) = .633, P > .05, C = .03] or faculties [χ2 (6, N = 600) = 11.13, P > .05, C = .14].

Perception and Action

According to an estimated consumption of fruits and vegetables, participants gave their perceptions on whether they had consumed enough fruits and vegetables (Table 2). In general, most of the participants perceived that they had consumed enough amounts of fruits and vegetables [χ2 (3, N = 600) = .72.89, P < .01, C = .33]. Only 6 (2.1%) participants had a consumption amount of less than 1 portion daily, 200 (70.7%) participants reported 1 to 4 portions daily, 75 (26.5%) participants reported consuming 5 to 7 portions daily and 2 (0.7%) more than 7 portions daily. Of those who perceived that they consumed inadequate amount of fruits and vegetables, 29 (9.1%) participants reported consuming less than 1 portion daily, 275 (86.8%) participants reported 1 to 4 portions daily, while 11 (3.5%) participants reported consumption to be 5 to 7 portions daily, and 2 (0.6%) more than 7 portions daily.

Table 2. Perceptions of university students (n = 600) on their sufficient consumption of fruits and vegetables, compared to actions on the consumption amount. These are tabulated into gender and faculty to analyze.

Demographic / Perception / Measurements	Gender				Faculty						Total	
	Male[b]		Female[c]		Sciences[d]		Arts[e]		Commerce[f]			
	Yes	No	Yes	No	Yes	No	Yes	No	Yes	No	Yes	No
n [a] (% of Total)	135 (51.9)	125 (48.1)	148 (43.5)	192 (56.5)	105 (46.5)	121 (53.5)	133 (51.0)	128 (49.0)	45 (39.8)	68 (60.2)	283 (47.2)	317 (52.8)
Amount												
< 1 Portion/day	4 (3.0)	12 (9.6)	2 (1.4)	17 (8.9)	3 (2.9)	10 (8.3)	3 (2.3)	16 (12.5)	0 (0)	3 (4.4)	6 (2.1)	29 (9.1)
1-4 Portions/day	99 (73.3)	103 (82.4)	101 (68.2)	172 (89.6)	77 (73.3)	104 (86)	88 (66.2)	108 (84.4)	35 (77.8)	63 (92.6)	200 (70.7)	275 (86.8)
5-7 Portions/day	32 (23.7)	8 (6.4)	4 (29.1)	3 (1.6)	25 (23.8)	7 (5.8)	40 (30.1)	2 (1.6)	10 (22.2)	2 (2.9)	75 (26.5)	11 (3.5)
> 7 Portions/day	0 (0)	2 (1.6)	2 (1.4)	0 (0)	0 (0)	0 (0)	2 (1.5)	2 (1.6)	0 (0)	0 (0)	2 (0.7)	2 (0.6)

[a] There are differences in between perception and action (χ^2 = 72.89, P < .01) in general
[b] There are differences in between perception of males and consumption amount (χ^2 = 20.12, P < .01)
[c] There are differences in between perception of females and consumption amount (χ^2 = 62.44, P < .01)
[d] There are differences in between perception of students in Sciences and consumption amount (χ^2 = 16.87, P < .01)
[e] There are differences in between perception of students in Arts and consumption amount (χ^2 = 45.24, P < .01)
[f] There are differences in between perception of students in Commerce and consumption amount (χ^2 = 12.16, P < .01)

Likelihood of Consumption

The major determinant for university students in Hong Kong to consume fruits and vegetables was related to the health beliefs associated with fruits and vegetables, followed by factors such as taste, family reasons, keeping fit and social reasons. According to the findings, of those who consumed fruits and vegetables, more than 80% of the consumption was explained by their associated health benefits for consumption. Over 41% of participants consumed fruits and vegetables for the reason of taste, more than 30% of the consumption preferences were affected by family reasons, and over 17% of the participants reported that they consumed fruits and vegetables to keep fit. Only a few participants (less than 8%) reported that social reasons were a determinant for their fruits and vegetable consumption.

The degree of preferences in fruits and vegetables were measured by using a 5-point Likert Scale as listed in Table 3. The degree of preferences in fruits and vegetables for males and females were analyzed by using an independent-samples t-test. Genders related to the score on the preference of fruits [$t(600) = -2.93$, $p = .004$, Cohen's $d = .24$] and vegetables [$t(600) = -3.66$, $p = .00$, Cohen's $d = .30$]. Female participants demonstrated higher scores on fruits and vegetables than male participants. The degree of preferences on fruits and vegetables consumption for faculty of Sciences, Arts and Commerce were analyzed by one-way ANOVA between groups. Tukey's post hoc comparisons examined differences between groups ($p > .05$). The mean values between each group did not differ ($p > .05$). However, it could be observed that the preference scores on fruits were always higher than vegetables.

REASON OF PREFERENCE BY FACULTY

As mentioned above, most of the participants (over 80%) were likely to consume fruits and vegetables because they knew the associated health benefits, which was also the major reason observed in the

Table 3. Preference degree on fruits and vegetables by gender and faculty

Demography / Measurements	Gender		Faculty		
	Male	Female	Sciences	Arts	Commerce
	Mean ± SE[a]	Mean ± SE	Mean ± SD	Mean ± SD	Mean ± SD
Preference on Fruits	3.88 ± .06*	4.10 ± .05*	3.96 ± .93	3.99 ± .85	4.12 ± .96
Preference on Vegetables	3.63 ± .06**	3.91 ± .05**	3.73 ± .92	3.78 ± .96	3.93 ± .94

[a] Mean ± Standard Error of the Mean, measured on a 5-point Likert scale (1 = Dislike, 5 = Like).
* P < .05, ** P < .01 indicate significant difference according to independent-samples t tests

categories of gender and academic disciplines. The second factor for males' consumption was taste (68.29%), and for females the consumption was actually due to avoiding constipation (67.07%). The third determinant for male was also to avoid constipation (59.76%), while for female was taste. The remaining factors were in the same order for both male and female: low calories, fullness after consumption, convenience, appearance of fruits and vegetables and mass media.

The second factor for students in the faculties of sciences and of arts was taste (70.80% & 64.43% respectively). Meanwhile students in the faculty of commerce believed that consuming fruits and vegetables would avoid constipation (61.61%). The third factor for students in the faculties of sciences and arts was to avoid constipation (64.16% & 60.87% respectively), but for students in faculty of commerce is was taste (58.93%). The remaining factors were in the same order for all academic faculties and gender, except for students in commerce who believed that convenience were more important than the feeling of satiety. The major determinants that led participants to prefer less consumption of fruits and vegetables were taste, texture and cooking method. These were the top three reasons, which were observed in both genders and different faculties.

KNOWLEDGE ON FRUITS AND VEGETABLES

The findings on minimum consumption versus the actual consumption by gender or faculty is shown in Tables 4 and 5. For males who reported the minimum consumption amount was 5 to 7 portions per day, approximately 72% of them only consumed 1 to 4 portions per day [χ^2 (9, N=600) = 65.69, p < .01, C=.45]. For females who reported the minimum consumption amount was 5 to 7 portions per day, approximately 77% of them only consumed 1 to 4 portions per day, [χ^2 (9, N=600) = 32.67, p < .01, C=.30].

For students in the faculties of science, arts and commerce who reported the minimum consumption amount was 5 to 7 portions per day, approximately 78% [χ^2 (6, N=600) = 15.66, p < .05, C=.26], 67%

Table 4. Comparison between the knowledge on the minimum consumption and action consumption of fruits and vegetables by gender. It measured by giving choices of different portions per day.

Demographic / Knowledge / Measurements	Gender								Total (M/F)
	Male				Female				
	1-4	5-7	8-10	>10	1-4	5-7	8-10	>10	
n (% of total)	95	152 (58.5)	11	2	142	186 (54.7)	10	2	260/340 (100/100)
Actual Consumption									
< 1 portion	7 (7.4)	8 (5.3)	1 (9.1)	0 (0)	13 (9.2)	6 (3.2)	0 (0)	0 (0)	16/19 (6.2/5.6)
1-4 portions	85 (89.5)	109 (71.7)	7 (63.6)	1 (50)	123 (86.6)	143 (76.9)	5 (50)	2 (100)	202/273 (77.7/80.3)
5-7 portions	3 (3.2)	35 (23.0)	1 (9.1)	1 (50)	6 (4.2)	35 (18.8)	5 (50)	0 (0)	40/46 (15.4/13.5)
7 portions	0 (0)	0 (0)	2 (18.2)	0 (0)	0 (0)	2 (1.1)	0 (0)	0(0)	2/2 (0.8/0.6)

Table 5. Comparison between the knowledge on the minimum consumption and action consumption of fruits and vegetables by faculty. It measured by giving choices of different portions per day.

Demographic Knowledge / Measurement	Faculty: Science[a] 1-4	Science[a] 5-7	Science[a] 8-10	Science[a] >10	Arts[b] 1-4	Arts[b] 5-7	Arts[b] 8-10	Arts[b] >10	Commerce[c] 1-4	Commerce[c] 5-7	Commerce[c] 8-10	Commerce[c] >10	Total (S/A/C)
n (% of total)	82	138	5	1	102	146	10	3	53	54	6	0	226/261/113 (100/100/100)
Actual Consumption													
< 1 portion	7 (8.5)	6 (4.3)	0 (0)	0 (0)	10 (9.8)	8 (5.5)	1 (10)	0 (0)	3 (5.7)	0 (0)	0 (0)	0 (0)	13/19/3 (8.5/7.3/ 2.7)
1-4 portions	70 (85.3)	108 (78.3)	2 (40)	1 (100)	90 (88.2)	98 (67.1)	6 (60)	2 (66.7)	48 (90.6)	46 (85.2)	4 (66.7)	0 (0)	181/196/98 (80.1/75.1/ 86.7)
5-7 portions	5 (6.1)	24 (17.4)	3 (60)	0 (0)	2 (2)	38 (26.0)	1 (10)	1 (33.3)	2 (3.8)	8 (14.8)	2 (33.3)	0 (0)	32/42/12 (14.2/16.1/ 10.6)
7 portions	0 (0)	0 (0)	0 (0)	0 (0)	0 (0)	2 (1.4)	2 (20)	0 (0)	0 (0)	0 (0)	0 (0)	0 (0)	0/4/0) (0/1.5/0)

[χ^2 (9, N=600) = 50.61, p < .01, C=.41], and 85% [χ^2 (4, N=600) = 9.93, p < .05, C=.28] of them only consumed 1 to 4 portions per day respectively. For students who reported the minimum consumption amount was 1 to 4 portions per day, more than 86% of all these students consumed equally 1 to 4 portions per day. These findings suggested that students who reported a higher consumption of fruits and vegetables tended to overestimate their actual consumption.

It was found that participants' knowledge on highest fiber-containing food was neither related to gender or the faculty students studied at, participants had similar responses. The highest fiber containing food was actually peas rather than carrots, cucumber, celery and lettuce. However, 232 (38.7%) participants answered celery was the vegetable that contained most fiber, followed by "I do not know" (20.8%), carrots (17.5%), lettuce (10.7%), peas (8.7%) and cucumber (3.7%). Only about 9% of the respondents had answered correctly.

HEALTH PROMOTION EFFECTS AFTER COMPLETING THE SURVEY

The tendency of gathering more information about fruits and vegetables after completion of the questionnaire was measured by using 5-point Likert Scale (Table 6) and analyzed by using an independent-samples t-test for gender.

The gender of participants was related to the score on the tendency of gathering more information about fruits and vegetables after completing the questionnaire [t(600) = -2.63, p = .016, Cohen's d = .22]. Female participants' mean was higher than male participants' mean. In other words, female participants had a higher tendency to gather more information about fruits and vegetables than male participants after completing the questionnaire. Using a one-way ANOVA, comparisons were made between students studying at each of the three faculties in relation to their likelihood of gathering more information about fruits and vegetables. Tukey's post hoc comparisons examined differences between the groups (p

Table 6. Tendency of gathering more information about fruits and vegetables

Measurements \ Demography		Gender*		Faculty			Total
		Male	Female	Sciences	Arts	Commerce	M/F, S/A/C
		Mean±SE	Mean±SE	Mean±SD	Mean±SD	Mean±SD	Mean±SD
n (% of Total)	600(100)						
Likelihood [a]							
1 Not likely at all	19(3.2)						
2 Not likely	29(4.8)	3.40 ± .05	3.58 ± .04	3.50 ± .75	3.48 ± .82	3.56 ± .87	3.50 ± .80
3 Same as before	215(35.8)						
4 Likely	306(51.0)						
5 Very likely	31(5.8)						

[a] Mean ± Standard Error of the Mean, measured on a 5-point Likert scale (1 = Not likely at all, 5 = Very likely).
* P < .05, ** P < .01 indicate significant difference according to independent-samples t tests

>.05) and there was no difference (p >.05). The sequence of mean from high to low was in the order of commerce, sciences and arts. In other words, commerce students had a slightly higher tendency for gathering more information about fruits and vegetables than students in sciences and arts. In general, the tendency mean of gathering more information in the future was 3.5 and the tendency mode was 4. More than 50% of total participants in this study selected '4' which suggested they were likely to gather more information related to fruits and vegetables in the future after completing the questionnaire.

DISCUSSION

From the above findings, it can be observed that most participants (85%) did not reach the minimum consumption of 5 portions of fruits and vegetables per day. It seemed that the "2 Plus 3 a day" intervention programs had not been as effective as projected. Most of the participants did not consume fruits or vegetables for every meal during the day. Half of the participants consumed fruits or vegetables once per day while 35% consumed these twice per day. Only about 15% of participants consumed fruits and vegetables more than 3 times per day. While there was significant difference between males and females in the frequency of consumption (females had a higher frequency for consumption of fruits and vegetables than males); this seemed to be consistent with other similar literature (Glynn, Emmett, & Rogers, 2005). Instead of promoting an increase in consumption amount only, university or government agencies could suggest everyone increases the frequency of consumption during every meal, which in return will increase the overall consumption. Meanwhile, more efforts can be focused on encouraging males to consume fruits and vegetables during each meal.

It was very interesting to find out that most participants perceived they were having an insufficient consumption of fruits and vegetables, and yet, approximately 96% of them still consumed less than 5 portions of fruits and vegetables per day. They knew that they were consuming an insufficient amount of fruits and vegetables, but they did not do anything to change that. They seemed to understand the general health benefits associated with the consumption of fruits and vegetables. While it was the main determinant that affected their consumption status, it was not a strong enough factor to motivate those with a lower consumption status to consume more. Advices from family members became the second reasons for their change in consumption; while convenience and time costs seemed to play a large role as well on consumption status. Future health promotion campaigns could focus efforts on encouraging families to have a higher availability of fruits and vegetables at home, which might increase the consumption of family members as indicated by other similar research (Cullen et. al., 2003; Rasmussen et al.,2006).

Barriers to consumption were found to include taste, texture, cooking methods, high price and potential residues of fruits and vegetables stuck between teeth. Cooking methods could alter the taste and texture of vegetables and further affect participants' preferences. Consuming other types of fruits and vegetables that are easier to chew and less expensive could solve the issues of residues of fruits and vegetables stuck between teeth, and high price respectively. Meanwhile, increasing the diversity of fruit and vegetable choices, as well as cooking method in normal diet could potentially increase the appetite of people.

In accordance with other research, this study found out that likelihood of consumption was related to the degree of preference and reasons of preference (Brug et. al., 2008). Taste preference was most positively related to the likelihood of consumption, followed by the availability and accessibility at home. Taste preference is an innate predisposition for sweet, salty, as well as energy-dense foods (Birch, 1999). The public has much more acceptance of fruits than vegetables because of the flavor. It is suggested that it would be better to have habitual changes in earlier life for less developed taste preference (William, Ball, & Crawford, 2010), in order to increase the consumption of both fruits and vegetables later in life.

According to a survey conducted by the Centre for Health Promotion (2010), over half of the respondents were eating every meal out-with the home. Eating outside frequently is significantly associated with insufficient consumption of fruit and vegetables. The availability and accessibility are general lower in outside settings. Restaurants, as well as cafeterias in universities, are encouraged to provide more options of fruits and vegetables to students. University students are also encouraged to carry fruits in bags for accessible consumption everywhere, especially for fruits that do not require much preparation, such as apples or bananas.

KNOWLEDGE RELATED TO THE SERVING SIZE AND NUTRIENTS

Only half of the respondents (56.3%) answered correctly on the daily minimum consumption of 5 to 7 portions of fruits and vegetables. 39.5% of participants answered correctly on the daily minimum consumption with 1 to 4 portions. This suggested that the awareness of the *"2 Plus 3 a day"* campaign among university students were rather low. Promotional health talks or events could be hosted at different universities on a regular basis in order raise the awareness and benefits of consuming sufficient fruits and vegetables among university students

On the other hand, in the question that asked participants to identify the highest fiber-containing food, 38.7% of participants incorrectly answered celery as the highest fiber-containing food and only 52 (8.7%) participants correctly indicated that it was peas. This suggested that participants might not have a clear concept on the amount fiber content within fruits and vegetables.

The Supplemental Nutrition Assistance Program Education and Evaluation Study (Wave II) conducted by Long et al. (2013) found that the nutrition education program could increase fruits and vegetables consumption. Efforts on nutritional education could help individuals to make healthier food choices, while correct knowledge on nutrition value of foods would contribute to proper eating and nutrition, which was directly associated with people's health. Hence, universities could incorporate appropriate concepts on fruit and vegetable consumption into their existing curricula in order to improve students' understanding in this aspect, which may have an overall beneficial effect on students' health status.

HEALTH PROMOTION EFFECT OF CONDUCTING QUESTIONNAIRE

One of the most interesting findings of the results was the participants' tendency to gathering more information about fruits and vegetables after completion of the questionnaire. The tendency mean of gathering more information in the future was 3.5 while mode was 4. 51% of the participants in this study reported that they were likely to gather more information related to fruits and vegetables in the future after completing the survey and 5.2% of participants indicated that they are very likely to gather information (e.g health benefits) related to fruits and vegetables in the future. It suggested that health promotion effects could be observed during the processes of conducting these health research studies, assuming the response bias is at a minimum. Administering questionnaires could potentially raise participants' awareness of the required amount of fruits and vegetables consumption. Completing questionnaires could elicit or enhance people' perception of fruits and vegetables intakes. Therefore, health promotion campaigns could be promoted along with scientific health research. For example, researchers could distribute health promotion leaflets after conducting in-person survey.

LIMITATIONS

The self-reporting nature of fruit and vegetable intake was one of the main limitations in this studying. Measurement error and recall bias may have impacted the data gathered (Moore, & Thompson, 2015). Overestimation and underestimation might occur in analysis and reporting data. Participants might not report or answer the questionnaire genuinely due to response bias or social desirability bias (Van de Mortel, 2008). Participants did not want to be perceived as unhealthy and reported a higher than actual amount of fruit and vegetable consumption and this may have skewed the findings. Gender was one of the variables that might have significant impact on the results. In this study, there were imbalanced proportions of male and female among the participants among the three faculties. To reduce error, stratified random sampling with grouping for male and female could be used in the future.

IMPLICATIONS AND WAY FORWARD

According to the present investigation, inadequate consumption of fruits and vegetables was reported among university students in Hong Kong. University students' basic knowledge towards fruits and vegetables was considered insufficient; for example, they understood that they should consume at least 5 portions of fruits and vegetables per day while they also knew that there were certain health benefits associated with fruits and vegetables consumption. Although they had the basic knowledge, the results demonstrated that most of them were still not consuming enough amounts of fruits and vegetables according to the standards. The study also revealed that there were barriers to consuming more fruits and vegetables, including factors such as taste, texture, accessibility and availability.

As mentioned earlier, this chapter does not aim at directly providing guidelines and suggestions for readers. Instead, it aims to provoke contemplation about what role higher education institutions should play in promoting healthy ageing in the future.

A study carried out by Mak et al. (2011) in Hong Kong had an objective to better understand how health care should be prioritized in light of the rapidly ageing population. The results showed that most people in Hong Kong would give priority to the young over the old in distributing a given amount of healthcare services. Among the findings, it was also revealed that health promotion and education services aimed at helping people lead healthy lives were ranked fifth. This was one of the highest priorities of health services, only trailing behind treatment for children with life threatening illness, high technology surgery and organ transplants, preventive screening, and surgery that helps people to carry out daily task such as a hip replacement. People with a tertiary education level perceived that health promotion and education services could possibly be even more important than psychiatric services for mental health illness patients, or long stay hospital care for elderly people.

Whether policy makers should follow such prioritization suggested by the Hong Kong study is a subject worthy of further research, the implications of how health promotion is perceived to be an important health service especially for the young should not be overlook. A similar study carried out by Bowling (1996) suggested that health promotion and education services were also perceived as important health services by UK citizens though the ranking was lower than the Hong Kong study. In a short summary, these studies revealed that the need for basic health promotion and education services exist and is growing stronger than expected. We need to have health promotion and education services that is not only theoretically sound but also practically effective; the current Chapter serve not as a guide for policy making or curriculum design, but as an impetus to arouse discussion among educators and policy makers to reflect on the effectiveness of our current efforts in promoting healthy lifestyles.

REFERENCES

Barnett, K., Mercer, S., Norbury, M., Watt, G., Wyke, S., & Guthrie, B. (2012). Epidemiology of multimorbidity and implications for health care, research, and medical education: A cross-sectional study. *Lancet*, *380*(9836), 37–43. doi:10.1016/S0140-6736(12)60240-2 PMID:22579043

Blanchette, L., & Brug, J. (2005). Determinants of fruit and vegetable consumption among 6–12years old children and effective interventions to increase consumption. *Journal of Human Nutrition and Dietetics*, *18*(6), 431–443. doi:10.1111/j.1365-277X.2005.00648.x PMID:16351702

Bowling, A. (1996). Health care rationing: The publics debate. *British Medical Journal*, *312*(7032), 670–674. doi:10.1136/bmj.312.7032.670 PMID:8597733

Brug, J., Tak, N. I., te Velde, S. J., Bere, E., & De Bourdeaudhuij, I. (2008). Taste preferences, liking and other factors related to fruit and vegetable intakes among schoolchildren: Results from observational studies. *The British Journal of Nutrition*, *99*(S1), 7–14. doi:10.1017/S0007114508892458 PMID:18257952

Census and Statistics Department. (2012). Retrieved from: www.censtatd.gov.hk

Centre for Health Protection. (2015). *Diet and Nutrition*. Retrieved from http://www.chp.gov.hk/en/content/9/25/8800.html

Chow, C., Jolly, S., Rao-Melacini, P., Fox, K., Anand, S., & Yusuf, S. (2010). Association of diet, exercise, and smoking modification with risk of early cardiovascular events after acute coronary syndromes. *Circulation, 121*(6), 750–758. doi:10.1161/CIRCULATIONAHA.109.891523 PMID:20124123

Chung, R. Y., Tin, K. Y. K., Cowling, B. J., Chan, K. P., Chan, W. M., Lo, S. V., & Leung, G. M. (2009). Long-term care cost drivers and expenditure projection to 2036 in Hong Kong. *BMC Health Services Research, 9*(1), 172. doi:10.1186/1472-6963-9-172 PMID:19775476

College of Medicine. (2013). *The crisis in costs.* Retrieved from: http://www.collegeofmedicine.org.uk/crisis-costs

Conn, V. (2011). Helping patients help themselves: Chronic disease self-management interventions. *Western Journal of Nursing Research, 33*(2), 159–160. doi:10.1177/0193945910386194 PMID:21252383

Cullen, K. W., Baranowski, T., Owens, E., Marsh, T., Rittenberry, L., & de Moor, C. (2003). Availability, accessibility, and preferences for fruit, 100% fruit juice, and vegetables influence childrens dietary behavior. *Health Education & Behavior, 30*(5), 615–626. doi:10.1177/1090198103257254 PMID:14582601

Department of Health. (2011). *Health Watch: Aim for "2 Plus 3 a day"*. Retrieved from http://www.change4health.gov.hk/en/whats_new/health_watch/index_id_2.html

Department of Health. (2014). *Student Health Service - About Student Health ServiceCentre / Special Assessment Centre.* Retrieved from http://www.studenthealth.gov.hk/english/aboutus/aboutus_shscsac/aboutus_shscsac.html

Department of Health. (2016). Retrieved from http://www.dh.gov.hk/cindex.html

Department of Health and Human Services National Institute on Aging. (2007). Growing Older in America: The Health and Retirement Study. Washington, DC: Author.

Elwood, P., Galante, J., Pickering, J., Palmer, S., Bayer, A., Ben-Shlomo, Y., & Gallacher, J. et al. (2013). Healthy Lifestyles Reduce the Incidence of Chronic Diseases and Dementia: Evidence from the Caerphilly Cohort Study. *PLoS ONE, 8*(12), 81877–81884. doi:10.1371/journal.pone.0081877 PMID:24349147

Fisher, J. O., Mitchell, D. C., Smiciklas-Wright, H., & Birch, L. L. (2002). Parental influences on young girls fruit and vegetable, micronutrient, and fat intakes. *Journal of the American Dietetic Association, 102*(1), 58–64. doi:10.1016/S0002-8223(02)90017-9 PMID:11794503

Glanz, K., Rimer, B. K., & Viswanath, K. (Eds.). (2008). *Health behavior and health education: theory, research, and practice.* John Wiley & Sons.

Glynn, L., Emmett, P., & Rogers, I. (2005). Food and nutrient intakes of a population sample of 7-year-old children in the southwest of England in 1999/2000–what difference does gender make? *Journal of Human Nutrition and Dietetics, 18*(1), 7–19. doi:10.1111/j.1365-277X.2004.00582.x PMID:15647094

Laitinen, T. T., Pahkala, K., Magnussen, C. G., Viikari, J. S., Oikonen, M., Taittonen, L., & Juonala, M. et al. (2012). Ideal cardiovascular health in childhood and cardiometabolic outcomes in adulthood: The Cardiovascular Risk in Young Finns Study. *Circulation, 125*(16), 1971–1978. doi:10.1161/CIRCULATIONAHA.111.073585 PMID:22452832

Liu, K., Daviglus, M. L., Loria, C. M., Colangelo, L. A., Spring, B., Moller, A. C., & Lloyd-Jones, D. M. (2012). Healthy lifestyle through young adulthood and the presence of low cardiovascular disease risk profile in middle age: The Coronary Artery Risk Development in (Young) Adults (CARDIA) study. *Circulation, 125*(8), 996–1004. doi:10.1161/CIRCULATIONAHA.111.060681 PMID:22291127

Mak, B., Woo, J., Bowling, A., Wong, F., & Chau, P. H. (2011). Health care prioritization in ageing societies: Influence of age, education, health literacy and culture. *Health Policy (Amsterdam), 100*(2-3), 219–233. doi:10.1016/j.healthpol.2010.08.015 PMID:20850194

McAleese, J. D., & Rankin, L. L. (2007). Garden-based nutrition education affects fruit and vegetable consumption in sixth-grade adolescents. *Journal of the American Dietetic Association, 107*(4), 662–665. doi:10.1016/j.jada.2007.01.015 PMID:17383272

Moore, L. V., & Thompson, F. E. (2015). Adults Meeting Fruit and Vegetable Intake Recommendations—United States, 2013. *Morbidity and Mortality Weekly Report, 64*(26), 709–713. PMID:26158351

Mossey, J. M., & Shapiro, E. (1982). Self-rated health: A predictor of mortality among the elderly. *American Journal of Public Health, 72*(8), 800–808. doi:10.2105/AJPH.72.8.800 PMID:7091475

Rasmussen, M., Krølner, R., Klepp, K. I., Lytle, L., Brug, J., Bere, E., & Due, P. (2006). Determinants of fruit and vegetable consumption among children and adolescents: a review of the literature. Part I: quantitative studies. *The International Journal of Behavioral Nutrition and Physical Activity, 3*(1), 22. doi:10.1186/1479-5868-3-22 PMID:16904006

Spring, B., Moller, A. C., Colangelo, L. A., Siddique, J., Roehrig, M., Daviglus, M. L., & Liu, K. et al. (2014). Healthy lifestyle change and subclinical atherosclerosis in young adults: Coronary Artery Risk Development in Young Adults (CARDIA) Study. *Circulation, 130*(1), 10–17. doi:10.1161/CIRCULATIONAHA.113.005445 PMID:24982115

Van de Mortel, T. F. (2008). *Faking it: Social desirability response bias in self-report research.* Academic Press.

Wang, X., Ouyang, Y., Liu, J., Zhu, M., Zhao, G., Bao, W., & Hu, F. B. (2014). Fruit and vegetable consumption and mortality from all causes, cardiovascular disease, and cancer: Systematic review and dose-response meta-analysis of prospective cohort studies. *British Medical Journal, 349*(3), 4490. doi:10.1136/bmj.g4490 PMID:25073782

World Health Organization. (2004, September 1). *Promoting fruit and vegetable consumption around the world.* Retrieved October 24, 2015, from http://www.who.int/dietphysicalactivity/fruit/en/

World Health Organization. (2015). Retrieved from http://www.who.int/dietphysicalactivity/fruit/en/index2.html

Yuen, P. P. (2014). Financing Health Care and Long-term Care in a Rapidly Ageing Context: Assessing Hong Kong's Readiness. *Public Administration and Policy – An Asia Pacific Journal, 17*(1), 56 – 64.

Compilation of References

AARP Public Policy Institute. (2015). *Caregiving - Public Policy Institute*. Retrieved April 14, 2016, from http://www.aarp.org/ppi/issues/caregiving/

Abate, L. E., Gomes, A., & Linton, A. (2011). Engaging students in active learning: Use of a blog and audience response system. *Medical Reference Services Quarterly*, *30*(1), 12–18. doi:10.1080/02763869.2011.540206 PMID:21271448

Abdolvand, N., Albadvi, A., & Ferdowsi, Z. (2008). Assessing readiness for business process reengineering. *Business Process Management Journal*, *14*(4), 497–511. doi:10.1108/14637150810888046

Abidi, S. S. R. (2001). Knowledge management in healthcare: Towards knowledge-driven decision-support services. *International Journal of Medical Informatics*, *63*(1), 5–18. doi:10.1016/S1386-5056(01)00167-8 PMID:11518661

Achenbaum, W. A., & Bengtson, V. L. (1994). Re-engaging the disengagement theory of aging: On the history and assessment of theory development in gerontology. *The Gerontologist*, *34*(6), 756–763. doi:10.1093/geront/34.6.756 PMID:7843604

Addicott, R. (2014). *Commissioning and contracting for integrated care*. London: The Kings Fund.

Addington-Hall, J., & Karlsen, S. (2000). Do home deaths increase distress in bereavement? *Palliative Medicine*, *14*(2), 161–162. doi:10.1191/026921600674991350 PMID:10829152

Agency for Volunteer Service. (2009). *Survey of NGOs and NGO Volunteers*. Retrieved May 20, 2016 from http://www.avs.org.hk/symposium/pdf/AVS_BOOKlet_21.pdf

Agency for Volunteer Service. (n.d.). *About AVS*. Retrieved July 24, 2016 from http://www.avs.org.hk/en/intro

Ahmadi, H., Ibrahim, O., & Nilashi, M. (2015). Investigating a new framework for hospital information system adoption: A case on Malaysia. *Journal of Soft Computing and Decision Support Systems*, *2*(2), 26–33.

Ahn, S. Y., & Park, D. J. (2016). Corporate Social Responsibility and Corporate Longevity: The Mediating Role of Social Capital and Moral Legitimacy in Korea. *Journal of Business Ethics*. doi:10.1007/s10551-016-3161-3

Al-Balushi, S., Sohal, A. S., Singh, P. J., Al Hajri, A., Al Farsi, Y. M., & Al Abri, R. (2014). Readiness factors for lean implementation in healthcare settings–a literature review. *Journal of Health Organization and Management*, *28*(2), 135–153. doi:10.1108/JHOM-04-2013-0083 PMID:25065107

Albarrak, A. (2011). E-learning in Medical Education and Blended learning approach. *Learning*, *13*, 14-20.

Althaus, F., Paroz, S., Hugli, O., Ghali, W. A., Daeppen, J. B., Peytremann-Bridevaux, I., & Bodenmann, P. (2011). Effectiveness of interventions targeting frequent users of emergency departments: A systematic review. *Annals of Emergency Medicine*, *58*(1), 41–52. doi:10.1016/j.annemergmed.2011.03.007 PMID:21689565

Amaeshi, K., Nnodim, P., & Osuji, O. (2013). *Corporate Social Responsibility, Entrepreneurship and Innovation*. New York: Routledge.

American Association of Colleges of Nursing. (2008). *The Essentials of Baccalaureate Education for Professional Nursing Practice*. Washington, DC: American Association of Colleges of Nursing.

Anderson, R. A., Issel, L. M., & McDaniel, R. R. Jr. (2003). Nursing homes as complex adaptive systems: Relationship between management practice and resident outcomes. *Nursing Research*, *52*(1), 12–21. doi:10.1097/00006199-200301000-00003 PMID:12552171

Antibiotic clinics provide 'incredible' community care. (2015). *Nursing Standard*, *29*(40), 10. doi: 10.7748/ns.29.40.10.s11

Applebaum, R., Bardo, A., & Robbins, E. (2013). International approaches to long-term services and supports. *Generations (San Francisco, Calif.)*, *37*(1), 59–65.

Aras, G., & Crowther, D. (2012). *Governance and social responsibility: international perspectives*. Hampshire, UK: Palgrave Macmillan.

Armitage, G. D., Suter, E., Oelke, N. D., & Adair, C. (2009). Health systems integration: State of the evidence. *International Journal of Integrated Care*, *9*(17), 1–11. PMID:19590762

Arnold, E., Finucane, A. M., & Oxenham, D. (2015). Preferred place of death for patients referred to a specialist palliative care service. *BMJ Supportive & Palliative Care*, *5*(3), 294–296. doi:10.1136/bmjspcare-2012-000338 PMID:24644165

Arnott, J., & Koubel, G. (2012). Interprofessional working and the community care conundrum. In G. Koubel & H. Bungay (Eds.), *Rights, risks and responsibilities: Interprofessional working in health and social care* (pp. 159–178). Basingstoke, UK: Palgrave Macmillan. doi:10.1007/978-0-230-36907-8_10

Aronow, W. S., Ahn, C., & Kronzon, I. (1997). Effect of propranolol versus no propranolol on total mortality plus nonfatal myocardial infarction in older patients with prior myocardial infarction, congestive heart failure, and left ventricular ejection fraction≥ 40% treated with diuretics plus angiotensin-converting enzyme inhibitors. *The American Journal of Cardiology*, *80*(2), 207–209. doi:10.1016/S0002-9149(97)00320-2 PMID:9230162

Aronow, W. S., Ahn, C., & Kronzon, I. (2001). Effect of beta blockers alone, of angiotensin-converting enzyme inhibitors alone, and of beta blockers plus angiotensin-converting enzyme inhibitors on new coronary events and on congestive heart failure in older persons with healed myocardial infarcts and asymptomatic left ventricular systolic dysfunction. *The American Journal of Cardiology*, *88*(11), 1298–1300. doi:10.1016/S0002-9149(01)02092-6 PMID:11728359

Asia Insurance Review. (2015). *China: 1 bln+ people to have state-run critical illness cover*. Retrieved June 12, 2016, from http://www.asiainsurancereview.com/News/View-NewsLetter-Article?id=33334&Type=edaily

Atchley, R. C. (1971). Retirement and leisure participation: Continuity or crisis? *The Gerontologist*, *11*(1), 13–17. doi:10.1093/geront/11.1_Part_1.13 PMID:5579223

Atchley, R. C. (1989). A continuity theory of normal aging. *The Gerontologist*, *29*(2), 183–190. doi:10.1093/geront/29.2.183 PMID:2519525

Atchley, R. C. (2000). *Continuity and adaptation in aging: Creating positive experiences*. Baltimore, MD: Johns Hopkins University Press.

Athauda, L. K., Wickremasinghe, A. R., Kumarendran, B., & Kasturiratne, A. (2015). An ecological study for Sri Lanka about health effects of coconut. *The Ceylon Medical Journal*, *60*(3), 97–99. doi:10.4038/cmj.v60i3.8188 PMID:26520863

Atun, R. (2004). *What are the advantages and disadvantages of restructuring a health care system to be more focused on primary care services?* Copenhagen: WHO Regional Office for Europe, Health Evidence Network report. Retrieved February 1, 2017, from http://www.euro.who.int/document/e82997.pdf

Atun, R. (2004). *What are the advantages and disadvantages of restructuring a health care system to be more focused on primary care services?* Copenhagen: WHO Regional Office for Europe. Retrieved from http://www.euro.who.int/document/e82997.pdf

Augustovski, F., Martí, S. G., Riviere, A. P., & Rubinstein, A. (2011). Universal coverage with rising healthcare costs; health outcomes research value in decision making in Latin America. *Expert Review of Pharmacoeconomics & Outcomes Research, 11*(6), 657–659. doi:10.1586/erp.11.83 PMID:22098279

Aungst, T. D. (2013). Medical applications for pharmacists using mobile devices. *The Annals of Pharmacotherapy, 47*(7-8), 1088–1095. doi:10.1345/aph.1S035 PMID:23821609

Auster, E. R., Wylie, K. K., & Valente, M. S. (2005). *Strategic organizational change: building change capabilities in your organization.* Basingstoke, UK: Palgrave Macmillan. doi:10.1057/9780230508064

Australian Government Aged Care Financing Authority. (2015). *Factors Influencing the Financial Performance of Residential Aged Care Providers.* Canberra: Australian Government Aged Care Financing Authority.

Australian Institute of Health and Welfare. (2015). *Use of aged care services before death. Data linkage series no. 19. Cat. no. CSI 21.* Canberra: AIHW.

Aylward, S., Stolee, P., Keat, N., & Johncox, V. (2003). Effectiveness of continuing education in long-term care: A literature review. *The Gerontologist, 43*(2), 259–271. doi:10.1093/geront/43.2.259 PMID:12677083

Babiarz, K. S., Miller, G., Yi, H., Zhang, L., & Rozelle, S. (2010). New evidence on the impact of Chinas New Rural Cooperative Medical Scheme and its implications for rural primary healthcare: Multivariate difference-in-difference analysis. *BMJ (Clinical Research Ed.), 341*(2), c5617. doi:10.1136/bmj.c5617 PMID:20966008

Bai, C., & Wu, B. (2014). Health insurance and consumption: Evidence from Chinas New Cooperative Medical Scheme. *Journal of Comparative Economics, 42*(2), 450–469. doi:10.1016/j.jce.2013.07.005

Bajorek, B., Magin, P., Hilmer, S., & Krass, I. (2014). A cluster-randomized controlled trial of a computerized anti-thrombotic risk assessment tool to optimize stroke prevention in general practice: A study protocol. *BMC Health Services Research, 14*(1), 55. doi:10.1186/1472-6963-14-55 PMID:24507462

Baldassar, L., Wilding, R., Boccagni, P., & Merla, L. (2017). Aging in place in a mobile world: New media and older peoples support networks. *Transnational Social Review, 7*(1), 2–9. doi:10.1080/21931674.2016.1277864

Banerjee, A. (2007). *An Overview of Long-Term Care in Canada in Selected Provinces and Territories, Women and Health Care Reform Group.* Toronto: York University.

Banister, J. (1987). *China's changing population.* Stanford, CA: Stanford University Press.

Barclay, J. S., Kuchibhatla, M., Tulsky, J. A., & Johnson, K. S. (2013). Association of hospice patients income and care level with place of death. *JAMA Internal Medicine, 173*(6), 450. doi:10.1001/jamainternmed.2013.2773 PMID:23420383

Bardsley, M., Steventon, A., Smith, J., & Dixon, J. (2013). *Evaluating integrated and community-based care: How do we know what works?* London, UK: Nuffield Trust. Retrieved March 20, 2017 from https://www.nuffieldtrust.org.uk/files/2017-01/evaluating-integrated-community-care-web-final.pdf

Barnett, K., Mercer, S., Norbury, M., Watt, G., Wyke, S., & Guthrie, B. (2012). Epidemiology of multimorbidity and implications for health care, research, and medical education: A cross-sectional study. *Lancet*, *380*, 37–43.

Barrett-Lennard, G. T. (1962). Dimensions of therapist response as causal factors in therapeutic change. *Psychological Monographs*, *76*(43), 1–36. doi:10.1037/h0093918

Batic-Mujanovic, O., Zildzic, M., & Beganlic, A. (2006). Secondary prevention of heart disease in primary health care. *Bosnian Journal of Basic Medical Sciences*, *6*(2), 37–41. PMID:16879111

Battilana, J., & Leca, B. (2009). The role of resources in institutional entrepreneurship: insights for an approach to strategic management that combines agency and institutions. In L. A. Costanzo & R. B. MacKay (Eds.), *Handbook of research on strategy and foresight* (pp. 260–274). Cheltenham, UK: Edward Elgar. doi:10.4337/9781848447271.00022

Baum, F. (2008). The social determinants of health inequity. In F. Baum (Ed.), *The new public health* (3rd ed.). Melbourne, Australia: Oxford University Press.

Beaulieu, R., Shamian, J., Donner, G., & Pringle, D. (1997). Empowerment and commitment of nurses in long-term care. *Nursing Economics*, *15*(1), 32–42. PMID:9087042

Beckett, N. S., Peters, R., Fletcher, A. E., Staessen, J. A., Liu, L., Dumitrascu, D., & Bulpitt, C. J. et al. (2008). Treatment of hypertension in patients 80 years of age or older. *The New England Journal of Medicine*, *358*(18), 1887–1898. doi:10.1056/NEJMoa0801369 PMID:18378519

Beckman, J. A., Creager, M. A., & Libby, P. (2002). Diabetes and atherosclerosis: Epidemiology, pathophysiology, and management. *Journal of the American Medical Association*, *287*(19), 2570–2581. doi:10.1001/jama.287.19.2570 PMID:12020339

Beijing Business Today. (2014a, December 9). *Price caps on drugs has little effectiveness,* Chinese version. Retrieved July 15, 2016, from http://finance.sina.com.cn/chanjing/cyxw/20141209/012021026167.shtml

Beijing Business Today. (2014b, December 9). *Some regions experience a deficit in the medical insurance fund,* Chinese version. Retrieved July 15, 2016, from http://www.cn-healthcare.com/article/20141209/content-465355.html

Béland, D. (2007). Ideas and institutional change in social security: Conversion, layering, and policy drift. *Social Science Quarterly*, *88*(1), 20–38. doi:10.1111/j.1540-6237.2007.00444.x

Béland, D., & Cox, R. H. (2011). Introduction: ideas and politics. In D. Béland & R. H. Cox (Eds.), *Ideas and Politics in Social Science Research* (pp. 3–20). New York: Oxford University Press.

Béland, F., Bergman, H., Lebel, P., Clarfield, A. M., Tousignant, P., Contandriopoulos, A. P., & Dallaire, L. (2006a). A system of integrated care for older persons with disabilities in Canada: Results from a randomized controlled trial. *The Journals of Gerontology. Series A, Biological Sciences and Medical Sciences*, *61*(4), 367–373. doi:10.1093/gerona/61.4.367 PMID:16611703

Béland, F., Bergman, H., Lebel, P., Dallaire, L., Fletcher, J., Tousignant, P., & Contandriopoulos, A. P. (2006b). Integrated services for frail elders (SIPA): A trial of a model for Canada. *Canadian Journal on Aging*, *25*(1), 25–42. doi:10.1353/cja.2006.0019 PMID:16770746

Béland, F., & Hollander, M. J. (2011). Integrated models of care delivery for the frail elderly: International perspectives. *Gaceta Sanitaria*, *25*, 138–146. doi:10.1016/j.gaceta.2011.09.003 PMID:22088903

Benefield, L. E., & Holtzclaw, B. J. (2014). Aging in Place: Merging Desire with Reality. *The Nursing Clinics of North America*, *19*(2), 123–131. doi:10.1016/j.cnur.2014.02.001 PMID:24846462

Bengtson, V. L., Burgess, E. O., & Parrott, T. M. (1997). Theory, explanation, and a third generation of theoretical development in social gerontology. *The Journals of Gerontology. Series B, Psychological Sciences and Social Sciences*, *52B*(2), S72–S88. doi:10.1093/geronb/52B.2.S72 PMID:9060987

Bennett, A. R. (2012). Accountable care organizations: Principles and implications for hospital administrators. *Journal of Healthcare Management*, *57*(4), 244–254. PMID:22905603

Bennett, A., & Taylor, J. (2012). Popular music and the aesthetics of ageing. *Popular Music*, *31*(2), 231–243. doi:10.1017/S0261143012000013

Benson, M., & O'Reilly, K. (Eds.). (2009). Lifestyle Migration: Expectations, Aspirations and Experiences. Ashgate, UK: Aldershot.

Berg, K., Wood-Dauphinee, S., Williams, J. I., & Makki, B. E. (1992). Measuring balance in the elderly: Validation of an instrument. *Canadian Journal of Public Health*, *83*, S7–S11. PMID:1468055

Bergman, H., Béland, F., Lebel, P., Contandriopoulos, A. P., Tousignant, P., Brunelle, Y., & Clarfield, M. et al. (1997). Care for Canada's frail elderly population: Fragmentation or integration? *Canadian Medical Association Journal*, *157*(8), 1116–1121. PMID:9347783

Bernard, M., & Phillips, J. (2000). The challenge of ageing in tomorrows Britain. *Ageing and Society*, *20*(1), 33–54. doi:10.1017/S0144686X99007576

Bernoth, M., Dietsch, E., Burmeister, O. K., & Schwartz, M. (2014). Information Management in Aged Care: Cases of Confidentiality and Elder Abuse. *Journal of Business Ethics*, *122*(3), 453–460. doi:10.1007/s10551-013-1770-7

Berry, W., Ringquist, E., Fording, R., & Hanson, R. (1998). Measuring citizen and government ideology in the American states, 19601993. *American Journal of Political Science*, *42*(1), 327–348. doi:10.2307/2991759

Berta, W., Teare, G. F., Gilbart, E., Ginsburg, L. S., Lemieux-Charles, L., Davis, D., & Rappolt, S. (2005). The contingencies of organizational learning in long-term care: Factors that affect innovation adoption. *Health Care Management Review*, *30*(4), 282–292. doi:10.1097/00004010-200510000-00002 PMID:16292005

Bharati, P., Zhang, W., & Chaudhury, A. (2015). Better knowledge with social media? Exploring the roles of social capital and organizational knowledge management. *Journal of Knowledge Management*, *19*(3), 456–475. doi:10.1108/JKM-11-2014-0467

Bhattacharya, M., & Wamba, S. F. (2015). A Conceptual Framework of RFID Adoption in Retail Using TOE Framework. *International Journal of Technology Diffusion*, *6*(1), 1–32. doi:10.4018/IJTD.2015010101

Bhatt, G. D. (2001). Knowledge management in organizations: Examining the interaction between technologies, techniques, and people. *Journal of Knowledge Management*, *5*(1), 68–75. doi:10.1108/13673270110384419

Billings, J., & Weger, E. (2015). Contracting for integrated health and social care: A critical review of four models. *Journal of Integrated Care*, *23*(3), 153–175. doi:10.1108/JICA-03-2015-0015

BIPAsia. (2016). *Actively Promoting Intellectual Property Trading HK PolyU's "Hand of Hope" gains international recognition*. Retrieved 20 July 2016, from http://bipasiaforum.com/en/success_stories/int_Actively_Promoting.html

Blanchette, L., & Brug, J. (2005). Determinants of fruit and vegetable consumption among 6–12years old children and effective interventions to increase consumption. *Journal of Human Nutrition and Dietetics*, *18*(6), 431–443. doi:10.1111/j.1365-277X.2005.00648.x PMID:16351702

Blaschke, C. M., Freddolino, P. P., & Mullen, E. E. (2009). Ageing and technology: A review of the research literature. *British Journal of Social Work*, *39*(4), 641–656. doi:10.1093/bjsw/bcp025

Bloom, D. E., Craig, P., & Mitchell, M. (2000). *Public and private roles in providing and financing social services: Health and education. In Public-Private Partnerships in the Social Sector: Issues and Country Experiences in Asia and the Pacific*. Tokyo: ADBI Publishing.

Blowfield, M. (2013). *Business and sustainability*. Oxford, UK: Oxford University Press.

Blyth, M. (2011). Ideas, uncertainty, and evolution. In D. Béland & R. H. Cox (Eds.), *Ideas and Politics in Social Science Research* (pp. 83–104). New York: Oxford University Press.

Bodenheimer, T., Lorig, K., Holman, H., & Grumbach, K. (2002). Patient self-management of chronic disease in primary care. *Journal of the American Medical Association*, *288*(19), 2469–2475. doi:10.1001/jama.288.19.2469 PMID:12435261

Bookman, A. (2008). Innovative models of aging in place: Transforming our communities for an aging population. *Community Work & Family*, *11*(4), 419–438. doi:10.1080/13668800802362334

Borchardt, G. (2000). Role Models for Health Promotion: The Challenge for Nurses. *Nursing Forum*, *35*(3), 29–32. doi:10.1111/j.1744-6198.2000.tb01002.x

Bordin, E. S. (1979). The generalizability of the psychoanalytic concept of the working alliance. *Psychotherapy (Chicago, Ill.)*, *16*(3), 252–260. doi:10.1037/h0085885

Bordoloi, P., & Islam, N. (2012). Knowledge management practices and health care delivery: A contingency framework. *Electronic Journal of Knowledge Management*, *10*(2), 110–120.

Bose, R. (2003). Knowledge management-enabled health care management systems: Capabilities, infrastructure, and decision-support. *Expert Systems with Applications*, *24*(1), 59–71. doi:10.1016/S0957-4174(02)00083-0

Boström, A. M., Slaughter, S. E., Chojecki, D., & Estabrooks, C. A. (2012). What do we know about knowledge translation in the care of older adults? A scoping review. *Journal of the American Medical Directors Association*, *13*(3), 210–219. doi:10.1016/j.jamda.2010.12.004 PMID:21450230

Boulos, M. N., Maramba, I., & Wheeler, S. (2006). Wikis, blogs and podcasts: A new generation of Web-based tools for virtual collaborative clinical practice and education. *BMC Medical Education*, *6*(1), 41. doi:10.1186/1472-6920-6-41 PMID:16911779

Bowling, A. (1996). Health care rationing: The publics debate. *British Medical Journal*, *312*(7032), 670–674. doi:10.1136/bmj.312.7032.670 PMID:8597733

Bowling, A., & Dieppe, P. (2005). What is successful ageing and who should define it? *British Medical Journal*, *331*(7531), 1548–1551. doi:10.1136/bmj.331.7531.1548 PMID:16373748

Brammer, S., Jackson, G., & Matten, D. (2012). Corporate Social Responsibility and Institutional Theory: New Perspectives on Private Governance. *Socio-economic Review*, *10*(1), 3–28. doi:10.1093/ser/mwr030

Bratton, J. (2015). *Introduction to work and organizational behaviour* (3rd ed.). New York: Palgrave Macmillan. doi:10.1007/978-1-137-43206-3

Bratton, K., & Haynie, K. (1999). Agenda setting and legislative success in state legislatures: The effects of gender and race. *The Journal of Politics*, *61*(3), 658–679. doi:10.2307/2647822

Brazil, K., Brink, P., Kaasalainen, S., Kelly, M. L., & McAiney, C. (2012). Knowledge and perceived competence among nurses caring for the dying in long-term care homes. *International Journal of Palliative Nursing*, *18*(2), 77–83. doi:10.12968/ijpn.2012.18.2.77 PMID:22399045

Brazil, K., Howell, D., Bedard, M., Krueger, P., & Heidebrecht, C. (2005). Preferences for place of care and place of death among informal caregivers of the terminally ill. *Palliative Medicine*, *19*(6), 492–499. doi:10.1191/0269216305pm1050oa PMID:16218162

Brenner, B. M., Cooper, M. E., de Zeeuw, D., Keane, W. F., Mitch, W. E., Parving, H.-H., & Shahinfar, S. et al. (2001). Effects of losartan on renal and cardiovascular outcomes in patients with type 2 diabetes and nephropathy. *The New England Journal of Medicine*, *345*(12), 861–869. doi:10.1056/NEJMoa011161 PMID:11565518

Brignote, M., Auricchio, A., & Baron-Esquivias, G. (2013). ESC guidelines on cardiac pacing and cardiac resynchronization therapy. *European Heart Journal*, *34*, 2281–2329. PMID:23801822

Bristol, N. (2014). *Global action toward universal health coverage*. Retrieved June 1, 2016, from https://www.ciaonet.org/attachments/24280/uploads

Brombal, D. (2014). Health sector reforms in contemporary China: a political perspective. In K. E. Brodsgaard (Ed.), *Globalization and Public Sector Reform in China* (pp. 100–124). Abingdon, UK: Routledge.

Brosnan, C., Chung, V. C., Zhang, A. L., & Adams, J. (2016). Regional Influences on Chinese Medicine Education: Comparing Australia and Hong Kong. *Evidence-Based Complementary and Alternative Medicine*. PMID:27379170

Brown, J., & Finkelstein, A. (2007). Why is the market for long-term care insurance so small? *Journal of Public Economics*, *91*(10), 1967–1991. doi:10.1016/j.jpubeco.2007.02.010

Brown, J., & Finkelstein, A. (2008). The interaction of public and private insurance: Medicaid and long-term care insurance market. *The American Economic Review*, *98*(3), 1083–1102. doi:10.1257/aer.98.3.1083

Brown, R. T., Kiely, D. K., Bharel, M., & Mitchell, S. L. (2012). Geriatric syndromes in older homeless adults. *Journal of General Internal Medicine*, *27*(1), 16–22. doi:10.1007/s11606-011-1848-9 PMID:21879368

Brug, J., Tak, N. I., te Velde, S. J., Bere, E., & De Bourdeaudhuij, I. (2008). Taste preferences, liking and other factors related to fruit and vegetable intakes among schoolchildren: Results from observational studies. *The British Journal of Nutrition*, *99*(S1), 7–14. doi:10.1017/S0007114508892458 PMID:18257952

Brühl, K. G., Luijendijk, H. J., & Muller, M. T. (2007). Nurses and nursing assistants recognition of depression in elderly who depend on long-term care. *Journal of the American Medical Directors Association*, *8*(7), 441–445. doi:10.1016/j.jamda.2007.05.010 PMID:17845946

Bryman, A., & Bell, E. (2007). *Business Research Method*. Oxford, UK: Oxford University Press.

Buckley, B., Byrne, M., & Smith, S. (2010). *Service organization for the secondary prevention of ischaemic heart disease in primary care*. Retrieved from: http://onlinelibrary.wiley.com/doi/10.1002/14651858.CD006772.pub2/full on 24.07.16

Burke, D. D. (2011). *Organization change: theory and practice* (3rd ed.). Thousand Oaks, CA: SAGE Publications.

Burns, P., Jones, S. C., Iverson, D. C., & Caputi, P. (2013). Where do older Australians receive their health information? Health information sources and their perceived reliability. *Journal of Nursing Education and Practice*, *3*(12), 60. doi:10.5430/jnep.v3n12p60

Busse, R., & Stahl, J. (2014). Integrated care experiences and outcomes in Germany, the Netherlands, and England. *Health Affairs*, *33*(9), 1549–1558. doi:10.1377/hlthaff.2014.0419 PMID:25201659

Buyukozkan, G., & Feyzioglu, O. (2008, July). A decision framework for the evaluation of the knowledge management tools. In *PICMET'08-2008 Portland International Conference on Management of Engineering & Technology* (pp. 1075-1084). IEEE. doi:10.1109/PICMET.2008.4599717

Cagney, K. A., & Cornwell, E. Y. (2010). Neighborhoods and health in later life: The intersection of biology and community. *Annual Review of Gerontology & Geriatrics*, *30*(1), 323–348. doi:10.1891/0198-8794.30.323

Cai, F. (2015). Demystifying China's Economy Development. Berlin: Springer Berlin Heidelberg. doi:10.1007/978-3-662-46103-7

Calasanti, T. (2004). New directions in feminist gerontology: An introduction. *Journal of Aging Studies*, *18*(1), 1–8. doi:10.1016/j.jaging.2003.09.002

Campbell, J. L. (2002). Ideas, politics, and public policy. *Annual Review of Sociology*, *28*(1), 21–38. doi:10.1146/annurev.soc.28.110601.141111

Campbell, J., Ikegami, N., Gori, C., Barbabella, F., Chomik, R., d'Amico, F., & Theobald, H. (2016). *Long-term care reforms in OECD countries: Successes and failures* (C. Gori, J.-L. Fernandez, & R. Wittenberg, Eds.). Bristol, UK: Policy Press.

Campbell, R. J. (2004). Older women and the Internet. *Journal of Women & Aging*, *16*(1-2), 161–174. doi:10.1300/J074v16n01_11 PMID:15149930

Canadian Association of Schools of Nursing. (2015). *National Nursing Education Framework*. Retrieved from: http://www.casn.ca/wp-content/uploads/2014/12/Framwork-FINAL-SB-Nov-30-20151.pdf

Cancer Expert Working Group on Cancer Prevention and Screening, & Department of Health of Hong Kong. (2016). *Prevention and screening for breast cancer: Information for women and their families*. Hong Kong: Department of Health. Retrieved March 20, 2017 from http://www.chp.gov.hk/files/pdf/breast_ca_en.pdf

Cárdenas-Turanzas, M., Torres-Vigil, I., Tovalín-Ahumada, H., & Nates, J. L. (2011). Hospital versus home death: Results from the Mexican Health and Aging Study. *Journal of Pain and Symptom Management*, *41*(5), 880–892. doi:10.1016/j.jpainsymman.2010.07.007 PMID:21146354

Cardoso, T., Oliveira, M. D., Barbosa-Póvoa, A., & Nickel, S. (2016). Moving towards an equitable long-term care network: A multi-objective and multi-period planning approach. *Omega*, *58*, 69–85. doi:10.1016/j.omega.2015.04.005

Carey, K., & Stefos, T. (2015). The cost of hospital readmissions: Evidence from the VA. *Health Care Management Science*, 1–8. PMID:25576391

CARP. (2013). *One patient: CARP's care continuum*. Retrieved from http://www.carp.ca/wp-content/uploads/2013/12/One-Patient-Paper-Dec-2013.pdf

Carrin, G., Mathauer, I., Xua, K., & Evans, D. B. (2008). Universal coverage of health services: Tailoring its implementation. *Bulletin of the World Health Organization*, *86*(11), 857–863. doi:10.2471/BLT.07.049387 PMID:19030691

Carroll, A. B. (1979). A Three-Dimensional Conceptual Model of Corporate Social Performance. *Academy of Management Review*, *4*(4), 497–505.

Carroll, A. B. (1991). The Pyramid of Corporate Social Responsibility: Toward the Moral Management of Organizational Stakeholders. *Business Horizons*, *34*(4), 39–48. doi:10.1016/0007-6813(91)90005-G

Carroll, A. B., & Shabana, K. M. (2010). The Business Case for Corporate Social Responsibility: A Review of Concepts, Research and Practice. *International Journal of Management Reviews*, *12*(1), 85–105. doi:10.1111/j.1468-2370.2009.00275.x

Cendan, J., & Lok, B. (2012). The use of virtual patients in medical school curricula. *Advances in Physiology Education*, *36*(1), 48–53. doi:10.1152/advan.00054.2011 PMID:22383412

Census and Statistics Department Hong Kong SAR. (2014). *Thematic Household Survey Report No. 58*. Retrieved March 28, 2016, from http://www.statistics.gov.hk/pub/B11302582015XXXXB0100.pdf

Census and Statistics Department Hong Kong SAR. (2015). *Hong Kong Population Projections*. Retrieved March 28, 2016, from http://www.censtatd.gov.hk/hkstat/sub/sp190.jsp?productCode=B1120015

Census and Statistics Department Hong Kong SAR. (2016). *Table 002: Population by Age Group and Sex*. Retrieved March 28, 2016, from http://www.censtatd.gov.hk/hkstat/sub/sp150.jsp?tableID=002&ID=0&productType=8

Census and Statistics Department of Hong Kong. (2015a). *Hong Kong populations projections 2015-2064*. Retrieved March 20, 2017 from http://www.statistics.gov.hk/pub/B1120015062015XXXXB0100.pdf

Census and Statistics Department of Hong Kong. (2015b). *Hong Kong monthly digest of statistics: January 2015*. Hong Kong: Author. Retrieved March 20, 2017 from http://www.statistics.gov.hk/pub/B71501FB2015XXXXB0100.pdf

Census and Statistics Department of Hong Kong. (2016a). *2016 population by-census: Summary results*. Hong Kong: Author. Retrieved March 20, 2017 from http://www.bycensus2016.gov.hk/data/16bc-summary-results.pdf

Census and Statistics Department of Hong Kong. (2016b). Statistics and you. Retrieved March 20, 2017 from http://www.censtatd.gov.hk/statistical_literacy/educational_materials/statistics_and_you/

Census and Statistics Department. (2012). *2011 Population Census - Summary Results. Census and Statistics Department*. Retrieved July 1, 2016 from http://www.census2011.gov.hk/pdf/summary-results.pdf

Census and Statistics Department. (2012). Retrieved from: www.censtatd.gov.hk

Census and Statistics Department. (2015). *Women and Men in Hong Kong Key Statistics*. Retrieved March 18, 2016 from http://www.statistics.gov.hk/pub/B11303032015AN15B0100.pdf

Census and Statistics Department. (2016a). *Press Release*. Hong Kong: Hong Kong Special Administrative Region Government. Retrieved March 2, 2017, from http://www.censtatd.gov.hk/press_release/pressReleaseDetail.jsp?charsetID=1&pressRID=3810

Census and Statistics Department. (2016b). *Hong Kong Population Projections 2015-2064*. Hong Kong: Hong Kong Special Administrative Region Government. Retrieved March 2, 2017, from http://www.statistics.gov.hk/pub/B1120015062015XXXXB0100.pdf

Census and Statistics Department. (2016c). *Demographics*. Hong Kong: Hong Kong Special Administrative Region Government. Retrieved March 2, 2017, from http://www.censtatd.gov.hk/hkstat/sub/so160.jsp

Census and Statistics Department. (2017). *Statistics on Hong Kong residents usually staying in Guangdong*. Hong Kong: Hong Kong Special Administrative Region Government. Retrieved February 1, 2017, from http://www.censtatd.gov.hk/hkstat/sub/sp150.jsp?productCode=D5320188

Center for American Women and Politics. (2014). *Women in state legislatures*. Retrieved July 15, 2014, from http://www.cawp.rutgers.edu

Center for Health Statistics and Information. (2015). *The 2013 Analysis Report of National Health Services Survey in China, Chinese version*. Retrieved February 26, 2017, from http://www.nhfpc.gov.cn/mohwsbwstjxxzx/s8211/201610/9f109ff40e9346fca76dd82cecf419ce.shtml

Centers for Disease Control and Prevention. (2013). *Healthy places terminology.* Retrieved March 18, 2017, from https://www.cdc.gov/healthyplaces/terminology.htm

Centers for Medicare & Medicaid Services, Office of the Actuary. (2014). *Report to congress. 2014 actuarial report on the financial outlook for Medicaid.* Retrieved July 5, 2016, from http://www.medicaid.gov/medicaid-chip-program-information/by-topics/financing-and-reimbursement/downloads/medicaid-actuarial-report-2014.pdf

Centers for Medicare & Medicaid Services. (2011). *Programs of all-inclusive care for the elderly (PACE).* Retrieved from https://www.cms.gov/Regulations-and-Guidance/Guidance/Manuals/downloads/pace111c01.pdf

Centers for Medicare and Medicaid Services. (2015). *Brief summaries of Medicare & Medicaid Title XVIII and Title XIX of the Social Security Act.* Retrieved July 5, 2016, from http://www.cms.gov/Research-Statistics-Data-and-Systems/Statistics-Trends-and-Reports/MedicareProgramRatesStats/Downloads/MedicareMedicaidSummaries2015.pdf

Central Health Education Unit of Hong Kong. (2015). *The Central Health Education Unit.* Retrieved March 20, 2017 from https://www.cheu.gov.hk/eng/aboutus/index.htm

Central Provident Fund Board. (2016). *Medisave.* Retrieved 1 July 2016, from https://www.cpf.gov.sg/Members/Schemes/schemes/healthcare/medisave

Centre for Health Protection of the Department of Health of Hong Kong. (2012). Brain health. *Non-communicable Diseases Watch, 5*(12), 1-6. Retrieved March 20, 2017 from http://www.chp.gov.hk/files/pdf/ncd_watch_dec2012.pdf

Centre for Health Protection. (2015). *Diet and Nutrition.* Retrieved from http://www.chp.gov.hk/en/content/9/25/8800.html

Centre for Health Protection. (2015). *Elderly vaccination subsidy scheme.* Retrieved 10 August 2016, from http://www.chp.gov.hk/en/view_content/21863.html

Centre of Health Protection. (2016). *Vital statistics.* Retrieved March 17, 2016 from http://www.chp.gov.hk/en/data/4/10/27/111.html

Cerrato, P., & Satish, M. (2015). *Study describes the UC Irvine experience with use of the iPad in medical education.* Retrieved 4 March 2017, from http://www.imedicalapps.com/2015/08/uc-irvine-ipad-medical-education-study/

Chan, A. C. M., & Phillips, D. R. (2002). Policies on ageing and long-term care in Hong Kong. In D. R. Phillips & A. C. M. Chan (Eds.), Ageing and long-term care: National policies in the Asia-Pacific (pp. 23-67). Singapore: Institute of Southeast Asian Studies.

Chan, S. Y., & Choy, K. M. (2011). Fostering PPP in the Hong Kong healthcare system. *The Quarterly.* Retrieved 8 August 2016, from http://racma.edu.au/index.php?option=com_content&view=article&id=352:fostering-ppp-in-the-hong-kong-healthcare-system&catid=146:the-quarterly-2011&Itemid=61

Chan, W. C. H., Chan, H. Y., Chan, F. M. Y., Tin, A., & Chan, C. L. W. (2004). *Perceptions of good death: how does it affect end-of-life care decisions?* Paper presented at the 11th Hong Kong International Cancer Congress, Hong Kong.

Chan, A. P., Lam, P. T., Chan, D. W., & Cheung, E. (2008). Application of public private partnership (PPP) in Hong Kong special administrative region – the critics' perspectives. *Proceedings of the First International Conference on Construction in Developing Countries,* 302-11.

Chan, A. P., Lam, P. T., Chan, D. W., Cheung, E., & Ke, Y. (2009). Potential obstacles to successful implementation of public-private partnerships in Beijing and the Hong Kong special administrative region. *Journal of Management Engineering, 26*(1), 30–40. doi:10.1061/(ASCE)0742-597X(2010)26:1(30)

Chan, A., & Cheung, E. (2014). *Public-private partnerships in international construction.* Routledge.

Chan, C. W., & Chang, A. M. (2000). Experience of palliative home care according to caregivers' and patients' ages in Hong Kong Chinese people. *Oncology Nursing Forum*, *27*(10), 1601–1605. PMID:11103379

Chan, E., Liu, X. X., Guo, D. J., Kwan, Y. W., Leung, G. P., Lee, S. M., & Chan, S. W. (2011). Extract of Scutellaria baicalensis Georgi root exerts protection against myocardial ischemia-reperfusion injury in rats. *The American Journal of Chinese Medicine*, *39*(04), 693–704. doi:10.1142/S0192415X11009135 PMID:21721150

Chang, W. (2013). *Legal Issues relating to End-of-life and Palliative Care*. Paper presented at the Asia Pacific Regional Conference on End-of-life and Palliative Care in Long Term Care Settings, Hong Kong.

Chan, G. H. H., Law, B. Y. K., Chu, J. M. T., Yue, K. K. M., Jiang, Z. H., Lau, C. W., & Wong, R. N. S. et al. (2013). Ginseng extracts restore high-glucose induced vascular dysfunctions by altering triglyceride metabolism and down-regulation of atherosclerosis-related genes. *Evidence-Based Complementary and Alternative Medicine*, *2013*, 1–13. doi:10.1155/2013/812096 PMID:24194784

Chan, H. M., & Pang, S. (2007). Long-Term Care: Dignity, Autonomy, Family Integrity, and Social Sustainability: The Hong Kong Experience. *The Journal of Medicine and Philosophy*, *32*(5), 401–424. doi:10.1080/03605310701631661 PMID:17924269

Chan, S. C. C., Siu, A. M. H., Poon, P. K. K., & Chan, C. C. H. (2005). Chronic disease self-management program for Chinese patients: A preliminary multi-baseline study. *International Journal of Rehabilitation Research. Internationale Zeitschrift fur Rehabilitationsforschung. Revue Internationale de Recherches de Readaptation*, *28*(4), 351–354. doi:10.1097/00004356-200512000-00008 PMID:16319561

Chan, W. C. H., Tse, H. S., & Chan, T. H. Y. (2006). What is Good Death: Bridging the Gap between Research and Intervention. In C. L. W. Chan & A. Y. M. Chow (Eds.), *Death, dying and bereavement -- A Hong Kong Chinese experience* (pp. 127–135). Hong Kong: Hong Kong University Press.

Chan, W. M. (2012). Policy implication and the way forward. *Asian Journal of Gerontology and Geriatrics*, *7*(1), 59–63.

Chappell, N. L., Dlitt, B. H., Hollander, M. J., Miller, J. A., & McWilliam, C. (2004). Comparative Costs of Home Care and Residential Care. *The Gerontologist*, *44*(3), 389–400. doi:10.1093/geront/44.3.389 PMID:15197293

Chatterjee, S., Patel, V., Chatterjee, A., & Weiss, H. A. (2003). Evaluation of a community-based rehabilitation model for chronic schizophrenia in rural India. *The British Journal of Psychiatry*, *182*(1), 57–62. doi:10.1192/bjp.182.1.57 PMID:12509319

Chatterji, P., Burstein, N. R., Kidder, D., & White, A. (1998). *Evaluation of the program of all-inclusive care for the elderly demonstration. The Impact of PACE on participant outcomes*. Retrieved from https://www.cms.gov/Medicare/Demonstration-Projects/DemoProjectsEvalRpts/downloads/PACE_Outcomes.pdf

Chau, P. H., Kwok, T., Woo, J., Chan, F., Hui, E., & Chan, K. C. (2010). Disagreement in preference for residential care between family caregivers and elders is greater among cognitively impaired elders group than cognitively intact elders group. *International Journal of Geriatric Psychiatry*, *25*(1), 46–54. PMID:19551703

Chen, C. H., Lin, Y. C., Liu, L. N., & Tang, S. T. (2014). Determinants of Preference for Home Death among Terminally Ill Patients with Cancer in Taiwan. *The Journal of Nursing Research*, *22*(1), 37–44. doi:10.1097/jnr.0000000000000016 PMID:24517898

Chen, D., Tang, K. K., Zhao, L., & Zhang, Y. (2015). Will China's Cooperative Medical System fail again? Insight from farmer satisfaction survey. *Health Promotion International*, *30*(2), 251–261. doi:10.1093/heapro/dat032 PMID:23669160

Chen, G., Liu, G. G., & Xu, F. (2014). The Impact of the urban resident basic medical insurance on health services utilisation in China. *PharmacoEconomics*, *32*(3), 277–292. doi:10.1007/s40273-013-0097-7 PMID:24178373

Cheng, P. F. (2009). *An analysis of public private partnership in Hong Kong: a study of West Kowloon Cultural District. HKU Theses Online*. HKUTO. doi:10.5353/th_b4676044

Cheng, S. T., & Chan, A. C. M. (2003). Regulating quality of care in nursing homes in Hong Kong: A Social-ecological Investigation. *Law & Policy*, *25*(4), 403–423. doi:10.1111/j.0265-8240.2003.00156.x

Cheng, S. T., Lum, T., Lam, L. C. W., & Fung, H. H. (2013). Hong Kong: Embracing a Fast Aging Society With Limited Welfare. *The Gerontologist*, *53*(4), 527–533. doi:10.1093/geront/gnt017 PMID:23528290

Cheng, T. (2015). Universal health coverage: An overview and lessons from Asia. *Harvard Public Health Review*, *4*, 1–12.

Chen, J. (2001). *Mao's China and the Cold War*. Chapel Hill, NC: University of North Carolina Press.

Chen, K. J., & Lu, A. P. (2006). Situation of integrative medicine in China: Results from a National Survey in 2004. *Chinese Journal of Integrative Medicine*, *12*(3), 161–165. doi:10.1007/BF02836514 PMID:17005073

Cheung, A. B. L. (2001). Health policy reform. In L. Wong & N. Flynn (Eds.), *The market in Chinese social policy* (pp. 63–87). Houndmills, UK: Palgrave. doi:10.1057/9781403919939_4

Cheung, E., Chan, A. P., & Kajewski, S. (2012). Factors contributing to successful public private partnership projects: Comparing Hong Kong with Australia and the United Kingdom. *Journal of Facilities Management*, *10*(1), 45–58. doi:10.1108/14725961211200397

Cheung, E., Chan, A. P., Lam, P. T., Chan, D. W., & Ke, Y. (2012). A comparative study of critical success factors for public private partnerships (PPP) between Mainland China and the Hong Kong Special Administrative Region. *Facilities*, *30*(13/14), 647–666. doi:10.1108/02632771211273132

Cheung, K. K. W., Au, K., Lam, W. W. S., & Jones, A. Y. M. (2008). Effects of a structured exercise programme on functional balance in visually impaired elderly living in a residential setting. *Hong Kong Physiotherapy Journal*, *26*(1), 45–28. doi:10.1016/S1013-7025(09)70007-7

Chief Executive of Hong Kong. (2005). *The 2005-06 policy address: Strong governance for the people*. Retrieved March 20, 2017 from http://www.policyaddress.gov.hk/05-06/eng/pdf/speech.pdf

Chief Executive of Hong Kong. (2007). *The 2007-08 policy address: A new direction for Hong Kong*. Retrieved March 20, 2017 from http://www.policyaddress.gov.hk/07-08/eng/docs/policy.pdf

Chief Executive of Hong Kong. (2008). *The 2008-09 policy address: Embracing new challenges*. Retrieved March 20, 2017 from http://www.policyaddress.gov.hk/08-09/eng/docs/policy.pdf

Chief Executive of Hong Kong. (2009). *The 2009-10 policy address: Breaking new ground together*. Retrieved March 20, 2017 from http://www.policyaddress.gov.hk/09-10/eng/docs/policy.pdf

Chief Executive of Hong Kong. (2014). *The 2014 policy address: Support the needy, let youth flourish, unleash Hong Kong's potential*. Retrieved March 20, 2017 from http://www.policyaddress.gov.hk/2014/eng/pdf/PA2014.pdf

Chief Executive of Hong Kong. (2015). *The 2015 policy address: Uphold the rule of law, seize the opportunities, make the right choices*. Retrieved March 20, 2017 from http://www.policyaddress.gov.hk/2015/eng/pdf/PA2015.pdf

Chief Executive of Hong Kong. (2016). *The 2016 policy address: Innovate for the economy, improve livelihood, foster harmony, share prosperity*. Retrieved March 20, 2017 from http://www.policyaddress.gov.hk/2016/eng/pdf/PA2016.pdf

Chief Executive of Hong Kong. (2017). *The 2017 Policy Address: Make best use of opportunities, develop the economy, improve people's livelihood, build an inclusive society*. Retrieved March 20, 2017 from http://www.policyaddress.gov.hk/2017/eng/pdf/PA2017.pdf

Chief Secretary for Administration's Office of Hong Kong. (2012). *Steering Committee on Population Policy – Progress report 2012* (File Ref.: CSO/ADM CR 1/3581/12). Retrieved March 20, 2017 from http://www.legco.gov.hk/yr08-09/english/hc/sub_com/hs52/papers/hs520605-csoadmcr1358112-e.pdf

Chi, I. (2002). Long-term care policy for elders in Hong Kong. *Journal of Aging & Social Policy*, *13*(2), 137–153. doi:10.1300/J031v13n02_10 PMID:12216352

Chi, I., Lam, Z., & Chan, P. (2011). *Consultancy Report on Community Support Services for the Elderly People in Hong Kong*. Hong Kong: The University of Hong Kong.

China Business News. (2015 November 30). *Expenditures of medical insurance funds exceeded revenues of medical insurance funds in many regions in China,* Chinese version. Retrieved July 14, 2016, from http://finance.sina.com.cn/china/20151130/005723882229.shtml

China Social Insurance Net. (2015). *Analysis on personal financial burden among inpatients who were covered by the Urban Resident Basic Medical Insurance Scheme*, Chinese version. Retrieved July 14, 2016, from http://www.spicezee.com/zhishi/yiliao/108433.html

Chin, C. W. W., & Phua, K. (2016). Long Term Care Policy: Singapores Experience. *Journal of Aging & Social Policy*, *28*(2), 113–129. doi:10.1080/08959420.2016.1145534 PMID:26808468

Chinese Community Nursing Home for Greater Toronto. (1989). *Health care needs of the Chinese elderly population: A needs assessment*. Toronto, ON: Author.

Chinese Medicine Ordinance, Cap 549, Laws of Hong Kong (2000).

Chippendale, T. L., & Bear-Lehman, J. (2010). Enabling aging in place for urban dwelling seniors: An adaptive or remedial approach? *Physical & Occupational Therapy in Geriatrics*, *28*(1), 57–62. doi:10.3109/02703180903381078

Chobanian, A. V., Bakris, G. L., Black, H. R., Cushman, W. C., Green, L. A., Izzo, J. L., et al. (2003). Seventh report of the joint national committee on prevention, detection, evaluation, and treatment of high blood pressure. *Hypertension*, *42*(6), 1206-1252.

Choi, B., & Lee, H. (2003). An empirical investigation of KM styles and their effect on corporate performance. *Information & Management*, *40*(5), 403–417. doi:10.1016/S0378-7206(02)00060-5

Choi, B., Poon, S. K., & Davis, J. G. (2008). Effects of knowledge management strategy on organizational performance: A complementarity theory-based approach. *Omega*, *36*(2), 235–251. doi:10.1016/j.omega.2006.06.007

Choice. (2016). *Failing standards in nursing homes and aged care*. Retrieved February 1, 2017, from https://www.choice.com.au/health-and-body/healthy-aging/aging-and-retirement/articles/nursing-home-problems

Choi, J. H., Byeon, J., & Lee, S., & Sh, H. (2001). Preferred place of death of elderly women in Seoul. *Journal of Korean Academy of Family Medicine*, *22*(6), 939–945.

Choi, K. S., Chae, Y. M., Lee, C. G., Kim, S., Lee, S., Heo, D. S., & Yun, Y. H. et al. (2005). Factors influencing preferences for place of terminal care and of death among cancer patients and their families in Korea. *Supportive Care in Cancer*, *13*(8), 565–572. doi:10.1007/s00520-005-0809-4 PMID:15812653

Chokkanathan, S., Morrow-Howell, N., & Chen, H. (2015). Older adults in the community: Capacities and engagement for aging in place. *Asia Pacific Journal of Social Work and Development*, *25*(4), 183–185. doi:10.1080/02185385.2015.1119534

Chong, A. Y. L., & Chan, F. T. (2012). Structural equation modeling for multi-stage analysis on radio frequency identification (RFID) diffusion in the health care industry. *Expert Systems with Applications*, *39*(10), 8645–8654. doi:10.1016/j.eswa.2012.01.201

Chou, K. L., Chow, N. W. S., & Chi, I. (2005). A Proposal for a Voucher System for Long-Term Care in Hong Kong. *Journal of Aging & Social Policy*, *17*(2), 85–106. doi:10.1300/J031v17n02_06 PMID:15911519

Chow, C., Jolly, S., Rao-Melacini, P., Fox, K., Anand, S., & Yusuf, S. (2010). Association of diet, exercise, and smoking modification with risk of early cardiovascular events after acute coronary syndromes. *Circulation*, *121*(6), 750–758. doi:10.1161/CIRCULATIONAHA.109.891523 PMID:20124123

Chu, L. W., McGhee, S. M., Luk, J. K., Kwok, T., Hui, E., Chui, P. K., ... Woo, J. (2011). Advance directive and preference of old age home residents for community model of end-of-life care in Hong Kong. *Hong Kong Medical Journal*, *17*(852), 13–5.

Chu, F. Y., Wang, J., Yao, K. W., & Li, Z. Z. (2010). Effect of Xuefu Zhuyu Capsule on the symptoms and signs and health-related quality of life in the unstable angina patients with blood-stasis syndrome after percutaneous coronary intervention: A randomized controlled trial. *Chinese Journal of Integrative Medicine*, *16*(5), 399–405. doi:10.1007/s11655-010-9999-9 PMID:20535581

Chui, W. E., Chan, K., Chong, M. A., Ko, S. L., ... Ng, Y. S. (2009). Elderly Commission's Study on Residential Care Services for the Elderly: Final Report. The University of Hong Kong.

Chui, W. T. E., Chan, K. S., Chong, M. L., Ko, S. F., Law, S. C. K., Law, C. K., . . . Ng, Y. T. (2009). *Elderly Commission's Study on Residential Care Services for the Elderly - Final Report*. Retrieved February 1, 2017, from http://www.elderlycommission.gov.hk/en/download/library/Residential%20Care%20Services%20-%20Final%20Report(eng).pdf

Chui, E. W. T. (2008). Ageing in Place in Hong Kong – Challenges and Opportunities in a Capitalist Chinese City. *International Ageing*, *32*(3), 167–182. doi:10.1007/s12126-008-9015-2

Chui, W. T., Chan, K. S., Chong, M. L., Ko, S. F., Law, C. K., Law, C. K., & Ng, Y. T. et al. (2009). *Elderly Commission's Study on Residential Care Services for the Elderly*. Hong Kong: The University of Hong Kong.

Chu, L. W., & Chi, I. (2006). Long-Term Care and Hospital Care for the Elderly. In G. M. Leung & J. Bacon-shone (Eds.), *Hong Kong's Health System* (pp. 223–252). Hong Kong: Hong Kong University Press.

Chu, L. W., Luk, J. K. H., Hui, E., Chiu, P. K. C., Chan, C. S. Y., Kwan, F., & Woo, J. et al. (2011). Advance Directive and End-of-Life Care Preferences Among Chinese Nursing Home Residents in Hong Kong. *Journal of the American Medical Directors Association*, *12*(2), 143–152. doi:10.1016/j.jamda.2010.08.015 PMID:21266291

Chu, L.-W., & Chi, I. (2006). Long-term care and hospital care for the elderly. In G. M. Leung & J. Bacon-Shone (Eds.), *Hong Kong's health system: Reflections, perspectives and visions* (pp. 223–252). Hong Kong: Hong Kong University Press.

Chu, M. L. S. C., Liu, K. Y., Ip, C. F., Leung, E., & Tsang, A. K. T. (2015). Transforming organizational culture using the SSLD system to address the taboo of sexuality and intimacy needs of seniors. *Journal of Contemporary Management*, *4*(4), 15–23.

Chung, R. Y., Tin, K. Y. K., Cowling, B. J., Chan, K. P., Chan, W. M., Lo, S. V., & Leung, G. M. (2009). Long-term care cost drivers and expenditure projection to 2036 in Hong Kong. *BMC Health Services Research*, *9*(1), 172. doi:10.1186/1472-6963-9-172 PMID:19775476

Chung, R. Y., Wong, E. L., Kiang, N., Chau, P. Y., Lau, J. Y., Wong, S. Y., & Woo, J. et al. (2017). Knowledge, Attitudes, and Preferences of Advance Decisions, End-of-Life Care, and Place of Care and Death in Hong Kong. A Population-Based Telephone Survey of 1067 Adults. *Journal of the American Medical Directors Association*, *18*(4), 367. doi:10.1016/j.jamda.2016.12.066 PMID:28214237

Clark, A., Davidson, P., Currie, K., Karimi, M., Duncan, A., & Thompson, D. (2010). Understanding and promoting self-care during heart failure. *Current Treatment Options in Cardiovascular Medicine*, *12*(1), 1–9. doi:10.1007/s11936-009-0053-1 PMID:20842477

Cleaver, S., & Nixon, S. (2014). A scoping review of 10 years of published literature on community-based rehabilitation. *Disability and Rehabilitation*, *36*(17), 1385–1394. doi:10.3109/09638288.2013.845257 PMID:24151820

Cline, K. (2003). Influences on intergovernmental implementation: The states and the superfund. *State Politics & Policy Quarterly*, *3*(1), 66–83.

Cohen, D., Manuel, D. G., Tugwell, P., Sanmartin, C., & Ramsay, T. (2014). Direct healthcare costs of acute myocardial infarction in Canadas elderly across the continuum of care. *The Journal of the Economics of Ageing*, *3*, 44–49. doi:10.1016/j.jeoa.2014.05.002

Cole, J., Smith, S., Hart, N., & Cupples, M. (2013). Do practitioners and friends support patients with coronary heart disease in lifestyle change? *BMC Family Practice*, *14*(1), 126. doi:10.1186/1471-2296-14-126 PMID:23984815

College of Medicine. (2013). *The crisis in costs*. Retrieved from: http://www.collegeofmedicine.org.uk/crisis-costs

Collier, R. B., & Collier, D. (1991). *Shaping the political arena: critical junctures, the labor movement, and regime dynamics in Latin America*. Princeton, NJ: Princeton University Press.

Collin, C., Wade, D. T., Davies, S., & Horne, V. (1988). The Barthel ADL Index: A Reliability Study. *International Disability Studies*, *10*(2), 61–63. doi:10.3109/09638288809164103 PMID:3403500

Colombo F. and J Mercier (2011). Balancing fair protection and financial sustainability in long-term care. *Eurohealth*, *17*(2–3), 3-6.

Community Care Access Centre. (2014). *Home first*. Retrieved from http://healthcareathome.ca/central/en/Getting-care/Getting-Care-at-Home/home-first

Connor, S. R., & Sepulveda Bermedo, M. C. (2014). *Global atlas of palliative care at the end of life*. World Health Organization.

Conn, V. (2011). Helping patients help themselves: Chronic disease self-management interventions. *Western Journal of Nursing Research*, *33*(2), 159–160. doi:10.1177/0193945910386194 PMID:21252383

Cook, D. A., & Triola, M. M. (2009). Virtual patients: A critical literature review and proposed next steps. *Medical Education*, *43*(4), 303–311. doi:10.1111/j.1365-2923.2008.03286.x PMID:19335571

Corrigan, P., & Hicks, N. (2012). *What organisation is necessary for commissioners to develop outcomes based contracts? The COBIC case study*. Right Care Casebook Series. London: NHS. Retrieved from: http://www.rightcare.nhs.uk/downloads/RC_Casebook_cobic_final.pdf

Cortell, A. P., & Peterson, S. (1999). Altered states: Explaining domestic institutional change. *British Journal of Political Science*, *29*(1), 177–203. doi:10.1017/S0007123499000083

Costa, V. (2014). The Determinants of Place of Death: An Evidence-Based Analysis. *Ontario Health Technology Assessment Series*, *14*(16), 1–78. PMID:26351550

Coulson, I., Minichiello, V., Kao, R. S., Lin, F., & Wan, C. C. (2000). Developing collaborative gerontology programs offshore: A case study. *Educational Gerontology*, *26*, 387–400. doi:10.1080/036012700407866

Cox, C. B. (2005). *Community care for an aging society*. New York, NY: Springer.

Cresci, M. K., & Novak, J. M. (2012). Information Technologies as Health Management Tools: Urban Elders Interest and Ability in Usingthe Internet. *Educational Gerontology*, *38*(7), 491–506. doi:10.1080/03601277.2011.567185

Cressman, M. D., & Gifford, R. W. Jr. (1983). Hypertension and stroke. *Journal of the American College of Cardiology*, *1*(2), 521–527. doi:10.1016/S0735-1097(83)80083-7 PMID:6826961

Cullen, K. W., Baranowski, T., Owens, E., Marsh, T., Rittenberry, L., & de Moor, C. (2003). Availability, accessibility, and preferences for fruit, 100% fruit juice, and vegetables influence childrens dietary behavior. *Health Education & Behavior*, *30*(5), 615–626. doi:10.1177/1090198103257254 PMID:14582601

Cumming, E., & Henry, W. E. (1961). *Growing old*. New York: Basic.

Daft, R. L., & Marcic, D. (2017). *Understanding Management* (10th ed.). Boston, MA: Cengage Learning.

Dahlöf, B., Hansson, L., Lindholm, L., Schersten, B., Ekbom, T., & Wester, P. (1991). Morbidity and mortality in the Swedish trial in old patients with hypertension (STOP-Hypertension). *Lancet*, *338*(8778), 1281–1285. doi:10.1016/0140-6736(91)92589-T PMID:1682683

Dahlöf, B., Pennert, K., & Hansson, L. (1992). Reversal of left ventricular hypertrophy in hypertensive patients a meta-analysis of 109 treatment studies. *American Journal of Hypertension*, *5*(2), 95–110. doi:10.1093/ajh/5.2.95 PMID:1532319

Dalkir, K., & Liebowitz, J. (2011). *Knowledge Management in Theory and Practice*. Cambridge, MA: MIT Press.

Dalleck, L., Schmidt, L., & Lueker, R. (2011). Cardiac rehabilitation outcomes in a conventional versus telemedicine-based programme. *Journal of Telemedicine in Healthcare*, *17*(5), 217–221. doi:10.1258/jtt.2010.100407 PMID:21508077

Dannefer, D., Uhlenberg, P., Foner, A., & Abeles, R. P. (2005). On the shoulders of a giant: The legacy of Matilda White Riley for gerontology. *The Journals of Gerontology. Series B, Psychological Sciences and Social Sciences*, *60*(6), S296–S304. doi:10.1093/geronb/60.6.S296 PMID:16260711

Das, J., Do, Q.-T., Friedman, J., & McKenzie, D. (2008). *Mental Health Patterns and Consequences: Results from Survey Data in Five Developing Countries*. Policy Research Working Paper; No. WPS 4495. World Bank, Washington. Retrieved from https://openknowledge.worldbank.org/handle/10986/6376

Davey, A., & Eggebeen, D. J. (1998). Patterns of intergenerational exchange and mental health. *The Journals of Gerontology. Series B, Psychological Sciences and Social Sciences*, *53*(2), 86–95. doi:10.1093/geronb/53B.2.P86 PMID:9520925

Davies, B., & Challis, D. (1986). *Matching resources to needs in community care: An evaluated demonstrations of a long-term care model*. Hants, UK: Gower Publishing.

Davies, J., & Davies, D. (2010). Origins and evolution of antibiotic resistance. *Microbiology and Molecular Biology Reviews*, *74*(3), 417–433. doi:10.1128/MMBR.00016-10 PMID:20805405 de Bakker, D. H., Struijs, J. N., Baan, C. A., Raams, J., de Wildt, J. E., Vrijhoef, H. J., & Schut, F. T. (2012). Early results from adoption of bundled payment for diabetes care in the Netherlands show improvement in care coordination. *Health Affairs*, *31*(2), 426–433. doi:10.1377/hlthaff.2011.0912 PMID:22323174

De Bruin, S., Heijink, R., Lemmens, L. C., Struijs, J. N., & Baan, C. A. (2011). Impact of disease management programs on healthcare expenditures for patients with diabetes, depression, heart failure or chronic obstructive pulmonary disease: A systematic review of the literature. *Health Policy (Amsterdam)*, *101*(2), 105–121. doi:10.1016/j.healthpol.2011.03.006 PMID:21592607

De Brún, C. (2007). Knowledge management and the national health service in England. In R. Bali & A. Dwivedi (Eds.), *Healthcare Knowledge Management* (pp. 179–188). New York, NY: Springer. doi:10.1007/978-0-387-49009-0_13

De Gagne, J. C. (2011). The impact of clickers in nursing education: A review of literature. *Nurse Education Today*, *31*(8), e34–e40. doi:10.1016/j.nedt.2010.12.007 PMID:21232831

De Meijer, C., Wouterse, B., Polder, J., & Koopmanschap, K. (2013). The effect of population aging on health expenditure growth: A critical review. *European Journal of Ageing*, *10*(4), 353–361. doi:10.1007/s10433-013-0280-x

Deber, R. B. (2003). Health Care Reform: Lessons from Canada. *American Journal of Public Health*, *93*(1), 20–24. doi:10.2105/AJPH.93.1.20 PMID:12511378

Deloitte and Touche Consulting Group. (1996). *Consultancy Study on Needs of Elderly in Hong Kong for Community Support and Residential Care Services*. Retrieved March 19, 2017, from http://www.legco.gov.hk/yr98-99/english/panels/ws/papers/ws14093d.pdf

Deloitte. (2014). *Fortune Favors the Bold Shifting to Private Health*. Deloitte.

Demiris, G., Oliver, D. P., Dickey, G., Skubic, M., & Rantz, M. (2008). Findings from a participatory evaluation of a smart home application for older adults. *Technology and Health Care*, *16*(2), 111–118. PMID:18487857

Department of Family and Community Services (DFCS), NSW Government. (2012). *The NSW Aging Strategy 2016-2020*. Retrieved February 1, 2017, from https://www.adhc.nsw.gov.au/__data/assets/file/0011/257276/1282_ADHC_NSW-AgeingStrategy_WEB.pdf

Department of Family and Community Services (DFCS), NSW Government. (2016). *The NSW Aging Strategy 2016-2020*. Retrieved February 1, 2017, from https://www.facs.nsw.gov.au/participation-and-inclusion/the-nsw-ageing-strategy-2016-2020

Department of Health and Human Services National Institute on Aging. (2007). Growing Older in America: The Health and Retirement Study. Washington, DC: Author.

Department of Health of Hong Kong. (2008). *Promoting health in Hong Kong: A strategic framework for prevention and control of non-communicable diseases*. Retrieved March 20, 2017 from http://www.change4health.gov.hk/filemanager/common/image/strategic_framework/promoting_health/promoting_health_e.pdf

Department of Health of Hong Kong. (2016a). *Common health problems*. Retrieved March 20, 2017 from http://www.elderly.gov.hk/english/common_health_problems/index.html

Department of Health of Hong Kong. (2016b). *Health facts of Hong Kong* (2016 edition). Retrieved March 20, 2017 from http://www.dh.gov.hk/english/statistics/statistics_hs/files/Health_Statistics_pamphlet_E.pdf

Department of Health. (2011). *Health Watch: Aim for "2 Plus 3 a day"*. Retrieved from http://www.change4health.gov.hk/en/whats_new/health_watch/index_id_2.html

Department of Health. (2014). *Student Health Service - About Student Health ServiceCentre / Special Assessment Centre*. Retrieved from http://www.studenthealth.gov.hk/english/aboutus/aboutus_shscsac/aboutus_shscsac.html

Department of Health. (2015). *Health Facts of Hong Kong*. Retrieved July 1, 2016 from http://www.dh.gov.hk/english/statistics/statistics_hs/files/Health_Statistics_pamphlet_E.pdf

Department of Health. (2016). Retrieved from http://www.dh.gov.hk/cindex.html

Development Bureau of Hong Kong. (2016). *Legislative Council Panel on Development: Extending the operation of Energizing Kowloon East Office* (Paper No. LC Paper No. CB(1)133/16-17(04)). Retrieved March 20, 2017 from http://www.ekeo.gov.hk/filemanager/content/public/en/dev20161122cb1-133-4-e.pdf

Dillaway, H., & Byrnes, M. (2009). Reconsidering successful aging. *Journal of Applied Gerontology*, *28*(6), 702–722. doi:10.1177/0733464809333882

DiMaggio, P. (1988). Interest and agency in institutional theory. In L. G. Zucker (Ed.), *Institutional patterns and organizations: culture and environment* (pp. 3–21). Cambridge, MA: Ballinger Pub. Co.

Dixon, B. E., Simonaitis, L., Goldberg, H. S., Paterno, M. D., Schaeffer, M., Hongsermeier, T., & Middleton, B. et al. (2013). A pilot study of distributed knowledge management and clinical decision support in the cloud. *Artificial Intelligence in Medicine*, *59*(1), 45–53. doi:10.1016/j.artmed.2013.03.004 PMID:23545327

Doh, J. P., & Quigley, N. R. (2014). Responsible Leadership and Stakeholder Management: Influence Pathways and Organizational Outcomes. *The Academy of Management Perspectives*, *28*(3), 255–274. doi:10.5465/amp.2014.0013

Dong, W. (2001). *Health care reform in urban China*. Retrieved July 7, 2016, from http://munkschool.utoronto.ca/cphs/wp-content/uploads/2012/03/Weizhen_Dong-2001-02.pdf

Dong, W. (2008). Cost containment and access to care: The Shanghai health care financing model. *The Singapore Economic Review*, *53*(1), 27–41. doi:10.1142/S0217590808002823

Donovan, T., Mooney, C., & Smith, D. (2013). *State and local politics: Institutions and Reforms* (3rd ed.). Stamford, CT: Cengage Learning.

Dotterweich-Bryan, L., & McNeal, R. (2004). *No child left behind: the report card—why are some states successfully implementing new law and others not?* Paper at the meeting of the Fourth Annual State Politics and Policy Conference, Cuyahoga Falls, OH.

Dowd, J. J. (1975). Aging as exchange: A preface to theory. *Journal of Gerontology*, *30*(5), 584–594. doi:10.1093/geronj/30.5.584 PMID:1181364

Dowd, J. J. (1988). The reification of age: Age stratification theory and the passing of the autonomous subject. *Journal of Aging Studies*, *1*(4), 317–335. doi:10.1016/0890-4065(87)90008-9 PMID:25195842

Drago, F., Ciccarese, G., Broccolo, F., Sartoris, G., Stura, P., Esposito, S., & Parodi, A. et al. (2016). A new enhanced antibiotic treatment for early and late syphilis. *Journal of Global Antimicrobial Resistance*, *5*, 64–66. doi:10.1016/j.jgar.2015.12.006 PMID:27436469

Drucker, P. F. (2008). *Management* (revised edition). New York: Harper Collins Publishers.

Duckett, J. (2001). Political interests and the implementation of China's urban health insurance reform. *Social Policy and Administration*, *35*(3), 290–306. doi:10.1111/1467-9515.00234

Duff, J. (2001). Financing to foster community health care: A comparative analysis of Singapore, Europe, North America and Australia. *Current Sociology*, *49*(3), 135–154. doi:10.1177/0011392101049003009

Dunn, H. L. (1959). What high-level wellness means. *Canadian Journal of Public Health*, *50*(11), 447–457. PMID:13818678

Du, S., & Yuan, C. (2010). Evaluations of patient self-management outcomes in healthcare: A systematic review. *International Nursing Review*, *57*(2), 159–167. doi:10.1111/j.1466-7657.2009.00794.x PMID:20579149

Dwivedi, A. N., Bali, R. K., & Naguib, R. N. (2007). Building new healthcare management paradigms: A case for healthcare knowledge management. In R. Bali & A. Dwivedi (Eds.), *Healthcare Knowledge Management* (pp. 3–10). New York, NY: Springer. doi:10.1007/978-0-387-49009-0_1

Education Bureau (EDB). (2016). *Economic analysis and evaluation of government policies: Health and healthcare in Hong Kong*. Retrieved 22 March 2016, from http://www.edb.gov.hk/attachment/en/curriculum-development/kla/pshe/references-and-resources/economics/health_eng.pdf

Edwards, M. P., McClement, S. E., & Read, L. R. (2013). Nurses responses to initial moral distress in long-term care. *Journal of Bioethical Inquiry*, *10*(3), 325–336. doi:10.1007/s11673-013-9463-6 PMID:23793936

eHealth HKSAR. (2016). *About eHR*. Retrieved 12 April, 2016, from http://www.ehealth.gov.hk/en/about_ehrss/index.html

Eisenegger, M., & Schranz, M. (2014). Reputation Management and Corporate Social Responsibility. In Ø. Ihlen, J. L. Barlett, & S. May (Eds.), *The Handbook of Communication and Corporate Social Responsibility* (pp. 128–146). Malden, MA: Wiley-Blackwell.

Elderly Commission of Hong Kong. (2009). *Minutes of the 56th meeting*. Retrieved March 20, 2017 from http://www.elderlycommission.gov.hk/en/download/meeting/Min-56(22.1.09)_e.pdf

Elkington, J. (1994). Towards the sustainable corporation: Win-win-win business strategies for sustainable development. *California Management Review*, *36*(2), 90–100. doi:10.2307/41165746

Elliott, W. J. (2000). Therapeutic trials comparing angiotensin converting enzyme inhibitors and angiotensin II receptor blockers. *Current Hypertension Reports*, *2*(4), 402–411. doi:10.1007/s11906-000-0045-8 PMID:10981176

Elwood, P., Galante, J., Pickering, J., Palmer, S., Bayer, A., Ben-Shlomo, Y., & Gallacher, J. et al. (2013). Healthy Lifestyles Reduce the Incidence of Chronic Diseases and Dementia: Evidence from the Caerphilly Cohort Study. *PLoS ONE*, *8*(12), 81877–81884. doi:10.1371/journal.pone.0081877 PMID:24349147

Emanuel, E. J., & Emanuel, L. L. (1996). What is accountability in health care? *Annals of Internal Medicine*, *124*(2), 229–239. doi:10.7326/0003-4819-124-2-199601150-00007 PMID:8533999

Enache, D., Winblad, B., & Aarsland, D. (2011). Depression in dementia. *Current Opinion in Psychiatry*, 462–472. doi:10.1097/yco.0b013e32834bb9d4 PMID:21926624

Erikson, E. H. (1950). *Childhood and society*. New York: Norton.

Erikson, E. H., & Erikson, J. M. (1982/1997). *The life cycle completed: Extended version*. New York: Norton.

Ernst and Young. (2015). *Megatrends 2015: Making sense of a world motion*. Ernst and Young.

Escobar Pinzon, L. C., Claus, M., Zepf, K. I., Letzel, S., Fischbeck, S., & Weber, M. (2011). Preference for place of death in Germany. *Journal of Palliative Medicine*, *14*(10), 1097–1103. doi:10.1089/jpm.2011.0136 PMID:22004148

European Commission. (2011). *A renewed EU strategy 2011-14 for Corporate Social Responsibility*. Brussels, 25.10.2011, COM (2011) 681 final. Retrieved August 28, 2016, from http://eurlex.europa.eu/LexUriServ/LexUriServ.do?uri1/4COM:2011:0681:FIN:EN:PDF

European Federation of Pharmaceutical Industries and Association. (2014). *Health & Growth: Working Together for a Healthy Europe*. Retrieved July 17, 2016, from www.efpai.eu

European Investment Bank. (2016). Royal London and Barts Hospital PPP Project. *The EU bank*. Retrieved from http://www.eib.org/projects/pipeline/2003/20030038.htm

Evangelical Lutheran Church Social Service-Hong Kong. (2017a). *Elderly Services*. Retrieved February 20, 2017 from http://service.elchk.org.hk/eng/unit_service3.php

Evangelical Lutheran Church Social Service-Hong Kong. (2017b). *Support Us*. Retrieved February 20, 2017 from http://service.elchk.org.hk/eng/partner.php

Evashwick, C. J. (1989). Creating a continuum. The goal is to provide an integrated system of care. *Health Progress (Saint Louis, Mo.)*, *70*(5), 36–39, 56. PMID:10293328

Executive Yuan of Taiwan. (2017). *Executive Yuan passes 10-year long-term care 2.0 plan*. Retrieved March 20, 2017 from http://english.ey.gov.tw/News_Hot_Topic.aspx?n=FE8C5966F81D8273&sms=BBB420E471DAF6C0

Fang, H. S., Liu, C. C., Jia, C. H., Chen, Y. H., & Li, C. Y. (2015). Risk of Developing Coronary Artery Disease in Patients with Type 2 Diabetes Receiving Traditional Chinese Medicine Therapy. *Journal of Alternative and Complementary Medicine (New York, N.Y.)*, *21*(10), 604–609. doi:10.1089/acm.2014.0079 PMID:26247098

Feldstein, P. J. (1993). *Health Care Economics*. Albany, NY: Delmar Publishers.

Feng, Y., Xiong, X., Xue, Q., Yao, L., Luo, F., & Xiang, L. (2013). The impact of medical insurance policies on the hospitalization services utilization of people with schizophrenia: A case study in Changsha, China. *Pakistan Journal of Medical Sciences*, *29*(3), 793–798. doi:10.12669/pjms.293.3273 PMID:24353630

Feng, Z. (2016). Marginalisation and health provision in transitional China. In H. X. Zhang, B. Wu, & R. Sanders (Eds.), *Marginalisation in China: perspectives on transition and globalization* (pp. 97–116). Aldershot, UK: Ashgate.

Fenton, S., & Draper, H. (2014). *Cultural differences in aging in the UK - A significant knowledge gap*. Birmingham Policy Commission. Retrieved March 13, 2017, from http://www.birmingham.ac.uk/Documents/research/policycommission/healthy-aging/2-Cultural-differences-in-aging-in-the-UK-a-significant-knowledge-gap.pdf

Ferlie, E., Crilly, T., Jashapara, A., Trenholm, S., Peckham, A., & Currie, G. (2015). Knowledge mobilization in healthcare organizations: A view from the resource-based view of the firm. *International Journal of Health Policy and Management*, *4*(3), 127–130. doi:10.15171/ijhpm.2015.35 PMID:25774369

finance.china.com.cn. (2016 March 8). *Li Bin: China's elderly population aged 60 and over passed 220 million in 2015*, Chinese version. Retrieved June 18, 2016, from http://finance.huanqiu.com/roll/2016-03/8672801.html

Financial Secretary of Hong Kong. (2015). *The 2015-16 budget*. Retrieved March 20, 2017 from http://www.budget.gov.hk/2015/eng/pdf/e_budgetspeech2015-16.pdf

Financial Secretary of Hong Kong. (2016a). *2016-17 budget (media sheet)*. Retrieved March 20, 2017 from http://www.budget.gov.hk/2016/eng/pdf/2016-17_Media_Sheet.pdf

Financial Secretary of Hong Kong. (2016b). *The 2016-17 budget*. Retrieved March 20, 2017 from http://www.budget.gov.hk/2016/eng/pdf/e_budgetspeech2016-17.pdf

Finkeflügel, H., Wolffers, I., & Huijsma, R. (2005). The evidence base for community-based rehabilitation: A literature review. *International Journal of Rehabilitation Research. Internationale Zeitschrift fur Rehabilitationsforschung. Revue Internationale de Recherches de Readaptation*, *28*(3), 187–201. doi:10.1097/00004356-200509000-00001 PMID:16046912

Firszt, D. (2015). Innovations and Their Diffusion Versus CSR Practices. In L. O'Riodan, P. Zmuda, & S. Heinemann (Eds.), *New Perspectives on Corporate Social Responsibility: Locating the Missing Link* (pp. 109–125). Essen, Germany: Springer Gabler. doi:10.1007/978-3-658-06794-6_6

Firuzi, O., Javidnia, K., Gholami, M., Soltani, M., & Miri, R. (2010). Antioxidant activity and total phenolic content of 24 Lamiaceae species growing in Iran. *Natural Product Communications, 5*(2), 261-264.

Fisher, J. O., Mitchell, D. C., Smiciklas-Wright, H., & Birch, L. L. (2002). Parental influences on young girls fruit and vegetable, micronutrient, and fat intakes. *Journal of the American Dietetic Association, 102*(1), 58–64. doi:10.1016/S0002-8223(02)90017-9 PMID:11794503

Fitbit. (2016). *Fitbit PurePulse Continuous Wrist-Based Heart Rate*. Retrieved 28 July 2016, https://www.fitbit.com/hk/purepulse

Flannery, R. B. (2002). Treating learned helplessness in the elderly dementia patient: Preliminary inquiry. *American Journal of Alzheimers Disease and Other Dementias, 17*(6), 345–349. doi:10.1177/153331750201700605 PMID:12501481

Flather, M. D., Shibata, M. C., Coats, A. J., Van Veldhuisen, D. J., Parkhomenko, A., & Borbola, J. (2005). Randomized trial to determine the effect of nebivolol on mortality and cardiovascular hospital admission in elderly patients with heart failure (SENIORS). *European Heart Journal, 26*(3), 215–225. doi:10.1093/eurheartj/ehi115 PMID:15642700

Fleg, J. L. (2008). Improving Exercise Tolerance in Chronic Heart Failure. *Journal of the American College of Cardiology, 51*(17), 1672–1674. doi:10.1016/j.jacc.2008.01.027 PMID:18436119

Fleg, J. L., Aronow, W. S., & Frishman, W. H. (2011). Cardiovascular drug therapy in the elderly: Benefits and challenges. *Nature Reviews. Cardiology, 8*(1), 13–28. doi:10.1038/nrcardio.2010.162 PMID:20978470

Fleg, J. L., O'connor, F., Gerstenblith, G., Becker, L., Clulow, J., & Schulman, S. et al.. (1995). Impact of age on the cardiovascular response to dynamic upright exercise in healthy men and women. *Journal of Applied Physiology, 78*(3), 890–900. PMID:7775334

Flynn, M. B. (2015). *Pharmaceutical autonomy and public health in Latin America: state, society, and industry in Brazil's AIDS program*. New York, NY: Routledge.

Folstein, M. F., Fostein, S. E., & McHugh, P. R. (1975). Mini-mental state: A practical method for grading the cognitive state of patients for the clinician. *Journal of Psychiatric Research, 12*(3), 189–198. doi:10.1016/0022-3956(75)90026-6 PMID:1202204

Food and Health Bureau of Hong Kong. (2008). *Environmental Report, 2007*. Retrieved from http://www.epd.gov.hk/epd/english/how_help/tools_epr/files/fhb_ER2007e.pdf

Food and Health Bureau of Hong Kong. (2010). *Legislative Council Panel on Health Services: Healthcare service reform – primary care development strategy* (Paper No. CB(2)1995/09-10(01)). Retrieved March 20, 2017 from http://www.legco.gov.hk/yr09-10/english/panels/hs/papers/hs0712cb2-1995-1-e.pdf

Food and Health Bureau of Hong Kong. (2013). *Legislative Council Panel on Health Services Subcommittee on Health Protection Scheme: Role and development of public and private healthcare services* (Paper No. CB(2)448/12-13(02)). Retrieved March 20, 2017 from http://www.legco.gov.hk/yr12-13/english/panels/hs/hs_hps/papers/hs_hps0114cb2-448-2-e.pdf

Food and Health Bureau of Hong Kong. (2014). *Consultation document on voluntary health insurance scheme*. Retrieved March 20, 2017 from http://www.vhis.gov.hk/doc/en/full_consultation_document/consultation_full_eng.pdf

Food and Health Bureau of Hong Kong. (2015a). *Legislative Council Panel on Health Services: 2015 Policy Address – Policy initiatives of the Food and Health Bureau* (LC Paper No. CB(2)612/14-15(03)). Retrieved March 20, 2017 from http://www.legco.gov.hk/yr14-15/english/panels/hs/papers/hs20150119cb2-612-3-e.pdf

Food and Health Bureau of Hong Kong. (2015b). *Report of the Steering Committee on Review of Hospital Authority.* Retrieved March 20, 2017 from http://www.legco.gov.hk/yr14-15/english/panels/hs/papers/hs20150720cb2-1907-1-e.pdf

Food and Health Bureau of Hong Kong. (2016). *Legislative Council Panel on Health Services: An update on public hospital developments* (LC Paper No. CB(2)652/15-16(04)). Retrieved March 20, 2017 from http://www.legco.gov.hk/yr15-16/english/panels/hs/papers/hs20160118cb2-652-4-e.pdf

Food and Health Bureau. (2012). *Hospital Authority: Public-private prartnership (PPP) programmes.* Retrieved 26 Feb 2017, from http://www.aud.gov.hk/pdf_e/e58ch03.pdf

Food and Health Bureau. (2016). *Executive Summary for Improving Hong Kong Health Care System.* Healthcare Planning and Development Office. Retrieved 25 Feb 2017, from http://www.hpdo.gov.hk/en/doc/improving_hk_healtcare_system_summary_eng.pdf

Food and Health Bureau. (2016). *Life expectancy at birth.* Retrieved March 28, 2016, from http://www.fhb.gov.hk/statistics/en/statistics/life_expectancy.htm

Food and Health Bureau. (2016). *Life Expectancy.* Retrieved May 18, 2016 from http://www.fhb.gov.hk/statistics/en/statistics/life_expectancy.htm

Ford, G. A., Choy, A. M., Deedwania, P., Karalis, D. G., Lindholm, C.-J., Pluta, W., & Olsson, S. B. et al. (2007). Direct Thrombin Inhibition and Stroke Prevention in Elderly Patients With Atrial Fibrillation. *Stroke*, *38*(11), 2965–2971. doi:10.1161/STROKEAHA.107.488007 PMID:17885258

Fording, R. (2012). *State ideology data.* Retrieved June 15, 2014, from http://rcfording.wordpress.com/state-ideology-data/

Foster, D., & Harkness, G. (2010). *Healthcare reform: pending changes to reimbursement for 30-day readmissions.* Healthcare reform: reimbursement. Thomson Reuters.

Francesca, C., Ana, L. N., Jérôme, M., & Frits, T. (2011). *OECD health policy studies help wanted? Providing and paying for long-term care: providing and paying for long-term care* (Vol. 2011). OECD Publishing.

Franco-Santosa, M., Lucianetti, L., & Bourne, M. (2012). Contemporary performance measurement systems: A review of their consequences and a framework for research. *Management Accounting Research*, *23*(2), 79–119. doi:10.1016/j.mar.2012.04.001

Franse, L. V., Pahor, M., Di Bari, M., Somes, G. W., Cushman, W. C., & Applegate, W. B. (2000). Hypokalemia associated with diuretic use and cardiovascular events in the Systolic Hypertension in the Elderly Program. *Hypertension*, *35*(5), 1025–1030. doi:10.1161/01.HYP.35.5.1025 PMID:10818057

Friedman, M. (1970, September 13). The Social Responsibility of Business Is to Increase Profits. *New York Times Magazine*, p. 13.

Fries, B. E., & Cooney, L. M. (1985). Validation and use of resource utilization groups as a case-mix measure for long-term care. *Medical Care*, *23*(2), 123–132. doi:10.1097/00005650-198502000-00003 PMID:3919223

Fries, B. E., Schneider, D. P., Foley, W. J., Gavazzi, M., Burke, R., & Cornelius, E. (1994). Redefining a case mix measure for nursing homes: Resouce utilization groups (RUG-III). *Medical Care*, *32*(7), 668–685. doi:10.1097/00005650-199407000-00002 PMID:8028403

Frishman, W. H., Chiu, R., Landzberg, B. R., & Weiss, M. (1998). Medical therapies for the prevention of restenosis after percutaneous coronary interventions. *Current Problems in Cardiology, 23*(10), 533–635. doi:10.1016/S0146-2806(98)80002-9 PMID:9805205

Fugate, B. S., Stank, T. P., & Mentzer, J. T. (2009). Linking improved knowledge management to operational and organizational performance. *Journal of Operations Management, 27*(3), 247–264. doi:10.1016/j.jom.2008.09.003

Fukui, S., Fukui, N., & Kawagoe, H. (2004). Predictors of place of death for Japanese patients with advanced-stage malignant disease in home care settings: A nationwide survey. *Cancer, 101*(2), 421–429. doi:10.1002/cncr.20383 PMID:15241842

Fukui, S., Yoshiuchi, K., Fujita, J., Sawai, M., & Watanabe, M. (2011). Japanese peoples preference for place of end-of-life care and death: A population-based nationwide survey. *Journal of Pain and Symptom Management, 42*(6), 882–892. doi:10.1016/j.jpainsymman.2011.02.024 PMID:21689901

Gage, H., Holdsworth, L. M., Flannery, C., Williams, P., & Butler, C. (2015). Impact of a hospice rapid response service on preferred place of death, and costs. *BMC Palliative Care, 14*(1), 75. doi:10.1186/s12904-015-0065-4 PMID:26701763

Gamroth, L. N., Semradek, J., & Tornquist, E. M. (Eds.). (1995). *Enhancing Autonomy in Long-term Care*. New York: Springer Publishing.

Gardner, C. D., Zehnder, J. L., Rigby, A. J., Nicholus, J. R., & Farquhar, J. W. (2007). Effect of Ginkgo biloba (EGb 761) and aspirin on platelet aggregation and platelet function analysis among older adults at risk of cardiovascular disease: A randomized clinical trial. *Blood Coagulation & Fibrinolysis, 18*(8), 787–793. doi:10.1097/MBC.0b013e3282f102b1 PMID:17982321

Gardner, J. (2011). Natural neighborhood networks: Important social networks in the lives of older adults aging in place. *Journal of Aging Studies, 25*(3), 263–271. doi:10.1016/j.jaging.2011.03.007

Garner, J. D. (1999). Feminism and feminist gerontology. *Journal of Women & Aging, 11*(2-3), 3–12. doi:10.1300/J074v11n02_02 PMID:10568093

Garrett, B. M., & Jackson, C. (2006). A mobile clinical e-portfolio for nursing and medical students, using wireless personal digital assistants (PDAs). *Nurse Education Today, 26*(8), 647–654. doi:10.1016/j.nedt.2006.07.020 PMID:17011674

Ge, B., Zhang, Z., & Zuo, Z. (2016). Radix Puerariae lobatae (Gegen) suppresses the anticoagulation effect of warfarin: A pharmacokinetic and pharmacodynamics study. *Chinese Medicine, 11*(1), 7. doi:10.1186/s13020-016-0078-9 PMID:26925159

Geiser, P., & Boersma, M. (2013). The role of the community in CBR. In G. Musoke & P. Geiser (Eds.), *Linking CBR, disability and rehabilitation* (pp. 24–35). Bangalore, India: CBR Africa Network.

General Medical Council. (2015). *Outcomes for Graduates (Tomorrow's Doctors)*. Manchester, UK: GMC.

General Office of the State Council. (2003). *Opinions on Establishing the New Rural Cooperative Medical System*, Chinese version. Retrieved July 12, 2016, from http://www.law-lib.com/law/law_view.asp?id=43058

Gerber, B., Maestas, C., & Dometrius, N. (2005). State legislative influence over agency rulemaking: The utility of ex ante review. *State Politics & Policy Quarterly, 5*(1), 24–46. doi:10.1177/153244000500500102

Ge, Y. (2014). Interpretation of 'Expert consensus on methicillin-resistant Staphylococcus aureus infection prevention and control'. *Chinese Clinical Oncology, 42*, 11–12.

Gibson, P., Powell, H., Wilson, A., Abramson, M., Haywood, P., Bauman, A., . . . Roberts, J. (2009). *Self-management education and regular practitioner review for adults with asthma.* Retrieved from: http://onlinelibrary.wiley.com/doi/10.1002/14651858.CD001117/pdf

Gibson, D. (1998). *Aged care: Old policies, new problems.* Melbourne: Cambridge University Press.

Girard, J. P. (2005). The Inukshuk: A Canadian knowledge management model. *KMPro Journal, 2*(1), 9–19.

Glanz, K., Rimer, B. K., & Viswanath, K. (Eds.). (2008). *Health behavior and health education: theory, research, and practice.* John Wiley & Sons.

Glied, S., & Smith, P. (2011). *The Oxford handbook of health economics.* Oxford, UK: Oxford University Press. doi:10.1093/oxfordhb/9780199238828.001.0001

Global Reporting Initiative. (n.d.). *GRI's History.* Retrieved July 7, 2016, from https://www.globalreporting.org/information/about-gri/gri-history/Pages/GRI's%20history.aspx

Glynn, L., Emmett, P., & Rogers, I. (2005). Food and nutrient intakes of a population sample of 7-year-old children in the southwest of England in 1999/2000–what difference does gender make? *Journal of Human Nutrition and Dietetics, 18*(1), 7–19. doi:10.1111/j.1365-277X.2004.00582.x PMID:15647094

Goggin, M. (1999). The use of administration discretion in implementing the State Childrens Health Insurance Program. *Publius, 29*(2), 35–51. doi:10.1093/oxfordjournals.pubjof.a030025

Goggin, M., Bowman, A., Lester, J., & O'Toole, L. (1990). *Implementation theory and practice: toward a third generation.* New York, N.Y.: Harper Collins Publishers.

Golant, S. M. (2015). *Aging in the right place.* Baltimore, MD: Health Professions Press.

Golmohammadi, D., & Radnia, N. (2016). Prediction modeling and pattern recognition for patient readmission. *International Journal of Production Economics, 171*(Part 1), 151–161. doi:10.1016/j.ijpe.2015.09.027

Gomes, B., Calanzani, N., Gysels, M., Hall, S., & Higginson, I. J. (2013). Heterogeneity and changes in preferences for dying at home: A systematic review. *BMC Palliative Care, 12*(1), 7. doi:10.1186/1472-684X-12-7 PMID:23414145

Gomes, B., Calanzani, N., Koffman, J., & Higginson, I. J. (2015). Is dying in hospital better than home in incurable cancer and what factors influence this? A population-based study. *BMC Medicine, 13*(1), 235. doi:10.1186/s12916-015-0466-5 PMID:26449231

Gomes, B., & Higginson, I. J. (2006). Factors influencing death at home in terminally ill patients with cancer: Systematic review. *BMJ (Clinical Research Ed.), 332*(7540), 515–521. doi:10.1136/bmj.38740.614954.55 PMID:16467346

Gomes-Schwartz, B. (1978, October). Effective ingredients in psychotherapy: Prediction of outcome from process variables. *Journal of Consulting and Clinical Psychology, 46*(5), 1023–1035. doi:10.1037/0022-006X.46.5.1023 PMID:701541

Gonzales, E., & Morrow-Howell, N. (2009). Productive engagement in aging-friendly communities. *Generations (San Francisco, Calif.), 33*(2), 51–58.

Gonzalez-Villanueva, L., Cagnoni, S., & Ascari, L. (2013). Design of a Wearable Sensing System for Human Motion Monitoring in Physical Rehabilitation. *Sensors (Basel, Switzerland), 13*(6), 7735–7755. doi:10.3390/s130607735 PMID:23774987

Goodwin, N., Smith, J., Davies, A., Perry, C., Rosen, R., Dixon, A., & Ham, C. (2012). *Integrated care for patients and populations: Improving outcomes by working together.* London: King's Fund.

Gordon, L. A., Morrison, E. Y., McGrowder, D. A., Young, R., Fraser, Y. T. P., Zamora, E. M., & Irving, R. R. et al. (2008). Effect of exercise therapy on lipid profile and oxidative stress indicators in patients with type 2 diabetes. *BMC Complementary and Alternative Medicine*, *8*(1), 21. doi:10.1186/1472-6882-8-21 PMID:18477407

Gotsadze, G., Zoidze, A., & Rukhadze, N. (2009). Household catastrophic health expenditure: Evidence from Georgia and its policy implications. *BMC Health Services Research*, *9*(1), 69. doi:10.1186/1472-6963-9-69 PMID:19400939

Government Office for Science, UK Government. (2016). *Future of an ageing population.* Retrieved from: https://www.gov.uk/government/uploads/system/uploads/attachment_data/file/535187/gs-16-10-future-of-an-ageing-population.pdf

GPnotebook. (2016). *Lead Time Bias*. General Practice Notebook-a UK medical reference. Retrieved 25 Feb 2017, from http://www.gpnotebook.co.uk/simplepage.cfm?ID=577437764

Graham, C., Scharlach, A. E., & Kurtovich, E. (2016). Do Villages Promote Aging in Place? Results of a Longitudinal Study. *Journal of Applied Gerontology*, 1–22. doi:10.1177/0733464816672046 PMID:27708072

Graybill, E. M., McMeekin, P., & Wildman, J. (2014). Can Aging in Place Be Cost Effective? A Systematic Review. *PLoS ONE*, *9*(7), e102705. doi:10.1371/journal.pone.0102705 PMID:25058505

Gray, V. (1973). Innovations in the states: A diffusion study. *The American Political Science Review*, *67*(4), 1174–1185. doi:10.2307/1956539

Greenfield, E. A., Scharlach, A. E., Graham, C., Davitt, J., & Lehning, A. (2012). *A national overview of Villages: Results from a 2012 organizational survey*. New Brunswick, NJ: Rutgers University. Retrieved March 21, 2017, from http://www.neighborsnetworkfl.org/media/2012-Village-Org-Survey.pdf

Greenfield, E. A., Scharlach, A. E., Lehning, A. J., Davitt, J. K., & Graham, C. L. (2013). A tale of two community initiatives for promoting aging in place: Similarities and differences in the national implementation of NORC programs and villages. *The Gerontologist*, *53*(6), 928–938. doi:10.1093/geront/gnt035 PMID:23626371

Grencavage, L. M., & Norcross, J. C. (1990). Where are the commonalities among the therapeutic common factors? *Professional Psychology, Research and Practice*, *21*(5), 372–378. doi:10.1037/0735-7028.21.5.372

Grossman, E., Messerli, F. H., & Neutel, J. M. (2000). Angiotensin II receptor blockers: Equal or preferred substitutes for ACE inhibitors? *Archives of Internal Medicine*, *160*(13), 1905–1911. doi:10.1001/archinte.160.13.1905 PMID:10888965

Gruson, D., Hilbert, G., Vargas, F., Valentino, R., Bebear, C., Allery, A., & Cardinaud, J. P. et al. (2000). Rotation and restricted use of antibiotics in a medical intensive care unit: Impact on the incidence of ventilator-associated pneumonia caused by antibiotic-resistant gram-negative bacteria. *American Journal of Respiratory and Critical Care Medicine*, *162*(3), 837–843. doi:10.1164/ajrccm.162.3.9905050 PMID:10988092

Guangzhou Daily. (2016 January 5). *Do retired employees need to pay premium contribution for health care?* Chinese version. Retrieved July 16, 2016, from http://jiankang.163.com/16/0105/08/BCI6N50N0038002S.html

Gu, D., Liu, G., Vlosky, D. A., & Yi, Z. (2007). Factors Associated With Place of Death Among the Chinese Oldest Old. *Journal of Applied Gerontology*, *26*(1), 34–57. doi:10.1177/0733464806296057

Gu, E. (2001). Market transition and the transformation of the health care system in urban China. *Policy Studies*, *22*(3/4), 197–215. doi:10.1080/01442870120112692

Gulliford, M., Naithani, S., & Morgan, M. (2006). What is continuity of care? *Journal of Health Services Research & Policy*, *11*(4), 248–250. doi:10.1258/135581906778476490 PMID:17018200

Guo, J. (2016 January 4). *How long does it last for 720 million retired employees not paying premium contribution for medical care?* Chinese version. Retrieved July 16, 2016, from http://www.yicai.com/news/4733894.html

Guptill, J. (2005). Knowledge management in health care. *Journal of Health Care Finance, 31*(3), 10–14. PMID:16080410

Haber, D. (2013). *Health promotion and aging: practical applications for health professionals* (6th ed.). New York, NY: Springer Publishing Company, LLC.

Hajhashemi, V., Sajjadi, S. E., & Heshmati, M. (2009). Anti-inflammatory and analgesic properties of Heracleum persicum essential oil and hydroalcoholic extract in animal models. *Journal of Ethnopharmacology, 124*(3), 475–480. doi:10.1016/j.jep.2009.05.012 PMID:19467316

Haller, C. A., & Benowitz, N. L. (2000). Adverse cardiovascular and central nervous system events associated with dietary supplements containing ephedra alkaloids. *The New England Journal of Medicine, 343*(25), 1833–1838. doi:10.1056/NEJM200012213432502 PMID:11117974

Hall, K., & Hardill, I. (2016). Retirement migration, the other story: Caring for frail elderly British citizens in Spain. *Ageing and Society, 36*(3), 562–585. doi:10.1017/S0144686X14001342 PMID:26962269

Hall, M. (2011). Do comprehensive performance measurement systems help or hinder managers mental model development? *Management Accounting Research, 22*(2), 68–83. doi:10.1016/j.mar.2010.10.002

Hall, P. A., & Taylor, R. C. R. (1996). Political science and the three new institutionalisms. *Political Studies, 44*(5), 936–957. doi:10.1111/j.1467-9248.1996.tb00343.x

Hamilton, K., Sullivan, F., Donnan, P., Taylor, R., Ikenwilo, D., Scott, A., & Wyke, S. et al. (2005). A managed clinical network for cardiac services: Set-up, operation and impact on patient care. *International Journal of Integrated Care, 5*(3), 1–13. doi:10.5334/ijic.135 PMID:16773161

Han, L., Cole, M., Bellavance, F., McCusker, J., & Primeau, F. (2000). Tracking cognitive decline in Alzheimers disease using the mini-mental state examination: A meta-analysis. *International Psychogeriatrics, 12*(2), 231–247. doi:10.1017/S1041610200006359 PMID:10937543

Hansen, M. T., Nohria, N., & Tierney, T. (1999). What's your strategy for managing knowledge? In J. A. Woods & J. Cortada (Eds.), *The Knowledge Management Yearbook 2000–2001* (pp. 55–69). Butterworth Heinemann.

Hanson, D., & Emlet, C. A. (2006). Assessing a communitys elder friendliness. *Family & Community Health, 29*(4), 266–278. doi:10.1097/00003727-200610000-00005 PMID:16980802

Hansson, L. (1990). How far should blood pressure be lowered? What is the importance of the J-curve phenomenon? *Giornale Italiano di Cardiologia, 20*(1), 1. PMID:2184071

Hansson, L., Lindholm, L. H., Niskanen, L., Lanke, J., Hedner, T., Niklason, A., & Björck, J.-E. et al. (1999). Effect of angiotensin-converting-enzyme inhibition compared with conventional therapy on cardiovascular morbidity and mortality in hypertension: The Captopril Prevention Project (CAPPP) randomised trial. *Lancet, 353*(9153), 611–616. doi:10.1016/S0140-6736(98)05012-0 PMID:10030325

Hao, P. P., Jiang, F., Chen, Y. G., Yang, J., Zhang, K., Zhang, M. X., & Zhang, Y. et al. (2015). Evidence for traditional Chinese medication to treat cardiovascular disease. *Nature Reviews. Cardiology, 12*(6), 374–374. doi:10.1038/nrcardio.2014.177-c2 PMID:25917155

Hardy, C., & Maguire, S. (2008). Institutional entrepreneurship. In R. Greenwood, C. Oliver, K. Sahlin, & R. Suddaby (Eds.), *The SAGE handbook of organizational institutionalism* (pp. 198–217). Los Angeles, CA: SAGE. doi:10.4135/9781849200387.n8

Harper, S. (2014). Economic and social implications of aging societies. *Science, 346*(6209), 587–591. doi:10.1126/science.1254405 PMID:25359967

Hartley, D., & Strupp, H. H. (1983). The therapeutic alliance: Its relationship to outcome in brief psychotherapy. In J. Masling (Ed.), *Empirical studies of psychoanalytic theories* (Vol. 1, pp. 1–38). Hillsdale, NJ: Lawrence Erlbaum.

Harvard Team. (1999). *Improving Hong Kong Health Care System: Why and for Whom?* Hong Kong: HKSAR Government Printer.

Harvath, T. A., Swafford, K., Smith, K., Miller, L. L., Volpin, M., Sexson, K., & Young, H. A. et al. (2008). Enhancing nursing leadership in long-term care: A review of the literature. *Research in Gerontological Nursing, 1*(3), 187–196. doi:10.3928/00220124-20091301-06 PMID:20077963

Haunschild, P., & Chandler, D. (2008). Institutional-level learning: learning as a source of institutional change. In R. Greenwood, C. Oliver, K. Sahlin, & R. Suddaby (Eds.), *The SAGE handbook of organizational institutionalism* (pp. 624–649). Los Angeles, CA: SAGE. doi:10.4135/9781849200387.n27

Havighurst, R. J. (1961). Successful Aging. *The Gerontologist, 1*(1), 8–13. doi:10.1093/geront/1.1.8

Health and Medical Development Advisory Committee of Hong Kong. (2005). *Building a healthy tomorrow: Discussion paper on the future service delivery model for our health care system.* Retrieved March 20, 2017 from http://www.info.gov.hk/archive/consult/2005/hmdac_paper_e.pdf

Health and Welfare Bureau of Hong Kong. (2000). *Lifelong investment in health: Consultation document on health care reform.* Hong Kong: Author. Retrieved March 20, 2017 from http://www.hpdo.gov.hk/en/doc/lifelong_investment_in_health_eng.pdf

Health Care Voucher. (2016). *Background of elderly health care voucher scheme.* Retrieved 24 March 2016, from http://www.hcv.gov.hk/eng/pub_background.htm

Health Reform Implementation Taskforce of Western Australia. (2007). *Ambulatory and community-based care: A framework for non-inpatient care.* Retrieved March 20, 2017 from http://zanran_storage.s3.amazonaws.com/www.health.wa.gov.au/ContentPages/19041594.pdf

Health, Welfare and Food Bureau of Hong Kong. (2007). *LegCo Panel on Welfare Services – 2007 rehabilitation programme plan* (LC Paper No. CB(2)2348/06-07(01)). Retrieved March 20, 2017 from http://www.legco.gov.hk/yr06-07/english/panels/ws/papers/ws0709cb2-2348-1-e.pdf

Heart Protection Study Collaborative Group. (2002). MRC/BHF Heart Protection Study of cholesterol lowering with simvastatin in 20 536 high-risk individuals: A randomised placebocontrolled trial. *Lancet, 360*(9326), 7–22. doi:10.1016/S0140-6736(02)09327-3 PMID:12114036

Hébert, R., Durand, P. J., Dubuc, N., & Tourigny, A. (2003). PRISMA: A new model of integrated service delivery for the frail older people in Canada. *International Journal of Integrated Care, 3*(1). Retrieved from http://www.ijic.org/articles/10.5334/ijic.73/ doi:10.5334/ijic.73 PMID:16896376

Hébert, R., Raîche, M., Dubois, M. F., NDeye, R. G., Dubuc, N., & Tousignant, M. (2009). Impact of PRISMA, a coordination-type integrated service delivery system for frail older people in Quebec (Canada): A quasi-experimental study. *The Journals of Gerontology. Series B, Psychological Sciences and Social Sciences, 65B*(1), 107–118. doi:10.1093/geronb/gbp027 PMID:19414866

Heidegger, M., & Stambaugh, J. (1996). *Being and time: a translation of Sein und Zeit.* Albany, NY: State University of New York Press.

Helander, E., Mendis, P., Nelson, G., & Goerdt, A. (1989). *Training in the community for people with disabilities*. Geneva, Switzerland: World Health Organization. Retrieved March 20, 2017 from http://www.who.int/disabilities/publications/cbr/training/en/

Helm, J. E., Alaeddini, A., Stauffer, J. M., Bretthauer, K. M., & Skolarus, T. A. (2016). Reducing Hospital Readmissions by Integrating Empirical Prediction with Resource Optimization. *Production and Operations Management*, *25*(2), 233–257. doi:10.1111/poms.12377

Henan Business Daily. (2013, December 31). *The reasons for cheap essential drugs disappearing from the market in China,* Chinese version. Retrieved July 15, 2016, from http://www.cb.com.cn/investigation/2013_1231/1031072.html

Henisz, W. J., Dorobantu, S., & Nartey, L. J. (2014). Spinning Gold: The Financial Returns to Stakeholder Engagement. *Strategic Management Journal*, *35*(12), 1727–1748. doi:10.1002/smj.2180

Henwood, B. F., Katz, M. L., & Gilmer, T. P. (2015). Aging in place within permanent supportive housing. *International Journal of Geriatric Psychiatry*, *30*(1), 80–87. doi:10.1002/gps.4120 PMID:24737594

He, Q. Y., Wang, J., Zhang, Y. L., Tang, Y. L., Chu, F. Y., & Xiong, X. J. (2010). Effect of Yiqi Yangyin Decoction on the quality of life of patients with unstable angina pectoris. *Chinese Journal of Integrative Medicine*, *16*(1), 13–18. doi:10.1007/s11655-010-0013-3 PMID:20131030

Hernández-Quevedo, C., Llano, R., & Mossialos, E. (2013). Paying for integrated care: an overview. *Euro Health Incorporating Euro Observer, 19*(2), 3-6.

Hibbert, P., Hannaford, N., Long, J., Plumb, J., & Braithwaite, J. (2013). *Final Report: Performance indicators used internationally to report publicly on healthcare organisations and local health systems*. Australian Institute of Health Innovation.

Hilton, R. W. & Platt, E. W. (2015). *Managerial Accounting: Creating Value in a Dynamic Business Environment*. Singapore: McGraw Hill Education.

Hinings, C. R., Greenwood, R., Reay, T., & Suddaby, R. (2004). Dynamics of change in organizational fields. In M. S. Poole & A. H. Van de Ven (Eds.), *Handbook of organizational change and innovation* (pp. 304–323). New York: Oxford University Press.

Hipgrave, D. (2011). Communicable disease control in China: From Mao to now. *Journal of Global Health*, *1*(2), 224–238. PMID:23198121

Hirst, S. P., Lane, A. M., & Miller, C. A. (2015). *Miller's Nursing for Wellness in Older Adults* (Canadian Edition). Philadelphia, PA: Wolters Kluwer.

Hirth, V., Baskins, J., & Dever-Bumba, M. (2009). Program of all-inclusive care (PACE): Past, present, and future. *Journal of the American Medical Directors Association*, *10*(3), 155–160. doi:10.1016/j.jamda.2008.12.002 PMID:19233054

Hoare, S., Morris, Z. S., Kelly, M. P., Kuhn, I., & Barclay, S. (2015). Do Patients Want to Die at Home? A Systematic Review of the UK Literature, Focused on Missing Preferences for Place of Death. *PLoS ONE*, *10*(11), e0142723. doi:10.1371/journal.pone.0142723 PMID:26555077

Hoeman, S. P. (1992). Community-based rehabilitation. *Holistic Nursing Practice*, *6*(2), 32–41. doi:10.1097/00004650-199206020-00007 PMID:1735743

Ho, L. A. (2008). What affects organizational performance? The linking of learning and knowledge management. *Industrial Management & Data Systems*, *108*(9), 1234–1254. doi:10.1108/02635570810914919

Hollinger-Smith, L., & Ortigara, A. (2004). Changing Culture: Creating a Long-Term Impact for a Quality Long-Term Care Workforce. *Alzheimer's Care Today*, *5*(1), 60–70.

Holman, H., & Lorig, K. (2000). Patients as partners in managing chronic disease. *British Medical Journal*, *320*(7234), 526–527. doi:10.1136/bmj.320.7234.526 PMID:10688539

Holman, H., & Lorig, K. (2004). Patient self-management: A key to effectiveness and efficiency in care of chronic disease. *Public Health Records*, *119*, 239–243. PMID:15158102

Holroyd, E. A., & Mackenzie, A. E. (1995). A review of the historical and social processes contributing to care and caregiving in Chinese families. *Journal of Advanced Nursing*, *22*(3), 473–479. doi:10.1046/j.1365-2648.1995.22030473.x PMID:7499614

Honda. (2004). *The Bronx Says "Hello" to ASIMO*! Retrieved 20 July 2016, from http://asimo.honda.com/event-details.aspx?XML=Events/PostEvent_0026.xml

Hon, E. K., Lee, K., Tse, H. M., Lam, L. N., Tam, K. C., Chu, K. M., & Leung, T. F. et al. (2004). A survey of attitudes to Traditional Chinese Medicine in Hong Kong pharmacy students. *Complementary Therapies in Medicine*, *12*(1), 51–56. doi:10.1016/j.ctim.2003.12.002 PMID:15130573

Hong Kong Community Nurses Association. (2012). *Newsletter 2012*. Retrieved July 14, 2016 from http://www.hkcnaltd.org.hk/2012.pdf

Hong Kong Fire Service Department Volunteer Team. (n.d.). *About Us*. Retrieved September 14, 2016 from http://www.hkfsdvt.org.hk/eng/establish.php

Hong Kong government. (2012a, June 5). *Opening ceremony held for Tin Shui Wai (Tin Yip Road) Community Health Centre (with photos)* [Press release]. Retrieved March 20, 2017 from http://www.info.gov.hk/gia/general/201206/05/P201206050459.htm

Hong Kong government. (2012b, June 7). *Transformation of Kowloon East in full swing with inception of Energizing Kowloon East Office* [Press release]. Retrieved March 20, 2017 from http://www.info.gov.hk/gia/general/201206/07/P201206070322.htm

Hong Kong government. (2013, April 9). *HK healthcare is a dual-track system*. Retrieved March 20, 2017 from http://www.news.gov.hk/en/record/html/2013/04/20130409_190409.shtml

Hong Kong government. (2016, July 16). *Medical platform to be formed*. Retrieved March 20, 2017 from http://www.news.gov.hk/en/categories/health/html/2016/07/20160716_111123.lin.shtml

Hong Kong government. (2017a, March 9). *LWB's response to Ombudsman's direct investigation report* [Press release]. Retrieved March 20, 2017 from http://www.info.gov.hk/gia/general/201703/09/P2017030900515.htm

Hong Kong government. (2017b, March 9). *Ombudsman recommendations noted* [Press release]. Retrieved March 20, 2017 from http://www.news.gov.hk/en/categories/health/html/2017/03/20170309_141809.shtml

Hong Kong Housing Society. (2017a). *"Aging in Place" Concept*. Retrieved March 13, 2017, from http://www.hkhselderly.com/en/aboutus

Hong Kong Housing Society. (2017b). *Universal Design Guidebook for Residential Development in Hong Kong*. Retrieved March 13, 2017, from http://www.hkhs.com/eng/wnew/udg.asp

Hong Kong S. A. R. Government (2017). *The 2017 Policy Address*. Retrieved March 18, 2017, from http://www.policyaddress.gov.hk/2017/eng/p173.html

Hong Kong S. A. R. Government. (2016a). *The 2016 Policy Address*. Retrieved March 13, 2017, from http://www.policyaddress.gov.hk/2016/eng/pdf/leaflet_community.pdf

Hong Kong S. A. R. Government. (2016b). *LCQ13: Housing for elderly*. Retrieved March 13, 2017, from http://www.info.gov.hk/gia/general/201604/13/P201604130432.htm

Hong Kong Society for Rehabilitation. (n.d.). *Community rehabilitation network* . Retrieved March 20, 2017 from http://www.rehabsociety.org.hk/dccs/crn/wp-content/uploads/sites/4/2016/01/crn_社區復康網絡服務介紹單張.pdf (in Chinese)

Hong, T. C., Yau, L. M., Ng, C. C., Au Yeung, H. Y., Ma, S. Y., Ng, H. Y., . . . Chao, D. V. K. (2010). *Attitudes and expectations of patients with advanced cancer towards community palliative care service in Hong Kong*. Paper presented at The 2010 Hospital Authority Convention, Hong Kong.

Hong, C. Y., Chow, K. Y., Poulose, J., Jin, A. Z., Devi, A., Chee, E. M. F., & Goh, C. (2011). Place of death and its determinants for patients with cancer in Singapore: An analysis of data from the Singapore Cancer Registry, 20002009. *Journal of Palliative Medicine*, *14*(10), 1128–1134. doi:10.1089/jpm.2011.0092 PMID:21966990

Hong, S. J., Wan, J. B., Zhang, Y., Hu, G., Lin, H. C., Seto, S. W., & Lee, S. M.-Y. et al. (2009). Angiogenic effect of saponin extract from Panax notoginseng on HUVECs in vitro and zebrafish in vivo. *Phytotherapy Research*, *23*(5), 677–686. doi:10.1002/ptr.2705 PMID:19107746

Hong, T. C., Lam, T. P., & Chao, D. V. (2013). Barriers facing family physicians providing palliative care service in Hong Kong - A questionnaire survey. *The Hong Kong Practitioner*, *35*(2), 36–51.

Hoorn, E. J., & Zietse, R. (2011). Hyponatremia and mortality: How innocent is the bystander? *Clinical Journal of the American Society of Nephrology; CJASN*, *6*(5), 951–953. doi:10.2215/CJN.01210211 PMID:21493744

Hospital Authority of Hong Kong. (2012). *Hospital Authority strategic plan 2012–2017*. Retrieved March 20, 2017 from http://www.ha.org.hk/upload/publication_29/359.pdf

Hospital Authority of Hong Kong. (2014). *Hospital Authority statistical report 2012-2013*. Retrieved March 20, 2017 from https://www.ha.org.hk/upload/publication_15/491.pdf

Hospital Authority of Hong Kong. (2016). *Update on Hospital Authority's public-private partnership programmes* (paper no. AOM-P1180). Retrieved March 20, 2017 from https://www.ha.org.hk/haho/ho/cad_bnc/AOM-P1180.pdf

Hospital Authority. (2003). *HA and Clinical Research - Support, Output & Direction*. Retrieved 20 July 2016, from http://www.ha.org.hk/ho/research_ethics/msdc_p181.pdf

Hospital Authority. (2005). *Highlights of Hospital Authority Annual Plan 2005/06*. Retrieved 20 July 2016, from http://www.ha.org.hk/haho/ho/cad_bnc/126135e.pdf

Hospital Authority. (2007). *Chief Executive's Progress Report on Strategic Priorities*. Retrieved 20 July 2016, from http://www.ha.org.hk/haho/ho/cad_bnc/131443e.pdf

Hospital Authority. (2010a). *Pilot project on enhancing radiological investigation services through collaboration with the private sector (Radi Collaboration)*. Retrieved 25 March 2016, from https://www3.ha.org.hk/ppp/radi.aspx

Hospital Authority. (2010b). *Haemodialysis public private partnership programme (HD PPP)*. Retrieved 23 March 2016, from https://www3.ha.org.hk/ppp/hdscp.aspx?lang=eng

Hospital Authority. (2016). *Home care*. Retrieved August 23, 2016 from http://www21.ha.org.hk/smartelder/en/home_care.html

Hospital Authority. (2016a). *PPI-ePR sharing pilot project & eHR sharing system.* Retrieved 10 August 2016, from http://www3.ha.org.hk/ppp/ppiepr_a.aspx

Hospital Authority. (2016b). *General Outpatient Clinic Public Private Partnership Programme (GOPC PPP).* Retrieved 12 Feb 2017, from http://www3.ha.org.hk/ppp/gopcppp.aspx?lang=eng

Howden-Chapman, P., Signal, L., & Crane, J. (1999). Housing and Health in Older People. *Social Policy Journal of New Zealand, 13.* Retrieved March 13, 2017, from http://www.msd.govt.nz/about-msd-and-our-work/publications-resources/journals-and-magazines/social-policy-journal/spj13/housing-and-health-in-older-people.html

Hsu, M., Huang, X., & Yupho, S. (2015). The development of universal health insurance coverage in Thailand: Challenges of population aging and informal economy. *Social Science & Medicine, 145*, 227–236. doi:10.1016/j.socscimed.2015.09.036 PMID:26452699

Hu, A. (2016). *China's social insurance in the twentieth century: a global historical perspective.* Leiden, Germany: Brill.

Huang, J., Su, D., Feng, Y., Liu, K., & Song, Y. (2014). Antiviral herbs-present and future. *Infectious Disorders-Drug Targets (Formerly Current Drug Targets-Infectious Disorders), 14*(1), 61-73.

Huang, Y. (2013). *Governing Health in Contemporary China. Milton Park.* Abingdon, UK: Routledge.

Hunter, S., & Levett-Jones, T. (2010). The practice of nurses working with older people in long term care: An Australian perspective. *Journal of Clinical Nursing, 19*(3-4), 527–536. doi:10.1111/j.1365-2702.2009.02967.x PMID:20500289

Hwang, S., & Gray, V. (1991). External limits and internal determinants of state public policy. *The Western Political Quarterly, 44*(2), 277–299. doi:10.2307/448779

Ichien, M. (2000). Introduction of Long-term Care Insurance in Japan. *International Review of Public Administration, 5*(2), 23–36. doi:10.1080/12294659.2000.10804953

Iemmi, V., Suresh Kumar, K., Blanchet, K., Gibson, L., Hartley, S., Murthy, G. V. S., & Kuper, H. et al. (2013). Community-based rehabilitation for people with physical and mental disabilities in low- and middle-income countries. *Cochrane Database of Systematic Reviews, 7*, 1–15. doi:10.1002/14651858.CD010617

Institute of Active Aging. (2017). *Project for the Third Age.* Retrieved March 13, 2017, from http://iaa.fhss.polyu.edu.hk/Project_Third_Age.html

Institute of Medicine. (2013). *Best care at lower cost: The path to continuously learning health care in America.* Washington, DC: The National Academies Press.

International Diabetes Federation. (2015). *IDF Diabetes Atlas* (7th ed.). Retrieved March 28, 2016, from http://www.diabetesatlas.org/

International Federation of Red Cross and Red Crescent Societies. (2011). *South Eastern Europe Home Care Conference.* Retrieved February 20, 2017 from https://www.cri.it/flex/cm/pages/ServeAttachment.php/L/IT/D/9%252F8%252Fe%252FD.ccbdf568ba9a2da44638/P/BLOB%3AID%3D10831/E/pdf

Ismail, S. (2013). Critical success factors of public private partnership (PPP) implementation in Malaysia. *Asia-Pacific Journal of Business Administration, 5*(1), 6–19. doi:10.1108/17574321311304503

ISO. (2010). *ISO 26000:2010 Guidelines on Social Responsibility.* Retrieved August 20, 2016, from http://www.iso.org/iso/catalogue_detail?csnumber=42546

ISO. (2014). *GRI G4 Guidelines and ISO 26000:2010 How to use the GRI G4 Guidelines and ISO 26000 in conjunction.* Retrieved July 7, 2016, from http://www.iso.org/iso/iso-gri-26000_2014-01-28.pdf

Ivey, S. L., Kealey, M., Kurtovich, E., Hunter, R., Prohaska, T. R., Bayles, C. M., & Satariano, W. A. (2015). Neighborhood characteristics and depressive symptoms in an older population. *Aging & Mental Health, 19*(8), 713–722. Retrieved from http://www.tandfonline.com/loi/camh20#.V0cWX1c01FI doi;10.1080/13607863.2014.962006

Jackson, B. S., Smith, S. P., Adams, R., Frank, B., & Mateo, M. A. (1999). Healthy life styles are a challenge for nurses. *Image, 31*, 196.

Jacob, K. S. (2001). Community care for people with mental disorders in developing countries: Problems and possible solutions. *The British Journal of Psychiatry, 178*(4), 296–298. doi:10.1192/bjp.178.4.296 PMID:11282806

Jadad, A. R., Haynes, R. B., Hunt, D., & Browman, G. P. (2000). The Internet and evidence-based decision-making: A needed synergy for efficient knowledge management in health care. *Canadian Medical Association Journal, 162*(3), 362–365. PMID:10693595

James, K. (2015). *The rise of the value-added tax*. New York, NY: Cambridge University Press. doi:10.1017/CBO9781107358522

Jamrozik, A. (2001). *Social policy in the post-welfare state: Australians on the threshold of the 21st century*. Frenchs Forest: Longman.

Jewell, A. J. (2014). Tornstams notion of gerotranscendence: Re-examining and questioning the theory. *Journal of Aging Studies, 30*, 112–120. doi:10.1016/j.jaging.2014.04.003 PMID:24984914

Jewell, A., & Nell, E. (2014). Gerotranscendence. *Rural Theology, 12*(2), 96–105. doi:10.1179/1470499414Z.00000000029

John, R. (1984). Prerequisites of an adequate theory of aging: A critique and reconceptualization. *Mid-American Review of Sociology, 9*(2), 79–108.

Joint Task Force of the European Society of Cardiology and Other Societies on Cardiovascular Disease Prevention in Clinical Practice. (2012). European guidelines on cardiovascular disease prevention in clinical practice. *European Heart Journal, 33*, 1635–1701. PMID:22555213

Jones, K. (1984). Psychological Problems in the Elderly. *Canadian Family Physician Medecin de Famille Canadien, 30*, 591–593. PMID:21279076

Jonsdottir, H. (2013). Self-management programmes for people living with chronic obstructive pulmonary disease. *Journal of Clinical Nursing, 22*(5-6), 621–637. doi:10.1111/jocn.12100 PMID:23398312

Joyce, B. T., & Bermanand, R. (2014). Formal and informal support of family caregivers managing medications for patients who receive end-of-life care t home: A cross –sectional survey of caregivers. *Palliative Medicine, 28*(9), 0269216314535963. doi:10.1177/0269216314535963 PMID:24854033

Joy, J. P., Carter, D. E., & Smith, L. (2000). The evolving educational needs of nurses caring for the older adult: A literature review. *Journal of Advanced Nursing, 31*(5), 1039–1045. doi:10.1046/j.1365-2648.2000.01392.x PMID:10840236

Jung, C., & Padman, R. (2014). Virtualized healthcare delivery: Understanding users and their usage patterns of online medical consultations. *International Journal of Medical Informatics, 83*(12), 901–914. doi:10.1016/j.ijmedinf.2014.08.004 PMID:25193501

Jütting, J. (2002). *Public-private partnerships in the health sector: experiences from developing countries. Social Security Policy and Development Branch*. International Labour Office.

Jyrkkä, J., Vartiainen, L., Hartikainen, S., Sulkava, R., & Enlund, H. (2006). Increasing use of medicines in elderly persons: A five-year follow-up of the Kuopio 75+ Study. *European Journal of Clinical Pharmacology*, *62*(2), 151–158. doi:10.1007/s00228-005-0079-6 PMID:16408226

Kaiser Family Foundation. (2013). *Cumulative percentage change in Medicaid fees, by type of service timeframe: 2008-2012*. Retrieved June 10, 2016, from http://kff.org/medicaid/state-indicator/change-in-medicaid-fees/

Kaiser Family Foundation. (2015a). *Distribution of Medicaid spending on long-term care*. Retrieved June 10, 2016, from http://kff.org/medicaid/state-indicator/spending-on-long-term-care/

Kaiser Family Foundation. (2015b). *State action on Medicaid expansion as of April 2015*. Retrieved June 10, 2016, from http://kff.org/health-reform/state-indicator/state-activity-around-expanding-medicaid-under-the-affordable-care-act/

Kaiser Family Foundation. (2015c). *Medicaid financing: how does it work and what are the implications?* Retrieved June 10, 2016, from http://kff.org/medicaid/issue-brief/medicaid-financing-how-does-it-work-and-what-are-the-implications/

Kaiser Family Foundation. (2015d). *Long-term care in the United States: a timeline*. Retrieved June 10, 2016, from http:// kff.org/medicaid/timeline/long-term-care-in-the-united-states-a-timeline/

Kaiser Family Foundation. (2015e). *Medicaid enrollment & spending growth: FY 2015 & 2016*. Retrieved June 10, 2016, from http:// kff.org/medicaid/issue-brief/medicaid-enrollment-spending-growth-fy-2015-2016/

Kaiser Family Foundation. (2015f). *Putting Medicaid in the larger budget context: an in-depth look at three states in FY 2015 and 2016, Alaska*. Retrieved June 10, 2016, from http://kff.org/report-section/putting-medicaid-in-the-larger-budget-context-an-in-depth-look-at-three-states-in-fy-2015-and-2016-alaska/

Kaiser Family Foundation. (2015g). *Putting Medicaid in the larger budget context: an in-depth look at three states in FY 2015 and 2016, California*. Retrieved June 10, 2016, from http://kff.org/report-section/putting-medicaid-in-the-larger-budget-context-an-in-depth-look-at-three-states-in-fy-2015-and-2016-california/

Kaiser Family Foundation. (2015h). *Medicaid and long-term services and supports: a primer*. Retrieved June 10, 2016, from http:// kff.org/medicaid/report/medicaid-and-long-term-services-and-supports-a-primer/

Kane, R. A. (2012). Thirty years of home- and community-based services: Getting closer and closer to home. *Generations (San Francisco, Calif.)*, *36*(1), 6–13.

Kankeu, H. T., Saksena, P., Xu, K., & Evans, D. B. (2013). The financial burden from non-communicable diseases in low- and middle-income countries: A literature review. *Health Research Policy and Systems*, *11*(1), 31. doi:10.1186/1478-4505-11-31 PMID:23947294

Karalliedde, L. D., & Kappagoda, C. T. (2009). The challenge of traditional Chinese medicines for allopathic practitioners. *American Journal of Physiology. Heart and Circulatory Physiology*, *297*(6), H1967–H1969. doi:10.1152/ajpheart.00944.2009 PMID:19855052

Karasik, R. J., & Kishimoto, K. (2016). Is gerontology ready for anti-racist pedagogy? A survey of educators practices and perspectives. *Gerontology & Geriatrics Education*, *37*(1), 1–18. doi:10.1080/02701960.2015.1115984 PMID:26886051

Kaufman, S. R., Livingston, J., Zhang, H., & Lock, M. (2013). Transforming concepts of ageing: three case studies from anthropology. In T. Dening & A. Thomas (Eds.), *Oxford Textbook of Old Age Psychiatry* (2nd ed.; pp. 39–56). Oxford University Press. doi:10.1093/med/9780199644957.003.0004

Kengne, F. G., Andres, C., Sattar, L., Melot, C., & Decaux, G. (2008). Mild hyponatremia and risk of fracture in the ambulatory elderly. *QJM*, *101*(7), 583–588. doi:10.1093/qjmed/hcn061 PMID:18477645

Kerr, C., Murray, E., Noble, L., Morris, R., Bottomley, C., Stevenson, F., & Nazareth, I. et al. (2010). The potential of web-based interventions for heart disease self-management: A mixed methods investigation. *Journal of Medical Internet Research*, *12*(4), 56. doi:10.2196/jmir.1438 PMID:21156471

Kespichayawattana, J., & Jitapunkul, S. (2008). Health and health care system for older persons. *Ageing International*, *33*(1), 28–49. doi:10.1007/s12126-009-9028-5

Kevelaitiene, S., & Slapikas, R. (2007). A new approach to the treatment of dyslipidemia. *Medicina (Kaunas, Lithuania)*, *44*(5), 407–413. PMID:18541958

Khalifa, M. (2013). Barriers to health information systems and electronic medical records implementation. A field study of Saudi Arabian hospitals. *Procedia Computer Science*, *21*, 335–342. doi:10.1016/j.procs.2013.09.044

Khan, S. A., Gomes, B., & Higginson, I. J. (2014). End-of-life care--what do cancer patients want? *Nature Reviews. Clinical Oncology*, *11*(2), 100–108. PMID:24281062

Khunti, K., Gray, L., Skinner, T., Carey, M., Realf, K., Dallosso, H., & Davies, M. et al. (2012). Effectiveness of a diabetes education and self-management programme (DESMOND) for people with newly diagnosed type 2 diabetes mellitus. *British Medical Journal*, *344*(apr26 2), 2333. doi:10.1136/bmj.e2333 PMID:22539172

Kim, T. H., Lee, J. N., Chun, J. U., & Benbasat, I. (2014). Understanding the effect of knowledge management strategies on knowledge management performance: A contingency perspective. *Information & Management*, *51*(4), 398–416. doi:10.1016/j.im.2014.03.001

King, G., Tomz, M., & Wittenberg, J. (2000). Making the most of statistical analysis: Improving interpretation and presentation. *American Journal of Political Science*, *44*(2), 347–361. doi:10.2307/2669316

Kingsley, D. E. (2015). Aging and health care costs: Narrative versus reality. *Poverty & Public Policy*, *7*(1), 3–21. doi:10.1002/pop4.89

Kinoshita, H., Maeda, I., Morita, T., Miyashita, M., Yamagishi, A., Shirahige, Y., & Eguchi, K. et al. (2015). Place of death and the differences in patient quality of death and dying and caregiver burden. *Journal of Clinical Oncology*, *33*(4), 357–363. doi:10.1200/JCO.2014.55.7355 PMID:25534381

Kirchner, S. (2013). How organizations become enduring: disentangling the organizational identity paradox. In J. Sydow & G. Schreoygg (Eds.), *Self-reinforcing processes in and among organizations* (pp. 33–54). Houndmills, UK: Palgrave Macmillan. doi:10.1057/9780230392830_3

Kirkpatrick, C., Clarke, R., & Polidano, C. (2003). *Handbook on development policy and management*. Cheltenham, UK: Edward Elgar.

Kitson, A. L. (2009). The need for systems change: Reflections on knowledge translation and organizational change. *Journal of Advanced Nursing*, *65*(1), 217–228. doi:10.1111/j.1365-2648.2008.04864.x PMID:19032518

Kjeldsen, S. E., Julius, S., Hedner, T., & Hansson, L. (2001). Stroke is more common than myocardial infarction in hypertension: Analysis based on 11 major randomized intervention trials. *Blood Pressure*, *10*(4), 190–192. doi:10.1080/08037050152669684 PMID:11800055

Knapp, M., Marks, I., Wolstenholme, J., Beecham, J., Astin, J., Audini, B., & Watts, V. et al. (1998). Home-based versus hospital-based care for serious mental illness. Controlled cost-effectiveness study over four years. *The British Journal of Psychiatry*, *172*(6), 506–512. doi:10.1192/bjp.172.6.506 PMID:9828991

Knickman, J. R., & Snell, E. K. (2002). The 2030 Problem: Caring for Aging Baby Boomers. *Health Services Research*, *37*(4), 849–884. doi:10.1034/j.1600-0560.2002.56.x PMID:12236388

Ko, W. M. (2014). *Steps address aging population, rising costs.* Hong Kong Information Services Department. Retrieved 10 June 2016, from http://www.news.gov.hk/en/record/html/2014/08/20140815_162410.shtml

Kodner, D. L. (2006). Whole-system approaches to health and social care partnerships for the frail elderly: An exploration of North American models and lessons. *Health & Social Care in the Community, 14*(5), 384–390. doi:10.1111/j.1365-2524.2006.00655.x PMID:16918830

Kong, H., & Hsieh, E. (2012). The social meanings of traditional Chinese medicine: Elderly Chinese immigrants health practice in the United States. *Journal of Immigrant and Minority Health, 14*(5), 841–849. doi:10.1007/s10903-011-9558-2 PMID:22160808

Kong, S.-T., Fang, C. M.-S., & Lou, V. W. Q. (2016, August 7). Solving the personhood jigsaw puzzle in residential care homes for the elderly in the Hong Kong Chinese context. *Qualitative Health Research, 27*(3), 421–433. doi:10.1177/1049732316658266

Kong, X., Li, Z., & Kong, Y. (2011). The formation basis of high drug prices, Chinese version. *China Pharmacy, 22*(12), 1069–1071.

Kononowicz, A. A., Zary, N., Edelbring, S., Corral, J., & Hege, I. (2015). Virtual patients-what are we talking about? A framework to classify the meanings of the term in healthcare education. *BMC Medical Education, 15*(1), 1. doi:10.1186/s12909-015-0296-3 PMID:25638167

Korhonen, I., & Bardram, J. (2004). Guest editorial introduction to the special section on pervasive healthcare. *IEEE Transactions on Information Technology in Biomedicine, 8*(3), 229–234. doi:10.1109/TITB.2004.835337 PMID:15484426

Kowloon Hospital. (2015). *Community Nursing Services.* Retrieved July 16, 2016 from http://www3.ha.org.hk/kh/ch/aboutus/introd.html

KPMG (2013). *An uncertain age: Reimaging long term care in the 21st century.* KPMG International.

Kua, E. H., & Tan, S. L. (1997). Stress of caregivers of dementia patients in the Sinagore Chinese family. *International Journal of Geriatric Psychiatry, 12*(4), 466–469. doi:10.1002/(SICI)1099-1166(199704)12:4<466::AID-GPS517>3.0.CO;2-U PMID:9178051

Kubesova, H. M., Weber, P., Meluzinova, H., Bielakova, K., & Matejovsky, J. (2013). Benefits and pitfalls of cardiovascular medication in seniors. *Wiener Klinische Wochenschrift, 125*(15-16), 425–436. doi:10.1007/s00508-013-0395-2 PMID:23846454

Kucukyazici, B., & Verter, V. (2013). Managing Community-based Care for Chronic Diseases: The Quantitative Approach. In G. S. Zaric (Ed.), Operations Research and Health Care Policy, (pp. 71–90). New York: Springer.

Kucukyazici, B., Verter, V., & Mayo, N. E. (2011). An Analytical Framework for Designing Community-Based Care for Chronic Diseases. *Production and Operations Management, 20*(3), 474–488. doi:10.1111/j.1937-5956.2011.01224.x

Kumar, V., Abbas, A. K., & Aster, J. C. (2013). *Robbins basic pathology.* Elsevier Health Sciences.

Kung, K. (2013). Family medicine and palliative care: Is there a missing link? *The Hong Kong Practitioner, 35*(2), 33–34.

Kwon, S. (2009). *Introduction of Long-Term Care Insurance in Korea.* Paper presented at the Asian Social Protection in Comparative Perspective Conference, Singapore.

Kwong, E. W. Y., & Kwan, A. Y. H. (2002). A Review of Private Residential Care in Hong Kong. *Journal of Aging & Social Policy, 13*(4), 73–89. doi:10.1300/J031v13n04_05 PMID:12418383

Labour and Welfare Bureau of Hong Kong. (2014). *Item for Establishment Subcommittee of Finance Committee Head 141– Government Secretariat: Labour and Welfare Bureau Subhead 000 Operational expenses* (Paper No. EC(2014-15)2). Retrieved March 20, 2017 from http://www.legco.gov.hk/yr13-14/english/fc/esc/papers/e14-02e.pdf

Labour and Welfare Bureau, & Social Welfare Department of Hong Kong. (2014). *Legislative Council Panel on Welfare Services: Home care and community support services for the elderly and persons with disabilities* (LC Paper No. CB(2)2077/13-14(05)). Retrieved March 20, 2017 from http://www.legco.gov.hk/yr13-14/english/panels/ws/papers/ws0725cb2-2077-5-e.pdf

Lai, D. W. (2000). Depression among the elderly Chinese in Canada. *Canadian Journal on Aging*, *19*(3), 409–429. doi:10.1017/S0714980800015063 PMID:10765589

Lai, I. K., Tam, S. K., & Chan, M. F. (2012). Knowledge cloud system for network collaboration: A case study in medical service industry in China. *Expert Systems with Applications*, *39*(15), 12205–12212. doi:10.1016/j.eswa.2012.04.057

Laitinen, T. T., Pahkala, K., Magnussen, C. G., Viikari, J. S., Oikonen, M., Taittonen, L., & Juonala, M. et al. (2012). Ideal cardiovascular health in childhood and cardiometabolic outcomes in adulthood: The Cardiovascular Risk in Young Finns Study. *Circulation*, *125*(16), 1971–1978. doi:10.1161/CIRCULATIONAHA.111.073585 PMID:22452832

Lai, W. W. L., Chan, J. P. Y., Choi, P. K. K., Ngai, L. C. T., Mar, C. S. F., Chan, E. Y. L., & Lam, F. N. Y. et al. (2009). Occupational therapy in the integrated elderly and community support services for the elderly in Hong Kong. *Hong Kong Journal of Occupational Therapy*, *19*(1), 27–30. doi:10.1016/S1569-1861(09)70041-5

Lakatta, E. G. (2003). Arterial and cardiac aging: Major shareholders in cardiovascular disease enterprises. *Circulation*, *107*(3), 490–497. doi:10.1161/01.CIR.0000048894.99865.02 PMID:12551876

Lam, A. C. Y. (2011). Quality healthcare for an aging population. *Improving Hong Kong*, *8*, 7–9.

Lambert, M. J., & Barley, D. E. (2002). Research summary on the therapeutic relationship and psychotherapy outcome. In J. C. Norcross (Ed.), *Psychotherapy relationships that work* (pp. 17–32). New York: Oxford University Press; doi:10.1037//0033-3204.38.4.357

Lam, C. L. K. (2005). The role of the family doctor in building a healthy tomorrow. *The Hong Kong Practitioner*, *27*, 363–367.

Lam, P. T. (2013). Practical challenges in ambulatory palliative care service in a regional hospital in Hong Kong. *The Hong Kong Practitioner*, *35*(2), 52–58.

Lam, T. P. (2001). Strengths and weaknesses of traditional Chinese medicine and Western medicine in the eyes of some Hong Kong Chinese. *Journal of Epidemiology and Community Health*, *55*(10), 762–765. doi:10.1136/jech.55.10.762 PMID:11553662

Langenbrunner, J. C., & Somanathan, A. (2011). *Financing health care in East Asia and the Pacific: best practices and remaining challenges*. Washington, DC: World Bank.

Larus, E. F. (2012). *Politics and society in contemporary China*. Boulder, CO: Lynne Rienner Publishers.

Lau, K. S. (2010). Facilitating home death. *HKSPM Newsletter,* (2), 24–25.

Lau-Walker, M., & Thompson, D. (2009). Self-management in long-term health conditions. *Patient Education and Counseling*, *75*(2), 290–292. doi:10.1016/j.pec.2009.02.001 PMID:19272746

Law, K. K. (2014). The problem with knowledge ambiguity. *European Management Journal*, *32*(3), 444–450. doi:10.1016/j.emj.2013.07.010

Lawrence, S. V., & Martin, M. F. (2013). *Understanding China's Political System*. Retrieved July 18, 2016, from https://www.fas.org/sgp/crs/row/R41007.pdf

Lawton, M. P., Weisman, G. D., Sloane, P., & Calkins, M. (1997). Assessing environments for older people with chronic illness. *Journal of Mental Health and Aging*, *3*, 83–100.

Lawton, M., & Brody, E. (1969). Assessment of older people: Self-maintaining and instrumental activities of daily living. *The Gerontologist*, *9*(3 Part 1), 179–186. doi:10.1093/geront/9.3_Part_1.179 PMID:5349366

Lazenby, J. M., & Olshvevski, J. (2012). Place of death among Botswana's oldest old. *Omega*, *65*(3), 173–187. PMID:23057243

Lecours, A. (2000). Theorizing cultural identities: Historical institutionalism as a challenge to the culturalists. *Canadian Journal of Political Science*, *33*(3), 499–522. doi:10.1017/S0008423900000172

Lee, V. (2005). *Public Private Partnerships*. Research and Library Services Division. Legislative Council Secretariat. Retrieved 12 Feb 2017, from http://www.legco.gov.hk/yr04-05/english/sec/library/0405rp03e.pdf

Lee, A. L., Chen, B. C., Mou, C. H., Sun, M. F., & Yen, H. R. (2016). Association of traditional Chinese medicine therapy and the risk of vascular complications in patients with type II diabetes mellitus: A nationwide, retrospective, Taiwanese-registry, cohort study. *Medicine*, *95*(3), e2536. doi:10.1097/MD.0000000000002536 PMID:26817897

Lee, A., & Pang, W. S. (1998). Preferred place of death--a local study of cancer patients and their relatives. *Singapore Medical Journal*, *39*(10), 447–450. PMID:9885706

Lee, H. C. B., Chiu, H. F., Kowk, W. Y., & Leung, C. M. (1993). Chinese elderly and the GDS short form: A preliminary study. *Clinical Gerontologist: The Journal of Aging and Mental Health*, *14*(2), 37–42.

Lee, S. H., Ahn, Y. M., Ahn, S. Y., Doo, H. K., & Lee, B. C. (2008). Interaction between warfarin and Panax ginseng in ischemic stroke patients. *Journal of Alternative and Complementary Medicine (New York, N.Y.)*, *14*(6), 715–721. doi:10.1089/acm.2007.0799 PMID:18637764

Lee, S.-D. (2002). Exploring policy and financing options for long-term care in Taiwan. *Journal of Aging & Social Policy*, *13*(2-3), 203–216. doi:10.1300/J031v13n02_14 PMID:12216356

Lee, S., Gon Kim, B., & Kim, H. (2012). An integrated view of knowledge management for performance. *Journal of Knowledge Management*, *16*(2), 183–203. doi:10.1108/13673271211218807

Lee, V. W., Lam, Y. Y., Yuen, A. C., Cheung, S. Y., Yu, C.-M., & Yan, B. P. (2013). Direct medical cost of newly diagnosed stable coronary artery disease in Hong Kong. *Heart Asia*, *5*(1), 1–6. doi:10.1136/heartasia-2012-010168 PMID:27326062

Legg, L., & Langhorne, P. (2004). Rehabilitation therapy services for stroke patients living at home: Systematic review of randomised trials. *Lancet*, *363*(9406), 352–356. doi:10.1016/S0140-6736(04)15434-2 PMID:15070563

Legislative Council Secretariat. (2015). *Challenges of population aging*. Retrieved March 13, 2017, from http://www.legco.gov.hk/research-publications/english/1516rb01-challenges-of-population-aging-20151215-e.pdf

Legislative Council Secretariat. (2015a). Challenges of population ageing. *Research Brief, 2015-2016*(1). Retrieved March 20, 2017 from http://www.legco.gov.hk/research-publications/english/1516rb01-challenges-of-population-ageing-20151215-e.pdf

Legislative Council Secretariat. (2015b). *Panel on Health Services – Updated background brief prepared by the Legislative Council Secretariat for the meeting on 16 March 2015: Private hospital development* (LC Paper No. CB(2)993/14-15(04)). Retrieved March 20, 2017 from http://www.legco.gov.hk/yr14-15/english/panels/hs/papers/hs20150316cb2-993-4-e.pdf

Legislative Council. (2015a). *Challenges of population ageing*. Research Brief, 1. Retrieved 25 Feb 2017, from http://www.legco.gov.hk/research-publications/english/1516rb01-challenges-of-population-ageing-20151215-e.pdf

Legislative Council. (2015b). *Proposed $10 billion endowment fund to the Hospital Authority for public-private partnership initiatives*. Panel on Health Services. Retrieved 22 March 2016, from http://www.legco.gov.hk/yr15-16/english/panels/hs/papers/hs20151116cb2-235-7-e.pdf

Lehning, A. J. (2012). City Governments and Aging in Place: Community Design, Transportation and Housing Innovation Adoption. *The Gerontologist*, *52*(3), 345–356. doi:10.1093/geront/gnr089 PMID:21900505

Lei, P., & Wu, Z. (2014). Analysis on over-medication in hospitals in China, Chinese version. *Chinese Health Economics*, *33*(5), 9–11.

Leung, P. Y. (2016). *Chief Executive Speech -- Travelling life's journeys together*. Paper presented at the Hospital Authority Convention 2016, Hong Kong.

Leung, E. M. F. (2002). Changing Needs and Changing Service Delivery for Long-term Care in Hong Kong. *Journal of Aging & Social Policy*, *13*(2-3), 155–168. doi:10.1300/J031v13n02_11 PMID:12216353

Leutz, W. N. (1999). Five laws for integrating medical and social services: Lessons from the United States and the United Kingdom. *The Milbank Quarterly*, *77*(1), 77–110. doi:10.1111/1468-0009.00125 PMID:10197028

Lewis, C. B. (2002). *Aging: The Health-Care Challenge*. Philadelphia: F. A. Davis Company.

Lewis, S. J., Moye, L. A., Sacks, F. M., Johnstone, D. E., Timmis, G., & Mitchell, J. et al.. (1998). Effect of pravastatin on cardiovascular events in older patients with myocardial infarction and cholesterol levels in the average range: Results of the Cholesterol and Recurrent Events (CARE) trial. *Annals of Internal Medicine*, *129*(9), 681–689. doi:10.7326/0003-4819-129-9-199811010-00002 PMID:9841599

Li, Q. (2009). The study on realizing the path to universal health insurance in China, Chinese version. Beijing: People's Publishing House.

Li, S. (2006, September 29). *Population aging brings three types of pressure to China*, Chinese version. Retrieved June 24, 2016, from http://www.huaxia.com/xw/zh/2006/00516600.html

Li, T. (2015, February 13). *Individual premium contribution of the New Rural Cooperative Medical System (NRCMS) will increase to Renminbi 120, but some regions still have the problem of expenditure exceeding revenue of the NRCMS fund,* Chinese version. Retrieved July 14, 2016, from http://news.xinhuanet.com/politics/2015-02/13/c_127491063.htm

Liamis, G., Filippatos, T., Liontos, A., & Elisaf, M. (2016). Hyponatremia in patients with liver diseases: not just a cirrhosis-induced hemodynamic compromise. *Hepatology International, 10*(5), 762-772.

Liang, W. (1991). *Empowering The Elderly: Direct Consumer Funding of Care Services. Choice in Welfare Series No. 6*. London: IEA Health & Welfare Unit.

Lian, J. W., Yen, D. C., & Wang, Y. T. (2014). An exploratory study to understand the critical factors affecting the decision to adopt cloud computing in Taiwan hospital. *International Journal of Information Management*, *34*(1), 28–36. doi:10.1016/j.ijinfomgt.2013.09.004

Liao, S. H., & Wu, C. C. (2009). The relationship among knowledge management, organizational learning, and organizational performance. *International Journal of Business and Management*, *4*(4), 64. doi:10.5539/ijbm.v4n4p64

Li, C., Hou, Y., Sun, M., Lu, J., Wang, Y., Li, X., & Hao, M. et al. (2015). An evaluation of China's new rural cooperative medical system: Achievements and inadequacies from policy goals. *BMC Public Health, 15*(1), 1079. doi:10.1186/s12889-015-2410-1 PMID:26494015

Lien, A. S. Y., Jiang, Y. D., Mou, C. H., Sun, M. F., Gau, B. S., & Yen, H. R. (2016). Integrative traditional Chinese medicine therapy reduces the risk of diabetic ketoacidosis in patients with type 1 diabetes mellitus. *Journal of Ethnopharmacology, 191*, 324–330. doi:10.1016/j.jep.2016.06.051 PMID:27340102

Li, M., Yu, S., Zheng, Y., Ren, K., & Lou, W. (2013). Scalable and secure sharing of personal health records in cloud computing using attribute-based encryption. *IEEE Transactions on Parallel and Distributed Systems, 24*(1), 131–143. doi:10.1109/TPDS.2012.97

Lim, C. K., Luo, Z., Chen, I. M., & Yeo, S. H. (2011). Wearable wireless sensing system for capturing human arm motion. *Sensors and Actuators. A, Physical, 166*(1), 125–132. doi:10.1016/j.sna.2010.10.015

Lim, M. K. (2004). Shifting the burden of healthcare finance: A case study of public-private partnership in Singapore. *Health Policy (Amsterdam), 69*(1), 83–92. doi:10.1016/j.healthpol.2003.12.009 PMID:15484609

Lin, C., Tan, B., & Chang, S. (2008). An exploratory model of knowledge flow barriers within healthcare organizations. *Information & Management, 45*(5), 331–339. doi:10.1016/j.im.2008.03.003

Lin, C., Wu, J. C., & Yen, D. C. (2012). Exploring barriers to knowledge flow at different knowledge management maturity stages. *Information & Management, 49*(1), 10–23. doi:10.1016/j.im.2011.11.001

Lindholm, L. H., Ibsen, H., Dahlöf, B., Devereux, R. B., Beevers, G., de Faire, U., & Snapinn, S. et al. (2002). Cardiovascular morbidity and mortality in patients with diabetes in the Losartan Intervention For Endpoint reduction in hypertension study (LIFE): A randomised trial against atenolol. *Lancet, 359*(9311), 1004–1010. doi:10.1016/S0140-6736(02)08090-X PMID:11937179

Lin, F. O. Y., Luk, J. K. H., Chan, T. C., Mok, W. W. Y., & Chan, F. H. W. (2015). Effectiveness of a discharge planning and community support programme in preventing readmission of high-risk older patients. *Hong Kong Medical Journal, 21*(3), 208–216. PMID:25904292

Lin, H. C., Lin, Y. J., Liu, T. C., Chen, C. S., & Lin, C. C. (2007). Urbanization and place of death for the elderly: A 10-year population-based study. *Palliative Medicine, 21*(8), 705–711. doi:10.1177/0269216307083033 PMID:18073257

Lin, H. F. (2014). A multi-stage analysis of antecedents and consequences of knowledge management evolution. *Journal of Knowledge Management, 18*(1), 52–74. doi:10.1108/JKM-07-2013-0278

Lin, N. (1999). Building a network theory of social capital. *Connections, 22*(1), 28–51.

Lin, P. H., Lin, S. K., Hsu, R. J., Cheng, K. C., & Liu, J. M. (2016). The Use and the Prescription Pattern of Traditional Chinese Medicine Among Urolithiasis Patients in Taiwan: A Population-Based Study. *Journal of Alternative and Complementary Medicine (New York, N.Y.), 22*(1), 88–95. doi:10.1089/acm.2015.0116 PMID:26359806

Lin, W., Liu, G. G., & Chen, G. (2009). The urban resident basic medical insurance: A landmark reform towards universal coverage in China. *Health Economics, 18*(S2), S83–S96. doi:10.1002/hec.1500 PMID:19551750

Liu, F. C. F. (2006). Community palliative care in Hong Kong. In C. L. W. Chan & A. Y. M. Chow (Eds.), Death, dying and bereavement -- A Hong Kong Chinese experience (pp. 183–193). Hong Kong: Hong Kong University Press.

Liu, G. G., Yuen, P., Hu, T., Li, L., & Liu, X. (2004). Urban health insurance reform: what can we learn from the pilot experiment? In A. Chen, G.G. Liu, & K.H. Zhang (Eds.), Urbanization and social welfare in China (pp. 38-62). Aldershot, UK: Ashgate.

Liu, F. C. F., & Lam, C. (2005). Preparing cancer patients to die at home. *Hong Kong Nursing Journal*, *4*(1), 7–14.

Liu, G. G., Zhao, Z., Cai, R., Yamada, T., & Yamada, T. (2002). Equity in health care access to: Assessing the urban health insurance reform in China. *Social Science & Medicine*, *55*(10), 1779–1794. doi:10.1016/S0277-9536(01)00306-9 PMID:12383462

Liu, H., & Zhao, Z. (2014). Does health insurance matter? Evidence from China's urban resident basic medical insurance. *Journal of Comparative Economics*, *42*(4), 1007–1020. doi:10.1016/j.jce.2014.02.003

Liu, K., Daviglus, M. L., Loria, C. M., Colangelo, L. A., Spring, B., Moller, A. C., & Lloyd-Jones, D. M. (2012). Healthy lifestyle through young adulthood and the presence of low cardiovascular disease risk profile in middle age: The Coronary Artery Risk Development in (Young) Adults (CARDIA) study. *Circulation*, *125*(8), 996–1004. doi:10.1161/CIRCULATIONAHA.111.060681 PMID:22291127

Liu, X., & Cao, H. (1992). China's cooperative medical systems: Its historical transformation and the trend of development. *Journal of Public Health Policy*, *13*(4), 501–511. doi:10.2307/3342538 PMID:1287043

Liu, X., & Mills, A. (2005). The effect of performance-related pay of hospital doctors on hospital behaviour: A case study from Shandong, China. *Human Resources for Health*, *3*(1), 11. doi:10.1186/1478-4491-3-11 PMID:16253137

Liu, X., Wong, H., & Liu, K. (2016). Outcome-based health equity across different social health insurance schemes for the elderly in China. *BMC Health Services Research*, *16*(1), 9. doi:10.1186/s12913-016-1261-5 PMID:26762146

Liu, Y. (2004). Development of the rural health insurance system in China. *Health Policy and Planning*, *19*(3), 159–165. doi:10.1093/heapol/czh019 PMID:15070864

Liu, Y. M., Sheu, S. J., Chiou, S. H., Chang, H. C., & Chen, Y. P. (1993). A comparative study of commercial samples of Ephedrae Herba. *Planta Medica*, *59*(04), 376–378. doi:10.1055/s-2006-959706 PMID:17235993

Liu, Y., Hsiao, W. C. L., Li, Q., Liu, X., & Ren, M. (1995). Transformation of China's rural health care financing. *Social Science & Medicine*, *41*(8), 1085–1093. doi:10.1016/0277-9536(95)00428-A PMID:8578331

Liu, Y., Li, N., Jia, Z., Lu, F., & Pu, J. (2014). Chinese medicine shensongyangxin is effective for patients with bradycardia: Results of a randomized, double-blind, placebo-controlled multicenter trial. *Evidence-Based Complementary and Alternative Medicine*. PMID:24527049

Li, Y. (2013). Analysis on high drug prices, the practice of drug kickbacks, and the centralized bidding and procurement for drugs, Chinese version. *Contemporary Economics*, *23*, 17–19.

Li, Y. Q., Jin, M., Qiu, S. L., Wang, P. L., Zhu, T. G., Wang, C. L., & Shi, D. Z. et al. (2009). Effect of Chinese drugs for supplementing Qi, nourishing yin and activating blood circulation on myocardial perfusion in patients with acute myocardial infarction after revascularization. *Chinese Journal of Integrative Medicine*, *15*(1), 19–25. doi:10.1007/s11655-009-0019-7 PMID:19271165

Li, Y., & Chui, W.-E. (2016). Community care for adults with severe mental disorders in rural China: A case study. *International Journal of Social Welfare*, *25*(3), 273–282. doi:10.1111/ijsw.12201

Li, Y., Kong, N., Chen, M., & Zheng, Q. P. (2016). Optimal physician assignment and patient demand allocation in an outpatient care network. *Computers & Operations Research*, *72*, 107–117. doi:10.1016/j.cor.2016.02.013

Llano, R. (2013). Bundled payments for integrated care in the Netherlands. In Incentivising 2013 Integrated Care (pp. 15-16). Quarterly of the European Observatory on Health Systems and Policies.

Lluch, M., & Abadie, F. (2013). Exploring the role of ICT in the provision of integrated care—evidence from eight countries. *Health Policy (Amsterdam)*, *111*(1), 1–13. doi:10.1016/j.healthpol.2013.03.005 PMID:23587547

Lo, M. F., & Ng, P. M. L. (2015). *Role of codification and personalization in organizational learning, innovation and performance: A conceptual framework and research propositions.* The 12th International Conference on Intellectual Capital, Knowledge Management & Organizational Learning, Bangkok, Thailand.

Lofqvist, C., Granbom, M., Himmelsbach, I., Iwarsson, S., Oswald, F., & Haak, M. (2013). Voices on Relocation and Aging in Place in Very Old Age - A Complex and Ambivalent Matter. *The Gerontologist*, *53*(6), 919–927. doi:10.1093/geront/gnt034 PMID:23626372

Loke, A. Y., Liu, C. F. F., & Szeto, Y. (2003). The difficulties faced by informal caregivers of patients with terminal cancer in Hong Kong and the available social support. *Cancer Nursing*, *26*(4), 276–283. doi:10.1097/00002820-200308000-00004 PMID:12886118

Longest, B. B. Jr, & Lin, C. J. (2005). Can Nonprofit Hospitals Do Both Well and Good? *Health Care Management Review*, *30*(1), 62–68. doi:10.1097/00004010-200501000-00009 PMID:15773255

Long, V., Cates, S., Blitstein, J., Deehy, K., Williams, P., Morgan, R., & Hersey, J. (2013). *Supplemental Nutrition Assistance Program Education and Evaluation Study (Wave II).* Ann Arbor, MI: Altarum Institute.

López-Nicolás, C., & Meroño-Cerdán, Á. L. (2011). Strategic knowledge management, innovation and performance. *International Journal of Information Management*, *31*(6), 502–509. doi:10.1016/j.ijinfomgt.2011.02.003

Lou, Kwan, & Chan. (2011). *A Study on the Effectiveness of Community Care Services in Hong Kong*. The University of Hong Kong.

Lou, V. W. Q. (2014). Case Management in Community-based Long-term Care: Good Practices and Challenges in Hong Kong. In K. W. Tong & K. N. K. Fong (Eds.), *Community Care in Hong Kong: Current Practices, Practice-research Studies and Future Directions* (pp. 17–36). Hong Kong: City University of Hong Kong Press.

Low, C., Chen, Y., & Wu, M. (2011). Understanding the determinants of cloud computing adoption. *Industrial Management & Data Systems*, *111*(7), 1006–1023. doi:10.1108/02635571111161262

Lowi, T. (1964). American business, public policy, case studies, and political theory. *World Politics*, *16*(4), 667–715. doi:10.2307/2009452

Lowi, T. (1979). *The end of liberalism: the second republic of the United States*. New York: W.W. Norton & Company, Inc.

Lu, X. P. (2015, February 10). *Government official from China Insurance Regulatory Commission: Individuals currently still have to bear a relatively high medical expenses*, Chinese version. Retrieved July 14, 2016, from http://finance.sina.com.cn/stock/t/20150210/111321518553.shtml

Luk, J. K., Chan, T. Y., & Chan, D. K. (2015). Falls prevention in the elderly: Translating evidence into practice. *Hong Kong Medical Journal*, *21*(2), 165–171. PMID:25722468

Luk, J., Liu, A., Ng, W., Beh, P., & Chan, F. (2011). End-of-life care in Hong Kong. *Asian Journal of Gerontology & Geriatrics*, *6*(2), 103–106.

Luk, S. (2014). *Health Insurance Reforms in Asia*. London: Routledge.

Lu, M. T., Lin, S. W., & Tzeng, G. H. (2013). Improving RFID adoption in Taiwans healthcare industry based on a DEMATEL technique with a hybrid MCDM model. *Decision Support Systems*, *56*, 259–269. doi:10.1016/j.dss.2013.06.006

Lump Sum Grant Independent Review Committee. (2008). *Review Report on the Lump Sum Grant Subvention System.* Retrieved March 20, 2017 from http://www.lwb.gov.hk/eng/consult_paper/Review%20Report%20on%20Lump%20Sum%20Grant%20Subvention%20System.pdf

Lussier, R. N. (2009). *Management fundamentals: concepts, applications, skill development* (4th ed.). South Western College.

Lu, Z., Kou, W., Du, B., Wu, Y., Zhao, S., Brusco, O. A., & Capuzzi, D. M. et al. (2008). Effect of Xuezhikang, an extract from red yeast Chinese rice, on coronary events in a Chinese population with previous myocardial infarction. *The American Journal of Cardiology, 101*(12), 1689–1693. doi:10.1016/j.amjcard.2008.02.056 PMID:18549841

Lynn, J., & Adamson, D. M. (2003). *Living well at the end of life. Adapting health care to serious chronic illness in old age.* Santa Monica, CA: RAND.

MacAdam, M. (2008). *Frameworks of integrated care for the elderly: A systematic review.* Toronto, ON: Canadian Policy Research Networks.

MacAdam, M. (2015). PRISMA: Program of research to integrate the services for the maintenance of autonomy. A system-level integration model in Quebec. *International Journal of Integrated Care, 15*(6). doi:10.5334/ijic.2246 PMID:26417212

MacLaughlin, E. J., Raehl, C. L., Treadway, A. K., Sterling, T. L., Zoller, D. P., & Bond, C. A. (2005). Assessing medication adherence in the elderly. *Drugs & Aging, 22*(3), 231–255. doi:10.2165/00002512-200522030-00005 PMID:15813656

Madore, O. (2004). *The Canada Health Act: Overview and Options.* Parliamentary Information and Research Service.

Magnus, G. (2012). *The age of aging: How demographics are changing the global economy and our world.* John Wiley & Sons. doi:10.1002/9781119207702

Mahoney, F. I., & Barthel, D. W. (1965). Functional evaluation: The barthel index. *Maryland State Medical Journal, 14*, 61–65. PMID:14258950

Mahoney, J. (2001). *The legacies of liberalism: path dependence and political regimes in Central America.* Baltimore, MD: Johns Hopkins University Press.

Mak, B., Woo, J., Bowling, A., Wong, F., & Chau, P. H. (2011). Health care prioritization in ageing societies: Influence of age, education, health literacy and culture. *Health Policy (Amsterdam), 100*(2-3), 219–233. doi:10.1016/j.healthpol.2010.08.015 PMID:20850194

Mak, M. H. J. (2010). Quality insights of university students on dying, death, and death education--a preliminary study in Hong Kong. *Omega, 62*(4), 387–405. PMID:21661541

Ma, N. (2007). *Political development in Hong Kong: State, political society, and civil society.* Hong Kong: Hong Kong University Press.

Manos, R., & Drori, I. (2016). *Corporate Responsibility: Social Action, Institutions and Governance.* Hampshire, UK: Palgrave Macmillan. doi:10.1057/9781137450722

Mao, W., & Chen, W. (2015). *China: The zero mark-up policy for essential medicines at primary level facilities.* Retrieved July 17, 2016, from http://www.who.int/health_financing/documents/Efficiency_health_systems_China/en/

March, J. G. (1991). Exploration and exploitation in organizational learning. *Organization Science, 2*(1), 71–87. doi:10.1287/orsc.2.1.71

Marek, K. D., Stetzer, F., Adams, S. J., Popejoy, L. L., & Rantz, M. (2012). Aging in place versus nursing home care: Comparison of costs to Medicare and Medicaid. *Research in Gerontological Nursing*, *5*(2), 123–129. doi:10.3928/19404921-20110802-01 PMID:21846081

Markell, D. (1993). The federal superfund program: Proposals for strengthening the federal/state relationship. *William and Mary Journal of Environmental Law*, *18*, 1–82.

MarketLine. (2014). *MarketLine Industry Profile: Healthcare Providers in Asia-Pacific*. London: MarketLine.

Martin, D. J., Garske, J. P., & Davis, M. K. (2000). Relation of the therapeutic alliance with outcome and other variables: A meta-analytic review. *Journal of Consulting and Clinical Psychology*, *68*(3), 438–450. doi:10.1037/0022-006X.68.3.438 PMID:10883561

Mason, D., & Pauleen, D. J. (2003). Perceptions of knowledge management: A qualitative analysis. *Journal of Knowledge Management*, *7*(4), 38–48. doi:10.1108/13673270310492930

Mathematica Policy Research. (2014). *The changing medical and long-term care expenditures of people who transition from institutional care to home- and community-based services*. Retrieved July 5, 2016, from https://www.mathematica-mpr.com/our-publications-and-findings/publications/the-changing-medical-and-long-term-care-expenditures-of-people-who-transition

Ma, Y., & Sun, S. (2014). Analysis on the medical insurance system for the elderly, Chinese version. *China Social Security*, *9*, 28–29.

McAleese, J. D., & Rankin, L. L. (2007). Garden-based nutrition education affects fruit and vegetable consumption in sixth-grade adolescents. *Journal of the American Dietetic Association*, *107*(4), 662–665. doi:10.1016/j.jada.2007.01.015 PMID:17383272

McArthur, G. (2016). *Melbourne grandfather's life saved by FitBit*. Herarld Sun. Retrieved 4 March 2017, from http://www.heraldsun.com.au/news/victoria/melbourne-grandfathers-life-saved-by-fitbit/news-story/cfcd28310c938a4de2811b97ad-b417af

McBride, A. B., Fagin, C. M., Franklin, P. D., Huba, G. J., & Quach, L. (2006). Developing geriatric nursing leaders via an annual leadership conference. *Nursing Outlook*, *54*(4), 226–230. doi:10.1016/j.outlook.2006.05.003 PMID:16890042

McCracken, S. S., & Edwards, J. S. (2015). Implementing a knowledge management system within an NHS hospital: a case study exploring the roll-out of an electronic patient record (EPR). *Knowledge Management Research & Practice*, 1-11

McDonald, S.M., Wagner, L.M., & Gruneir, A. (2015). Accreditation and Resident Safety in Ontario Long-Term Care Homes. *Healthcare quarterly (Toronto, Ont.)*, *18*(1), 54-9.

McGill, H. C., McMahan, C. A., Herderick, E. E., Malcom, G. T., Tracy, R. E., & Strong, J. P. et al.. (2000). Origin of atherosclerosis in childhood and adolescence. *The American Journal of Clinical Nutrition*, *72*(5), 1307s–1315s. PMID:11063473

McKay, K., Kuntz, J. R., & Naswall, K. (2013). The effect of affective commitment, communication and participation on resistance to change: The role of change readiness. *New Zealand Journal of Psychology*, *42*(2), 29–40.

McNeal, R. (2012). State response to Obama's broadband access policy: a study in policy implementation. In V. Weerakkody & C. Reddick (Eds.), *Public sector transformation through e-government: experiences from Europe and North America*. Routledge.

Mead, H., Andres, E., Ramos, C., Siegel, B., & Regenstein, M. (2010). Barriers to effective self-management in cardiac patients. *Patient Education and Counseling*, *79*(1), 69–76. doi:10.1016/j.pec.2009.08.003 PMID:19748205

Means, R., Richards, R., & Smith, R. (2008). *Community care: policy and practice* (4th ed.). Basingstoke, UK: Palgrave Macmillan. doi:10.1007/978-1-137-07383-9

Medicaid and CHIP Payment and Access Commission (MACPAC). (2014). *Report to Congress on Medicaid and CHIP*. Retrieved July 14, 2016, from http://www.macpac.gov/reports

Meier, K. (1994). *The politics of sin: drugs, alcohol and public policy*. New York: Sharpe.

Melchart, D., Hager, S., Dai, J., & Weidenhammer, W. (2016). Quality control and complication screening programme of Chinese medicinal drugs at the first German hospital of traditional Chinese medicine-a retrospective analysis. *Forschende Komplementärmedizin/Research in Complementary Medicine, 23*(Suppl. 2), 21-28.

Melchart, D., Linde, K., Weidenhammer, W., Hager, S., Liao, J., Bauer, R., & Wagner, H. (1999). Use of traditional drugs in a hospital of Chinese medicine in Germany. *Pharmacoepidemiology and Drug Safety*, *8*(2), 115–120. doi:10.1002/(SICI)1099-1557(199903/04)8:2<115::AID-PDS412>3.0.CO;2-I PMID:15073936

Meng, Q., Rehnberg, C., Zhuang, N., Bian, Y., Tomson, G., & Tang, S. (2004). The impact of urban health insurance reform on hospital charges: A case study from two cities in China. *Health Policy (Amsterdam)*, *68*(2), 197–209. doi:10.1016/j.healthpol.2003.09.010 PMID:15063019

Metaxiotis, K. S. (2011). Healthcare Knowledge Management. In D. G. Schwartz (Ed.), *Encyclopedia of Knowledge Management* (pp. 204–210). London, UK: Idea Group Inc.

Metha, K. K. (2005). A critical review of Singapore's policies aimed at supporting families caring for older members. *Journal of Aging & Social Policy*, *18*, 43–57. PMID:17135094

Micheletti, J., & Shlala, T. J. (1986). RUGsII: Implications for management and quality in long-term care. *Quality Review Bulletin*, *12*(7), 236–242. doi:10.1016/S0097-5990(16)30049-5 PMID:3092161

Miettinen, T. A., Pyörälä, K., Olsson, A. G., Musliner, T. A., Cook, T. J., Faergeman, O., & Group, S. S. S. et al. (1997). Cholesterol-lowering therapy in women and elderly patients with myocardial infarction or angina pectoris. *Circulation*, *96*(12), 4211–4218. doi:10.1161/01.CIR.96.12.4211 PMID:9416884

Miller, R. G., Ashar, B. H., & Getz, K. J. (2003). Evaluation of an audience response system for the continuing education of health professionals. *The Journal of Continuing Education in the Health Professions*, *23*(2), 109–115. doi:10.1002/chp.1340230208 PMID:12866330

Ministry of Health, Singapore. (2015). *Public-private partnerships*. Retrieved 3 July 2016, from https://www.moh.gov.sg/content/moh_web/home/pressRoom/Parliamentary_QA/2016/public-private-partnerships-.html

Ministry of Health. (2000). Eldercare Fund. *Ministry of Health*. Retrieved from: https://www.moh.gov.sg/content/moh_web/home/pressRoom/pressRoomItemRelease/2000/establishment_of_eldercare_fund.html

Ministry of Health. (2008). *Medifund Silver*. Retrieved February 26, 2017, from https://www.moh.gov.sg/content/moh_web/home/pressRoom/pressRoomItemRelease/2008/medifund_silver.html

Ministry of Health. (2012). Community Silver Trust. *Ministry of Health*. Retrieved from: https://www.moh.gov.sg/content/moh_web/home/pressRoom/Parliamentary_QA/2012/community_silvertrust.html

Ministry of Health. (2016). *ElderShield Fast Facts*. Retrieved February 26, 2017, from https://www.moh.gov.sg/content/dam/moh_web/Publications/Educational%20Resources/2016/ElderShield%20Fast%20Facts%20Brochure.pdf

Ministry of Human Resources and Social Security. (2014). *Opinions on Further Strengthening the Supervision and Management of Medical Services for the Basic Medical Insurance*, Chinese version. Retrieved July 17, 2016, from http://www.law-lib.com/law/law_view.asp?id=460883

Min, Y., Jiang, L., Yan, L. L., Wang, L., Basu, S., Wu, Y., & Stafford, R. S. (2015). Tackling China's noncommunicable diseases: Shared origins, costly consequences and the need for action. *Chinese Medical Journal*, *128*(6), 839–843. doi:10.4103/0366-6999.152690 PMID:25758283

Mission of the Statistics and Census Service (DSEC). (2016). *Population Statistics 2016 1st Quarter Report*. Macau: Statistics and Census Service.

Mitchell, M. (2008). *An overview of public private partnerships in health. International Health Systems Program Publication*. Harvard School of Public Health.

Mitton, C., Adair, C. E., McKenzie, E., Patten, S. B., & Perry, B. W. (2007). Knowledge transfer and exchange: Review and synthesis of the literature. *The Milbank Quarterly*, *85*(4), 729–768. doi:10.1111/j.1468-0009.2007.00506.x PMID:18070335

Miyagawa, S., Yamasaki, S., Uchiyama, E., & Amoroso, D. L. (2014). Framework for information sharing with privacy and priority control in long-term care in Japan. *International Journal of E-Health and Medical Communications*, *5*(1), 46–62. doi:10.4018/ijehmc.2014010103

Mjelde-Mossey, L., & Chan, C. (2007). Survey on death and dying in Hong Kong: Attitudes, beliefs, and preferred end-of-life care. *Social Work in Health Care*, *45*(1), 49–65. doi:10.1300/J010v45n01_04 PMID:17804347

Moberg, D. O. (2008). Spirituality and aging: Research and Implications. *Journal of Religion, Spirituality and Aging*, *20*(1-2), 95–134. doi:10.1080/15528030801922038

Mok, E., Chan, F., Chan, V., & Yeung, E. (2002). Perception of empowerment by family caregivers of patients with a terminal illness in Hong Kong. *International Journal of Palliative Nursing*, *8*(3), 137–145. doi:10.12968/ijpn.2002.8.3.10250 PMID:11923742

Mooney, C., & Lee, M. (1995). Legislating morality in the American states: The case of pre-Roe abortion regulation reform. *American Journal of Political Science*, *39*(3), 599–627. doi:10.2307/2111646

Moore, B. (1966). *Social origins of dictatorship and democracy: lord and peasant in the making of the modern world*. Boston: Beacon Press.

Moore, L. V., & Thompson, F. E. (2015). Adults Meeting Fruit and Vegetable Intake Recommendations—United States, 2013. *Morbidity and Mortality Weekly Report*, *64*(26), 709–713. PMID:26158351

Moran, D. (2014). What does Heidegger mean by the transcendence of Dasein? *International Journal of Philosophical Studies*, *22*(4), 491–514. doi:10.1080/09672559.2014.948717

Morgan, L. A., & Kunkel, S. R. (2016). *Aging, society, and the life course* (5th ed.). New York, NY: Springer.

Morris, S., Wilmot, A., Hill, M., Ockenden, N., & Payne, S. (2013). A narrative literature review of the contribution of volunteers in end-of-life care services. *Palliative Medicine*, *27*(5), 428–436. doi:10.1177/0269216312453608 PMID:22833474

Morse, J. M., Morse, B. M., & Tylko, S. (1986). Development of a scale to identify the fall-prone patient. *Canadian Journal on Aging*, *8*, 66–77.

Mor, V., Berg, K., Angelelli, J., Gifford, D., Morris, J., & Moore, T. (2003). The Quality of Quality Measurement in U.S. Nursing Homes. *The Gerontologist*, *43*(2Supplement 2), 37–46. doi:10.1093/geront/43.suppl_2.37 PMID:12711723

Mossey, J. M., & Shapiro, E. (1982). Self-rated health: A predictor of mortality among the elderly. *American Journal of Public Health*, *72*(8), 800–808. doi:10.2105/AJPH.72.8.800 PMID:7091475

Moustaghfir, K., & Schiuma, G. (2013). Knowledge, learning, and innovation: Research and perspectives. *Journal of Knowledge Management*, *17*(4), 495–510. doi:10.1108/JKM-04-2013-0141

Movement, V. (n.d.). *About Volunteer Service*. Retrieved May 14, 2016 from http://www.volunteering-hk.org/aboutvs

Mui, A. C. (2002). The program of all-inclusive care for the elderly (PACE): An innovative long-term care model in the United States. *Journal of Aging & Social Policy*, *13*(2–3), 53–67. doi:10.1300/J031v13n02_05 PMID:12216362

Mulani, T. T., & Pingle, S. V. (2016). Internet of Things. *International Research Journal of Multidisciplinary Studies*, *2*(3).

Munir, F., Khan, H., Yarker, J., Haslam, C., Long, H., Bains, M., & Kalawsky, K. (2009). Self-management of health behaviours among older and younger workers with chronic illness. *Patient Education and Counseling*, *77*(1), 109–115. doi:10.1016/j.pec.2009.02.014 PMID:19356885

Muoio, D. (2015). *Japan is running out of people to take care of the elderly, so it's making robots instead.* Retrieved 20 July 2016, from http://www.techinsider.io/japan-developing-carebots-for-elderly-care-2015-11

Murchie, P., Campbell, N., Ritchie, L., Simpson, J., & Thain, J. (2003). secondary prevention clinics for coronary heart disease: Four year follow up of a randomised controlled trial in primary care. *British Medical Journal*, *326*(7380), 84–87. doi:10.1136/bmj.326.7380.84 PMID:12521974

Murphy, E. (1987). Community care I: Problems. *British Medical Journal*, *295*(6612), 1505–1508. doi:10.1136/bmj.295.6612.1505-a PMID:3122879

Nagel, H., Baehring, T., & Scherbaum, W. A. (2008). Disease management programmes for diabetes in Germany. *Diabetes Voice*, *53*(3), 17–19.

Nakanishi, M., Shimizu, S., Murai, T., & Yamaoka, A. (2015). Ageing in place policy in Japan: Association between the development of an integrated community care system and the number of nursing home placements under the public long-term care insurance program among municipal governments. *Ageing International*, *40*(3), 248–261. doi:10.1007/s12126-014-9215-x

Nanfang Metropolis Daily. (2015 February 10). *Green Book of Health Reform and Development 2014 said that medical insurance funds are faced with risks and will have a deficit in 2017*, Chinese version. Retrieved July 12, 2016, from http://www.nandu.com/html/201502/10/1050767.html

National Bureau of Statistics of China. (2014). *China Statistical Yearbook 2014*. Retrieved July 12, 2016, from http://www.stats.gov.cn/tjsj/ndsj/2014/indexch.htm

National Conference of State Legislatures. (2011). *Long-term care provisions in health reform*. Retrieved June 10, 2016, from http://www.ncsl.org/research/health/long-term-care-provisions-in-health-reform.aspx

National Conference of State Legislatures. (2017). *Children's health insurance program overview*. Retrieved February 15, 2017, from http://www.ncsl.org/research/health/childrens-insurance-program-overview.aspx

National Council on Aging. (2016). *Facts about healthy aging*. Retrieved 8 August 2016, from https://www.ncoa.org/news/resources-for-reporters/get-the-facts/healthy-aging-facts/

National Development and Reform Commission, Ministry of Health, Ministry of Finance, Ministry of Human Resources and Social Security, Ministry of Civil Affairs, and China Insurance Regulatory Commission. (2012). *The Guiding Opinions on the Launch of the Work on Critical Illness Insurance for Urban and Rural Residents,* Chinese version. Retrieved July 12, 2016, from http://www.gov.cn/gzdt/2012-08/31/content_2214223.htm

National Development and Reform Commission, National Health and Family Planning Commission, Ministry of Human Resources and Social Security, Ministry of Industry and Information Technology, Ministry of Finance, Ministry of Commerce, and China Food and Drug Administration. (2015). *Opinions on Proceeding with the Reform on Drug Pricing,* Chinese version. Retrieved July 17, 2016, from http://www.sdpc.gov.cn/zcfb/zcfbtz/201505/W020150505398057890638.pdf

National Health Service of the UK. (2014). *Five-year forward view for the NHS.* Retrieved March 20, 2017 from https://www.england.nhs.uk/wp-content/uploads/2014/10/5yfv-web.pdf

National Institute for Health and Care Excellence. (2011). *Management of stable angina.* Retrieved from: http://www.nice.org.uk/guidance/cg126/chapter/1-recommendations#information-and-support-for-people-with-stable-angina

National Institute for Health and Care Excellence. (2013). *Cardiac rehabilitation services.* Retrieved from: http://publications.nice.org.uk/cardiac-rehabilitation-services-cmg40/43-delivery-of-programme on 26.07.16

National Institute on Aging, National Institutes of Health, & World Health Organization. (2011). *Global health and aging.* Retrieved March 20, 2017 from http://www.who.int/ageing/publications/global_health.pdf

National PACE Association. (2016). *PACE services.* Retrieved from http://www.npaonline.org/pace-you/pace-services

National Records of Scotland. (2015). *Life expectancy for areas within Scotland.* Retrieved from http://www.nrscotland.gov.uk/files//statistics/life-expectancy-areas-in-scotland/12-14/life-exp-in-scotland-2012-to-2014.pdf

National Treasury PPP Unite of South Africa. (2007). *Public private partnership manual.* Retrieved 24 March 2016, from http://www.treasury.gov.za/organisation/ppp/default.htm

National University of Singapore. (2016). *Research team led by NUS scientists develop plastic flexible magnetic memory device.* Singapore: National University of Singapore.

Naylor, C. D. (1999). Health care in Canada: Incrementalism under fiscal duress. *Health Affairs, 18*(3), 9–26. doi:10.1377/hlthaff.18.3.9 PMID:10388197

Ndandiko, C., & Ibanda, S. (2016). *Public private partnerships guidelines for local governments.* United Nation Development Programme. Retrieved 27 May 2016, from http://www.undp.org/content/dam/uganda/img/Research%20and%20Publications/PPP%20Guidelines%20Final.pdf

Newgarten, B. L. (1964). *Personality in the middle and late life.* New York: Atherton Press.

Ng, M., Sha, K., & Tong, B. (2011). *Bridging the Gap: Win-win from Integrated Discharge Support for Elderly Patients.* Presentation, HA Convention 2011.

Ngai, E. W., & Chan, E. W. C. (2005). Evaluation of knowledge management tools using AHP. *Expert Systems with Applications, 29*(4), 889–899. doi:10.1016/j.eswa.2005.06.025

NHS England. (2016). *NHS England Patient Online.* Retrieved 11 April 2016, from https://www.england.nhs.uk/our-work/pe/patient-online/

NHS Foundation Trust, United Kingdom. (2014). *Strategic plan document for 2014-19 Alder Hey Children's NHS Foundation Trust.* Retrieved 27 May 2016, from https://www.gov.uk/government/uploads/system/uploads/attachment_data/file/389689/Alderhey_Publishable_Summary_Strategic_Plan_1415.pdf

NHS. (2010). *Do Once and Share Factsheet*. Retrieved 20 July 2016, from http://webarchive.nationalarchives.gov.uk/20130502102046/http://www.connectingforhealth.nhs.uk/resources/systserv/do-once-and

Nieboer, A. P., & Strating, M. M. (2012). Innovative culture in long-term care settings: The influence of organizational characteristics. *Health Care Management Review*, *37*(2), 165–174. doi:10.1097/HMR.0b013e318222416b PMID:21720249

Nimrod, G., & Kleiber, D. A. (2007). Reconsidering change and continuity in later life: Toward an innovation theory of successful aging. *International Journal of Aging & Human Development*, *65*(1), 1–22. doi:10.2190/Q4G5-7176-51Q2-3754 PMID:17703747

Nolte, E., Knai, C., Hofmarcher, M., Conklin, A., Erler, A., Elissen, A., Vrijhoef, H. J. M. (2012). Overcoming fragmentation in health care: chronic care in Austria, Germany and the Netherlands. *Health Economics, Policy and Law*, *7*(S1), 125–146.

Nonaka, I., & Takeuchi, H. (1995). *The knowledge-creating company: How Japanese companies create the dynamics of innovation*. Oxford University Press.

Norcross, J. C. (2010). The therapeutic relationship. In B. L. Duncan, S. D. Miller, B. E. Wampold, & M. A. Hubble (Eds.), *The heart & soul of change: Delivering what works in therapy* (2nd ed.; pp. 113–141). Washington, DC: American Psychological Association; doi:10.1037/12075-004

Norton, D., McLaren, R., & Exton-smith, A. N. (1979). *An investigation of Geriatric problems in hospital* (3rd ed.). London: Churchill Livingstone.

Noruzy, A., Dalfard, V. M., Azhdari, B., Nazari-Shirkouhi, S., & Rezazadeh, A. (2013). Relations between transformational leadership, organizational learning, knowledge management, organizational innovation, and organizational performance: An empirical investigation of manufacturing firms. *International Journal of Advanced Manufacturing Technology*, *64*(5-8), 1073–1085. doi:10.1007/s00170-012-4038-y

Nownes, A., Thomas, C., & Hrebenar, R. (2008). Interest groups in the states. In V. Grey & R. Hanson (Eds.), *Politics in the American states: A comparative analysis* (9th ed.; pp. 98–126). Washington, DC: CQ Press.

Nursing and Midwifery Council. (2010). *Standards for Pre-Registration Nursing Education*. London: Nursing and Midwifery Council.

Nygren, C., & Iwarsson, S. (2009). Negotiating and effectuating relocation to sheltered housing in old age: A Swedish study over 11 years. *European Journal of Ageing*, *6*(3), 177–189. doi:10.1007/s10433-009-0121-0

O'Flynn, J., Dickinson, H., O'Sullivan, S., Gallet, W., Currie, K., Pettit, M., . . . Robinson, T. (2014), *The Prime Provider Model. An Opportunity for Better Public Service Delivery?* Social Policy Working Paper No. 18, published report. Melbourne: University of Melbourne and Brotherhood of St Laurence.

OECD. (2001a). *Private long term care insurance: A niche or a "Big Tent"?* OECD.

OECD. (2011b). *Public Long-term Care Financing Arrangements in OECD Countries in Help Wanted. Providing and Paying for Long Term Care*. OECD.

OECD. (2015). *Health at a glance 2015: OCED indicators*. Paris: OECD Publishing.

OECD. (2016). *Corporate responsibility: Frequently asked questions*. Retrieved May 2, 2016, from http://www.oecd.org/corporate/mne/corporateresponsibilityfrequentlyaskedquestions.htm

OECD. (2016). *OECD Health Statistics 2015*. Retrieved May 14, 2016, from http://stats.oecd.org/index.aspx?DataSetCode=HEALTH_STAT

Office of Policy Development and Research (PD&R). (2016). *Community-Centered Solutions for Aging at Home*. Retrieved February 1, 2017, from https://www.huduser.gov/portal/periodicals/em/fall13/highlight3.html#title

Oh, J. H., & Kim, S. (2009). Aging, neighborhood attachment, and fear of crime: Testing reciprocal effects. *Journal of Community Psychology*, *37*(1), 21–40. doi:10.1002/jcop.20269

Okapara, J. O., & Idowu, S. O. (Eds.). (2013). *Corporate Social Responsibility: Challenges, Opportunities and Strategies for 21st Century Leaders*. New York: Springer. doi:10.1007/978-3-642-40975-2

Okereke, C. E., & Messerli, F. H. (2001). Efficacy and safety of angiotensin II receptor blockers in elderly patients with mild to moderate hypertension. *The American Journal of Geriatric Cardiology*, *10*(1), 42–49. doi:10.1111/j.1076-7460.2001.90855.x PMID:11413935

Oliveira, V., Ferreira, P., Maher, C., Pinto, R., Refshauge, K., & Ferreira, M. (2012). Effectiveness of self-management of low back pain. *Arthritis Care and Research*, *64*(11), 1739–1748. doi:10.1002/acr.21737 PMID:22623349

Oliver, C. (2007). Imagined communitas: older migrants and aspirational mobility. In V. Amit (Ed.), *Going First Class? New Approaches to Privileged Travel and Movement* (pp. 126–143). Oxford: Berghahn.

Oliver, D., Foot, C., & Humphries, R. (2014). *Making our health and care systems fit for an ageing population*. London: The King's Fund.

Olmstead v. L.C. (98-537) 527 U.S. 581 (1999)

Olsson, S. B., & Halperin, J. L. (2005). Prevention of stroke in patients with atrial fibrillation. *Seminars in Vascular Medicine*, *5*(03), 285–292. doi:10.1055/s-2005-916168 PMID:16123916

Ouwens, M., Wollersheim, H., Hermens, R., Hulscher, M., & Grol, R. (2005). Integrated care programmes for chronically ill patients: A review of systematic reviews. *International Journal for Quality in Health Care*, *17*(2), 141–146. doi:10.1093/intqhc/mzi016 PMID:15665066

Ozdalga, E., Ozdalga, A., & Ahuja, N. (2012). The smartphone in medicine: A review of current and potential use among physicians and students. *Journal of Medical Internet Research*, *14*(5), e128. doi:10.2196/jmir.1994 PMID:23017375

Pallassana, R. B., & Patchner, M. A. (1987). *Quality Assurance in Nursing Homes: Jane Addams School of Social Work*. Urbana, IL: Illinois University.

Pamela Youde Nethersole Eastern Hospital. (2013). *Scope of Hospital Services*. Retrieved July 16, 2016 from http://www.ha.org.hk/pyneh/internet/Eng/scope/CNS/DOC/CNS.pdf

Panahi, Y., Pishgoo, B., Beiraghdar, F., Araghi, Z. M., Sahebkar, A., & Abolhasani, E. (2011). Results of a randomized, open-label, clinical trial investigating the effects of supplementation with Heracleum persicum extract as an adjunctive therapy for dyslipidemia. *TheScientificWorldJournal*, *11*, 592–601. doi:10.1100/tsw.2011.43 PMID:21403978

Panahi, Y., Pishgoo, B., & Sahebkar, A. (2015). Angiographic findings after supplementation with Heracleum persicum extract: Results of a randomized controlled trial. *Heart Views: The Official Journal of the Gulf Heart Association*, *16*(3), 85. doi:10.4103/1995-705X.164462 PMID:27326348

Pang, S. M. (2003). *Nursing ethics in modern China: conflicting values and competing role requirements*. Amsterdam: Rodopi.

Pan, M. J., & Jang, W. Y. (2008). Determinants of the adoption of enterprise resource planning within the technology-organization-environment framework: Taiwan's communications industry. *Journal of Computer Information Systems*, *48*(3), 94–102.

Papadopoulos, T., Stamati, T., & Nopparuch, P. (2013). Exploring the determinants of knowledge sharing via employee weblogs. *International Journal of Information Management*, *33*(1), 133–146. doi:10.1016/j.ijinfomgt.2012.08.002

Pasupathy, K. (2016). *Knowledge Management in Long-term Care: What You Need to Now*. Accessed at: http://www.ltlmagazine.com/article/knowledge-management-long-term-care-what-you-need-know

Paudel, S., Bhandari, L., & Bhandari, D. B. (2017). Disability: A case screening program approach. *Journal of Biosciences and Medicines*, *5*(2), 10–21. doi:10.4236/jbm.2017.52002

Peckham, S., Hann, A., & Boyce, T. (2011). Health promotion and ill-health prevention: The role of general practice. *Quality in Primary Care*, *19*, 317–323. PMID:22186174

Pentland, D., Forsyth, K., Maciver, D., Walsh, M., Murray, R., Irvine, L., & Sikora, S. (2011). Key characteristics of knowledge transfer and exchange in healthcare: Integrative literature review. *Journal of Advanced Nursing*, *67*(7), 1408–1425. doi:10.1111/j.1365-2648.2011.05631.x PMID:21466576

Permanent Mission of the People's Republic of China to the United Nations. (2008). *Preventing neglect and abuse in a rapidly ageing society*. Retrieved June 18, 2016, from http://www.china-un.org/eng/chinaandun/socialhr/aging_disabilities/t531015.htm

Perrels, A. J., Fleming, J., Zhao, J., Barclay, S., Farquhar, M., Buiting, H. M., & Brayne, C. (2014). Place of death and end-of-life transitions experienced by very old people with differing cognitive status: Retrospective analysis of a prospective population-based cohort aged 85 and over. *Palliative Medicine*, *28*(3), 220–233. doi:10.1177/0269216313510341 PMID:24317193

Peterson, E. R. (2006). *Between Hopes and Realities: Reflections on the Promises and Practices of Corporate Social Responsibility (CSR)*. PhD School of Technologies of Managing/Copenhagen Business School.

Pew Charitable Trusts. (2014). *State health care spending on Medicaid: a 50-state study of trends and drivers of cost*. Retrieved June 12, 2016, from http://www.pewtrusts.org/en/Multimedia/Data-Visualizations/2014/Medicaid-Spending-Growth

Pew Charitable Trusts. (2015). *For first time, tax revenue has recovered in majority of states*. Retrieved June 12, 2016, from http:// www.pewtrusts.org/en/research-and-analysis/analysis/2015/12/10/for-first-time-tax-revenue-has-recovered-in-majority-of-states

Pew Charitable Trusts. (2016a). *Reserves remain short of pre-recession levels in most states*. Retrieved June 12, 2016, from http://www.pewtrusts.org/en/research-and-analysis/analysis/2016/01/05/reserves-remain-short-of-pre-recession-levels-in-most-states

Pew Charitable Trusts. (2016b). *Is Medicaid expansion near a tipping point?* Retrieved June 12, 2016, from http://www.pewtrusts.org/en/research-and-analysis/blogs/stateline/2016/01/26/is-medicaid-expansion-near-a-tipping-point

Pew Charitable Trusts. (2016c). *Revenue is up in most states; but weak forecasts prompt caution*. Retrieved June 12, 2016, from http://www.pewtrusts.org/en/research-and-analysis/blogs/stateline/2016/01/27/revenue-is-up-in-most-states-but-weak-forecasts-prompt-caution

Pew Charitable Trusts. (2016d). *Fiscal 50*. Retrieved June 12, 2016, from http:// www.pewtrusts.org/en/multimedia/data-visualizations/2014/fiscal-50

Pfeffer, M. A., Braunwald, E., Moyé, L. A., Basta, L., Brown, E. J. Jr, Cuddy, T. E., & Hawkins, C. M. et al. (1992). Effect of captopril on mortality and morbidity in patients with left ventricular dysfunction after myocardial infarction: Results of the Survival and Ventricular Enlargement Trial. *The New England Journal of Medicine, 327*(10), 669–677. doi:10.1056/NEJM199209033271001 PMID:1386652

Pierson, P., & Skocpol, T. (2002). Historical institutionalism in contemporary political science. In I. Katznelson, & H. V. Milner (Eds.), Political science: The state of the discipline (pp.693-721). New York: American Political Science Association.

Pierson, P. (2000a). Not just what, but when: Timing and sequence in political processes. *Studies in American Political Development, 14*(1), 72–92. doi:10.1017/S0898588X00003011

Pierson, P. (2000b). Increasing returns, path dependence, and the study of politics. *The American Political Science Review, 94*(2), 251–267. doi:10.2307/2586011

Pinquart, M., & Sörensen, S. (2003). Differences between caregivers and noncaregivers in psychological health and physical health: A meta-analysis. *Psychology and Aging, 18*(2), 250–267. doi:10.1037/0882-7974.18.2.250 PMID:12825775

Plaice, C., & Kitch, P. (2003). Embedding knowledge management in the NHS south-west: Pragmatic first steps for a practical concept. *Health Information and Libraries Journal, 20*(2), 75–85. doi:10.1046/j.1471-1842.2003.00417.x PMID:12786906

Plouffe, L., & Kalache, A. (2010). Towards global age-friendly cities: Determining urban features that promote active aging. *Journal of Urban Health, 87*(5), 733–739. doi:10.1007/s11524-010-9466-0 PMID:20549569

Po Leung Kok. (2011). *Our Services.* Retrieved May 20, 2016 from http://www.poleungkuk.org.hk/en/201408153461/social-services-department/Service.html

Pollock, K. (2015). Is home always the best and preferred place of death? *BMJ (Clinical Research Ed.), 351*(October), h4855. PMID:26446163

Poon, P. K.-k., So, A., & Loong, E. L.-c. (2014). Self-management in community-based rehabilitation programmes for persons with chronic disease. In K.-w. Tong & K. N.-k. Fong (Eds.), *Community care in Hong Kong: Current practice, practice research studies, and future directions* (pp. 53–73). Hong Kong: City University of Hong Kong Press.

Popejoy, L. L., Stetzer, F., Hicks, L., Rantz, M. J., Galambos, C., Popescu, M., & Marek, K. D. (2015). Comparing Aging in Place to Home Health Care: Impact of Nurse Care Coordination on Utilization and Costs. *Nursing Economics, 33*(6), 306–313. PMID:26845818

Pourhamidi, M. (2013). Prioritisation of knowledge management strategies in the learning organisation: An integrated Shannons entropy-TOPSIS methodology. *International Journal of Learning and Intellectual Capital, 10*(3-4), 213–227. doi:10.1504/IJLIC.2013.057431

Prabhakaran, B., Dowling, E. A., Branch, J. D., Swain, D. P., & Leutholtz, B. C. (1999). Effect of 14 weeks of resistance training on lipid profile and body fat percentage in premenopausal women. *British Journal of Sports Medicine, 33*(3), 190–195. doi:10.1136/bjsm.33.3.190 PMID:10378072

Pratt, J. R. (2010). *Long-term Care: Managing Across the Continuum* (3rd ed.). Sudbury, MA: Jones & Barlett Publishers.

Primary Care Office, Hong Kong. (2016). *Primary care initiatives.* Retrieved 8 August 2016, from http://www.pco.gov.hk/english/initiatives/projects.html

Prince, M., Wimo, A., Guerchet, M., Ali, G. C., Wu, Y. T., & Prina, M. (2015). World Alzheimer's Report. The Global Impact of Dementia: An Analysis of Prevalence, Incidence, Cost and Trends. London: Alzheimer's Disease International (ADI).

PRISMA. (2016). *Overview*. Retrieved from http://www.prisma-qc.ca/cgi-cs/cs.waframe.content?topic=5796&lang=2

Public Law 101-336. (1990). *Americans with Disability Act of 1990.*

Public Law 105-33. (1997). *The Children's Health Insurance Program.*

Public Law 109-171. (2005). *Deficit Reduction Act of 2005.*

Public Law 111–148. (2010). *Patient Protection and Affordable Care Act.*

Public Law 111-5. (2009). *American Recovery and Reinvestment Act of 2009.*

Public Law 74-271. (1935). *Social Security Act of 1935.*

Public Law 89-97. (1965). *Social Security Amendments of 1965.*

Pudjianto, B., Zo, H., Ciganek, A. P., & Rho, J. J. (2011). Determinants of e-government assimilation in Indonesia: An empirical investigation using a TOE framework. *Asia Pacific Journal of Information Systems*, *21*(1), 49–80.

Purdy, S. (2010). Avoiding hospital admissions: what does the research evidence say? London: The King's Fund. Retrieved from https://www.kingsfund.org.uk/sites/files/kf/Avoiding-Hospital-Admissions-Sarah-Purdy-December2010.pdf

Qiu, Y. (2015). The impact of aging population on health care expenditures in China, Chinese version. *Journal of Nanjing College for Population Programme Management*, *31*(2), 95–102.

Quadagno, J. (2014). *Aging and The Life Course: An Introduction to Social Gerontology* (6th ed.). New York: McGraw-Hill.

Racherla, P., & Hu, C. (2008). eCRM system adoption by hospitality organizations: A technology-organization-environment (TOE) framework. *Journal of Hospitality & Leisure Marketing*, *17*(1-2), 30–58. doi:10.1080/10507050801978372

Rajani, F. (2015). Theory of Gerotranscendence: An Analysis. *European Psychiatry*, *30*, 1467. doi:10.1016/S0924-9338(15)31138-X

Raman, A. V., & Björkman, J. W. (2009). *Public/Private partnership in healthcare services in India.* Research study funded by the Indo-Dutch Programme on Alternatives in Development (project 5.3.96). Retrieved 27 May 2016, http://www.pppinharyana.gov.in/ppp/sector/health/report-healthcare.pdf

Rasmussen, M., Krølner, R., Klepp, K. I., Lytle, L., Brug, J., Bere, E., & Due, P. (2006). Determinants of fruit and vegetable consumption among children and adolescents: a review of the literature. Part I: quantitative studies. *The International Journal of Behavioral Nutrition and Physical Activity*, *3*(1), 22. doi:10.1186/1479-5868-3-22 PMID:16904006

Ravera, A., Carubelli, V., Sciatti, E., Bonadei, I., Gorga, E., Cani, D., & Lombardi, C. et al. (2016). Nutrition and cardiovascular disease: Finding the perfect recipe for cardiovascular health. *Nutrients*, *8*(6), 363. doi:10.3390/nu8060363 PMID:27314382

Reich, M. R., Harris, J., Ikegami, N., Maeda, A., Cashin, C., Araujo, E. C., & Evans, T. G. et al. (2016). Moving towards universal health coverage: Lessons from 11 country studies. *Lancet*, *387*(10020), 811–816. doi:10.1016/S0140-6736(15)60002-2 PMID:26299185

Reker, G. T., & Chamberlain, K. (Eds.). (2000). *Exploring existential meaning: Optimizing human development across the life span*. Thousand Oaks, CA: Sage.

Resnick, H. E., & Alwan, M. (2010). Use of health information technology in home health and hospice agencies: United States, 2007. *Journal of the American Medical Informatics Association*, *17*(4), 389–395. doi:10.1136/jamia.2010.005504 PMID:20595305

Ricci-Cabello, I., Ruiz-Perez, I., Rojas-Garcia, A., Pastor, G., Rodriguez-Barranco, M., & Goncalves, D. (2014). *Characteristics and effectiveness of diabetes self-management educational programmes targeted to racial / ethnic minority groups.* Retrieved from: http://www.biomedcentral.com/content/pdf/1472-6823-14-60.pdf

Riley, M. W. (1973). Aging and cohort succession: Interpretations and misinterpretations. *Public Opinion Quarterly*, *37*(1), 35–49. doi:10.1086/268058

Riley, M. W. (1974). The perspective of age stratification. *The School Review*, *83*(1), 85–91. doi:10.1086/443174

Riley, M. W. (1994). Aging and society: Past, present, and future. *The Gerontologist*, *34*(4), 436–446. doi:10.1093/geront/34.4.436 PMID:7959099

Ripley, R., & Franklin, G. (1980). *Congress, the bureaucracy, and public policy*. Homewood, IL: The Dorsey Press.

Robert, L., & Fulop, T. (Eds.). (2014). *Aging: Facts and theories*. Basel, Switzerland: Karger. doi:10.1159/isbn.978-3-318-02653-5

Rockefeller Institute of Government. (2016). *State revenue report no. 102. softening third-quarter growth in state taxes, weak forecasts for fiscal 2016 and 2017*. Retrieved July 1, 2016, from http://www.rockinst.org

Rolden, H. J. A., van Bodegom, D., & Westendorp, R. G. J. (2014). RGJ. Variation in the costs of dying and the role of different health services, socio-demographic characteristics, and preceding health care expenses. *Social Science & Medicine*, *120*, 110–117. doi:10.1016/j.socscimed.2014.09.020 PMID:25238558

Röling, N. G., & Engel, P. G. (1990). Information technology from a knowledge system perspective: Concepts and issues. *Knowledge, Technology & Policy*, *3*(3), 6–18.

Roski, J., Bo-Linn, G. W., & Andrews, T. A. (2014). Creating value in health care through big data: Opportunities and policy implications. *Health Affairs*, *33*(7), 1115–1122. doi:10.1377/hlthaff.2014.0147 PMID:25006136

Rosli, K., Yeow, P. H., & Siew, E. G. (2012). Factors influencing audit technology acceptance by audit firms: A new I-TOE adoption framework. *Journal of Accounting and Auditing*, *2012*, 1–11.

Rowe, J. W., & Kahn, R. L. (1998). *Successful aging*. New York: Pantheon Book.

Rowles, G. D. (1993). Evolving images of place in aging and 'Aging in Place'. *Generations (San Francisco, Calif.)*, *17*(2), 65–70.

Royal College of Nursing of the UK. (2014). *Moving care to the community: An international perspective* (Policy briefing 12/13 March 2013 (updated December 2014)). RCN Policy and International Department, Royal College of Nursing. Retrieved March 20, 2017 from https://www2.rcn.org.uk/__data/assets/pdf_file/0006/523068/12.13_Moving_care_to_the_community_an_international_perspective.pdf

Rudner, J., McDougall, C., Sailam, V., Smith, M., & Sacchetti, A. (2016). Interrogation of Patient Smartphone Activity Tracker to Assist Arrhythmia Management. *Annals of Emergency Medicine*, *68*(3), 292–294. doi:10.1016/j.annemergmed.2016.02.039 PMID:27045694

Ruggeri, K., Maguire, Á., Andrews, J. L., Martin, E., & Menon, S. (2016). Are We There Yet? Exploring the Impact of Translating Cognitive Tests for Dementia Using Mobile Technology in an Aging Population. *Frontiers in Aging Neuroscience*, *8*, 21. doi:10.3389/fnagi.2016.00021 PMID:27014053

Rupp, D. E., Shao, R., Thornton, M. A., & Skarlicki, D. P. (2013). Applicants and Employees Reactions to Corporate Social Responsibility: The Moderating Effect of First-party Justice Perceptions and Moral Identity. *Personnel Psychology, 66*(4), 895–933. doi:10.1111/peps.12030

Saleh, N. (2010). The value of virtual patients in medical education. *Annals of Behavioral Science and Medical Education, 16*(2), 29–31. doi:10.1007/BF03355129

Samuelson, P. A. (1976). *Economics.* Tokyo: McGraw Hill.

Sandars, J. (2009). Twelve tips for using podcasts in medical education. *Medical Teacher, 31*(5), 387–389. doi:10.1080/01421590802227958 PMID:19140038

Sau Po Center on Ageing, & Department of Social Work & Social Administration, the University of Hong Kong. (2011). *Consultancy study on community care services for the elderly: Final report.* Hong Kong: Authors. Retrieved March 20, 2017 from http://www.elderlycommission.gov.hk/en/download/library/Community%20Care%20Services%20Report%20 2011_eng.pdf

Sau Po Center on Aging and Department of Social Work & Social Administration, The University of Hong Kong. (2011). *Consultancy Study on Community Care Services for the Elderly: Final Report* (Elderly Commission report). Retrieved February 1, 2017, from http://www.elderlycommission.gov.hk/en/download/library/Community%20Care%20 Services%20Report%202011_eng.pdf

Saurugger, S. (2014). *Theoretical approaches to European integration.* Basingstoke, UK: Palgrave Macmillan.

Savedoff, W. D., & Smith, A. L. (2011). *Achieving universal health coverage: learning from Chile, Japan, Malaysia and Sweden.* Retrieved June 5, 2016, from http://www.resultsfordevelopment.org/knowledge-center/achieving-universal-health-coverage-learning-chile-japan-malaysia-and-sweden

Savings Working Group Final Report to the Minister of Finance. (2011). *Saving New Zealand: Reducing Vulnerabilities and Barriers to Growth and Prosperity.* Retrieved from http://purl.oclc.org/nzt/r-1348

Scandinavian Simvastatin Survival Study Group. (1994). Randomised trial of cholesterol lowering in 4444 patients with coronary heart disease: The Scandinavian Simvastatin Survival Study (4S). *Lancet, 344*(8934), 1383–1389. PMID:7968073

Schaller, S., Mauskopf, J., Kriza, C., Wahlster, P., & Kolominsky-Rabas, P. L. (2015). The main cost drivers in dementia: A systematic review. *International Journal of Geriatric Psychiatry, 30*(2), 111–129. doi:10.1002/gps.4198 PMID:25320002

Schlenker, R. E. (1986). Case mix reimbursement for nursing homes. *Journal of Health Politics, Policy and Law, 11*(3), 445–461. doi:10.1215/03616878-11-3-445 PMID:3098827

Schmeida, M. (2005). *Telehealth innovation in the American states.* Ann Arbor, MI: ProQuest.

Schmeida, M., & McNeal, R. (2015). Online health information: home caregiver population driving cyberspace searches in the United States. In M. Khosrow-Pour (Ed.), *Public affairs and administration: concepts, methodologies, tools, and applications* (pp. 1664–1683). Hershey, PA: Information Science Reference. doi:10.4018/978-1-4666-8358-7.ch085

Schofield, J. (2014, 3 July). What tech can I use to keep an eye on an ageing parent? *The Guardian.*

Schou-Andersen, M., Ullersted, M. P., Jensen, A. B., & Neergaard, M. A. (2015). Factors associated with preference for dying at home among terminally ill patients with cancer. *Scandinavian Journal of Caring Sciences, 2015*(Sept), 22. PMID:26395354

Schreiber, B. E., Fukuta, J., & Gordon, F. (2010). Live lecture versus video podcast in undergraduate medical education: A randomised controlled trial. *BMC Medical Education, 10*(1), 1. doi:10.1186/1472-6920-10-68 PMID:20932302

Scottish Government. (2015). *Long-term monitoring of health inequalities*. Retrieved from http://www.gov.scot/Publications/2015/10/6061

Scott, S. (2011). A tripartite learning partnership in health promotion. *Nursing Praxis in New Zealand Inc*, *27*(2), 16–23. PMID:21957557

Scott, S. D., Albrecht, L., OLeary, K., Ball, G. D., Hartling, L., Hofmeyer, A., & Thompson, D. (2012). Systematic review of knowledge translation strategies in the allied health professions. *Implementation Science; IS*, *7*(1), 1–17. doi:10.1186/1748-5908-7-70 PMID:22831550

Scott, T., Mannion, R., Davies, H., & Marshall, M. (2003). The quantitative measurement of organizational culture in health care: A review of the available instruments. *Health Services Research*, *38*(3), 923–945. doi:10.1111/1475-6773.00154 PMID:12822919

Senior Citizen Home Safety Association. (2015). *Volunteer Service*. Retrieved July 16, 2016 from https://www.schsa.org.hk/en/support_schsa/community_volunteer/volunteer/index.html

Sergeant, J. F., Ekerdt, D. J., & Chapin, R. (2008). Measurement of late-life residential relocation: Why are rates for such a manifest event so varied? *The Journals of Gerontology. Series B, Psychological Sciences and Social Sciences*, *63*(2), S92–S98. doi:10.1093/geronb/63.2.S92 PMID:18441274

Seto, S., Lam, T., Tam, H., Au, A., Chan, S., Wu, J., & Kwan, Y. W. et al. (2009). Novel hypoglycemic effects of Ganoderma lucidum water-extract in obese/diabetic (+ db/+ db) mice. *Phytomedicine*, *16*(5), 426–436. doi:10.1016/j.phymed.2008.10.004 PMID:19109000

Shah, A. B., Morrissey, R. P., Baraghoush, A., Bharadwaj, P., Phan, A., & Hamilton, M. et al.. (2012). Failing the failing heart: A review of palliative care in heart failure. *Reviews in Cardiovascular Medicine*, *14*(1), 41–48. PMID:23651985

Sharkey, P. (2007). *The essentials of community care* (2nd ed.). New York, NY: Palgrave.

Sharma, A. (2016). Attitudes of medical students toward use of clickers for assessment in classrooms: A cross-sectional study. *International Journal (Toronto, Ont.)*, *2*(1), 60.

Sharma, M. (2007). Evaluation in community based rehabilitation programmes: A strengths, weaknesses, opportunities and threats analysis. *Asia Pacific Disability Rehabilitation Journal*, *18*(1), 46–62.

Sharp, D. (2003). Knowledge management today: Challenges and opportunities. *Information Systems Management*, *20*(2), 32–37. doi:10.1201/1078/43204.20.2.20030301/41468.6

Shea, C. M., Jacobs, S. R., Esserman, D. A., Bruce, K., & Weiner, B. J. (2014). Organizational readiness for implementing change: A psychometric assessment of a new measure. *Implementation Science; IS*, *9*(1), 1. doi:10.1186/1748-5908-9-7 PMID:24410955

Shen, C., Zhao, X., & Zou, H. (2014). Fiscal decentralization and public services provision in China. *Annals of Economics and Finance*, *15*(1), 135–160.

Sheng, M. L., Chang, S. Y., Teo, T., & Lin, Y. F. (2013). Knowledge barriers, knowledge transfer, and innovation competitive advantage in healthcare settings. *Management Decision*, *51*(3), 461–478. doi:10.1108/00251741311309607

Shennib, A. (2014). *Programmable ECG sensor patch*. Google Patents.

Shenzhen News. (2013, October 18). *Shenzhen will implement new medical insurance measure starting on January 1 next year; Local Supplementary Medical Insurance Scheme will cover migrant workers*, Chinese version. Retrieved July 16, 2016, from http://www.sznews.com/news/content/2013-10/18/content_8641375.htm

Shepherd, J. (2002). Resource management in prevention of coronary heart disease: Optimising prescription of lipid-lowering drugs. *Lancet*, *359*(9325), 2271–2273. doi:10.1016/S0140-6736(02)09299-1 PMID:12103306

Sheppard, L., & Ko, K. F. (2009). A new stroke unit: Implementation issues. *The Hong Kong Physiotherapy Journal*, *27*(1), 7–10. doi:10.1016/S1013-7025(10)70003-8

Shrivastava, S., Shrivastava, P., & Ramasamy, J. (2015). Exploring the scope of community-based rehabilitation in ensuring the holistic development of differently-abled people. *African Health Sciences*, *15*(1), 278–280. doi:10.4314/ahs.v15i1.36 PMID:25834559

Sica, D. A. (1999). Old antihypertensive agents-diuretics and β-Blockers: Do we know how and in whom they lower blood pressure? *Current Hypertension Reports*, *1*(4), 296–304. doi:10.1007/s11906-999-0037-2 PMID:10981081

Sim, J., Liddle, J., Bernard, M., Scharf, T., & Bartlam, B. (2012). Home from home? A mixed-methods study of relocation within a purpose built retirement community. *Journal of Housing for the Elderly*, *26*(4), 372–394. doi:10.1080/02763893.2012.724375

Singapore Government. (2016). *Pioneer generation package: Know the benefits*. Retrieved 20 May 2016, from https://www.ecitizen.gov.sg/Topics/Pages/Pioneer-Generation-Package-Know-the-benefits.aspx

Singh, D. A. (2016). *Effective Management of Long-term Care Facilities* (3rd ed.). Burlington, MA: Jones & Bartlett Learning.

Smith, R., Gaser, L., Harrison, L., Martin, L., Means, R., & Thistlethwaite, P. (1993). *Working together for better community care*. Bristol, UK: School for Advanced Urban Studies.

Social and Welfare Department. (2013). *Legislative Council Paper CB(2)673/12-13(01) Long-term Care Policy for the Elderly and Persons with Disabilities*. Paper presented to the Joint Subcommittee on Long Term Care Policy.

Social and Welfare Department. (2017). *Overview of Residential Care Services for Elders*. Retrieved February 1, 2017, from http://www.swd.gov.hk/en/index/site_pubsvc/page_elderly/sub_residentia/id_overviewon/

Social Welfare Department of Hong Kong. (2012). *List of self-financing day care centres for the dementia elderly* (June 2012). Retrieved March 20, 2017 from http://www.swd.gov.hk/doc/elderly/List%20of%20Self-financing%20Day%20Care%20Centre%20for%20the%20Dementia%20Elderly_Jun%202012(1).pdf

Social Welfare Department of Hong Kong. (2016a). *Enhanced home and community care services*. Retrieved March 20, 2017 from http://www.swd.gov.hk/en/index/site_pubsvc/page_elderly/sub_csselderly/id_enhancedho/

Social Welfare Department of Hong Kong. (2016b). *Integrated home care services*. Retrieved March 20, 2017 from http://www.swd.gov.hk/en/index/site_pubsvc/page_elderly/sub_csselderly/id_618/

Social Welfare Department of Hong Kong. (2016c). *Pilot scheme on living allowance for low-income carers of persons with disabilities*. Retrieved March 20, 2017 from http://www.swd.gov.hk/en/index/site_pubsvc/page_supportser/sub_PWD/

Social Welfare Department of Hong Kong. (2016d). *Waiting list for subsidised residential care services for the elderly*. Retrieved March 20, 2017 from http://www.swd.gov.hk/doc/elderly/ercs2/LTC%20statistics%20HP-Eng(201607).pdf

Social Welfare Department of Hong Kong. (2017). *Standardised care need assessment mechanism for elderly services*. Retrieved March 20, 2017 from http://www.swd.gov.hk/en/index/site_pubsvc/page_elderly/sub_standardis/

Social Welfare Department of Hong Kong. (n.d.). *Community rehabilitation day centre*. Retrieved March 20, 2017 from http://www.swd.gov.hk/doc/rehab/Service%20brief_CRDC_Eng.pdf

Social Welfare Department, Hong Kong: Hong Kong Special Administrative Region Government. (2016a). *Services for the Elderly.* Retrieved August 23, 2016, from http://www.swd.gov.hk/en/index/site_pubsvc/page_elderly/

Social Welfare Department, Hong Kong: Hong Kong Special Administrative Region Government. (2016b). *Service Quality Standards (SQSs) and Criteria.* Retrieved March 10, 2017, from http://www.swd.gov.hk/doc/ngo/_SQSs%20 and%20Criteria%20(Dec%2001)(Eng).pdf

Social Welfare Department. (2005). *Care and Attention Homes for the Elderly. Residential Care Services for the Elderly.* Retrieved 25 Feb 2017, from http://www.swd.gov.hk/en/index/site_pubsvc/page_elderly/sub_residentia/id_careandatt/

Social Welfare Department. (2005). *Central Office for Volunteer Service.* Retrieved May 14, 2016 from http://www.swd.gov.hk/en/index/site_pubsvc/page_supportser/sub_centraloff/

Social Welfare Department. (2013). *Legislative Council Paper CB(2)673/12-13(01) Long-term Care Policy for the Elderly and Persons with Disabilities.* Paper presented to the Joint Subcommittee on Long Term Care Policy.

Social Welfare Department. (2016). *Overview on residential care services for elders.* Retrieved 6 August 2016, from http://www.swd.gov.hk/en/index/site_pubsvc/page_elderly/sub_residentia/id_overviewon/

Social Welfare Department. (2016). *Services for Prevention and Handling of Elder Abuse.* Retrieved February 20, 2017 from http://www.swd.gov.hk/en/index/site_pubsvc/page_family/sub_listofserv/id_serabuseelder/

Society for the Promotion of Hospice Care. (2011). *Opinion on End-of-life Care and Advance Care (Chinese version).* Retrieved March 1, 2017 from http://www2.hospicecare.org.hk/wp-content/uploads/2011/10/20111003acpsurvey-whd11.pdf

Soderberg, M., Stahl, A., & Emilsson, U. M. (2012). Independence as a stigmatizing value for older people considering relocation to a residential home. *European Journal of Social Work*, *16*(3), 1–16.

Solana, J., Cáceres, C., García-Molina, A., Chausa, P., Opisso, E., Roig-Rovira, T., & Gómez, E. J. et al. (2014). Intelligent Therapy Assistant (ITA) for cognitive rehabilitation in patients with acquired brain injury. *BMC Medical Informatics and Decision Making*, *14*(1), 58. doi:10.1186/1472-6947-14-58 PMID:25038823

Songyuan, Z., Shuxiang, G., Baofeng, G., Hideyuki, H., & Hidenori, I. (2015). Design of a Novel Telerehabilitation System with a Force-Sensing Mechanism. *Sensors*, *15*(5), 11511-11527. doi:10.3390/s150511511

Sørensen, K., & Brand, H. (2011). Health Literacy - A Strategic Asset for Corporate Social Responsibility in Europe. *Journal of Health Communication*, *16*(supp. 3), 322–327. doi:10.1080/10810730.2011.606072 PMID:21951261

South China Morning Post. (2014). *Hong Kong faces challenge ensuring the elderly feel right at home.* Retrieved 10 August 2016, from http://www.scmp.com/news/hong-kong/article/1433787/hong-kong-faces-challenge-ensuring-elderly-feel-right-home

South China Morning Post. (2014). *Hong Kong faces challenge ensuring the elderly feel right at home.* Retrieved from http://www.scmp.com/news/hong-kong/article/1433787/hong-kong-faces-challenge-ensuring-elderly-feel-right-home

Spalding, K. L., Williams, A. P., & Watkins, J. R. (2006). *Self managed care programs in Canada: A report to Health Canada.* Retrieved from http://healthycanadians.gc.ca/publications/health-system-systeme-sante/2006-self-managed-soins-autogeres/index-eng.php#a1

Spector, W. D., & Fleishman, J. A. (2001). *The Characteristics of Long-Term Care Users.* U.S. Department of Health and Human Services, Agency for Healthcare Research and Quality Research Report.

Speklé, R. F., & Verbeeten, F. H. M. (2014). The use of performance measurement systems in the public sector: Effects on performance. *Management Accounting Research*, *25*(2), 131–146. doi:10.1016/j.mar.2013.07.004

Špinar, J. (2012). Hypertension and ischemic heart disease. *Cor et Vasa, 54*(6), e433-e438.

Spring, B., Moller, A. C., Colangelo, L. A., Siddique, J., Roehrig, M., Daviglus, M. L., & Liu, K. et al. (2014). Healthy lifestyle change and subclinical atherosclerosis in young adults: Coronary Artery Risk Development in Young Adults (CARDIA) Study. *Circulation, 130*(1), 10–17. doi:10.1161/CIRCULATIONAHA.113.005445 PMID:24982115

Squire, P. (1992). Legislative professionalism and membership diversity in state legislatures. *Legislative Studies Quarterly, 17*(1), 69–79. doi:10.2307/440081

St. John, P. D., Tyas, S. L., & Montgomery, P. R. (2013). Depressive symptoms and frailty. *International Journal of Geriatric Psychiatry, 28*(6), 607–614. doi:10.1002/gps.3866 PMID:22961757

Steinmo, S. (2008). Historical institutionalism. In D. D. Porta & M. Keating (Eds.), *Approaches and methodologies in the social sciences: a pluralist perspective* (pp. 118–138). Cambridge, UK: Cambridge University Press. doi:10.1017/CBO9780511801938.008

Stephenson, A. K. (2009). The pursuit of CSR and business ethics policies: Is it a source of competitive advantage for organizations? *Journal of American Academy of Business, 14*(2), 251–262.

Stern, S., Behar, S., & Gottlieb, S. (2003). Aging and diseases of the heart. *Circulation, 108*(14), e99–e101. doi:10.1161/01.CIR.0000086898.96021.B9 PMID:14530186

Steves, C. J., Spector, T. D., & Jackson, S. H. (2012). Ageing, genes, environment and epigenetics: What twin studies tell us now, and in the future. *Age and Ageing, 41*(5), 581–586. doi:10.1093/ageing/afs097 PMID:22826292

Stewart, M. J., Georgiou, A., & Westbrook, J. I. (2013). Successfully integrating aged care services: A review of the evidence and tools emerging from a long-term care program. *International Journal of Integrated Care, 13*(1), e003. doi:10.5334/ijic.963 PMID:23687475

Stock, S., Drabik, A., Büscher, G., Graf, C., Ullrich, W., Gerber, A., & Lüngen, M. (2010). German Diabetes Management Programs Improve Quality Of Care And Curb Costs. *Health Affairs, 29*(12), 2197–2205. doi:10.1377/hlthaff.2009.0799 PMID:21134920

Stoeckel, K. J., & Porell, F. (2010). Do older adults anticipate relocation? *Journal of Applied Gerontology, 29*(2), 231–250. doi:10.1177/0733464809335595

Strategies & Skills Learning & Development. (2014). *Background.* Retrieved from http://ssld.kttsang.com/html/introduction/background.html

Straus, S. E., Tetroe, J. M., & Graham, I. D. (2009). Defining knowledge translation. *Canadian Medical Association Journal, 181*(3-4), 165–168. doi:10.1503/cmaj.081229 PMID:19620273

Straus, S. E., Tetroe, J. M., & Graham, I. D. (2011). Knowledge translation is the use of knowledge in health care decision making. *Journal of Clinical Epidemiology, 64*(1), 6–10. doi:10.1016/j.jclinepi.2009.08.016 PMID:19926445

Strawbridge, W. J., Wallhagen, M. I., & Cohen, R. D. (2002). Successful aging and well-being: Self-rated compared with Rowe and Kahn. *The Gerontologist, 42*(6), 727–733. doi:10.1093/geront/42.6.727 PMID:12451153

Streeck, W., & Thelen, K. (2005). Introduction: institutional change in advanced political economies. In W. Streeck & K. Thelen (Eds.), *Beyond continuity: institutional change in advanced political economies* (pp. 3–39). Oxford, UK: Oxford University Press.

Struijs, J. N., & Baan, C. A. (2011). Integrating care through bundled payments—lessons from the Netherlands. *The New England Journal of Medicine, 364*(11), 990–991. doi:10.1056/NEJMp1011849 PMID:21410368

Stuck, A.E., Egger, M., Hammer, A., Minder, C.E., & Beck, J.C. (2002). Home visits to prevent nursing home admission and functional decline in elderly people: systematic review and meta-regression analysis. *JAMA, 287*(8), 1022–8.

Subcommittee of Palliative Medicine, Hong Kong College of Physicians. (2008). *Palliative Care: Setting the scene for the future. A position paper of Hong Kong College of Physicians*. Retrieved July 1, 2016 from http://www.hkcp.org/docs/News/Position%20paper%20in%20Palliative%20Medicine.pdf

Sullivan-Marx, E. M., & Gray-Miceli, D. (Eds.). (2008). *Leadership and Management Skills for Long-term Care*. New York: Springer Publishing.

Sultan, N. (2014). Making use of cloud computing for healthcare provision: Opportunities and challenges. *International Journal of Information Management, 34*(2), 177–184. doi:10.1016/j.ijinfomgt.2013.12.011

Sun, J., Guo, Y., Wang, X., & Zeng, Q. (2016). mHealth For Aging China: Opportunities and Challenges. *Aging and Disease, 7*(1), 53. doi:10.14336/AD.2015.1011 PMID:26816664

Sun, Q., Liu, X., Meng, Q., Tang, S., Yu, B., & Tolhurst, R. (2009). Evaluating the financial protection of patients with chronic disease by health insurance in rural China. *International Journal for Equity in Health, 8*(1), 42. doi:10.1186/1475-9276-8-42 PMID:20003188

Surve, M. B. A., & Natarajan, G. (2015). Knowledge Management Tools: Recognition for The Support To Healthcare Practitioners. *International Journal of Advanced Information and Communication Technology, 1*(12), 923–927.

Susic, D., & Frohlich, E. D. (2008). The aging hypertensive heart: A brief update. *Nature Clinical Practice. Cardiovascular Medicine, 5*(2), 104–110. doi:10.1038/ncpcardio1091 PMID:18223542

Su, T. T., Kouyaté, B., & Flessa, S. (2006). Catastrophic household expenditure for health care in low–income society: A study from Nouna District, Burkina Faso. *Bulletin of the World Health Organization, 84*(1), 21–27. doi:10.2471/BLT.05.023739 PMID:16501711

Szulanski, G., Ringov, D., & Jensen, R. J. (2016). Overcoming Stickiness: How the Timing of Knowledge Transfer Methods Affects Transfer Difficulty. *Organization Science, 27*(2), 304–322. doi:10.1287/orsc.2016.1049

Tadevosyan, A., MacLaughlin, E. J., & Karamyan, V. T. (2011). Angiotensin II type 1 receptor antagonists in the treatment of hypertension in elderly patients: focus on patient outcomes. *Patient Related Outcome Measures, 2*, 27.

Tang, F., & Pickard, J. G. (2008). Aging in place or relocation: Perceived awareness of community-based long-term care and services. *Journal of Housing for the Elderly, 22*(4), 404–422. doi:10.1080/02763890802458429

Tang, S. T. (2000). Meanings of dying at home for Chinese patients in Taiwan with terminal cancer: A literature review. *Cancer Nursing, 23*(5), 367–370. doi:10.1097/00002820-200010000-00007 PMID:11037957

Tang, S., Ehiri, J., & Long, Q. (2013). Chinas biggest, most neglected health challenge: Non-communicable diseases. *Infectious Diseases of Poverty, 2*(1), 7. doi:10.1186/2049-9957-2-7 PMID:23849054

Task Force on Conceptual Model and Preventive Protocols, Working Group on Primary Care, & Food and Health Bureau of Hong Kong. (2012a). *Hong Kong reference framework for preventive care for children in primary care settings 2012*. Retrieved March 20, 2017 from http://www.pco.gov.hk/english/resource/files/ref_framework_children.pdf

Task Force on Conceptual Model and Preventive Protocols, Working Group on Primary Care, & Food and Health Bureau of Hong Kong. (2012b). *Hong Kong reference framework for preventive care for older adults in primary care settings 2012*. Retrieved March 20, 2017 from http://www.pco.gov.hk/english/resource/files/ref_framework_adults.pdf

Taylor, E. J., Ensor, B., & Stanley, J. (2012). Place of death related to demographic factors for hospice patients in Wellington, Aotearoa New Zealand. *Palliative Medicine*, *26*(4), 342–349. doi:10.1177/0269216311412229 PMID:21697264

Taylor, G., & Hawley, H. (2010). *Health and society: Key debates in health care*. New York, NY: Open University Press.

Taylor, S. A. P. (2001). Place identification and positive realities of aging. *Journal of Cross-Cultural Gerontology*, *16*(1), 5–20. doi:10.1023/A:1010673000367 PMID:14617990

Team, V., Canaway, R., & Manderson, L. (2011). Integration of complementary and alternative medicine information and advice in chronic disease management guidelines. *Australian Journal of Primary Health*, *17*(2), 142–149. doi:10.1071/PY10013 PMID:21645469

Tennant, B., Stellefson, M., Dodd, V., Chaney, B., Chaney, D., Paige, S., & Alber, J. (2015). eHealth literacy and Web 2.0 health information seeking behaviors among baby boomers and older adults. *Journal of Medical Internet Research*, *17*(3), e70. doi:10.2196/jmir.3992 PMID:25783036

Teo, K. K., Yusuf, S., & Furberg, C. D. (1993). Effects of prophylactic antiarrhythmic drug therapy in acute myocardial infarction: An overview of results from randomized controlled trials. *Journal of the American Medical Association*, *270*(13), 1589–1595. doi:10.1001/jama.1993.03510130095038 PMID:8371471

The ARC Centre of Excellence in Population Ageing Research (CEPAR). (2014). *Aged care in Australia: Part I - policy, demand and funding*. Australian Research Council.

The China Health Care Study Group. (1974). *Health Care in China, an introduction: The report of a study group in Hong Kong*. Geneva: Christian Medical Commission.

The Community Care Fund. (2016). *Assistance programmes under the fund*. Retrieved March 20, 2017 from https://www.communitycarefund.hk/en/assistance.asp

The Conference Board of Canada. (2012). *Home and community care in Canada: An economic footprint*. Ottawa, Canada: Author. Retrieved March 20, 2017 from http://carewatchtoronto.org/wp-content/uploads/2012/05/12-306_HomeandCommunityCare_PRT.pdf

The Convention on the Rights of Persons with Disabilities (2006).

The Declaration of Alma-Ata (1978).

The Exchange and Clearing Limited. (2015). *Corporate Social Responsibility Report*. Retrieved September 14, 2016 from http://www.hkexgroup.com/-/media/HKEX-Group-Site/ssd/Investor-Relations/Regulatory-Reports/documents/2016/e160321csr.pdf

The Food and Health Bureau. (2008). The need for Change. *Your Health Your Life*. Retrieved from http://www.fhb.gov.hk/beStrong/files/consultation/chapter1_eng.pdf

The Food and Health Bureau. (2010). Healthcare Reform- Progress to Date. *My Health My Choice*. Retrieved 11 August 2016, from http://www.myhealthmychoice.gov.hk/pdf/chapter2_eng.pdf

The Food and Health Bureau. (2016). Promote Public Private Partnership in Healthcare. *Your Health, Your Life*. Retrieved 22 March 2016, from http://www.fhb.gov.hk/beStrong/files/consultation/chapter3_eng.pdf

The Government of Hong Kong. (2017). *2017 Policy Address*. Retrieved 1 March 2017, from http://www.policyaddress.gov.hk/2017/eng/p195.html

The Government of United Kingdom. (2013). *Healthcare: Public Private Partnerships. Promotional material*. Retrieved 3 July 2016, from https://www.gov.uk/government/publications/public-private-partnerships/public-private-partnerships

The Hong Kong Census and Statistics Department. (2009b). *Thematic household survey* report - Report No. 40. Retrieved 12 July, 2016, from http://www.censtatd.gov.hk/products_and_services/products/publications/statis tical_report/social_data/index_cd_B1130240_dt_latest.jsp

The Hong Kong Council of Social Service. (2017). *Social indicators of Hong Kong*. Retrieved March 20, 2017 from http://www.socialindicators.org.hk/en/indicators/elderly/31.12

The Hong Kong Council of Social Service. (n.d.). *Organization structure*. Retrieved July 14, 2016 from http://www.hkcss.org.hk/e/fc_detail1.asp?fc_id=25

The Hong Kong Jockey Club. (n.d.). *Staff Volunteer Activities*. Retrieved September 14, 2016 from http://charities.hkjc.com/charities/english/connect-and-join/staff-volunteer-activities.aspx

The Hong Kong Polytechnic University. (2008). *Robotic hand responds to intention signals*. Retrieved 20 July 2016, from https://www.polyu.edu.hk/ife/corp/upload/docs/8_publication/KT_Eng_2012/pdf/06_4.pdf

The Hong Kong Social Welfare Department. (2001). *Legislative Council Panel On Welfare Services - Allocation of New Social Welfare Service Units, Provision of Residential Care Home Services for the Elders through Open Tender*. Hong Kong: Social Welfare Department.

The Hong Kong Social Welfare Department. (2016). *Provision of Residential Care Services for Elders (Subsidised versus Non-subsidised Places)*. Hong Kong: Social Welfare Department.

The Hospital Authority Ordinance (Cap 113) of Hong Kong.

The International Labour Organization, the United Nations Educational, Scientific and Cultural Organization, & the World Health Organization. (2004). *CBR: A strategy for rehabilitation, equalization of opportunities, poverty reduction and social inclusion of people with disabilities*. Joint position paper 2004. Geneva, Switzerland: World Health Organization. Retrieved March 20, 2017 from http://apps.who.int/iris/bitstream/10665/43060/1/9241592389_eng.pdf

The Macau SAR Government. (2016). *Consultative Paper on the 5 Year Development Plans (2016-2020)*. Macau: The Macau SAR Government.

The National Committee of the Chinese People's Political Consultative Conference. (2014). *Integrating medical and nursing care for the elderly*, Chinese version. Retrieved February 26, 2017 from http://www.cppcc.gov.cn/zxww/2014/12/30/ARTI1419900481141424.shtml

The Ombudsman of Hong Kong. (2014, November 20). *Ombudsman probes government regulation of rehabilitation transport services to persons with mobility difficulties* [Press release]. Retrieved March 20, 2017 from http://ofomb.ombudsman.hk/abc/en-us/press_releases/detail/45

The Ombudsman of Hong Kong. (2017). *Executive summary: Direct investigation into government regulation of special transport services to persons with mobility difficulties*. Retrieved March 20, 2017 from http://ofomb.ombudsman.hk/abc/files/IR360_ES_E-9_3_2017.pdf

The Patient Protection and Affordable Care Act 2010 of the United States.

The Samaritan Befrienders Hong Kong. (2016). *About us*. Retrieved May 20, 2016 from http://www.sbhk.org.hk/aboutus.php?lang=en

The Social Welfare Department. (2017). *First Phase of the Pilot Scheme on Community Care Service Voucher for the Elderly (Pilot Scheme)*. Retrieved 11 Feb 2017, from http://www.swd.gov.hk/en/index/site_pubsvc/page_elderly/sub_csselderly/id_firstphase/

The State Council. (1998). *The Decision of the State Council Concerning the Establishment of the Urban Employee Basic Medical Insurance,* Chinese version. Retrieved July 8, 2016, from http://www.gov.cn/banshi/2005-08/04/content_20256.htm

The State Council. (2007). *The Guiding Opinions on Piloting Urban Resident Basic Medical Insurance,* Chinese version. Retrieved July 13, 2016, from http://www.gov.cn/zwgk/2007-07/24/content_695118.htm

The State Council. (2016). *Opinions on Integrating the Basic Medical Insurance Systems for Urban and Rural Residents,* Chinese version. Retrieved July 16, 2016, from http://www.gov.cn/zhengce/content/2016-01/12/content_10582.htm

The United Nations. (2015). *World Population Prospects: The 2015 Revision, Key Findings & Advance Table.* New York: The United Nations.

The United Nations Population Fund. (2015). *World Population Ageing in 2015.* New York: The United Nations.

The World Bank. (2010). *Fixing the public hospital system in China.* Retrieved June 26, 2016, from http://siteresources.worldbank.org/HEALTHNUTRITIONANDPOPULATION/Resources/281627-1285186535266/FixingthePublicHospitalSystem.pdf

The World Health Organization (WHO). (2000). Health Systems: Improving Performance. Geneva: The World Health Organization.

The World Health Organization (WHO). (2015). China country assessment report on ageing and health. Geneva: Department of Ageing and Life Course, The World Health Organization.

Thelen, K. (1999). Historical institutionalism in comparative politics. *Annual Review of Political Science, 2*(1), 369–404. doi:10.1146/annurev.polisci.2.1.369

Thielke, S. M., Mattek, N. C., Hayes, T. L., Dodge, H. H., Quiñones, A. R., Austin, D., . . . Kaye, J. A. (2014). Associations Between Observed In-Home Behaviors and Self-Reported Low Mood in Community-Dwelling Older Adults. *Journal of the American Geriatrics Society, 62*(4), 685-689 685. doi:10.1111/jgs.12744

Time-weekly. (2014). *The Zero-mark-up Policy for Drugs in Public Hospitals in Zhejiang,* Chinese version. Retrieved July 17, 2016, from http://money.163.com/14/0410/07/9PF0NPUI00252G50.html

Tin, K. Y. K., Song, W., Tsoi, P. K. O., Lee, Y. H., Chong, D. S. Y., Lam, D. W. S., & Maw, C. K. C. et al. (2016). Hong Kong domestic health spending: Financial years 1989/90 to 2012/13. *Hong Kong Medical Journal, 22*(Supplement 3), S2–S23. PMID:27389870

Tong, A. Y., & Man, D. W. (2002). The validation of the Hong Kong Chinese version of Lawton instrumental activities of daily living scale for institutionalized elderly persons. *The Occupational Therapy Journal of Research, 22,* 132–142.

Tong, K.-w., & Fong, K. N.-k. (2014). Introduction: Challenges in healthcare and community care in Hong Kong. In K.-w. Tong & K. N.-k. Fong (Eds.), *Community care in Hong Kong: Current practice, practice research studies, and future directions* (pp. 3–16). Hong Kong: City University of Hong Kong Press. doi:10.1142/9789814566582_0016

Topaz, M., Troutman-Jordan, M., & MacKenzie, M. (2014). Construction, deconstruction, and reconstruction: The roots of successful aging theories. *Nursing Science Quarterly, 27*(3), 226–233. doi:10.1177/0894318414534484 PMID:24951524

Torjesen, I. (2012). Go with the flow. *The Health Service Journal, 122*(6303), 2–3. PMID:22741355

Tornstam, L. (1989). Gero-transcendence; A Meta-theoretical Reformulation of the Disengagement Theory. *Aging: Clinical and Experimental Research (Milano), 1*(1), 55–63.

Tornstam, L. (1996). Gerotranscendence – a theory about maturing into old age. *Journal of Aging and Identity, 1,* 37–50.

Tornstam, L. (1997). Gerotranscendence: The contemplative dimension of aging. *Journal of Aging Studies*, *11*(2), 143–154. doi:10.1016/S0890-4065(97)90018-9

Tornstam, L. (2005). *Gerotranscendence: A developmental theory of positive aging*. New York: Springer Pub. Co.

Torres, S. (2015). Expanding the gerontological imagination on ethnicity: Conceptual and theoretical perspectives. *Ageing and Society*, *35*(5), 935–960. doi:10.1017/S0144686X14001330

Tourangeau, A., Cranley, L., Spence Laschinger, H. K., & Pachis, J. (2010). Relationships among leadership practices, work environments, staff communication and outcomes in long-term care. *Journal of Nursing Management*, *18*(8), 1060–1072. doi:10.1111/j.1365-2834.2010.01125.x PMID:21073577

Trybou, J., Spaepen, E., Vermeulen, B., Porrez, L., & Annemans, L. (2013). Hospital-acquired infections in Belgian acute-care hospitals: Financial burden of disease and potential cost savings. *Acta Clinica Belgica*, *68*(3), 199–205. doi:10.2143/ACB.3258 PMID:24156220

Tsang, A. K. T. (2014). Managing sexuality and intimacy issues among seniors: The SSLD approach. Toronto: Yee Hong Centre for Geriatric Care.

Tsang, J. C. (2014). The 2014-15 Budget. Speech by the Financial Secretary, the Hon John C Tsang moving the Second Reading of the Appropriation Bill 2014, 26 February 2014, Hong Kong.

Tsang, A. K. T. (2013). *Learning to change lives: The strategies and skills learning and development system*. Toronto, ON: University of Toronto Press.

Tsang, A. K. T., Choi, C., Liu, K. Y., Chu, M., Wong, C., & Fung, K. K. (2013). *The changing needs of Chinese seniors in the Greater Toronto area*. Toronto, ON: Yee Hong Centre for Geriatric Care.

Tsang, A. K. T., & Li, B. (in press). Building a practice system for working with immigrants and refugees: The SSLD approach. In M. C. Yan & U. Anucha (Eds.), *Working with immigrants and refugees: A handbook for social work and human services*. Toronto: Oxford University Press.

Tsiachristas, A., Dikkers, C., Boland, M. R. S., & Rutten-van Mölken, M. P. M. H. (2013). Exploring payment schemes used to promote integrated chronic care in Europe. *Health Policy (Amsterdam)*, *113*(3), 296–304. doi:10.1016/j.healthpol.2013.07.007 PMID:23937868

Tully, P. J., Hanon, O., Cosh, S., & Tzourio, C. (2016). Diuretic antihypertensive drugs and incident dementia risk: A systematic review, meta-analysis and meta-regression of prospective studies. *Journal of Hypertension*, *34*(6), 1027–1035. doi:10.1097/HJH.0000000000000868 PMID:26886565

Tynkkynen, L. K., Hakari, K., Koistinen, T., Lehto, J., & Miettinen, S. (2012). Integrating public and private home care services: The Kotitori model in Tampere, Finland. *Journal of Integrated Care*, *20*(5), 284–295. doi:10.1108/14769011211270738

UK Self-Management. (2013). *What is self-management?* Retrieved from: http://www.selfmanagementuk.org/what-is-self-management

UK Trade & Investment. (2013). *Public private partnership*. HealthcareUK. Retrieved from https://www.gov.uk/government/uploads/system/uploads/attachment_data/file/266818/07_PPP_28.11.13.pdf

Unit, E. (2015). *Private sector involvement: Management consultancy*. Retrieved 20 March 2016, from http://www.eu.gov.hk/en/our-work/management-consultancy/private-sector-involvement.html

Unit, K. M. (2016). *eKG Home Page*. Retrieved 20 July 2016, from https://www.ekg.org.hk

United Christian Nethersole Community Health Service. (2016). *Comprehensive Diabetes Mellitus Management Service*. Retrieved May 20, 2016 from http://www.ucn.org.hk/?l=e&c=comprehensive#

United Nations Economic Commission for Europe / European Commission. (2015). *Active ageing index 2014: Analytical report*. Report prepared by Asghar Zaidi of Centre for Research on Ageing, University of Southampton and David Stanton, under contract with United Nations Economic Commission for Europe (Geneva), co-funded by European Commission's Directorate General for Employment, Social Affairs and Inclusion (Brussels). Retrieved March 20, 2017 from http://www.age-platform.eu/images/stories/Publications/AAI_2014_Report.pdf

United Nations Population Division. (2001). New York: World Population Ageing.

United Nations. (1991). *Principles for Older Persons*. Retrieved March 19, 2017, from http://www.ohchr.org/Documents/ProfessionalInterest/olderpersons.pdf

United States Census Bureau. (2012a). *2010 Census urban and rural classification and urban area criteria*. Retrieved November 7, 2013, from http://www.census.gov/geo/reference/ua/urban-rural-2010.html

United States Census Bureau. (2012b). *2012 statistical abstract*. Retrieved December 9, 2013, from http://www.census.gov/compendia/statab/

United States Census Bureau. (2014). *Statistical abstracts in the United States*. Washington, DC: U.S. Government Printing Office.

United States Department of Commerce, Bureau of Economic Analysis. (2015). *GSP missions of current 2014 dollars*. Retrieved June 1, 2016, from http://www.bea.gov

United States Department of Health and Human Services, Administration of Aging. (2014). *A profile of older Americans: 2014*. Retrieved June 12, 2016, from http://www.aoa.acl.gov/aging_statistics/profile/2014/docs/2014-profile.pdf

United States Government Accountability Office. (2011). *Medicaid improving responsiveness of federal assistance to states during economic downturns. Report GAO-11-395*. Retrieved June 12, 2016, from http:// www.gao.gov/assets/320/317275.pdf

United States Government Accountability Office. (2015a). *Medicaid key issues facing the program. report to congressional addressees. Report GAO-15-677*. Retrieved June 12, 2016, from http:// www.gao.gov/assets/680/671761.pdf

United States Government Accountability Office. (2015b). *Medicaid managed care trends in federal spending and state oversight of costs and enrollment. Report GAO-16-77*. Retrieved June 12, 2016, from http://gao.gov/assets/680/674307.pdf

Urban Institute. (2014). *Reversing the Medicaid fee bump: how much could Medicaid physician fees for primary care fall in 2015?* Retrieved July 5, 2016, from http://www.urban.org/sites/default/files/alfresco/publication-pdfs/2000025-Reversing-the-Medicaid-Fee-Bump.pdf

Van de Mortel, T. F. (2008). *Faking it: Social desirability response bias in self-report research*. Academic Press.

Van Marrewijk, M. (2003). Concept and Definitions of CSR and Corporate Sustainability: Between Agency and Communion. *Journal of Business Ethics, 44*(2-3), 95 & 105.

Vasunilashorn, S., Steinman, B. A., Liebig, P. S., & Pynoos, J. (2012). Aging in place: Evolution of a research topic whose time has come. *Journal of Aging Research, 2012*, 1–6. doi:10.1155/2012/120952 PMID:22175020

Ventola, C. L. (2014). Mobile devices and apps for health care professionals: Uses and benefits. *Pharmacy and Therapeutics, 39*(5), 356. PMID:24883008

Veras, R. P., Caldas, C. P., Motta, L. B. D., Lima, K. C. D., Siqueira, R. C., Rodrigues, R. T., & Guerra, A. C. et al. (2014). Integration and continuity of care in health care network models for frail older adults. *Revista de Saude Publica, 48*(2), 357–365. doi:10.1590/S0034-8910.2014048004941 PMID:24897058

Vidal-Alaball, J. (2011). *Health services evaluation.* Academic Press.

Virdun, C., Luckett, T., Davidson, P. M., & Phillips, J. (2015). Dying in the hospital setting: A systematic review of quantitative studies identifying the elements of end-of-life care that patients and their families rank as being most important. *Palliative Medicine, 29*(9), 774–796. doi:10.1177/0269216315583032 PMID:25921707

Vladeck, F. (2004). *A good place to grow old: New York's model for NORC supportive service programs.* New York: United Hospital Fund.

Voelker, K. E., Rakich, J. S., & French, G. R. (2001). The balanced scorecard in healthcare organizations: A performance measurement and strategic planning methodology. *Hospital Topics, 79*(3), 13–24. doi:10.1080/00185860109597908 PMID:11794940

Volunteer Movement. (2008). *Volunteer Movement Volunteer GuideBook.* Retrieved May 20, 2016 from http://www.volunteering-hk.org/swdwebdata/tc_chi/resource/userguide/guidelines.pdf

Volunteer Movement. (2016). *Volunteer Movement Participating Organizations & Registered Volunteers.* Retrieved May 14, 2016 from http://www.volunteering-hk.org/aboutvs/vs_intro/vs_stat

Vos, T., Goss, J., Begg, S., & Mann, N. (2007). *Projection of health care expenditure by disease: a case study from Australia.* New York: United Nations.

Wagstaff, A., Lindelow, M., Gao, J., Xu, L., & Qian, J. (2009). Extending health insurance to the rural population: An impact evaluation of Chinas new cooperative medical scheme. *Journal of Health Economics, 1*(1), 1–19. doi:10.1016/j.jhealeco.2008.10.007 PMID:19058865

Wahl, H. W., Schmitt, M., Danner, D., & Coppin, A. (2010). Is the emergence of functional ability decline in early old age related to change in speed of cognitive processing and also to change in personality? *Journal of Aging and Health, 22*(2), 691–712. doi:10.1177/0898264310372410 PMID:20495152

Wakefield, J. (2012). Virtual patient under the knife on hi-tech operating table. *BBC.* Retrieved from http://www.bbc.com/news/technology-18088337

Walder, A. G. (2015). *China under Mao: a revolution derailed.* Cambridge, MA: Harvard University Press. doi:10.4159/9780674286689

Walker, J. (1969). The diffusion of innovation among the American states. *The American Political Science Review, 63*(3), 880–899. doi:10.2307/1954434

Walker, L. (2012). The future of femme: Notes on femininity, aging and gender theory. *Sexualities, 15*(7), 795–814. doi:10.1177/1363460711417482

Wallace, S., Clark, M., & White, J. (2012). Its on my iPhone: Attitudes to the use of mobile computing devices in medical education, a mixed-methods study. *BMJ Open, 2*(4), e001099. doi:10.1136/bmjopen-2012-001099 PMID:22923627

Wang, J., & Chen, G. (2015 October 12). *Cheap essential drugs disappear from the market: 342 of more than 500 drugs are in severe shortage,* Chinese version. Retrieved July 15, 2016, from http://news.sciencenet.cn/htmlnews/2015/10/328428.shtm

Wang, J., Zhou, H., Lei, Y., & Wang, X. (2012). Financial protection under the New Rural Cooperative Medical Schemes in China. *Medical Care, 50*(8), 700–704. doi:10.1097/MLR.0b013e318249d8bf PMID:22354207

Wang, M. M., Xue, M., Xu, Y. G., Miao, Y., Kou, N., Yang, L., & Shi, D. et al. (2016). Panax notoginseng saponin is superior to aspirin in inhibiting platelet adhesion to injured endothelial cells through COX pathway in vitro. *Thrombosis Research, 141*, 146–152. doi:10.1016/j.thromres.2016.03.022 PMID:27043068

Wang, X., He, X., Zheng, A., & Ji, X. (2014). The effects of Chinas New Cooperative Medical Scheme on accessibility and affordability of healthcare services: An empirical research in Liaoning Province. *BMC Health Services Research, 14*(1), 388. doi:10.1186/1472-6963-14-388 PMID:25217224

Wang, X., Ouyang, Y., Liu, J., Zhu, M., Zhao, G., Bao, W., & Hu, F. B. (2014). Fruit and vegetable consumption and mortality from all causes, cardiovascular disease, and cancer: Systematic review and dose-response meta-analysis of prospective cohort studies. *British Medical Journal, 349*(3), 4490. doi:10.1136/bmj.g4490 PMID:25073782

Warner, M. E., Homsy, G. C., & Morken, L. J. (2017). Planning for Aging in Place: Stimulating a Market and Government Response. *Journal of Planning Education and Research, 37*(1), 29–42. doi:10.1177/0739456X16642824

Watson, D. (2003). The rise and rise of public private partnerships: Challenges for public accountability. *Australian Accounting Review, 13*(31), 2–14. doi:10.1111/j.1835-2561.2001.tb00167.x

Weiner, B., Amick, H., & Lee, S. Y. (2008). Conceptualization and measurement of organizational readiness for change: A review of the literature in health services research and other fields. *Medical Care Research and Review, 65*(4), 379–436. doi:10.1177/1077558708317802 PMID:18511812

Weir, M. (2006). When does politics create policy? The organizational politics of change. In I. Shapiro, S. Skowronek, & D. Galvin (Eds.), *Rethinking political institutions: the art of the state* (pp. 171–186). New York: New York University Press.

Weiss, P. L. T., Whiteley, C. P., Treviranus, J., & Fels, D. I. (2001). PEBBLES: A personal technology for meeting educational, social and emotional needs of hospitalised children. *Personal and Ubiquitous Computing, 5*(3), 157–168. doi:10.1007/s007790170006

Weller, C. (2013). Robotic Butt Offers Prostate Exam Training For Medical Students: How "Patrick" Teaches Empathy, Proper Technique. *Medical Daily*. Retrieved 4 March 2017, from http://www.medicaldaily.com/robotic-butt-offers-prostate-exam-training-medical-students-how-patrick-teaches-empathy-proper

West, D. (2012). How mobile devices are transforming healthcare. *Issues in Technology Innovation, 18*(1), 1-11.

WHO. (2015). *World Report on Aging and Health*. Retrieved from: http://www.who.int/ageing/events/world-report-2015-launch/en/

Wiles, J. L., Leibing, A., Guberman, N., Reeve, J., & Allen, R. E. S. (2012). The Meaning of Aging in Place to Older People. *The Gerontologist, 52*(3), 357–366. doi:10.1093/geront/gnr098 PMID:21983126

Williams, E. L. (n.d.). *Effective Hospital Visitation*. Retrieved May 20, 2016 from http://enrichmentjournal.ag.org/200403/200403_112_hospitalvisitation.cfm

Williams, A. P., Challis, D., Deber, R., Watkins, J., Kuluski, K., Lum, J. M., & Daub, S. (2009). Balancing institutional and community-based care: Why some older persons can age successfully at home while others require residential long-term care. *Healthcare Quarterly, 12*(2), 95–105. doi:10.12927/hcq.2009.3974 PMID:19369817

Williams, A. P., Lum, J., Morton-Chang, F., Kuluski, K., Peckham, A., Warrick, N., & Ying, A. (2016). *Integrating long-term care into a community-based continuum*. Montreal, QB: Institute for Research on Public Policy.

Wilson, A. A. (2005). Impact of management development on nurse retention. *Nursing Administration Quarterly, 29*(2), 137–145. doi:10.1097/00006216-200504000-00008 PMID:15923977

Wimo, A., Jonsson, L., & Winblad, B. (2006). An estimate of the worldwide prevalence and direct costs of dementia in 2003. *Dementia and Geriatric Cognitive Disorders*, *21*(3), 175–181. doi:10.1159/000090733 PMID:16401889

Wing, L. M., Reid, C. M., Ryan, P., Beilin, L. J., Brown, M. A., Jennings, G. L., & West, M. J. et al. (2003). A comparison of outcomes with angiotensin-converting–enzyme inhibitors and diuretics for hypertension in the elderly. *The New England Journal of Medicine*, *348*(7), 583–592. doi:10.1056/NEJMoa021716 PMID:12584366

Winters, S. (2006). Implementation. In B. Peters & J. Pierre (Eds.), *The SAGE handbook of public policy* (pp. 151–166). London: Sage. doi:10.4135/9781848608054.n9

Wolf, P. A., Abbott, R. D., & Kannel, W. B. (1991). Atrial fibrillation as an independent risk factor for stroke: The Framingham Study. *Stroke*, *22*(8), 983–988. doi:10.1161/01.STR.22.8.983 PMID:1866765

Wong, A. (2016). *Innovations in Health Education-M-Learning Facilitated Multimodal Learning using Clickable Images and Virtual Patients*. Paper presented at the CPCE Health Conference 2016, Hong Kong.

Wong, K. K. (2012). *Aging in place for the Hong Kong Housing Society public rental housing elderly* (Unpublished Master of Housing Management dissertation). University of Hong Kong, Hong Kong.

Wong, C., Lo, V. I., & Tang, K. (2006). *China's urban health care reform: from state protection to individual responsibility*. Lanham, MD: Lexington Books.

Wong, E. L., Yeoh, E. K., Chau, P. Y., Yam, C. H., Cheung, A. W., & Fung, H. (2015). How shall we examine and learn about public-private partnerships (PPPs) in the health sector? Realist evaluation of PPPs in Hong Kong. *Social Science & Medicine*, *147*, 261–269. doi:10.1016/j.socscimed.2015.11.012 PMID:26605970

Wong, Y. C., & Leung, J. (2012). Long-term care in China: Issues and Prospects. *Journal of Gerontological Social Work*, *55*(7), 570–586. doi:10.1080/01634372.2011.650319 PMID:22963116

Woo, K. W., Kwok, O. L. A., Ng, K. H. D., Khemlani, M. H., Yau, W. S. C., Poon, Y. C., & Tse, M. W. D. (2013). *The preferred place of care and death in advanced cancer patients under palliative care services*. Paper presented at the 10th Hong Kong Palliative Care Symposium, Hong Kong.

Woo, J. (2007). Development of elderly care services in Hong Kong: Challenges and creative solutions. *Clinical Medicine*, *6*(6), 548–550. doi:10.7861/clinmedicine.7-6-548 PMID:18193700

Woo, J., Ho, S. C., Chan, S. G., Yu, A. L., Yuen, Y. K., & Lau, J. (1997). An estimate of chronic disease burden and some economic consequences among the elderly Hong Kong population. *Journal of Epidemiology and Community Health*, *51*(5), 486–489. doi:10.1136/jech.51.5.486 PMID:9425456

Woo, K. S., Chook, P., Raitakari, O. T., McQuillan, B., Feng, J. Z., & Celermajer, D. S. (1999). Westernization of Chinese adults and increased subclinical atherosclerosis. *Arteriosclerosis, Thrombosis, and Vascular Biology*, *19*(10), 2487–2493. doi:10.1161/01.ATV.19.10.2487 PMID:10521379

Working Party on Primary Health Care of Hong Kong. (1990). *Health for all – The way ahead*. Hong Kong: Government Printer.

World Bank Group. (2015). *What are Public Private Partnership*. About PPPs. Retrieved 25 Feb 2017, from http://ppp.worldbank.org/public-private-partnership/overview/what-are-public-private-partnerships

World Health Organization, & Swedish Organizations of Disabled Persons International Aid Association. (2002). *Community-based rehabilitation as we have experienced it ... voices of persons with disabilities*. Geneva, Switzerland: World Health Organization. Retrieved March 20, 2017 from http://apps.who.int/iris/bitstream/10665/42629/1/9241590432.pdf

World Health Organization, & the Gulbenkian Global Mental Health Platform. (2015). *Promoting rights and community living for children with psychosocial disabilities*. Geneva, Switzerland: World Health Organization. Retrieved March 20, 2017 from http://apps.who.int/iris/bitstream/10665/184033/1/9789241565004_eng.pdf

World Health Organization. (1946/ 2016). *Constitution of WHO: Principles*. Retrieved from http://www.who.int/about/mission/en/

World Health Organization. (1986). *Ottawa Charter for Health Promotion*. Retrieved March 20, 2017 from http://www.who.int/healthpromotion/conferences/previous/ottawa/en/

World Health Organization. (1994). *Community-based rehabilitation and the health care referral services* (WHO/RHB/94.1). Retrieved March 20, 2017 from http://www.who.int/management/community/services/CommunityBase-dRehabilitation.pdf

World Health Organization. (2002). *Active ageing: A policy framework*. Geneva, Switzerland: World Health Organization Noncommunicable Disease Prevention and Health Promotion Ageing and Life Course. Retrieved March 20, 2017 from http://apps.who.int/iris/bitstream/10665/67215/1/WHO_NMH_NPH_02.8.pdf

World Health Organization. (2003). *Community contribution to TB care: Practice and policy* (WHO/CDS/TB/2003.312). Geneva: Author. Retrieved March 20, 2017 from http://apps.who.int/iris/bitstream/10665/67865/1/WHO_CDS_TB_2003.312.pdf

World Health Organization. (2004). *A glossary of terms for community health care and services for older persons* (WHO Centre for Health Development: Ageing and Health Technical Report, Volume 5, WHO/WKC/Tech.Ser./04.2). Retrieved March 20, 2017 from http://www.who.int/kobe_centre/ageing/ahp_vol5_glossary.pdf

World Health Organization. (2004, September 1). *Promoting fruit and vegetable consumption around the world*. Retrieved October 24, 2015, from http://www.who.int/dietphysicalactivity/fruit/en/

World Health Organization. (2005). *Sustainable health financing, universal coverage and social health insurance: World Health Assembly Resolution 58.33*. Retrieved March 20, 2017 from http://apps.who.int/iris/bitstream/10665/20383/1/WHA58_33-en.pdf?ua=1

World Health Organization. (2005a). *World Health Organization Knowledge Management Strategy*. Retrieved 20 July 2016, from http://www.who.int/kms/about/strategy/kms_strategy.pdf

World Health Organization. (2005b). *Knowledge Management in WHO: Bridging the Know–Do Gap*. Retrieved 20 July 2016, from http://www.who.int/kms/en/kms_leaflet.pdf

World Health Organization. (2007). *Global Age-friendly Cities: A Guide*. Retrieved March 13, 2017, from http://www.who.int/aging/publications/Global_age_friendly_cities_Guide_English.pdf

World Health Organization. (2008). *Primary health care: now more than ever*. Retrieved February 19, 2016, from http://www.who.int/whr/2008/whr08_en.pdf

World Health Organization. (2013). *Global action plan for the prevention and control of NCDs 2013-2020*. Retrieved March 20, 2017 from http://apps.who.int/iris/bitstream/10665/94384/1/9789241506236_eng.pdf?ua=1

World Health Organization. (2013). *The world health report 2013: research for universal health coverage*. Retrieved June 1, 2016, from http://apps.who.int/iris/bitstream/10665/85761/2/9789240690837_eng.pdf?ua=1

World Health Organization. (2014). *"Ageing well" must be a global priority*. Retrieved July 5, 2016, from http://www.who.int/mediacentre/news/releases/2014/lancet-ageing-series/en/

World Health Organization. (2014). *WHO traditional medicine strategy: 2014-2023.* Retrieved July 14, 2016, from http://www.who.int/medicines/publications/traditional/trm_strategy14_23/en/

World Health Organization. (2015). Retrieved from http://www.who.int/dietphysicalactivity/fruit/en/index2.html

World Health Organization. (2015). *WHO global strategy on people-centred and integrated health services: Interim report.* Geneva, CH: Author.

World Health Organization. (2015). *World Report on Ageing and Health 2015.* Retrieved March 19, 2017, from http://apps.who.int/iris/bitstream/10665/186463/1/9789240694811_eng.pdf

World Health Organization. (2016). *Ageing and health.* Retrieved August 23, 2016, from http://www.who.int/mediacentre/factsheets/fs404/en/

World Health Organization. (2016). *Mental health and older adults.* Retrieved February 1, 2017, from http://www.who.int/mediacentre/factsheets/fs381/en/

World Health Organization. (2016a). *Knowledge management and health.* Retrieved 20 July 2016, from http://www.who.int/kms/en/

World Health Organization. (2016b). *WHO knowledge management strategy.* Retrieved 20 July 2016, from http://www.who.int/kms/about/strategy/en/

World Health Organization. (2017). *Equity.* Health Systems. Retrieved 25 Feb 2017, from http://www.who.int/healthsystems/topics/equity/en/

World Health Organization. (n.d.a). *Disabilities and rehabilitation: Community-based rehabilitation (CBR).* Retrieved March 20, 2017 from http://www.who.int/disabilities/cbr/en/

World Health Organization. (n.d.b). *Disabilities and rehabilitation: Community-based rehabilitation guidelines.* Retrieved March 20, 2017 from http://www.who.int/disabilities/cbr/guidelines/en/

Wright, A. A., Keating, N. L., Balboni, T. A., Matulonis, U. A., Block, S. D., & Prigerson, H. G. (2010). Place of death: Correlations with quality of life of patients with cancer and predictors of bereaved caregivers mental health. *Journal of Clinical Oncology, 28*(29), 4457–4464. doi:10.1200/JCO.2009.26.3863 PMID:20837950

Wright, A. A., Zhang, B., Ray, A., Mack, J. W., Trice, E., Balboni, T., & Prigerson, H. G. et al. (2008). Associations between end-of-life discussions, patient mental health, medical care near death, and caregiver bereavement adjustment. *Journal of the American Medical Association, 300*(14), 1665–1673. doi:10.1001/jama.300.14.1665 PMID:18840840

Wu, C. (1991). *The aging of population in China.* Retrieved June 21, 2016, from http://www.cicred.org/Eng/Publications/pdf/c-d16.pdf

Wu, G., & Li, W. (2006). New Health Revolution, Chinese version. Beijing: Tsinghua University Press.

Wu, L., & Kuo, Y. Z. (2012). A balanced scorecard approach in assessing IT value in healthcare sector: An empirical examination. *Journal of Medical Systems, 36*(6), 3583–3596. doi:10.1007/s10916-012-9834-2 PMID:22366918

Wyller, T. B., Holmen, J., Laake, P., & Laake, K. (1998). Correlates of subjective well-being in stroke patients. *Stroke, 29*(2), 363–367. doi:10.1161/01.STR.29.2.363 PMID:9472875

Xinhua Net. (2013, March 28). *Mass media in the West said that the presence of structural defects in China's health insurance system had pushed migrant workers to visit black clinics,* Chinese version. Retrieved July 14, 2016, from http://news.qq.com/a/20130328/000824.htm

Xinhua Net. (2016, February 1). *China to orderly urbanize migrant workers: Premier Li.* Retrieved July 16, 2016, from http://news.xinhuanet.com/english/2016-02/01/c_135065434.htm

Xinhua Net. (2016, January 15). *The Chinese Communist Party's newspaper reported that migrant workers find it difficult to see a doctor,* Chinese version. Retrieved July 16, 2016, from http://finance.sina.com.cn/china/2016-01-15/doc-ifxnrahr8315304.shtml

Yam, C. H., Wong, E. L., Chan, F. W., Leung, M. C., Wong, F. Y., Cheung, A. W., & Yeoh, E. K. (2010). Avoidable readmission in Hong Kong-system, clinician, patient or social factor? *BMC Health Services Research, 10*(1), 1. doi:10.1186/1472-6963-10-311 PMID:21080970

Yan Oi Tong Limited. (2016). *Yan Oi Tong Annual Report 2015 – 2016.* Retrieved July 24, 2016 from http://www.yot.org.hk/download/annual-report/2015-16/2015_2016_Final.zip

Yan, Y. Y. (2010). Online health information seeking behavior in Hong Kong: An exploratory study. *Journal of Medical Systems, 34*(2), 147–153. doi:10.1007/s10916-008-9226-9 PMID:20433053

Yao, C. A., Hu, W. Y., Lai, Y. F., Cheng, S. Y., Chen, C. Y., & Chiu, T. Y. (2007). Does Dying at Home Influence the Good Death of Terminal Cancer Patients? *Journal of Pain and Symptom Management, 34*(5), 497–504. doi:10.1016/j.jpainsymman.2007.01.004 PMID:17629664

Yao, W., Chu, C. H., & Li, Z. (2012). The adoption and implementation of RFID technologies in healthcare: A literature review. *Journal of Medical Systems, 36*(6), 3507–3525. doi:10.1007/s10916-011-9789-8 PMID:22009254

Yarnell, J., Patterson, C., Sweetnam, P., Thomas, H., Bainton, D., Elwood, P. C., & Miller, N. E. et al. (2001). Do total and high density lipoprotein cholesterol and triglycerides act independently in the prediction of ischemic heart disease? *Arteriosclerosis, Thrombosis, and Vascular Biology, 21*(8), 1340–1345. doi:10.1161/hq0801.093505 PMID:11498463

Yee Hong Centre for Geriatric Care. (2016). *Mission & vision.* Retrieved from http://www.yeehong.com/centre/mission.php

Yen, I. H., Michael, Y. L., & Perdue, L. (2009). Neighborhood environment in studies of health of older adults: A systematic review. *American Journal of Preventive Medicine, 37*(5), 455–463. doi:10.1016/j.amepre.2009.06.022 PMID:19840702

Yeo, B., & Huang, S. (2009). Foreign domestic workers and home-based care for elders in Singapore. *Journal of Aging & Social Policy, 22*(1), 69–88. doi:10.1080/08959420903385635 PMID:20390713

Yesavage, J. A., Brink, T. L., Rose, T. L., Lum, O., Huang, V., Adey, M., & Leirer, V. O. (1983). Development and validation of a geriatric depression screening scale: A preliminary report. *Journal of Psychiatric Research, 17*(1), 37–49. doi:10.1016/0022-3956(82)90033-4 PMID:7183759

Yi-Jung, L. (2010). Long-term Care Residents 'View About the Contributions of Christian-based Volunteer in Taiwan: A Pilot Study. *Journal of Religion and Health, 51*(3), 709–722.

Yin, R. K. (2003). *Case Study Research: Design and Methods.* SAGE Publication. Inc.

Yip, P., Lee, J., & Law, C. K. (2006). Implications of the demographic transition. In G. M. Leung & J. Bacon-Shone (Eds.), *Hong Kong's health system: Reflections, perspectives and visions* (pp. 61–80). Hong Kong: Hong Kong University Press.

Yip, W., & Eggleston, K. (2004). Addressing government and market failures with payment incentives: Hospital reimbursement reform in Hainan, China. *Social Science & Medicine, 58*(2), 267–277. doi:10.1016/S0277-9536(03)00010-8 PMID:14604613

Yi, Y., Maynard, A., Liu, G., Xiong, X., & Lin, F. (2005). Equity in health care financing: Evaluation of the current urban employee health insurance reform in China. *Journal of the Asia Pacific Economy, 10*(4), 506–527. doi:10.1080/13547860500291745

Youdin, R. (2014). *Clinical gerontological social work practice.* New York, NY: Springer.

Yu, R., Chau, P. H., McGhee, S. M., Chau, J., Lee, C. H., Chan, M. Y., . . . Woo, J. (2012). *Trends of disease burden consequent to stroke in older persons in Hong Kong: Implications of population ageing.* Hong Kong: The Hong Kong Jockey Club. Retrieved March 20, 2017 from https://hub.hku.hk/bitstream/10722/161124/1/Content.pdf?accept=1

Yu, R., Chau, P. H., McGhee, S. M., Cheung, W. L., Chan, K. C., Cheung, S. H., . . . Woo, J. (2010). *Dementia trends: Impact of the ageing population and societal implications for Hong Kong.* Hong Kong: The Hong Kong Jockey Club. Retrieved March 20, 2017 from https://hub.hku.hk/bitstream/10722/138520/1/Content.pdf

Yu, R., Chau, P. H., McGhee, S. M., Cheung, W. L., Chan, K. C., Cheung, S. H., ... Woo, J. (2012). Trends in prevalence and mortality of dementia in elderly Hong Kong population: Projections, disease burden, and implications for long-term care. *International Journal of Alzheimer's Disease, 2012.* doi: 10.1155/2012/406852

Yuen, P. P. (1992). The Privatization of Hospital Services: An Empirical Study of the Determinants of the Public/Private Mix. Hong Kong Public Administration, 1(1), 24-64.

Yuen, P. P. (2014). Financing Health Care and Long-term Care in a Rapidly Ageing Context: Assessing Hong Kong's Readiness. *Public Administration and Policy – An Asia Pacific Journal, 17*(1), 56 – 64.

Yuen, P. P. (2014). Financing Health and Long Term Care in a Rapidly Aging Context: Assessing Hong Kong's Readiness. *Public Policy and Administration, 17*(1), 56–64.

Yuen, P. P. (2014). Financing Health Care and Long-term Care in a Rapidly Ageing Context: Assessing Hong Kong's Readiness. *Public Policy and Administration, 17*(1), 56–64.

Yuen, P. P. (2014). Financing health care and long-term care in a rapidly ageing context: Assessing Hong Kong's readiness. *Public Policy and Administration, 17*(1), 56–64.

Yuen, P. P., & Ng, A. W. (2012). Towards a balanced performance measurement system in a public health care organization. *International Journal of Health Care Quality Assurance, 25*(5), 421–430. doi:10.1108/09526861211235919 PMID:22946241

Yuen, R. M. F. (2014). The challenges of an ageing society from a health care perspective. *Public Policy and Administration, 17*(1), 1–14.

Yun, E. K. (2013). Predictors of attitude and intention to use knowledge management system among Korean nurses. *Nurse Education Today, 33*(12), 1477–1481. doi:10.1016/j.nedt.2013.05.018 PMID:23806194

Yun, Y. H., Lim, M. K., Choi, K. S., & Rhee, Y. S. (2006). Predictors associated with the place of death in a country with increasing hospital deaths. *Palliative Medicine, 20*(4), 455–461. doi:10.1191/0269216306pm1129oa PMID:16875117

Yusuf, S., Pepine, C. J., Garces, C., Pouleur, H., Rousseau, M., Salem, D., & Pitt, B. et al. (1992). Effect of enalapril on myocardial infarction and unstable angina in patients with low ejection fractions. *Lancet, 340*(8829), 1173–1178. doi:10.1016/0140-6736(92)92889-N PMID:1359258

Zack, M., McKeen, J., & Singh, S. (2009). Knowledge management and organizational performance: An exploratory analysis. *Journal of Knowledge Management, 13*(6), 392–409. doi:10.1108/13673270910997088

Zang, J., & Ng, S. W. (2016). Age, period and cohort effects on adult physical activity levels from 1991 to 2011 in China. *The International Journal of Behavioral Nutrition and Physical Activity, 13*(1), 40. doi:10.1186/s12966-016-0364-z PMID:27094983

Zetta, S., Smith, K., Jones, M., Allcoat, P., & Sullivan, F. (2011). Evaluating the Angina Plan in patients admitted to hospital with angina. [PubMed]. *Cardiovascular Therapeutics, 29*, 112–124.

Zhang, Y. (2013). Meeting the ageing challenge: China's social care policy for the elderly. In G. Wang, & Y. Zheng (Eds.), China: Development and governance (pp. 343-350). Singapore: World Scientific Pub. Co.

Zhang, R., Wang, Z., Fei, Y., Zhou, B., Zheng, S., Wang, L., & Yu, Y. et al. (2015). The difference in nutrient intakes between Chinese and Mediterranean, Japanese and American diets. *Nutrients, 7*(6), 4661–4688. doi:10.3390/nu7064661 PMID:26066014

Zhang, Y. C., Chen, R. M., Lu, B. J., Zhao, M. H., & Rong, Y. Z. (2009). Influence of Shengmai Capsule on recovery of living capacity in patients after myocardial infarction. *Chinese Journal of Integrative Medicine, 15*(5), 333–336. doi:10.1007/s11655-009-0333-3 PMID:19802535

Zheng, G. C. (2009). *The development of social security system with Chinese characteristics*. Beijing: China Labour & Social Security Publishing House.

Zhou, Q. (2016, February 1). *The zero mark-up policy leads to hospitals having difficulty in earning revenues,* Chinese version. Retrieved July 17, 2016 from http://news.youth.cn/sh/201602/t20160201_7591716.htm

Zhou, J., & Walker, A. (2016). The need for community care among older people in China. *Ageing and Society, 36*(6), 1312–1332. doi:10.1017/S0144686X15000343

Zhou, Z., Zhu, L., Zhou, Z., Li, Z., Gao, J., & Chen, G. (2014). The effects of Chinas urban basic medical insurance schemes on the equity of health service utilization: Evidence from Shaanxi Province. *International Journal for Equity in Health, 13*(1), 23. doi:10.1186/1475-9276-13-23 PMID:24606592

Zhu, C., Sun, X., Geng, Q. F. R., Yang, H., & Jiang, W. (2015). Self-rated chronic conditions and 2-week prevalence in adults in Zhongshan, China: An epidemiological survey. *BMJ Open, 5*(11), e008441. doi:10.1136/bmjopen-2015-008441 PMID:26560055

Zhu, Z. (2011). Whither China in the 21st century? In Z. Zhu (Ed.), *The People's Republic of China Today: Internal and External Exchanges* (pp. 429–440). Hackensack, NJ: World Scientific.

Zubair, M., & Norris, M. (2015). Perspectives on ageing, later life and ethnicity: Ageing research in ethnic minority contexts. *Ageing and Society, 35*(5), 897–916. doi:10.1017/S0144686X14001536 PMID:25937682

About the Contributors

Ben Yuk Fai Fong is a Family Doctor and a Specialist in Community Medicine, currently a Senior Lecturer and the Award Leader in Health Studies at the School of Professional Education and Executive Development in the College of Professional Education and Continuing Education at The Hong Kong Polytechnic University. Ben had his medical training and Public Health education at the University of Sydney, Australia. He has served in public, private and university healthcare facilities both in Hong Kong and in Sydney, and has commissioned and managed two hospitals in Hong Kong, including a new private hospital. He has also served as the Director of University Health Service of The Chinese University of Hong Kong. Academically, Ben holds Honorary Associate Professorship at both local medical schools, and a local school of Chinese Medicine in Hong Kong. He has published books, and is a reviewer of a local medical journal.

Artie W. Ng is currently Principal Lecturer and Deputy Director with School of Professional Education & Executive Development at The Hong Kong Polytechnic University (PolyU). Dr. Ng has a research interest in sustainability performance of knowledge-intensive organizations. He has published with international academic and professional journals, including International Journal of Health Care Quality Assurance, Journal of Intellectual Capital, Journal of Sustainable Finance & Investment as well as Thunderbird International Business Review. He obtained his Ph.D. degree from the Adam Smith School of Business at the University of Glasgow, MBA from Rotman School of Management at the University of Toronto and M.Eng. in Technology Management at the University of Waterloo. He is a qualified accountant and a fellow member with Chartered Institute of Management Accountants (UK) and Hong Kong Institute of Certified Public Accountants. He is also a Senior Member with Institute of Industrial and Systems Engineers.

Peter P. Yuen is Dean of the College of Professional and Continuing Education of The Hong Kong Polytechnic University (PolyU). He is also Professor in the Department of Management and Marketing of PolyU. He received his Bachelor of Arts degree in Cellular and Molecular Biology and Master in Business Administration degree from the State University of New York at Buffalo, and his Doctor of Philosophy degree in Health Economics from the University of Birmingham. Professor Yuen's research involves public policy formulation and evaluation, and health services management. He is an Editor of Public Administration and Policy and an Editorial Committee member of Asia Pacific Journal of Health Management. Professor Yuen is currently the Chairman of the Federation for Self-financing Tertiary Education (Hong Kong). He is a founding Fellow of the Hong Kong College of Health Services Executives, and an Honorary Fellow of the Australian College of Health Services Management.

* * *

Tsoi Ming Au Yeung is a graduate of The Hong Kong Polytechnic University and her major study is Applied Biology with Biotechnology. She is interested in Protein Biotechnology and studying drug-cell interactions in human cells. She believes biotechnology and medical research can ultimately promote the quality of life for human. After completion of her undergraduate studies, she worked as a part-time researcher in a healthcare-related study. Currently, Ms. Au Yeung is working in a testing laboratory for neonatal genetic diseases, where she gained an interest in the diagnostic technology in which the genetic defects in a fetus can be detected through the maternal blood during the course of pregnancy. This technology is highly advantageous for pregnant women, because it is a non-invasive technique. Ms. Au Yeung endeavours further work in this field and help bring about diagnostic methods with improved accuracy and efficiency.

Enoch Chan has great interest in biomedical science research and education. Dr. Chan completed his undergraduate studies in the Hong Kong Polytechnic University, major in Applied Biology with Biotechnology. He then completed a Masters by Research and PhD in Pathology at the School of Medical Sciences, UNSW Sydney (University of New South Wales). His primary research interests are the role of monocytes/macrophages and neutrophils in promoting cardiovascular diseases such as hypertension, atherosclerosis and aortic aneurysm; and the anti-inflammatory and immuno-modulatory functions of Chinese medicinal herbs. Dr Chan is currently a biomedical education developer at the Office of Pro-Vice Chancellor (Education), UNSW Sydney, responsible for digital uplifting and promoting blended learning in biomedical education. His teaching interest is the use of cloud-based applications and virtual lab practicals in aiding blending learning in the context of biomedical education.

Gabriel Chan Hoi-huen graduated from The Chinese University of Hong Kong where she received a BSc in Biochemistry (with a minor in Psychology) and an MPhil in Physiology. Besides, she obtained a Postgraduate Diploma in Education in Liberal Studies and a PhD in Biology from Hong Kong Baptist University. Dr. Chan is currently a lecturer of Health and Life Sciences in Hong Kong Community College, The Hong Kong Polytechnic University. Dr. Chan's research interests lie mainly in cardiovascular physiology and traditional Chinese medicine, and she has recently published research papers in international journals and conference proceedings.

Chan Kin-yee, of school of Professional Education and Executive Development, The Hong Kong Polytechnic University, majoring in health studies, is also a student research assistant in the Department of Family Medicine and Primary Health of The University of Hong Kong, where she conducts health assessments, helps in health literacy programs and recruits participants for new researches, so as to run the processes more effectively and efficiently. Studying in Health Studies and getting involved in voluntary works among different NGOs to achieve a better understanding on the issues of local primary and long-term healthcare industry are her inspirations. She has contributed to working papers and presentations at conferences within and outside the University.

Cheuk Wing Chau is a senior research associate in the Department of Management Sciences at CityU. She gained her master's degree in Sociology and Social Research from University of Newcastle. Her research interests lie in integrated care and healthcare management. As a member of the healthcare team, she supports in planning, liaise, and coordinate with different parties from community and academia. Her expertise is in Hong Kong's healthcare system, in particular social and community services.

Youhua (Frank) Chen is Chair Professor of and Head of Department of Management Sciences at City University of Hong Kong. His current research interests include healthcare management, supply-chain modeling, analysis of inventory systems, and sustainable supply chains. His recent papers appeared in Operations Research and POM. Prior to joining City University of Hong Kong in 2012, Prof. Chen was on the faculty of NUS Business School at National University of Singapore (1997-2001) and the Department of Systems Engineering and Engineering Management at the Chinese University of Hong Kong (2001-2012). He holds a bachelor degree in Engineering, master degree in Economics, and doctoral degree in Management from Tsinghua University (Beijing), the University of Waterloo, and the University of Toronto, respectively. He is currently Project Coordinator for a Theme-Based Research Scheme project on healthcare management: Delivering 21st Century Healthcare in Hong Kong – Building a Quality-and-Efficiency Driven System (11.2014-10.2019).

Simon T. Cheung is a lecturer at the Hong Kong Polytechnic University (PolyU); Fellow of the Australasian College of Health Services Management and Fellow of the Hong Kong College of Health Services Executives. He is responsible for teaching and conducting research in areas of health sciences and health services management. Dr. Cheung had received his doctorate from the University of Bristol in UK, he had also taken up executive and research positions at the Chinese University of Hong Kong and the University of British Columbia in Canada, where he had obtained his Master and Bachelor's degree respectively.

Maria Chu is the Deputy Executive Director of Social Services at the Yee Hong Centre for Geriatric Care, a multi-service centre for seniors. She has a Master Degree and Bachelor Degree in Social Work and is currently a Master Trainer of Stanford University's Chronic Disease Self-Management Program (CDSMP), Pain Self-Management Program, and the Diabetes Self-Management Program. At present, Maria is one of the only five T-Trainers of Stanford's CDSMP Program in Ontario, Canada. Maria is also a published author of her book, "Life with Love and Blessing" and is the first author of the article "Transforming Organizational Culture Using the SSLD System to Address the Taboo of Sexuality and Intimacy needs of seniors" that was published in the Oct 2015 issue of Journal of Contemporary Management - Academic Research Centre of Canada. In her spare time, Maria is a passionate volunteer Radio Program Host for the Chinese community in Toronto.

Susan Dawkes is a registered nurse who has spent over twenty years working in acute cardiology units and as a specialist cardiac rehabilitation nurse. Susan began her career in higher education at the University of Edinburgh and went on to join the School of Health and Social Care at Edinburgh Napier University in 2004 where she is now the Director of Learning, Teaching and Assessment. Susan is an Executive member of the Cardiac Rehabilitation Interest Group Scotland, and a member of: British Association for Cardiovascular Prevention and Rehabilitation, British Heart Foundation Alliance, Canadian Council of Cardiovascular Nurses and Council on Cardiovascular Nursing and Allied Professions (European Society of Cardiology). Her research interests include care of patients with coronary heart disease (CHD), self-management and secondary prevention of long-term conditions and how technology can support patients in managing long-term conditions.

Kenneth N. K. Fong is Associate Professor in the Department of Rehabilitation Sciences of the Hong Kong Polytechnic University. He is an occupational therapist by training. He has been the editor-in-chief of the Hong Kong Journal of Occupational Therapy (HKJOT) (5-year Impact Factor: 0.554) for more than 10 years, and honorary advisor of several self-help organizations for people with chronic diseases and disabilities in Hong Kong. He had received the Department Outstanding Teaching Award and the Faculty Team Teaching Award of the Faculty of Health and Social Sciences. He had been awarded several public competitive research grants from, among others, the General Research Fund, and Health and Medical Research Fund in order to develop innovative neurorehabilitation intervention and studies in the ageing population. In the past 10 years, he has published more than 50 journal papers and book chapters in the fields of neurorehabilitation and ageing.

Jacky Ho received his Ph.D. from the University of Sydney (Australia) specialized in gerontology and sleep science, he is currently an Assistant Professor and Program Director of Social Science and Social Work, and Director of Macau Healthy Lifestyles Research Centre at the City University of Macau. His research interests are in chronic disease development and management, its impact on the healthcare system. His recent project is to investigate the health impacts of Vitamin D intervention in school children using a cost effective model. Dr. Ho is a peer reviewer for Australasian Journal of Ageing, Journal of Aging and Physical Activity.

Ho Wing Tung is a graduate of the School of Professional Education and Executive Development, The Hong Kong Polytechnic University, with the Bachelor of Science (Honours) in Applied Science (Health Studies). She is currently a candidate in the Master of Public Health course in the Jockey Club School of Public Health and Primary Care at The Chinese University of Hong Kong. She has served in public and private healthcare organizations, academic organizations as well as non-government organizations in Hong Kong. Miss Ho has published papers in the Working Paper Series of the College of Professional and Continuing Education, and has had poster presentations at the Annual Scientific Meeting of the Hong Kong College of Community Medicine and the CPCE Health Conference 2016.

Annie Kwok is a specialist in Palliative Medicine, currently the Consultant & Team Head of Palliative Care Unit of Caritas Medical Centre. She is also an accredited trainer in Palliative Medicine and Advanced Internal Medicine under Hong Kong College of Physicians. Dr KWOK contributes to the development of palliative care in Hong Kong and Asia Pacific region through participation in various professional organizations. She currently serves as vice-chairman of Hong Kong Society of Palliative Medicine, council members of Hong Kong Pain Society and Asia Pacific Hospice Palliative Care network. She has been frequently invited as speaker in local and international conference in palliative care, pain management and end-of-life care.

Chui Fan Linus Ip is an experienced clinician who works with seniors and caregivers living with dementia, grief, addiction, pain and sleep disorders. Being a social worker/yoga instructor/community artist, her clinical practice combines body-mind principles with psychotherapeutic procedures, which engages clients in a creative and collaborative process of self discovery, learning and growth. Linus currently works at Baycrest Health Sciences in Toronto, Canada, where she provides behaviour support service for clients with dementia and family caregivers in the community, case consultation and training for helping professionals and organizations.

Lau Ting-leung, Staff Officer of the Auxiliary Medical Service (AMS), joined the AMS in 1980. By profession, he is a Registered Nurse. Apart from obtaining a Diploma in Disaster Management from the Asian Disaster Preparedness Center in Thailand, Mr Lau has completed a disaster medicine training programme organised by the Australian Emergency Management Institute. With his background and work experience, Mr LAU has been actively involved in formulating training and operational strategies for the emergency response of the AMS. The AMS Emergency Response Task Force and the AMS Health Protection Unit were set up in 1993 and 2007 respectively to respond to the needs of the community. Mr Lau is one of the key figures who lead the volunteers to expand the capacity and scope of its services to meet the changing demands in relation to the protection of Hong Kong citizens. In addition to his day-to-day administration duties, Mr Lau is one of the chief editors of "AMS Disaster Medical Assistant" handbook and "Our Victory Over Infections" manual.

Vincent T. Law, BSc (HKU), MBA (City University of Hong Kong), DBA (PolyU(H.K.)), is a Lecturer of the School of Professional Education and Executive Development (SPEED) of The Hong Kong Polytechnic University. Dr. Law received Doctor of Business Administration (DBA) from The Hong Kong Polytechnic University, Master of Business Administration (MBA) with distinction (human resource management concentration) from City University of Hong Kong, and Bachelor of Science from The University of Hong Kong. He authored three Chinese books on Confucianism and its contemporary application: "Governance Wisdom of Daxue" (published in July 2015), "Annotations to Daxue and Zhongyong" (published in August 2016), and "Management Wisdom of Zhongyong" (published in February 2017).

Alison Lee is currently working as a research assistant in the Department of Management Sciences at CityU. She received her Bachelor's degree in Psychology from University of St. Andrews. Ms. Lee has been actively involved in various community projects. Her research interests include elderly healthcare and community care.

Diana Lee is Chairman of the Nursing Council of Hong Kong and Professor of Nursing at the Chinese University of Hong Kong. She is a fellow of the American Academy of Nursing and Visiting Professor of various international and national universities. She is also Director of the Y.K. Pao Foundation Centre for Chronic Illness Care and Deputy Director of the CUHK Jockey Club Institute of Ageing. She is a member of various boards and councils such as the Hong Kong Hospital Authority Board and Elderly Commission. Professor Lee has researched and published widely in the area of gerontology. She has been honored with an excellent research award in health services research by the Food and Health Bureau of the HKSAR in 2007. In 2016, Professor Lee is appointed as the 'Justice of Peace'. Professor Lee has published over 160 refereed journal articles and delivered over 90 international and national keynote addresses.

Eman Leung joined the Department of Management Sciences, College of Business, CityU in December 2014. He received his PhD and undergraduate degrees from the University of Toronto, Canada. His research interests include biostatistics, public health, healthcare management sciences and implementation sciences. His program of research bridges between public health research in clinical risk analytics and operations research on data-driven resource allocation.

Tiffany C. H. Leung is a Lecturer in School of Professional Education & Executive Development, College of Professional & Continuing Education, The Hong Kong Polytechnic University (PolyU). She gained her doctorate and master's degree from the School of Management at the University of St Andrews, UK. Her research interests are in Corporate Social Responsibility, Corporate Social Disclosure, Environmental, Social and Governance, Controversial Industries, and Business Ethics. She has published her research papers in Journal of Business Ethics, Sustainability Accounting, Management and Policy Journal, and Meditari Accountancy Research. She is a peer reviewer for a number of international journals, such as Journal of Business Ethics, Sustainability Accounting, Management and Policy Journal, and International Gambling Studies.

William Y. W. Leung has been working in the social service sector for more than a decade in both Canada and Hong Kong. He currently leads Programs & Services Development at the Yee Hong Centre for Geriatric Care, a multi-service centre for seniors and caregivers of Chinese origin in Canada. William has a Master of Social Work from the University of Toronto and has strong interest on issues surrounding identity and cultural diversity as well as cross-cultural comparisons in social work practice. His work experience ranges from direct services in mental health counselling and group work for sex offenders to broader community work in youth development, community engagement of ethnic minorities in Hong Kong, and senior services. Current services development initiatives that he is working on include: Play Intervention for Dementia (PID) and Managing sexuality and intimacy issues among seniors.

Kwong Yuen Liu is the Executive Director - Social Services of the Yee Hong Centre for Geriatric Care, a multi-service centre for seniors of Chinese origin in Canada, overseeing all community-based social services of the Centre since 1994. He received social work training at the University of Hong Kong and worked in the Hong Kong Government for 19 years, specializing in working with community youth, young offenders and social work training. After moving to Canada in 1990, K.Y. worked a few years as drug addiction therapist before joining Yee Hong in 1994 to develop its community based social service programs for Chinese seniors.

Man Fung Lo received his doctoral degree from University of Newcastle, Australia. He is the Lecturer from the School of Professional Education and Executive Development, The Hong Kong Polytechnic University. His research interests are in the areas of knowledge management, absorptive capacity, quality management and learning technology. Besides, he serves as the editorial board member and reviewer of several international journals, including Journal of Management Research, Case Studies in Business and Management, Journal of Information Technology Education: Innovations in Practice, Computer and Information Science and International Journal of Statistics and Probability. Furthermore, he is the Fellow of several professional societies, including British Computer Society, The Institution of Analysts and Programmers, Irish Computer Society, Australian Institute of Management, Chartered Institute of Logistics and Transport, Strategic Planning Society, Royal Society of Arts, Manufactures and Commerce, The Higher Education Academy, Chartered Institute of Educational Assessors and The College of Teachers.

Sabrina Ching Yuen Luk is Assistant Professor in the School of Social Sciences, Nanyang Technological University. She previously worked at Open University of Hong Kong as Adjunct Associate Professor and Kunming University of Science and Technology as Associate Professor. She was awarded her PhD from the Department of Political Science and International Studies, University of Birmingham.

She is the author of Health Insurance Reforms in Asia (2014, Routledge) and Financing Healthcare in China: Towards Universal Health Insurance (2017, Routledge). She is the co-author of The Logic of Chinese Politics: Cores, Peripheries and Peaceful Rising (2016, Edward Elgar).

Ramona McNeal is an associate professor in the Department of Political Science at the University of Northern Iowa. Her chief research interests include e-government, telehealth, campaign finance reform and telecommunications policy. She also studies the impact of technology on participation, including its relationship to voting, elections, and public opinion. She has published work in a number of journals including Journal of Information Technology & Politics, Social Science Quarterly, Policy Studies Journal, Public Administration Review, Political Research Quarterly and State Politics and Policy Quarterly. She is a co-author of Digital Citizenship: The Internet, Society and Participation (MIT Press, 2007) with Karen Mossberger and Caroline Tolbert.

Candace W. Ng, BA (PolyU SPEED), MA (PolyU(H.K.)), is a tutor of the School of Professional Education and Executive Development (SPEED) of The Hong Kong Polytechnic University. Miss Ng obtained Bachelor of Arts in Public Administration with Distinction and Master of Arts in Social Policy and Social Development with Distinction. Her research interests are in the areas of government, policy and politics, social and political development in East-Asian regions.

Peggy Ng works as a Senior Lecturer at the School of Professional Education and Executive Development, The Hong Kong Polytechnic University. Her research interests include strategic enrolment management, student satisfaction, higher education, strategic planning, and knowledge management. In 2015 and 2016, Dr. Ng has publications in Higher Education, Asia Pacific Education Review, and Public Administration and Policy, an Asia-Pacific Journal. Besides, Dr. Ng is the principal investigator of "Strategic Enrolment, Graduation and Articulation (SEGA)" project and the co-investigator of "A study to identify the commonalities and differences in the perceived graduating students' competencies between UGC-funded and self-financing tertiary institutions in Hong Kong" project, the Federation for Self-Financing Tertiary Education (FSTE) funded research projects. She is also the co-investigator of "Learning analytics and higher education development: Towards a research agenda" project, RGC (Research Grant Council) Inter-Institutional Development Scheme (IIDS).

Mary Schmeida has served in several key research positions in the U.S. She holds a Ph.D. in Political Science, Public Policy from Kent State University, U.S.A. Her chief research interests include e-government and public administration, public opinion, health and social welfare policy, environmental and security policy. She also studies the relationship of technology on government participation. Her works are published in multiple books and journals including Journal of Health Policy and Technology, Administration and Policy in Mental Health and Mental Health Services Research, Journal of Health Care for the Poor and Underserved, International Journal of Computational Models and Algorithms in Medicine, and Government Information Quarterly.

Sai Wang Seto has strong and continuing interest in cardiovascular physiology and pharmacology research aiming at identifying new treatments for cardiovascular diseases such as hypertension, atherosclerosis, aortic aneurysm and stroke. Dr. Seto completed his PhD in Cardiovascular Pharmacology at the Chinese University of Hong Kong and received his postdoctoral training from the Department of

Physiology of the Royal College of Surgeons. He worked as a Senior Scientist in the Queensland Research Centre for Peripheral Vascular Disease, James Cook University. Dr. Seto joined the National Institute of Complementary Medicine, Western Sydney University in 2015. His works focus on the development of Chinese herbal formulation for cerebrovascular diseases, including stroke and vascular dementia. Dr Seto was a recipient of the Australian Government National Health and Medical Research Council Research Fellowship and National Heart Foundation of Australia Fellowship.

Kar-wai Tong has had multi-disciplinary exposure to the fields of health care, law and education. He has had over a decade's practical experience working in hospitals as a management staff. He holds the degree of Doctor of Juridical Science conferred by the City University of Hong Kong and was called to the Bar in England and Wales as an unregistered barrister. He is a solicitor and barrister in New Zealand, an accredited general mediator in Hong Kong, and also a member of the Chartered Institute of Arbitrators in the UK. He has been teaching at universities on a part-time basis for years. He volunteers himself in a few NGOs and is an editor/reviewer of international journals. His research interests include human rights, medico-legal liabilities in health care environments, legal issues in the context of education, and happiness.

K. T. Tsang, PhD (Toronto), is the Factor-Inwentash Chair in Social Work in the Global Community. His scholarship focuses on the development of a knowledge base for human services in a global context, through active integration of theory, practice and research. He is the founder of the SSLD (Strategies and Skills Learning and Development) System, which supports a wide range of human service applications in Canada and internationally. These applications cover personal, family, group, organizational, and community interventions. Recent R&D initiatives include intervention for dementia, social inclusion, and online learning regarding interpersonal relationships.

Doris Tse is the Hospital Chief Executive of Caritas Medical Centre and Clinical Stream Coordinator (Medical) of Kowloon West Cluster of the Hospital Authority. Being a physician by background and a specialist in Advanced Internal Medicine, Critical Care Medicine and Palliative Medicine, Dr Tse is dedicated in promotion of palliative and end-of-life care for both cancer and non-cancer patients. Dr. Tse is currently the Council member of Hong Kong College of Physicians (HKCP), the Chair of the Professional and General Affairs Committee, HKCP and a member of the Subcommittee in Palliative Medicine. Dr Tse is appointed by the Government of Hong Kong to join the Elderly Commission in 2015. She has published in peer reviewed journals in the areas of palliative care for cancer and non-cancer and bereavement, and contributed as co-authors of books including the Oxford Textbook of Palliative Medicine.

Adam Ka Lok Wong has over 20 years of experience in the Information Technology industry. Before joining PolyU SPEED in 2002, he had worked for international companies such as Acer, Philips, Hewlett-Packard, and PCCW. His professional experiences include system development, database support, and electronic-commerce and project management. He has over 10 years of teaching in various areas covering strategy, human resources management, research workshops, computer programming, computer security and e-commerce; from undergraduate to master programmes; from local universities to overseas universities. His research interests are the use of information technology in training and education, and digital marketing. He is an Associate Fellow of The Higher Education Academy, a certified Java programmer, a Microsoft Certified Systems Engineer and a full member of the Hong Kong Computer Society.

Bonnie H. Y. Wong is a Senior Coordinator at the Yee Hong Centre for Geriatric Care, a multi-service agency for Chinese seniors and caregivers living in Canada. At a young age, Bonnie volunteered at an orphanage and a retirement home in China, allowing her to develop an interest in helping others. Bonnie completed a Master of Social Work degree at the University of Toronto, specializing in gerontology. Since joining Yee Hong in 2011, she has helped to develop the Caregiver Education & Support Services, and helped to launch an e-learning platform for caregivers. She currently co-chairs the Chinese Caregiver Network and is a Master Trainer of the Stanford University model of the Chronic Disease Self-Management Program.

Raymond Kam-wing Woo, being a specialist in Palliative Medicine, serves as Associate Consultant in the Department of Medicine and Geriatrics in Caritas Medical Centre. He is active in both undergraduate and postgraduate palliative medicine and internal medicine training. He is currently appointed as Clinical Assistant Professor (Honorary) by the Department of Medicine and Therapeutics, Chinese University of Hong Kong. Dr. Woo is active in research and has received research grants from local academic faculties. His research results have been presented in both local and international academic conferences and attracted media attention. He serves as editor in the Newsletter of Hong Kong Society of Palliative Medicine.

Index

I

K

L

M

N

O

P

Q

R

S

T

U

V

W

Y

www.ingramcontent.com/pod-product-compliance
Lightning Source LLC
LaVergne TN
LVHW062108300926
849161LV00010B/2406